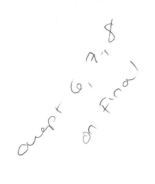

Chap. 6, 7, 8
on Final

Assessment and Treatment of Articulation and Phonological Disorders in Children

Assessment and Treatment of Articulation and Phonological Disorders in Children

A Dual-Level Text

Adriana Peña-Brooks
M. N. Hegde

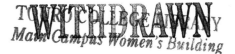
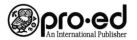

pro·ed
An International Publisher

8700 Shoal Creek Boulevard
Austin, Texas 78757-6897
800/897-3202   Fax 800/397-7633
Order online at http://www.proedinc.com

WB

pro·ed
An International Publisher

© 2000 by PRO-ED, Inc.
8700 Shoal Creek Boulevard
Austin, Texas 78757-6897
800/897-3202   Fax 800/397-7633
Order online at http://www.proedinc.com

Library of Congress Cataloging-in-Publication Data

Peña-Brooks, Adriana.
    Assessment and treatment of articulation and phonological disorders in children: a dual-
level text / Adriana Peña-Brooks, M. N. Hegde.
        p.   cm.
    Includes bibliographical references and indexes.
    ISBN 0-89079-846-x (alk. paper)
    1. Articulation disorders in children.   2. Children—Language.   I. Hegde, M. N.
    (Mahabalagiri N.)   II. Title.
RJ496.S7 P397   2000
618.92'855 — dc21
                                                                                    99-049459
                                                                                    CIP

Printed in the United States of America

  2 3 4 5 6 7 8 9 10   04 03 02 01

7/24/02

*I dedicate this book to God for supplying me
with the strength and courage to accomplish this
project and to Ryan for his genuine love and support.*

—APB

Contents

◆ ◆ ◆ ◆ ◆ ◆ ◆ ◆ ◆ ◆ ◆ ◆ ◆ ◆ ◆ ◆ ◆ ◆ ◆ ◆

Chapter 2: Perspectives in Articulation and Phonology

Basic Unit

Advanced Unit

Chapter 3: Development of Articulation and Phonological Skills

Basic Unit

Chapter 4: Variables Associated with Articulation and Phonological Development and Performance

Basic Unit

Advanced Unit

Chapter 7: Treatment of Articulation and Phonological Disorders

Basic Unit

Advanced Unit

Chapter 8: Specific Treatment Programs and Approaches

References ◆ *529*

Appendixes ◆ *551*

Glossary ◆ *653*

Index ◆ *681*

About the Authors ◆ *689*

Preface

◆ ◆ ◆ ◆ ◆ ◆ ◆ ◆ ◆ ◆ ◆ ◆ ◆ ◆ ◆ ◆ ◆ ◆ ◆

All speech, written or spoken, is a dead language, until it finds a willing and prepared hearer.

—ROBERT LOUIS STEVENSON

Thank you for listening to what we have to say. We hope that this text does not become "dead" and that it finds many who are willing and prepared to hear. We are excited to offer you a text that reviews the basic and advanced information on articulation and phonological disorders. A unique feature of this book is its modular organization. It is organized to serve both as an introduction to articulation and phonology and as an advanced text for graduate seminars. In most university programs in speech–language pathology, students take an introductory undergraduate course and a graduate course on articulation and phonological disorders.

Instructors often use different books at the undergraduate and graduate levels of instruction. If those books are vastly different, some students fail to see continuity from their undergraduate knowledge base to the more advanced graduate information. Also, for most students, several years will lapse between undergraduate study and the graduate seminar on articulation and phonology. Practically all students need to review the undergraduate material before they can effectively participate in a graduate seminar and understand and integrate the material presented at the two levels of instruction. Unfortunately, not all graduate texts summarize the basic information for a review at the graduate level. Also, sometimes opinions differ as to what is basic and what is advanced. Omitting certain materials from a text because it is judged basic or advanced may make it hard for instructors to use if they disagree with that judgment.

The modular organization of this text helps resolve that problem to some extent. To supplement a text, graduate seminar instructors typically use multiple sources, including other books and journal articles. We do not pretend that our distinction between basic and advanced information will be acceptable to all instructors. However, we do hope that the organization of the book will make it easier for students and instructors to use material as they see fit, at either level of instruction. For example, those who wish to avoid theoretical or more complicated information in their undergraduate classes can easily skip the advanced units or use the information in the units selectively. Graduate students can find the basic information in the text to review the assigned chapters before their participation in graduate seminars. We hope that this will better integrate information presented at the two levels.

Besides giving the book a two-tier organization, we have tried to use a student-friendly writing style. We have minimized the use of jargon, and all relevant technical terms are introduced and defined. Our goal was to write the book in such a way as to make it easier for students to understand phonology's basic vocabulary, approaches, perspectives, theories, and assessment and treatment techniques.

We have also included an extensive appendix that includes various sound establishment techniques for all English consonants. We have created several other appendixes that we believe will be clinically useful in the assessment and treatment of articulation and phonological disorders. These were developed with the student in mind. We hope that we have achieved our goal of writing this text in a readable and understandable manner, without sacrificing important technical and theoretical information.

We would like to extend our sincere appreciation to Allen Willard, an excellent student of ours at California State University at Fresno, for his help in researching the sound-evoking techniques included in Appendix M and other aspects of this textbook. We greatly appreciate his enthusiasm toward and dedication to this project. We would also like to thank the many undergraduate and graduate students who inspired us to write this textbook.

Introduction: Articulation and Phonological Disorders

◆ ◆ ◆ ◆ ◆ ◆ ◆ ◆ ◆ ◆ ◆ ◆ ◆ ◆ ◆ ◆ ◆ ◆ ◆

Speech is the mother, not the handmaid of thought.

—KARL KRAUS

Disorders of communication include articulation and phonological disorders, language disorders, fluency disorders, and voice disorders. Articulation and phonological disorders are among the most common communication disorders found in children. It is estimated that nearly 10% of the population has a disorder of communication. Of this percentage, 50 to 80% may have an articulation and phonological disorder. In certain professional settings, especially in public schools, clinicians serve a large number of children with articulation and phonological disorders. Therefore, students in speech–language pathology programs typically are offered extensive coursework and clinical practicums on articulation and phonological disorders.

A severe articulation or phonological disorder tends to have negative effects on a child's social and academic life. If the disorder persists into adult life, occupational choices may be limited. Although many children with articulation disorders do not have significant language disorders, the two coexist in a certain number of children. When they do, the negative consequences are magnified.

The most pervasive effect of an articulation or phonological disorder is reduced intelligibility of speech. The more severe the disorder, the greater the effect on intelligibility. Reduced speech intelligibility decreases everyday communicative effectiveness. The child or the speaker may be negatively evaluated in all aspects simply because of the problem of speech production. Articulation and phonological disorders are speech disorders. Speech disorders include such fluency disorders as stuttering and cluttering. Speech disorders are contrasted with language disorders. Speech is a part of a larger system called language; hence, articulation and phonological disorders may be technically considered disorders within this larger system. In fact, all problems of communication can be considered within the larger system of language. However, for the pragmatic sake of understanding and treating different disorders of communication, such classifications as speech disorders and language disorders are useful.

In the past, the communication problems we call articulation and phonological disorders in this book were all referred to as articulation disorders. Changing perspectives in the study of speech sound systems across languages, speech sound production, and the errors children make in learning the sounds of their language have necessitated the additional category of phonological disorders.

As defined and described in Chapter 2, *articulation* refers to the actual production of speech sounds. It involves the movement of the appropriate speech production mechanisms (e.g., the jaw, the lips, the tongue, and the soft palate). Listeners can see and hear articulation. Speakers can feel their own articulatory movements and hear the result: sound. Articulation thus involves physical movement of speech structures and the audible and physically measurable acoustic product that such movements generate. In the past, articulation was somewhat narrowly thought of as speech sound production; children's difficulties with speech sound productions were described as articulation disorders.

A broader view of articulation and its disorders emerged mostly because of developments in the linguistic study of language. As language was conceived as a system of rules that help organize patterns of communication, sounds of language, too, came to be viewed as subjected to rules of organization. Instead of viewing each speech sound as an entity unto itself, resulting from certain isolated physical movements, experts began to view sounds of languages as organized systems. This concept of a sound system (instead of a collection of sounds) led to the development of a new field of study called phonology. Again, as defined and discussed in Chapter 2, *phonology* is the study of sound systems of languages. It is concerned with the rules of organizing sounds into larger systems of communication: language. Thus, the study of articulation became a subfield of the study of language.

The different ways of making a distinction between articulation and phonological disorders are described in Chapter 2. By way of introduction, it may be stated here that there are finer and more fundamental distinctions that are theoretical, and less fine and more gross distinctions that are clinically pragmatic. Most clinicians tend to make a distinction between articulation and phonological disorders based on the presence or absence of identifiable patterns in the errors. If a child produces only a few errors that cannot be organized into a system of apparent rules, or if the errors are obviously due to organic, structural, or neurological factors, the term *articulation disorder* is more likely to be used. If a child produces multiple errors that can be organized into patterns that seem to follow certain rules of sound changes, the term *phonological disorder* is more likely to be used. Although the view that phonology includes articulation is widely accepted, the use of both terms continues in the profession. Which way the experts and clinicians will go in the use of these two terms in the future is difficult to judge. Therefore, we have used both terms in our discussion of speech sound production problems. Future editions of this book will reflect scientific and professional changes and preferences.

Chapter 1

◆ ◆ ◆ ◆ ◆ ◆ ◆ ◆ ◆ ◆ ◆ ◆ ◆ ◆ ◆ ◆ ◆ ◆ ◆

Anatomy and Neuroanatomy of Speech Production

Basic Unit

◆ ◆ ◆ ◆ ◆ ◆ ◆ ◆ ◆ ◆ ◆ ◆ ◆ ◆ ◆ ◆ ◆ ◆ ◆

The Structural Mechanisms of Speech Production

If the tongue had not been framed for articulation, man would still be a beast in the forest.

—RALPH WALDO EMERSON

Before proceeding with the units on articulation and phonological development and its disorders, it is essential to review the anatomy and physiology of speech. Knowledge of the anatomical and physiological aspects of speech production is critical in understanding disordered articulation and phonological skills. This is especially important when considering disorders with an organic, structural, or neurological origin. Anatomic, neurologic, physiologic, and sensory variables associated with articulatory-phonological development will be reviewed with great detail in the Advanced Units of Chapters 4 and 6. As a matter of introduction, it is well established that the integrity of at least some anatomical structures and the neuromuscular mechanism is essential for the typical acquisition and production of speech sounds.

In this Basic Unit we will review the structural processes of speech production and the related auditory mechanism. It is the authors' assumption that students at this level have taken a course on speech and hearing anatomy in which this information was reviewed at length. However, as even a short period of time can fog knowledge that was once crystal clear, we felt strongly that a reexamination was appropriate. A more in-depth presentation can be found in Palmer (1993), Perkins and Kent (1986), Seikel, King, and Drumright (1997), and Zemlin (1998).

On the surface, the production of speech appears to be a simple process. However, this seemingly effortless activity requires the complex interaction of several mechanisms or functional systems. The basic systems of speech are: (a) respiration, (b) phonation, (c) resonation, and (d) articulation. In addition, adequate hearing sensitivity is necessary for the natural development of speech and language and the continual monitoring of our own verbal output. An intact, or nearly intact, central nervous system is also essential for the neurological control and integration of these processes. The four basic speech systems along with the auditory and central nervous systems are schematically represented in Figure 1.1.

For simplicity in our review, the neuromotor control of speech will be examined in the Advanced Unit of this chapter. In this Basic Unit we will focus on the four structural processes of speech and the auditory mechanism. We emphasize that each process will be examined according to its contribution to speech rather than its pri-

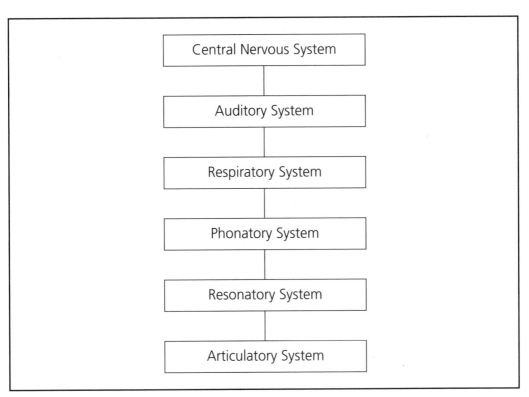

Figure 1.1. Schematic of the major systems (structures) of hearing, speech, and language.

mary biological purpose. Likewise, our review of the auditory mechanism will be limited to its interconnection with speech.

Overview

Each of the speech processes bears individual responsibilities that when intertwined contribute to a final product: speech. *Respiration* is the basic subsystem that provides the air supply necessary for speech. *Phonation* occurs when the **vocal folds** are adducted under tension, resulting in the production of voice. *Resonation* takes place when the vibrated air travels past the vocal folds to the pharyngeal, oral, and nasal cavities. The sounds are resonated as the tone of the noise from the vocal cords is modified according to the size and shape of the resonating cavities. The resonated sound is then shaped into specific speech sounds through various structures in the mouth (e.g., tongue, lips, teeth, and hard palate). This final process is called *articulation*.

Although we will review each process separately for simplification, the reader should bear in mind that this separation is merely arbitrary. Speech production is the result of the successive and simultaneous interactions of these four mechanisms. Their interaction is continuous and synchronized. Furthermore, the auditory system plays a crucial role in monitoring the verbal output created by the speech mechanism.

Respiratory Mechanism

The respiratory mechanism is an essential component of speech production. Without an adequate supply of air, talking would be extremely difficult, if not impossible. Respiration is the driving force behind the extraordinary act of vocalizing and verbalizing that provides human beings the special gift of talking to communicate.

Structures of the Respiratory Mechanism

To manage the adequate supply of air for speech, an individual must be able to breathe in (inhale) and breathe out (exhale) in a coordinated manner. Several structures play a key role in making this process possible, including the thoracic cavity, the abdomen, the lungs, and the diaphragm and other muscles.

The **diaphragm** is the chief muscle of inhalation. It is a thick, dome-shaped muscle that separates the abdomen from the thoracic cavity. The **abdomen** is the section below the diaphragm that houses important organs such as the kidneys, liver, and intestines. The works of various abdominal muscles provide an important active force in exhalation.

The **thoracic cavity** is the portion above the diaphragm that also shelters vital structures, such as the lungs and the heart. The thoracic cavity contains a bony structure, a muscular portion, and the respiratory passages. The bony framework is known as the **rib cage** or **thoracic cage.**

The rib cage has 12 **thoracic vertebrae** in its posterior surface, the **sternum** in its anterior surface, and 12 pairs of bony **ribs.** The ribs run in a curved lateral fashion from the spinal column vertebrae in the back to their own **costal cartilage** in the front. For each of the first seven ribs, the corresponding costal cartilage articulates directly with the sternum. Ribs 8 through 10 have their costal cartilage attached to the rib cage, and the lower two ribs (11 and 12) remain unattached or "floating." The last five ribs are sometimes called false ribs since they do not have a direct medial attachment to the sternum (Palmer, 1993, p. 148). This bony and cartilaginous framework is shown in Figure 1.2.

The muscular portion of the thoracic cavity includes the external and internal intercostal muscles and the subcostal muscles. The 11 paired **external intercostals** raise the ribs up and out to increase the diameter of the cavity for inhalation. The 11 paired **internal intercostals** are responsible for pulling the ribs down to decrease the diameter of the cavity for exhalation. Along with the internal intercostals, the **subcostals** also pull the lower ribs down and apart to decrease the cavity size. The thoracic nerves 1 to 11 supply the internal and external intercostals for neuromotor control.

The **external intercostals** fill up the space between the ribs on the **outside** of the thoracic cage.

The **internal intercostals** fill up the space between the ribs on the **inside** of the thoracic cage.

The **subcostal muscles** are located along the **lower inside back wall** of the thoracic cage.

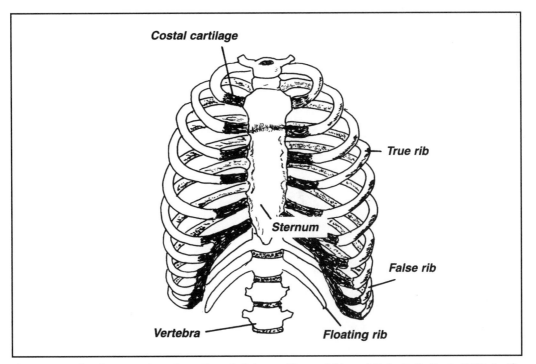

Figure 1.2. The rib cage. *Note.* From *Speech Sciences* (Figure 4.11, p. 81), by R. D. Kent, 1997, Pacific Grove, CA: Delmar. Copyright 1997 by Delmar, a division of Thomson Learning (Fax 800/730-2215). Reprinted with permission.

The respiratory passages are located within the thoracic cavity. These include the **trachea,** the **bronchial tubes,** and the **lungs.** The trachea is a tube formed by about 20 rings of **cartilage.** Its length is approximately 11 centimeters in the adult, and it serves as the main conductor chamber for air. The trachea, which lies just beneath the **larynx,** is the starting point of the lower airway. As it proceeds downward, it eventually **bifurcates** (divides) into the right and the left primary **bronchi.** As the bronchi enter the lungs, they further subdivide into **bronchioles.** The lungs, located inside the thoracic cavity and protected by the thoracic cage, are the organs responsible for the exchange of carbon dioxide and oxygen. Figure 1.3 shows the lungs and the bronchi.

Major and Minor Muscles of the Respiratory Mechanism

Adequate respiratory control requires the actions of various muscles. Some muscles have a more direct contribution to respiration, while others serve as auxiliary or stabilizing muscles. Palmer (1993) separates these into major and minor muscle groups. The major muscles include the diaphragm, the external intercostals, and the internal intercostals. Some of the minor muscle groups include the scalene, transverse thoracic, quadratus lumborum, pectoralis major, and pectoralis minor muscles.

We previously described the diaphragm as the chief muscle of respiration. It is instrumental in elevating the ribs and increasing the vertical dimension of the thoracic cage. The diaphragm is innervated by the cervical spinal nerves 3 to 5, which are collectively known as the **phrenic nerves.** The external intercostals assist in

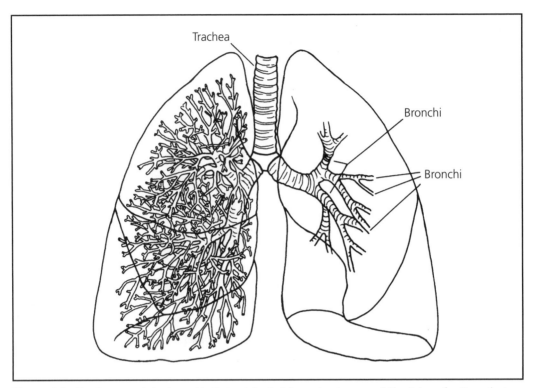

Figure 1.3. The lungs and the bronchi. *Note.* Adapted from *Anatomy and Physiology for Speech, Language, and Hearing* (Figure 3.19a, p. 68), by J. A. Seikel, D. W. King, and D. G. Drumright, 1997, Pacific Grove, CA: Delmar. Copyright 1997 by Delmar, a division of Thomson Learning (Fax 800/730-2215). Reprinted with permission.

elevating the ribs in inhalation, while the internal intercostals help in depressing the ribs in exhalation.

The minor muscles assist the major muscles in the inhalation and exhalation processes. The **scalene muscles,** which originate from the cervical vertebrae and insert into the upper surface of ribs 1 and 2, help to elevate and fixate the ribs for inhalation. Two other minor muscles help to elevate the ribs: pectoralis major and pectoralis minor. **Pectoralis major** originates at the head of the **humerus bone** and inserts to the anterior end of the **clavicle,** sternum, and costal cartilages 2 to 6. **Pectoralis minor**'s point of origin is the **scapula,** and its insertion is the bony ends of ribs 2 to 5.

The **transverse thoracic** and **quadratus lumborum muscles** assist in depressing the ribs for exhalation. The transverse thoracic muscles originate in the internal surface of the sternum and **xiphoid process** and insert into the **costal cartilages** and bony end of ribs 2 to 6. Quadratus laborum has several points of origin including the posterior part of the **iliac crest,** the **iliolumbar ligament,** and the transverse processes of lumbar vertebrae 3, 4, and 5. Its point of insertion is the lower border of rib 12 and the tendons of the abdominal muscles. It helps depress rib 12 and aids in fixing the origin of the diaphragm. Table 1.1 summarizes the point of origin and insertion of these muscles, their major action or function, and the nerves that supply them for neuromotor control.

Table 1.1. Major and Minor Muscles of Respiration

Muscle	Origin	Insertion	Function	Nerve Supply
Diaphragm	Xiphoid process of sternum, inferior margin of rib cage, corpus of L1, transverse processes of L1–L5	Central tendon of diaphragm	Primary muscle of inspiration; depresses central tendon of diaphragm, enlarges thorax vertically; distends abdomen	Phrenic nerves arising from cervical plexus of spinal nerves C3–C5
Scalenes (anterior, medial, and posterior portions)	Mastoid process of temporal bone (anterior); transverse processes of vertebrae C3 through C6 (medial); transverse processes of C5 through C7	Upper surface of ribs 1 and 2	Assist with inspiration; elevate ribs 1 and 2	Cervical nerves C3–C8
Pectoralis minor	Coracoid process of the scapula	Bony ends of ribs 2–5	Assists with forced inspiration; increases transverse dimension of rib cage	Superior branch of the brachial plexus (spinal nerves C4 through C7 and Tl)
Pectoralis major	Head of the humerus bone	Clavicle, sternum, costal cartilages 2–6	Assists with forced inspiration; elevates sternum, increases transverse dimension of rib cage	Superior branch of the brachial plexus (spinal nerves C4 through C7 and T1)
Quadratus lumborum	Posterior portion of iliac crest, iliolumbar ligament, and transverse processes of L3–L5	Lower border of rib 12 and the tendons of the abdominal muscles	Assists with exhalation; helps depress rib 12 and aids in fixing the origin of the diaphragm	Thoracic nerve T12 and L1–L4 lumbar nerves
Transverse thoracic	Inner thoracic lateral margin of sternum	Inner chondral surface of ribs 2–6	Assists with expiration; depresses rib cage	Intercostal nerves from T9 through T11 and subcostal nerves from T12

Breathing Patterns During Speech Production

Breathing for speech requires a systematic coordination of the structures previously described. Inhalation and exhalation must create a rhythmic cycle of respiration. The structural respiratory system must supply moving air that can set the vocal cords into vibration. Also, the production of lengthy sentences necessitates the duration of the exhalation portion of the respiratory cycle to be sustained for approximately 15 seconds (Hulitt & Howard, 1997).

At rest, during quiet breathing, the pressure inside and outside the thoracic cavity may be equal. However, for speech production, the pressure inside the thoracic cavity must be greater than the pressure outside to allow air to rush into the lungs. For this to happen, the thoracic cavity must expand in size.

Expansion of the thoracic cavity occurs primarily by contraction or flattening of the diaphragm. As the diaphragm, which is usually in a **concave** position, flattens, the size of the thoracic cavity increases. This creates a negative air pressure inside the lungs. This now negative air pressure inside the lungs and positive air pressure outside the lungs cause air to be inhaled through the mouth and the nose as pressure equalization is sought.

As air rushes through the trachea and into the lungs (inhalation), the thoracic cavity expands even more through the actions of other respiratory muscles. This causes the air pressure inside the lungs to become greater (positive) than the air pressure outside the cavity (negative).

The diaphragm then relaxes and returns to its dome-shaped position, decreasing the size of the thoracic cavity. As the ribs lower due to the actions of various muscles, the size of the thoracic cavity decreases even further. These motions act to expel the air from the lungs (exhalation) in a forced manner, creating sufficient air pressure to vibrate the vocal folds.

Compared to quiet breathing, breathing for speech is more consciously monitored and adjusted to meet the demands for speech. For example, in situations when an unusually strong burst of air is needed, as when special emphasis or loudness is required, the respiratory muscles can act to provide this additional pulse of energy by forceful squeezing of the thoracic cavity.

Phonatory Mechanism

As the respiratory system supplies the air needed for speech, the phonatory system is responsible for producing sound or voice. The **larynx,** also known as the voice box, is the chief structure involved in the production of sound. Like the respiratory mechanism, the phonatory mechanism is a complex and dynamic system.

Structures of the Phonatory System

The larynx, resting just above the trachea in the anterior portion of the neck, is a muscular, membranous, and cartilaginous structure. It is suspended by muscles and ligaments attached to a U-shaped bone called the hyoid. Although the **hyoid bone** is not part of the larynx, it bears an important laryngeal function in that various laryngeal muscles are attached to it.

Cartilaginous Framework of the Larynx

The structural framework of the larynx consists of nine cartilages and their connecting membranes and ligaments. This structural framework without the connecting membranes and ligaments is illustrated in Figure 1.4. Three cartilages are unpaired and rather large in size, while the remaining cartilages are paired and relatively smaller. The unpaired cartilages are the **thyroid, cricoid,** and **epiglottis** and the paired cartilages are the **arytenoids, corniculates,** and **cuneiforms**

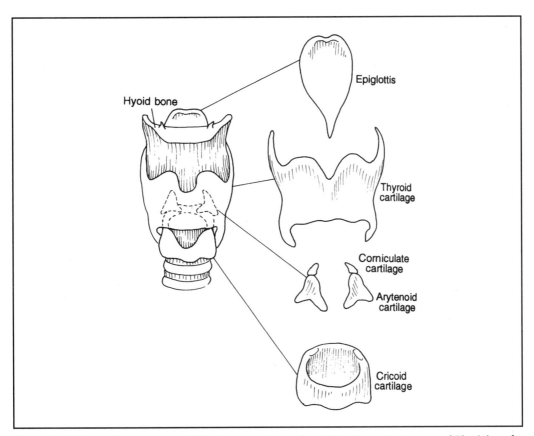

Figure 1.4. The major structures of the larynx, anterior view. *Note.* From *Anatomy and Physiology for Speech, Language, and Hearing* (Figure 5.4, p. 166), by J. A. Seikel, D. W. King, and D. G. Drumright, 1997, Pacific Grove, CA: Delmar. Copyright 1997 by Delmar, a division of Thomson Learning (Fax 800/730-2215). Reprinted with permission.

(not shown in Figure 1.4, as they reside within the aryepiglottic folds). Of these, the unpaired thyroid and cricoid and the paired arytenoids play the most significant role in speech production.

The **thyroid,** a large and butterfly-shaped cartilage, forms the frontal and lateral (side) walls of the larynx. It consists of two quadrilateral plates fused in front in a V shape. The open portion faces toward the back and the fused portion, named the **thyroid prominence,** projects toward the front. The thyroid prominence is the protruding part of the neck commonly known as the **Adam's apple.** Just above the thyroid prominence is an unfused portion of the plates known as the **thyroid notch.** This V-shaped notch marks the approximate anterior attachment of the vocal folds.

Below the thyroid cartilage and above the uppermost tracheal ring sits the **cricoid cartilage.** The cricoid is ring shaped with a plate on the posterior side (**posterior quadrate laminae**) and a narrower band forming the front and lateral sides (**anterior arch**). The anterior arch of the cricoid contains small oval **articular facets** on each side, which connect with the **inferior horns** of the thyroid. The articulation between the thyroid and cricoid results in a pivot joint, which permits the thyroid and the cricoid to rotate. This pivotal connection is important for shortening and elongating the vocal folds.

The paired arytenoid cartilages, despite their small size, play a significant role in laryngeal function. They are pyramid shaped and are connected to the top portion of the posterior plate of the cricoid through the **cricoarytenoid joint.** Each arytenoid contains a **vocal process** and a **lateral** or **muscular process.** The vocal processes extend anteriorly, and the vocal folds are attached to them. The lateral processes have several muscles attached to them that help the vocal folds open and close. These structures, seen from anterior, lateral, and posterior angles, are illustrated in Figure 1.5.

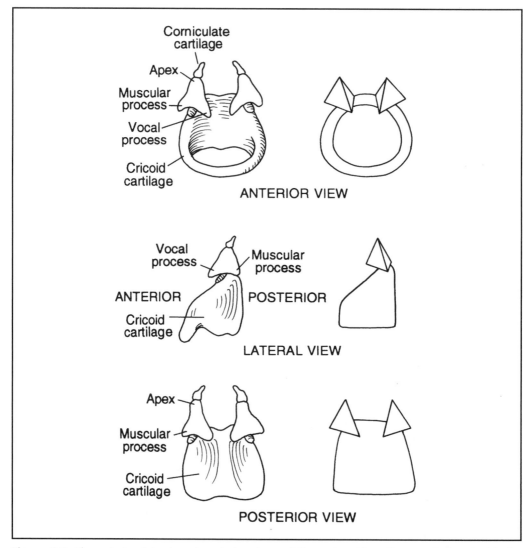

Figure 1.5. The anterior, lateral, and posterior views of the arytenoid cartilages articulated with the cricoid cartilage, along with the muscular and vocal processes of the arytenoid cartilages. *Note.* From *Anatomy and Physiology for Speech, Language, and Hearing* (Figure 5.11, p. 177), by J. A. Seikel, D. W. King, and D. G. Drumright, 1997, Pacific Grove, CA: Delmar. Copyright 1997 by Delmar, a division of Thomson Learning (Fax 800/730-2215). Reprinted with permission.

Muscles of the Larynx

The muscles of the larynx are classified as either extrinsic or intrinsic. The differentiating feature between the two is that **extrinsic muscles** have one attachment to structures outside of the larynx, while **intrinsic muscles** have both attachments confined to the larynx. Extrinsic muscles primarily provide a supportive framework for the larynx. However, they do have some laryngeal function in that they fix the larynx in place: their actions can lower or raise the larynx and thus indirectly influence sound production. The intrinsic musculature is directly responsible for the production of sound.

Although several muscles are part of the laryngeal mechanism, our focus will be only on the intrinsic muscles that have a leading role in phonation (production of voice). We will focus on the muscles that form the vocal folds, muscles that **adduct** the vocal folds (adductors), muscles that **abduct** the vocal folds (abductors), and muscles that tense and elongate the vocal folds.

The vocal folds comprise two separate muscle masses, the **thyrovocalis** and the **thyromuscularis,** which together form the **thyroarytenoid muscle.** The vocalis muscle mass forms the vibrating (sound producing) portion of the vocal folds. The vocal folds attach to the cartilaginous framework of the larynx in two places. The anterior portion of the vocal folds attaches to the inside angle of the thyroid notch. The posterior portion of the vocal folds attaches to the vocal process of the arytenoid cartilages. These attachments form a muscular band extending from the thyroid to the arytenoids on each side. The space between the vocal folds is named the **glottis.** The glottis is open when the vocal folds are apart and is closed or nearly so when they are approximated. During quiet breathing, the glottis is in an open position. It is important to remember that the glottis is not a bony or muscular structure, but a space formed by the muscles of the vocal folds. Figure 1.6 shows the thyromuscularis and thyrovocalis portions of the vocal folds.

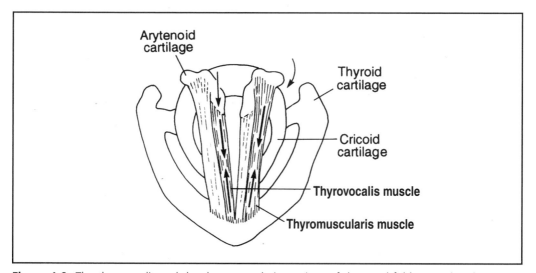

Figure 1.6. The thyrovocalis and the thyromuscularis portions of the vocal folds, superior view. *Note.* From *Anatomy and Physiology for Speech, Language, and Hearing* (Figure 5.19, p. 191), by J. A. Seikel, D. W. King, and D. G. Drumright, 1997, Pacific Grove, CA: Delmar. Copyright 1997 by Delmar, a division of Thomson Learning (Fax 800/730-2215). Reprinted with permission.

Adduction or approximation of the vocal folds is accomplished through the interaction of the **lateral cricoarytenoid muscles,** the **transverse arytenoid muscles,** and the **oblique arytenoid** muscles. See Figure 1.7 for an illustration of these muscles. The lateral cricoarytenoid muscles are responsible for swiveling the arytenoid cartilages toward the middle of the larynx (medially). Because the vocal folds are attached to the arytenoid cartilages, they will also move medially, and partially close off the glottis (partial adduction). To achieve complete adduction, the transverse and oblique arytenoid muscles must take part. As these

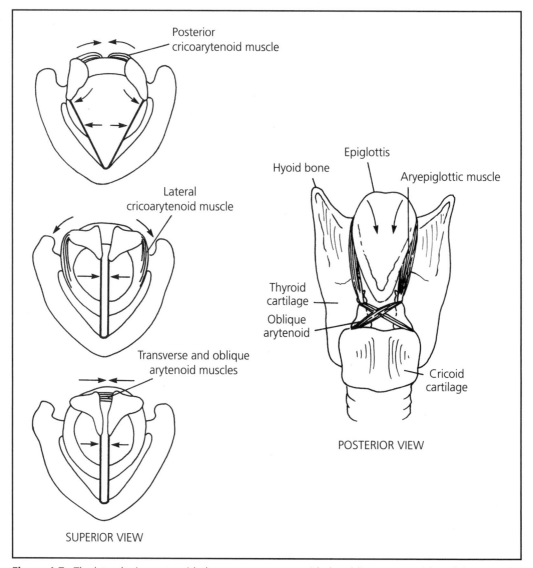

Figure 1.7. The lateral cricoarytenoid, the transverse arytenoid, the oblique arytenoid, and the posterior cricoarytenoid muscles. *Note.* From *Anatomy and Physiology for Speech, Language, and Hearing* (Figure 5.20a, p. 192), by J. A. Seikel, D. W. King, and D. G. Drumright, 1997, Pacific Grove, CA: Delmar. Copyright 1997 by Delmar, a division of Thomson Learning (Fax 800/730-2215). Reprinted with permission.

muscles contract, they pull the arytenoids and the vocal folds together, which assists the lateral cricoarytenoid muscles in completely closing off the glottis. Adduction of the vocal folds is essential for vibration of the air supplied by the respiratory mechanism in the production of voiced consonants and vowels.

To abduct or separate the vocal cords after they have been successfully adducted, an antagonistic action must take place. The **posterior cricoarytenoids** (see Figure 1.7), acting in opposition to the major vocal fold adductors, are the muscles responsible for abducting the vocal folds. They originate on both sides of the posterior plate of the cricoid cartilage and attach to the lateral processes of the arytenoid cartilages. As they contract, they pull the arytenoids in a rotating fashion, making them swivel laterally. This lateral movement pulls apart (abducts) the vocal folds attached to the vocal processes of the arytenoids. With the vocal folds in an abducted position, the air supplied by the respiratory mechanism travels past the level of the vocal folds in an unvibrated manner. This is essential for the production of unvoiced consonants.

Adduction and abduction of the vocal folds lead to the production or the absence of voice, respectively. Another laryngeal muscle is responsible for tensing and elongating the vocal folds, actions leading to pitch variation. This is the **cricothyroid muscle.** It is a fan-shaped muscle originating at the cricoid cartilage and inserting into the thyroid cartilage. The cricothyroid muscle consists of two parts: *pars oblique* and *pars recta.* With the cricoid cartilage in place and as the pars recta (erect portion) contracts, the thyroid cartilage tilts downward. Contraction of the oblique portion (pars oblique) slides the thyroid forward. These actions cause the vocal folds to elongate and become tense. Figure 1.8 illustrates the two parts of the cricothyroid muscle.

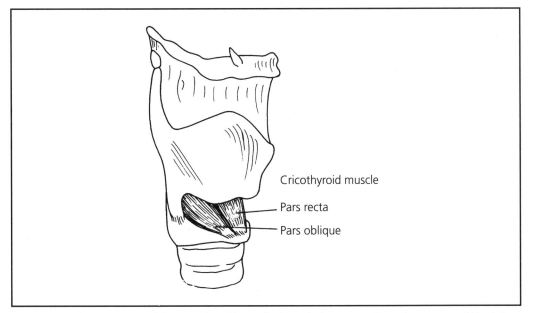

Cricothyroid muscle

Pars recta

Pars oblique

Figure 1.8. The two parts of the cricothyroid muscle, lateral view. *Note.* From *Anatomy and Physiology for Speech, Language, and Hearing* (Figure 5.18, p. 189), by J. A. Seikel, D. W. King, and D. G. Drumright, 1997, Pacific Grove, CA: Delmar. Copyright 1997 by Delmar, a division of Thomson Learning (Fax 800/730-2215). Reprinted with permission.

Physiology of Phonation

We have reviewed the cartilages that provide a supportive framework for the laryngeal musculature. We have also outlined the muscles that make up the vocal folds, the muscles that abduct and adduct the vocal folds, and the muscles that tense and elongate the vocal folds. We have previously stated that vibration of the vocal folds in a tensely adducted position leads to voice production. Adduction and tensing of the vocal folds are not sufficient for vibration to occur, however. At this point, the vocal folds are merely in position for a physiological effort to begin.

When the vocal folds are closed (adducted), the flow of air supplied by the respiratory mechanism is stopped. Stopping the rush of air being forcefully expelled from the lungs to the upper airway builds up air pressure below the vocal folds. This **subglottic** air pressure is higher than the pressure above the vocal folds (**supraglottic** pressure). As the subglottic air pressure becomes too great to contain, the vocal folds are forced apart in a vibrated manner. Opening of the vocal folds begins posteriorly, with the open space (**glottal chink**) moving anteriorly. This is the opening phase. Closing of the vocal folds begins when the opening phase reaches the most anterior portion of the vocal folds. The closing process also travels from the posterior to anterior portion of the vocal folds. Complete closure of the vocal folds again causes subglottic air pressure to build, restarting the cycle of opening and closing.

The building of pressure below the glottis can explain opening of the vocal folds. However, the **Bernoulli effect** is responsible for closing the vocal folds after they have been forcefully abducted. In short, the theory states that as gases or liquids move through a constricted passage, velocity increases and pressure decreases. During phonation, the air (gas) traveling from the lungs passes through the slightly abducted vocal folds (constricted passage). As the vocal folds are momentarily abducted, a puff of air is quickly released, causing a drop of air pressure directly between the vocal folds. This drop of air pressure causes a suction action to draw the vocal folds together.

The elasticity of the vocal folds is another factor that has been attributed to their opening and closing. The vocal folds are very strong and can resist the air pressure that builds under them, but they are also sufficiently elastic to go back to their original position after they have been blown apart to close again. Therefore, vocal fold opening and closing are more fully explained by considering the buildup of air pressure, the supra- and subglottic pressure differences (positive and negative), and the elasticity of the muscles. This thorough explanation is known as the **myoelastic-aerodynamic theory** of phonation.

Resonatory Mechanism

The sound produced by vibration of the vocal folds does not have the differential qualities perceived by the listener. The process by which the voiced breathstream (sound produced by the vocal folds) is modified to enhance and dampen certain frequency components is called resonation. The laryngeal tone is modified into perceptibly different voice qualities by the structures that serve as vocal sound resonators: the **pharyngeal cavity,** the **oral cavity,** and the **nasal cavity** (see Figure 1.9 in the next section, "Articulatory Mechanism").

Structures of the Resonatory System

The pharynx, often referred to as the throat, is part of the upper airway located superiorly and posteriorly to the larynx. The pharynx is not a very dynamic structure; its size and shape are modified by the vertical positioning of the larynx in the neck (high or low) and by the position of the tongue in the mouth (forward or back). Because the base of the tongue is attached to the pharynx, a retracted tongue position will dampen sound production at the pharyngeal level and thus decrease the effectiveness of oral voice projection. A forward tongue position is more effective because it allows a frontal resonation of sound.

The nasal cavity is important in the resonation of sound. Although many sounds can be produced with a nasal quality, only three sounds of English should be fully nasalized: /m/, /n/, and /ŋ/. This is possible through *coupling* (a coming together) of the oral and nasal cavities. The opening and closing control mechanism for the nasal cavity is the soft palate or **velum.** During speech production, the velum will elevate and make contact with the posterior pharynx, separating the nasal cavity from the pharynx and oral cavity. If the soft palate does not elevate to contact the posterior pharynx, the nasal and oral cavities are coupled, resulting in nasal resonation of the vibrated sound.

The oral cavity is the resonating structure for all sounds except /m/, /n/, and /ŋ/. Several structures within the oral cavity play a role in modifying oral resonance: the movement, excursion, and mass of the mandible; the size, shape, and positioning of the tongue; and the height, length, and width of the hard palate. The teeth, the cheekbones, and the contact of the velum with the posterior pharynx also play a part in oral resonance.

In describing the oral cavity and its role in resonation of the laryngeal tone, it is inevitable to initiate discussion of articulation. In fact, resonation is intricately involved with articulation in that the resonating cavities mold, shape, and modify the airstream coming from the larynx to help produce articulated speech sounds. Considering resonation apart from articulation is most important in understanding nasal versus oral resonance in the production of certain speech sounds.

Articulatory Mechanism

The final process involved in speech production is articulation. Simply stated, articulation is the molding of the airstream into recognizable speech sounds by several structures in the mouth, the **articulators.** Weiss, Gordon, and Lillywhite (1987) subclassify the various articulators into two major categories: *movable* and *immovable*. This subclassification helps distinguish articulators that are more static from those that are more dynamic.

The most important movable articulators include the tongue, the lips, the soft palate, and the jaw; and the most important immovable articulators include the teeth, the hard palate, and the **alveolar ridge.** Figure 1.9 shows the various movable and immovable articulators and the resonating cavities. The movable articulators move toward and away from the immovable articulators. At times the contact between the mobile and fixed articulators is complete, while at other times it is only approximate.

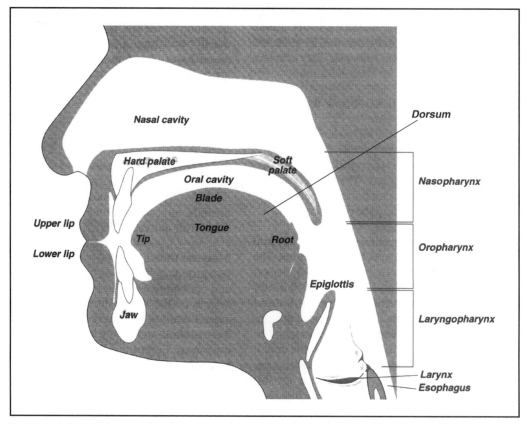

Figure 1.9. The major speech articulators and the resonating oral and nasal cavities. *Note.* Adapted from *Speech Sciences* (Figure 5.28, p. 167), by R. D. Kent, 1997, Pacific Grove, CA: Delmar. Copyright 1997 by Delmar, a division of Thomson Learning (Fax 800/730-2215). Reprinted with permission.

Movable Articulators

The tongue is generally considered the most important articulator due to its vital role in shaping the majority of speech sounds. This large and highly mobile and flexible muscle mass fills a large part of the oral cavity. It is typically divided into various anatomical sections including the *tip, blade, dorsum,* and *root.* The tip is the thinnest part of the tongue; it usually rests behind the lower front teeth. The blade is next to the tongue tip and lies just below the alveolar ridge. The dorsum is the largest area of the tongue, making contact with both the hard and soft palates. The root of the tongue makes up its very back portion.

Several **intrinsic** and **extrinsic** muscles make up the bulk of the tongue. The four intrinsic muscles (**superior** and **inferior longitudinal, transverse,** and **vertical**) shape the tongue into various contours. Four extrinsic muscles (**genio-glossus, hyoglossus, palatoglossus,** and **styloglossus**) help move the tongue into various positions within the oral cavity. Due to a rich supply of nerves, the intrinsic and extrinsic muscles allow the tongue to make rapid and precise movements, to lengthen, shorten, curl up, pull down, and flatten. These movements are extremely important in the production of consonant and vowel speech sounds.

The lips are made up primarily of the **orbicularis oris** muscle. Several other muscles of the mid and lower face connect to the orbicularis oris, allowing the lips also to make a variety of movements. Although not as vital as the tongue, the lips do play an important role in the production of the **bilabials** /p/, /b/, and /m/, the **labiodentals** /f/ and /v/, and other consonants and vowels requiring varying degrees of lip movement. Firm closure of the lips also allows the buildup of intra-oral pressure, which is then released in a plosive manner necessary for the production of many sounds.

The jaw or **mandible** is a large bone of the face that acts as a facilitator of articulation and resonance. It forms the floor of the mouth and houses the lower set of teeth. It also provides a bony framework for many tongue and lip muscles. The mandible can increase or decrease the size of the oral cavity according to its various movements.

The **velum** or **soft palate,** previously described under the section on resonatory mechanism, also plays an important role in the articulation of sounds. It begins at the end of the **hard palate** (roof of the mouth) and extends back toward the pharynx. A small cone-shaped structure hanging from the velum is called the **uvula.**

The velum contains several muscles including the **levator veli palatini, tensor veli palatini, palatoglossus, palatopharyngeus,** and **uvulae,** which acting in synchrony allow it to move superiorly and posteriorly to make firm contact against the pharyngeal wall. Firm contact of the soft palate against the pharyngeal wall is important to achieve **velopharyngeal closure** in the production of all sounds except /m/, /n/, and /ŋ/. Opening of the **velopharyngeal port** allows the breathstream to continue to the nasal cavity, where it is resonated for the nasal sounds /m/, /n/, and /ŋ/. The velum also is the site of articulatory contact for the back sounds /k/, /g/, and /ŋ/.

Immovable Articulators

The hard palate is a bony structure separating the oral cavity from the nasal cavity as it forms the floor of the nose and the roof of the mouth. It is primarily made up of two paired bones called the **maxilla** and the **palatine bones.** The maxillary bones (maxillae) form the bulk of the hard palate, while the palatine bones form its posterior portion.

The maxilla is subdivided into the **palatine process,** the **alveolar process,** and the **premaxilla.** The palatine process is made up of two pieces of bone that grow and fuse together during the fetal stage. They make up most of the hard palate. The alveolar process, also called the **alveolar ridge,** contains the sockets that house the upper molar, bicuspid, and cuspid teeth. The most anterior portion of the maxillary bone is called the premaxilla. It is a small wedge of bone that houses the four upper front teeth. In the fetal stage, the premaxilla begins as a separate structure that eventually fuses with the maxillary bone. See Figure 1.10 for a schematic and photographic representation of the inferior view of the hard palate.

The alveolar ridge or alveolar process is the place of lingual (tongue) contact for several front sounds, including /t/, /d/, /s/, /z/, /n/, and /l/. The palatine process, most commonly referred to as the hard palate, is the place of lingual contact for the palatal sounds /ʃ/, /ʒ/, /tʃ/, /dʒ/, /r/, and /j/.

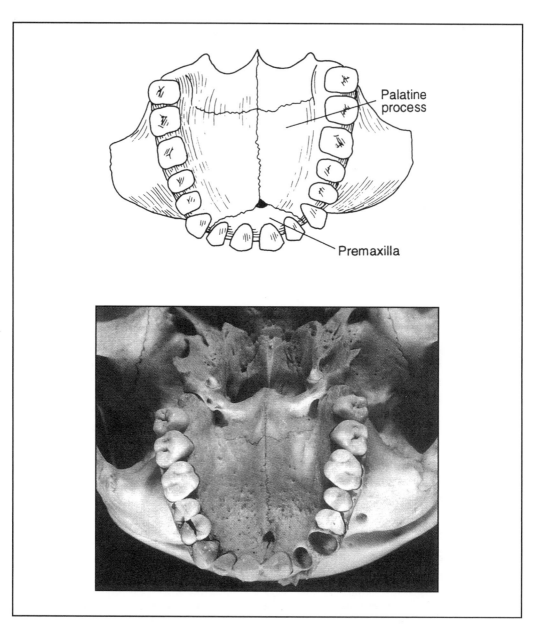

Figure 1.10. Schematic and photographic representation of the inferior view of the hard palate. *Note.* Adapted from *Anatomy and Physiology for Speech, Language, and Hearing* (Figure 7.12, p. 276), by J. A. Seikel, D. W. King, and D. G. Drumright, 1997, Pacific Grove, CA: Delmar. Copyright 1997 by Delmar, a division of Thomson Learning (Fax 800/730-2215). Reprinted with permission.

The teeth, apart from serving an important cosmetic purpose, also play a part in the articulation of speech sounds. Along with the tongue, they are directly involved in the production of the /f/, /v/, /θ/, and /ð/ sounds. They also help to produce the friction quality in many of the fricative sounds as the breathstream passes over the lower edges of the incisor (front) teeth.

Auditory Mechanism

Speaking and hearing are interrelated activities. The natural development of speech and language requires normal audition or hearing. Children learn verbal language through hearing what is said to them. Hearing is also important for individuals who are beyond the speech and language acquisition process, since this mechanism allows speakers to monitor and regulate their own speech production. Through the auditory feedback loop, speakers can often determine if they are speaking with appropriate speed, loudness, and clarity and can make modifications as needed.

The anatomy of the auditory mechanism includes mucous and fibrous membranes, bones, ligaments, muscles, fluid-filled canals, nerve fibers, and other supporting tissues that together make up a complex system. The gross anatomy of the human ear is typically divided into three parts: the outer ear, the middle ear, and the inner ear. The basic anatomy of the ear and its main structures is illustrated in Figure 1.11

Outer Ear

The most visible part of the outer ear is the **auricle** or **pinna.** As sound travels from the environment to the outer ear in the form of waves, those waves are collected by the pinna and directed into the **external auditory meatus,** also known

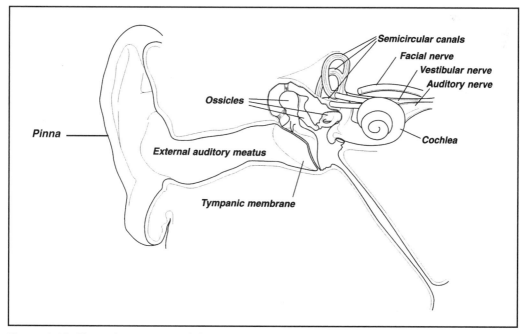

Figure 1.11. The major structures of the ear. *Note.* Adapted from *Speech Sciences* (Figure 6.2, p. 211), by R. D. Kent, 1997, Pacific Grove, CA: Delmar. Copyright 1997 by Delmar, a division of Thomson Learning (Fax 800/730-2215). Reprinted with permission.

as the **ear canal.** The pinna also helps humans localize the sources of sound coming from in front, behind, below, and above the head.

The external auditory meatus is a curved tube-like structure approximately 2.5 cm (1 inch) long. It resonates the sound waves that enter it. Martin (1986) indicates that the external auditory meatus serves as a resonator for frequencies between 2,000 and 5,500 Hz (p. 207). It ends at the point where the tympanic membrane (eardrum) is located.

Middle Ear

The middle ear is an air-filled space lined with mucous membrane. The structures of the middle ear include the tympanic membrane, the ossicular chain (three small bones), and the eustachian tube.

The **tympanic membrane** is a semitransparent, luminescent structure that is pearl gray in appearance when it is healthy. It is cone shaped and attached to the first bone of the ossicular chain. This trilayered membrane absorbs the acoustic energy traveling through the ear canal and transforms it into mechanical energy. It is sensitive to different sound frequencies, particularly low frequencies. However, some portions of the membrane can respond to specific high frequencies. Through its vibrations, the tympanic membrane transmits sound energy to the auditory ossicles.

Various ligaments sustain the ossicular chain in the middle ear. The ossicular chain, illustrated in Figure 1.12, is made up of three tiny bones. The first bone, called the **malleus,** resembles a hammer. It is the largest of the three bones and is attached to the tympanic membrane. The second (middle) bone of the chain is called the **incus;** it resembles an anvil. The incus is connected to the malleus in a tight joint, permitting little movement. The third and last bone is called the **stapes,** which resembles a stirrup on an English saddle. The incus articulates with the stapes. All three bones are thus intricately interconnected.

The malleus and the incus receive the sound energy traveling from the vibrating tympanic membrane. This sound energy is then transmitted to the stapes.

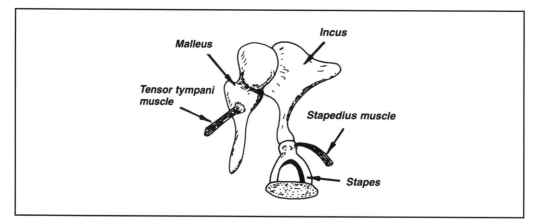

Figure 1.12. The ossicles of the middle ear. *Note.* Adapted from *Speech Sciences* (Figure 6.5, p. 215), by R. D. Kent, 1997, Pacific Grove, CA: Delmar. Copyright 1997 by Delmar, a division of Thomson Learning (Fax 800/730-2215). Reprinted with permission.

Finally, the stapes conducts the sound to an opening called the **oval window** of the inner ear.

Two small muscles in the middle ear dampen vibrations of the eardrum and the ossicular chain: the tensor tympani and the stapedius. The **tensor tympani** tenses the eardrum so that its vibrations are reduced. The **stapedius muscle** stiffens the ossicular chain so that its vibrations also are reduced. These reactions are reflexive and are known as the **acoustic reflex.** This reflex protects the ear from very loud sounds and noises that could damage it.

Inner Ear

The **oval window** is a small opening in the bone of the inner ear. It marks the beginning of the inner ear. It helps the foot of the stapes position itself to receive sound vibrations. The foot of the stapes also acts like a door to the inner ear.

A complex system of interconnecting canals and passages called the **labyrinth** is located within the temporal bone in the inner ear. The passages are filled with a special fluid called **perilymph,** and they house the sensitive organs of the inner ear. They also house three important structures that aid in the maintenance of balance or equilibrium. These structures are called the **semicircular canals.**

The main inner ear structure of hearing is known as the **cochlea.** When fully stretched, the human cochlea measures approximately 3.8 cm (1.5 inches). It is shaped like the shell of a snail or a coiled hose, and it is filled with a special fluid called **endolymph,** which gets moved around as the stapes pushes into the inner ear. The floor of the cochlea is called the **basilar membrane.** The cochlea and the semicircular canals are illustrated in Figure 1.13.

The inner ear's most important structure of hearing, which is called the **organ of Corti,** is located within the basilar membrane; it bathes in the endolymph. It

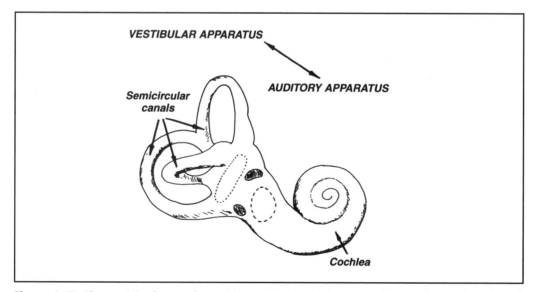

Figure 1.13. The semicircular canals and the cochlea in the inner ear. *Note.* Adapted from *Speech Sciences* (Figure 6.6, p. 216), by R. D. Kent, 1997, Pacific Grove, CA: Delmar. Copyright 1997 by Delmar, a division of Thomson Learning (Fax 800/730-2215). Reprinted with permission.

contains thousands of **cilia** that respond to sound. Cilia, also known as **hair cells,** are hairlike structures that are sensitive to sound vibrations.

As the vibrations delivered by the foot plate of the stapes reach the inner ear's oval window, wavelike movements are created in the perilymph. Those movements are transmitted to the endolymph through **Reissner's membrane,** which in turn transmits them to the basilar membrane. The hair cells of the organ of Corti respond to the shearing force created by the vibration of the basilar membrane.

At this point the mechanical forces or vibrations (wavelike movements of the fluids and membranes) are transformed into electrical energy. This energy transformation within the organ of Corti is essential, because the nerve fibers that carry the sound to the central nervous system can respond only to electrical impulses, not to mechanical vibrations.

The electrical or neural impulses created by the movement of the hair cells of the cochlea are picked up by the **vestibuloacoustic nerve,** which is also known as **cranial nerve VIII.** This nerve has two primary divisions, a vestibular division and an auditory division. The **vestibular division** is concerned with body equilibrium, and as the name implies the **auditory division** is concerned with hearing. The neural function of the auditory nerve will be addressed in the Advanced Unit of this chapter.

Summary of the Basic Unit

• The speech production mechanism can be divided into four major subsystems: respiration, phonation, resonation, and articulation.

• The auditory mechanism plays an integral role in the normal development of speech and language and the continual monitoring of our verbal output.

• Respiration is the basic subsystem that provides the air supply necessary for speech. Without air, speech production would be extremely difficult, if not impossible.

• The diaphragm, the external and internal intercostals, and other minor muscles make up the muscular framework of the respiratory mechanism.

• The thoracic vertebrae, the sternum, the ribs, and the costal cartilages make up the bony framework of the respiratory mechanism.

• The respiratory passages include the trachea, the bronchial tubes, and the lungs. These are located within the thoracic cavity.

• Compared to quiet breathing, breathing for speech is more consciously monitored and adjusted to meet the continually changing demands for speech.

• The phonatory system (i.e., the larynx) is responsible for producing the sound or voice that can eventually be modified to create voiced consonants and vowels.

• The thyroid, cricoid, epiglottis, arytenoids, corniculates, and cuneiforms form the cartilaginous framework of the larynx.

• The larynx contains several extrinsic and intrinsic muscles. The intrinsic muscles are directly implicated in the production of voice, while the extrinsic muscles primarily provide a supportive framework for the larynx.

• The Bernoulli effect and the myoelastic-aerodynamic theory of phonation can explain closing and opening of the vocal folds for voice production.

• The voiced and unvoiced sound produced by the respiratory and phonatory systems resonates in the pharynx, oral cavity, and nasal cavity.

• Nasal sounds are resonated in the nasal cavity. These include /m/, /n/, and /ŋ/.

• Non-nasal sounds are primarily resonated in the oral cavity. These include all sounds except the nasals.

• The velum moves in an upward and backward position to assist in velopharyngeal closure for non-nasal sounds.

• The final process involved in speech production is articulation. Articulation is the molding of the airstream into recognizable speech sounds by several structures in the mouth.

• The tongue, lips, velum, and mandible are the movable or dynamic articulators.

• The alveolar ridge, hard palate, and teeth make up the immovable or static articulators.

• The auditory mechanism allows human beings to learn speech and language initially and to monitor verbal output on a constant basis.

• The auditory mechanism has three peripheral divisions: the outer ear, middle ear, and inner ear.

• The tympanic membrane, ossicular chain, cochlea, and oval window are extremely important structures of the auditory mechanism.

• The mechanical vibrations from the middle ear are converted to electrical energy in the inner ear. This electrical information is picked up by the vestibulo-acoustic nerve in each ear and transmitted to the primary auditory cortex in the cerebral hemispheres of the brain.

Advanced Unit

◆ ◆ ◆ ◆ ◆ ◆ ◆ ◆ ◆ ◆ ◆ ◆ ◆ ◆ ◆ ◆ ◆ ◆ ◆

The Neuroanatomical Bases of Speech Production

The brain's power and function have fascinated human beings for centuries. Countless books have been written about the wonders of this relatively small human structure. Although the average adult brain weighs only about 3 pounds, all major bodily functions (speech and language included) are initiated, regulated, and integrated by its various structures.

In the Basic Unit of this chapter, we summarized the speech production mechanism according to four structural subsystems: respiration, phonation, resonation, and articulation. However, to fully understand the complexity of speech, it is necessary to also analyze it in relation to the nervous system that initiates, integrates, coordinates, and regulates all the movements necessary for the production of sounds, words, and sentences.

We do not claim to offer an extensive literary review on this topic since a comprehensive and detailed description of the neuroanatomy of speech cannot be well done in a single chapter. The reader may consult several outstanding textbooks for a more comprehensive presentation (Bhatnagar & Andy, 1995; Kuehn, Lemme, & Baumgartner, 1989; Love & Webb, 1996; Palmer, 1993; Perkins & Kent, 1986; Seikel et al., 1997; Zemlin, 1998). Our intent is to offer a basic introduction for students who are unfamiliar with the neuromotor control of speech and a general review for those readers who already have some foundational knowledge.

Overview

Speech production is a voluntary behavior that necessitates the coordination of various systems. As we reviewed earlier, the production of speech requires an appropriate supply of air that can eventually be shaped into specific sounds to form words and sentences. However, the anatomical structures that help us create speech are essentially useless without the neural impulses generated in the central nervous system.

A simple analogy can illustrate this point. If we buy the most rapid computer system available in today's market, we have the potential to do great things. However, even though such a computer may have all the necessary parts to generate countless projects (i.e., hard drive, memory, keyboard, mouse, and monitor), it is essentially a worthless appliance if electricity is not available. The complex neural impulses generated by the central nervous system are to the human body and all of its parts what electricity is to a computer, the most basic, essential, and driving force.

We emphasize that although we have used a brain-computer analogy, the two systems are not identical. A computer may bewilder and intimidate many of us because of its intricate functions, but in no way is it completely analogous to the human brain. Remember that a computer needs a human to have many of its special programs initiated and updated, whereas our brain seems to be able to do it all on its own. As the new millennium approached, countless television, magazine, radio, and Internet reports warned companies and consumers of the devastating effects that would be created by computer systems that were not programmed to identify the coming of a new century. Luckily, our brains did not require such reprogramming.

If you stop reading for a second and say the word *cat,* you see that the word can be uttered in about a millisecond. The relative ease with which we can utter words and sentences often makes us take this special gift for granted. However, the complexity of the interconnections between our anatomical structures and the nervous system in producing speech cannot be overstated. The example of people who suffer a cerebrovascular accident (a stroke) and subsequently cannot put sounds and words together to convey their most basic needs and wants best highlights this important interconnection. An ability that is so often taken for granted (talking) can be quickly lost or impaired if the nervous system is damaged.

Major Divisions of the Nervous System

The anatomy of the human nervous system is often divided into two major subsystems: the central nervous system and the peripheral nervous system. Both of these systems are directly implicated in the motor control of speech. Simply stated, the **central nervous system** is made up of the brain and the spinal cord. It is entirely encased in bone — the brain is inside the cranium (skull) and the spinal cord is surrounded by the spinal column (backbone). The peripheral nervous system consists of the various cranial and spinal nerves that serve as the final common pathway in carrying messages to and from the central nervous system (brain and spinal cord). To better understand the intertwined workings of these subsystems, it is essential to first review the building blocks of the nervous system: nerve cells.

Basic Units of Life: Neurons

While on the surface the central nervous system (CNS) can appear to be one cohesive anatomical structure, it is actually made up of billions of specialized nerve cells called **neurons.** Neurons are the most basic building blocks in the CNS and are responsible for (a) receiving, (b) transmitting, and (c) synthesizing information (Bhatnagar & Andy, 1995).

Parts of a Neuron

Each neuron (also known as a nerve cell) consists of three major parts: the cell body, dendrites, and a single axon. The **soma** or **cell body** of the nerve cell is made up of the nucleus and surrounding cytoplasm. The **nucleus** serves as the controlling center of the neuron. **Cytoplasm** is a water-based substance that surrounds the nucleus and helps metabolize protein essential for the maintenance and growth of the nerve cell. Extending from the cytoplasmic material are many dendrites and a single axon. **Dendrites** are receptive (afferent) processes that help transmit neural impulses generated from other nerve cells to the cell body. **Axons** are motor (efferent) processes that transmit information away from the cell body to other nerve cells. The neural messages conveyed from one nerve cell to another through these specialized extensions can be inhibitory or excitatory. Figure 1.14 highlights the parts of a neuron.

Note on Terminology

When referring to the communication between nerve cells, the term **efferent** generally refers to fiber extensions that conduct neural impulses away from the nerve cell body; thus, axons are efferent in function. **Afferent** refers to fiber extensions that transmit neural impulses toward the nerve cell body. By definition, dendrites are afferent cell structures. Sometimes the word **central** is used in reference to extensions that transmit information from the cell body (axons), and **peripheral** is used for those that convey information toward the cell body (dendrites).

- **Motor = efferent = transmitter = central** → **axons (or other fibers that serve the same function)**

- **Sensory = afferent = receptor = peripheral** → **dendrites (or other fibers that serve the same function)**

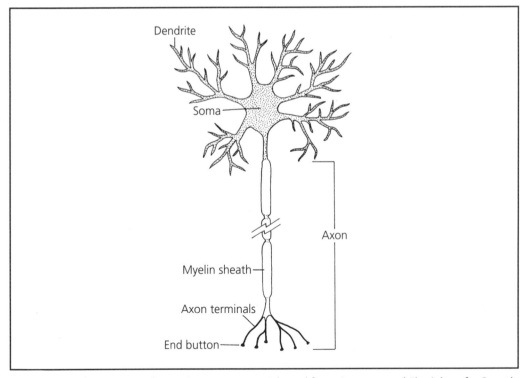

Figure 1.14. The neuron and its major parts. *Note.* Adapted from *Anatomy and Physiology for Speech, Language, and Hearing* (Figure 9.2, p. 389), by J. A. Seikel, D. W. King, and D. G. Drumright, 1997, Pacific Grove, CA: Delmar. Copyright 1997 by Delmar, a division of Thomson Learning (Fax 800/730-2215). Reprinted with permission.

Dendrites, which are only a few millimeters in length, tend to be shorter than axons. Each dendrite has many branchlike extensions that cover a large surface area. The dendrites from a single nerve cell can receive input from thousands of other nerve cells.

Although generally longer than dendrites, some axons may be only millimeters in length, while others can be up to several feet long. At its terminal end, the axon divides into several small branches called **axon terminals.** The axon terminals are covered with **end buttons** or **terminal knobs,** which are miniscule protuberances that release an important chemical called a neurotransmitter. A protective and insulating material known as **myelin** covers the length of the axon. The term **nerve fiber** is sometimes used in reference to an axon and its **myelin sheath.** Axons can communicate with various targets including a muscle, a gland, or other nerve cells.

It is important to note that the information above described the characteristics of a typical nerve cell; the size, shape, and biochemical property of nerve cells, and their resultant specialized functions, do vary.

**Nerve Cell Types
(Bhatnagar & Andy, 1995)**

Multipolar: nerve cells that have many dendrites and one axon. Most are located within the central nervous system.

Bipolar: nerve cells that have two processes extending from each pole of the body, an afferent process (**dendrite**) and an efferent process (**axon**).

Unipolar: nerve cells that are T-shaped and contain one divided process that extends from the body. The efferent division serves the function of the **axon,** while the afferent division serves the function of the **dendrite.**

Golgi Type I: nerve cells that have a long axon ranging from inches to feet; because of their length, these can exit the central nervous system toward the body.

Golgi Type II: nerve cells that have a short axonal process; these generally stay within the central nervous system.

Transmission of Neural Impulses

Within the brain, neural impulses typically travel from the cell body of one neuron via its axon to the cell body of another neuron through its dendrites. In the most common type of connection, the tip of an axon (**terminal knob**) of one nerve cell makes close contact with a dendrite of another. In another type of connection, the terminal knob of an axon actually makes contact with the cell body.

You may have noticed the use of the words *close contact* when describing the connection between nerve cells. These words are used because the axon of one neuron and the dendrite of another do not actually touch during the transmission of neural information. Rather, as the neural impulse that was generated from the cell body of one neuron reaches the end of its axon, it "jumps" to the dendrite of another neuron through a microscopic space. This tiny space is called the synapse (synaptic junction).

The **synapse,** or point of junction between two neurons, is not a single anatomical structure. Rather, it consists of the terminal knob of one neuron, the receptive site of another neuron, and the **synaptic cleft (space)** between the two. As indicated earlier, the terminal (synaptic) knobs of an axon contain and release an important chemical substance called a **neurotransmitter.** When released, neurotransmitters chemically activate the **receptive sites** of the neuron and help generate the electrical nerve impulses necessary for stimulation of the nerve cell body.

The communication between nerve cells is a complex process that is not yet completely understood. For simplification, we have presented the most essential information necessary to grasp the communication process between these basic functional units. Because the central nervous system contains literally billions of nerve cells and trillions of neural connections, it is no wonder that motor movements can be initiated, transmitted, regulated, and synthesized so quickly. See Figure 1.15 for an illustration of nerve cell interconnections.

**Note on Terminology
(Kuehn, Lemme, and Baumgartner, 1989)**

Neuron: single nerve cell.

Nerve: a bundle of neuron fibers traveling in the peripheral nervous system.

Nerve tract: a bundle of neuron fibers traveling in the central nervous system

Ganglion: a group of cell bodies that lie in the peripheral nervous system and form a nerve center or point of intercommunication. There is one exception to this, the **basal ganglia** located in the central nervous system. **Ganglia** is plural.

Nucleus: collection of cell bodies in the central nervous system that forms a nerve center or point of intercommunication. **Nuclei** is plural.

Gray matter: parts of the nervous system that actually look gray and are composed primarily of dendrites, cell bodies, and neuroglia (protective cells).

White matter: parts of the nervous system that appear whiter in color, composed primarily of myelinated axons.

Central Nervous System

Now that we have reviewed the basic function of the nerve cell, we are ready to begin our discussion of the central nervous system. As indicated earlier, the CNS is made up of the brain and spinal cord. The brain can be further subdivided into five major components: (1) cerebrum, (2) basal ganglia, (3) thalamus, (4) cerebellum, and (5) brain stem. These anatomical divisions are important for discussion of their specific functions. However, it should be recognized that all of the parts of the nervous system act as a rapid and integrated process that allows human beings to think, write, read, walk, dance, and, most important for our purposes, *talk* without difficulty.

Cerebrum

Of all the structures that make up the brain, the cerebrum is the largest and most important for speech. It is within the cerebrum that the voluntary motor movements for the production of sounds and words are initiated. This large portion of the brain is made up of billions of nerve cells that are densely packed within the cranium

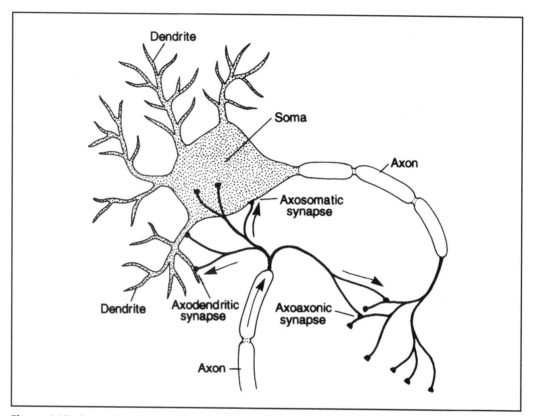

Figure 1.15. Synaptic connections between nerve cells. *Note.* From *Anatomy and Physiology for Speech, Language, and Hearing* (Figure 9.4, p. 391), by J. A. Seikel, D. W. King, and D. G. Drumright, 1997, Pacific Grove, CA: Delmar. Copyright 1997 by Delmar, a division of Thomson Learning (Fax 800/730-2215). Reprinted with permission.

(skull). Its outermost surface is called the **cerebral cortex,** a highly convoluted portion that can be seen best in an undissected brain. The cortex is organized in six layers, each consisting of different cell types. The convolutions of the cortex are often described as ridges and valleys that fold up and down, respectively. Technically, the ridges are called **gyri,** and the valleys are called **sulci** or **fissures. Sulcus** refers to a shallow valley, while **fissure** refers to a deeper convolution.

> **Note on Terminology**
>
> A mnemonic device can be used to remember whether a convolution is a gyrus or a sulcus. The word **gyrus** begins with a *g*, and a gyrus is a fold that *goes up;* whereas the word **sulcus** begins with an *s*, and a sulcus is a fold that *sinks down*. **Gyri** and **sulci** are plural.

The cerebrum consists of two **cerebral hemispheres** that are almost identical in appearance but very different in function. A large and deep central fissure called the **longitudinal** or **interhemispheric fissure** creates a boundary between the left and right **cerebral hemispheres.** However, the two hemispheres are interconnected by a thick bundle of myelinated fibers called the **corpus callosum.** Communication between the two hemispheres occurs through this relatively large structure.

Each cerebral hemisphere controls the opposite side of the body. This is the neurological principle of **contralateral motor control.** For almost 95% of the population, speech and language are initiated and processed in the left hemisphere. This means that the majority of people are left lateralized for speech and language. Recent studies, however, highlight the important role of the right hemisphere for certain aspects of speech and language (e.g., prosody and pragmatics).

Each cerebral hemisphere is anatomically divided into four major lobes: frontal, temporal, parietal, and occipital. The lobes are named after the major bones of the skull. Various sulci and fissures create the boundaries for these lobes on the lateral (outermost) surface of the cerebral cortex.

The **central sulcus,** also known as the **fissure of Rolando,** is a deep cortical valley that primarily serves as the boundary between the frontal lobe and the parietal lobe. The temporal lobe is separated from the frontal lobe on its anterior surface and the parietal lobe on its superior surface by the **lateral fissure** or the **fissure of Sylvius.** As the name implies, the **parieto-occipital sulcus** separates the parietal lobe from the occipital lobe on is posterior surface. Figure 1.16 illustrates the four lobes of the cerebral cortex and the important sulci that create their boundaries.

Frontal Lobe. The major portion of the frontal lobe sits in front of the central sulcus; a smaller inferior section lies above the lateral fissure. It is the largest of all lobes, occupying about one third of the cerebral hemisphere. Several landmarks

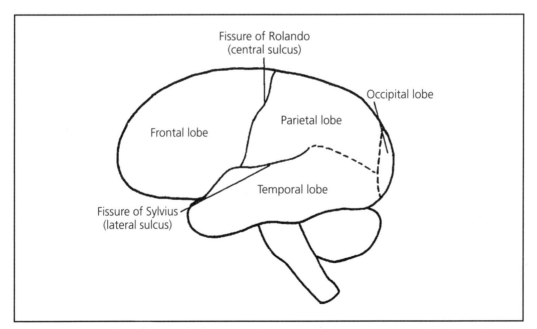

Figure 1.16. The lobes of the cerebral cortex and its major sulci. *Note.* From *Introduction to Communicative Disorders* (2nd ed., Figure 3.21, p. 96), by M. N. Hegde, 1995, Austin, TX: PRO-ED. Copyright 1995 by PRO-ED, Inc. Reprinted with permission.

important for speech and language are housed within the frontal lobe, typically in the dominant hemisphere. These include the primary motor cortex, the premotor cortex, and Broca's area.

The **primary motor cortex** is located on the precentral gyrus, a large ridge just anterior to the central sulcus. The function of this important neuroanatomical structure is to convey instructions to the opposite side of the body for voluntary movements. All muscles of the body, including those of speech production, are connected to the primary motor cortex through descending motor nerve cells. This connection is typically illustrated through a **homunculus** — a point-for-point representation of muscles of the body in the motor cortex (see Figure 1.17). You will notice the disproportionate representation of various body parts on the homunculus. As compared to other body structures, a large area of the primary motor cortex controls the lips, jaw, tongue, and larynx. Damage to the lower one third of the primary motor cortex may result in impaired movements of the articulators and other structures of speech production.

The **premotor cortex,** also called the **supplementary motor cortex,** lies just anterior to the precentral sulcus, a fissure situated in front of the primary motor cortex. Electrical stimulation studies have implicated this area in the planning of complex and skilled motor movements such as playing the piano and propositional speech.

Another important motor planning center for speech is **Broca's area.** Named after Paul Broca, a 19th-century French neurosurgeon, this area is typically located in the lower section of the frontal lobe just anterior to the portion of the primary motor cortex that controls jaw, lip, tongue, and laryngeal movements. This section

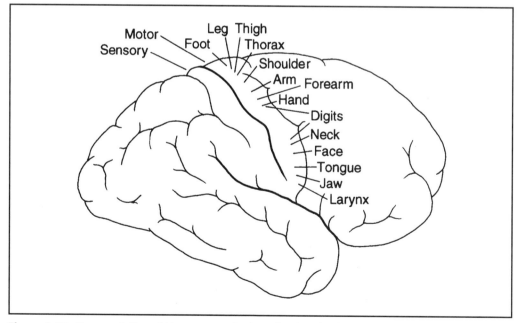

Figure 1.17. Representation of the motor activation of various body parts on the primary motor cortex (right hemisphere). *Note.* From *Anatomy and Physiology for Speech, Language, and Hearing* (Figure 9.40, p. 456), by J. A. Seikel, D. W. King, and D. G. Drumright, 1997, Pacific Grove, CA: Delmar. Copyright 1997 by Delmar, a division of Thomson Learning (Fax 800/730-2215). Reprinted with permission.

is specifically called the **inferior frontal gyrus.** Love and Webb (1996) indicate that Broca's area is important for the production of fluent and well-articulated speech (p. 22). It is found in the cerebral hemisphere that is dominant for language, which is the left hemisphere for most people. While damage to Broca's area in the dominant hemisphere typically leads to speech production problems, injury to the equivalent area in the nondominant hemisphere does not.

Temporal Lobe. The temporal lobe — roughly shaped like a thumb — is situated below the frontal and temporal lobes. The lateral fissure demarcates its superior boundary. An imaginary inferior extension of the parieto-occipital sulcus separates it from the occipital lobe posteriorly. It contains three prominent gyri: the superior, middle, and inferior temporal gyri. These are also called the first, second, and third temporal gyri, respectively. Like the frontal lobe, the temporal lobe houses important areas for speech and language. It also has important specialization centers for hearing. These include the primary auditory cortex, the auditory association area, and Wernicke's area.

The **primary auditory cortex** is situated on the superior temporal gyrus, which marks the lower surface of the lateral sulcus. Posterior to the primary auditory cortex is the auditory association area. The collective term **Heschl's gyri** is sometimes used in reference to the transverse convolutions that make up the primary auditory cortex and the auditory association cortex (Kuehn, Lemme, & Baumgartner, 1989).

The primary auditory cortex receives auditory stimuli from the vestibulo-acoustic nerve bilaterally (from both ears). This information is then synthesized in the auditory association area so that it can be recognized as whole units. In the language dominant hemisphere, the auditory association area is typically concerned with the analysis of speech sounds for the recognition of whole words and sentences. The auditory association area in the nondominant hemisphere primarily analyzes nonverbal material such as music and environmental noises.

The auditory association area in the language dominant hemisphere is typically called **Wernicke's area,** named after the now famous neurologist who first discovered its function, Carl Wernicke. In most people, Wernicke's area is located in the posterior superior portion of the first temporal gyrus in the left hemisphere. It is a relatively large area that is now believed to help humans both understand and formulate speech and language, since a person who suffers damage in this area generally has difficulty in both the comprehension and production of speech.

Parietal Lobe. Posterior to the frontal lobe and superior to the temporal lobe lies another large lobe called the **parietal lobe.** The parietal lobe is considered the primary somatic sensory area. It integrates contralateral body sensations such as pain, touch, temperature, and pressure in the **primary sensory cortex (PSC).** The major portion of the PSC is located on the **postcentral gyrus,** a large ridge just posterior to the central sulcus. The primary sensory cortex receives sensory **somatic** information from all the muscles of the body, including those of the face, neck, and head. This sensory control can be illustrated by a sensory homunculus, which is similar to the motor homunculus described for the primary motor cortex.

This lobe also houses some structures important for language: the **supra-marginal gyrus** and the **angular gyrus.** Damage to these areas in the language-dominant hemisphere may lead to word-finding problems, reading and writing deficits, and arithmetic problems.

Occipital Lobe. The occipital lobe is located posterior to the parietal lobe and superior to the cerebellum. It makes up the most posterior portion of the cerebrum. It is primarily concerned with vision and has very little relation to speech, language, and hearing.

Basal Ganglia

The **basal ganglia** are deep structures that cannot be observed in an undissected brain since they are completely surrounded by the cerebral hemispheres. Because of this, they are referred to as **subcortical** structures; they are primarily made up of gray matter. The term *ganglia* by definition refers to a group of nerve cell bodies that form a nerve center or point of intercommunication (Kuehn, Lemme, & Baumgartner, 1989). The basal ganglia certainly can be thought of as a point of intercommunication for various neurological subsystems. Although textbooks and researchers differ on which subcortical structures are part of the basal ganglion, it consists of at least three nuclear masses: the caudate nucleus, putamen, and globus pallidus. Sometimes these are collectively termed the **corpus striatum** (Love & Webb, 1996). Figure 1.18 illustrates the basal ganglia and its individual components: head of caudate nucleus, body of caudate nucleus, tail of caudate nucleus, putamen, and globus pallidus (not visible in lateral view shown in Figure 1.18).

Functionally, the basal ganglia are part of the *extrapyramidal system* (to be discussed in a later section of this chapter), a system that helps modify and regulate cortically initiated motor movements, including speech. A structure that is functionally related to—although not anatomically part of—the basal ganglia is the **substantia nigra.** Thus, the substantia nigra is considered an important part of the extrapyramidal system.

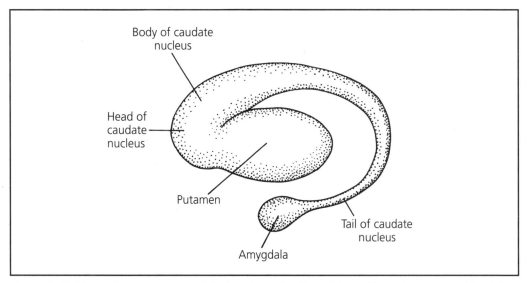

Figure 1.18. The major components of the basal ganglia. *Note.* Adapted from *Anatomy and Physiology for Speech, Language, and Hearing* (Figure 9.44, p. 463), by J. A. Seikel, D. W. King, and D. G. Drumright, 1997, Pacific Grove, CA: Delmar. Copyright 1997 by Delmar, a division of Thomson Learning (Fax 800/730-2215). Reprinted with permission.

Because motor movements are not directly controlled in the basal ganglia, the extrapyramidal system is considered an indirect activation system. It primarily makes its impact on motor movements by communicating with the cerebral cortex via other subcortical structures (e.g., the thalamus). Bhatnagar and Andy (1995) describe the basal ganglia as a set of interconnected feedback circuits (p. 220). Love and Webb (1996) indicate that the basal ganglia may function to influence movements related to posture, automatic movements, and skilled motor movements (p. 124).

Because the exact nature and function of the basal ganglia is not clearly understood, knowledge of the effects of the extrapyramidal system (basal ganglia) on motor movement comes primarily from studying people who have suffered damage to this area of the central nervous system. People with basal ganglia lesions have presented with the following movement disorders:

- *involuntary motor movements* — bizarre postures and unusual movements that cannot be brought under voluntary control (e.g., tremors, jerking, writhing, and flailing).

- *hyperkinesia* — involuntary movements that are characterized by too much movement (e.g., chorea, athetosis).

- *hypokinesia* — involuntary movements that are characterized by too few movements.

- *bradykinesia* — slowness of movements and movements that have limited range of motion.

- *altered posture* — typically the presence of a stooped or abnormal posture.

- *changes in body tone* — either hypertonicity (too much tone) or hypotonicity (too little tone).

- *dysarthria* — either hypokinetic dysarthria, a motor speech disorder typically associated with Parkinson's disease, or hyperkinetic dysarthria, a speech disorder of various etiologies (e.g., Huntington's disease).

Cerebellum

The cerebellum is a very important structure of the central nervous system, which sits below the occipital lobe of the cerebrum and just behind the brain stem (see Figure 1.19). Functionally, the cerebellum serves as the coordinator of fine motor movements, body posture, and balance. Included in the fine and skilled motor movements regulated by the cerebellum are *talking,* running, typing, writing, dancing, and playing the piano.

It is important to note that the cerebellum does not initiate or integrate motor movements; rather, it coordinates and regulates neural impulses that it receives from other centers in the brain. Bhatnagar and Andy (1995) describe the cerebellum as "an error control center" that "constantly monitors all motor outputs to muscles receiving projections from the motor cortex and sensory signals from joint receptors and muscle spindles" (p. 207). In essence, the cerebellum compares the outgoing motor movements with the sensory information that it receives and alters the movements accordingly. For example, when lifting a box that our system perceives as heavy, it is the cerebellum that regulates the outgoing motor movement initiated cortically so that we use the range of motion, force, and strength necessary to effectively accomplish the task. However, our sensory system sometimes

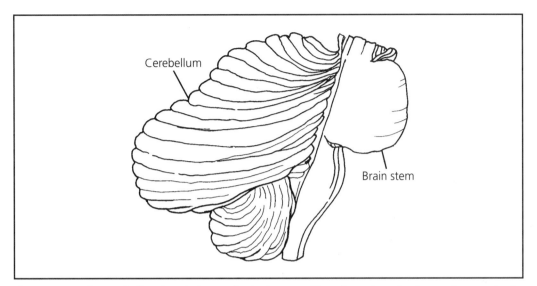

Figure 1.19. The cerebellum in relation to the brain stem. *Note.* From *Introduction to Communicative Disorders* (2nd ed., Figure 3.20, p. 95), by M. N. Hegde, 1995, Austin, TX: PRO-ED. Copyright 1995 by PRO-ED, Inc. Reprinted with permission.

deceives us. Have you ever gone to pick up a box that you believed to be heavy only to find out that it was empty? Did you fall over because of the excessive force that you were prepared to use? It is the cerebellum that helps us alter our original movements so that we use less strength and force than we originally intended.

As with the basal ganglia, the function of the cerebellum is most clearly understood by studying the problems that arise when it is damaged. Damage to the cerebellum may lead to various impairments, including:

- *ataxia*—a general term that refers to the incoordination of motor movements.

- *dysdiadochokinesia*—the inability to perform rapid alternating muscle movements.

- *dysmetria*—the inability to gauge the distance, velocity, and strength of movement. Both overshooting and undershooting of the target movement may be observed.

- *intention tremor*—an involuntary movement that is typically present when a person intends to reach a target. This differentiates it from the tremor typically associated with basal ganglia damage, which usually occurs at rest.

- *disequilibrium*—balance problems that predominantly involve the legs. People typically walk as if they were drunk; their gait is unsteady and their bodies waver. The person affected may try to compensate for these balance difficulties by using a *broad-based gait,* a gait characterized by feet that are wide apart.

- *nystagmus*—a term that refers to rapid, oscillating movements of the pupils; the movements may be vertical, horizontal, or rotary.

- *ataxic dysarthria*—a motor speech disorder present with some but not all cerebellar lesions.

Brain Stem

Phylogenetically, the **brain stem** is said to be the oldest part of the brain. This diagonally oriented structure connects the brain with the spinal cord through the diencephalon. The brain stem also serves as the bridge between the cerebellum and all other central nervous system structures (i.e., cerebrum, basal ganglia, thalamus, and spinal cord). Three important structures—the midbrain, pons, and medulla—make up the brain stem. The midbrain is the most superior portion, followed by the pons and the medulla. The medulla is the portion of the brain stem that directly attaches to the uppermost portion of the spinal cord. The parts of the brain stem are illustrated in Figure 1.20. Internally, the brain stem consists of the *reticular formation, cranial nerve nuclei,* and *longitudinal fiber tracts.* Among the important life-supporting functions of the brain stem are breathing, swallowing, and heart beat regulation.

Midbrain. The midbrain, also called the **mesencephalon,** sits below the diencephalon and above the pons. It contains the **superior peduncles,** which help connect the brain stem to the cerebellum. The substantia nigra, a cellular structure connected in function to the basal ganglia, runs the vertical length of the midbrain at the level of the peduncles. The midbrain also contains the **corpora quadrigemina,** made up of the paired **inferior** and **superior colliculi.** The inferior colliculi serve as relay stations for the transmission of auditory neural impulses from the ear to the auditory cortex. The superior colliculi help in reflex control of the eye

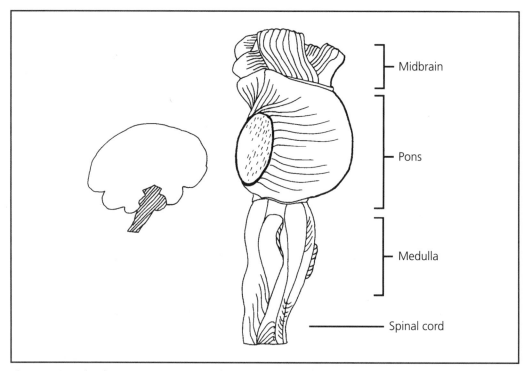

Figure 1.20. The three major structures of the brain stem. *Note.* From *Introduction to Communicative Disorders* (2nd ed., Figure 3.18, p. 93), by M. N. Hegde, 1995, Austin, TX: PRO-ED. Copyright 1995 by PRO-ED, Inc. Reprinted with permission.

movements, visual reflexes, and coordination of vestibular-generated head and eye movements. The midbrain houses the cranial nerve nuclei for the oculomotor and trochlear nerves. These are not implicated in speech production.

Pons. The pons, which has a bulging appearance on its anterior surface, is located just below the midbrain. Along with the midbrain, it serves as a connection point between various cerebral structures and the cerebellum through the **middle** and **inferior peduncles.** The Latin term for "bridge" is *pons,* which highlights one of the functions of this structure. The pons contains numerous descending motor fibers and it houses various cranial nerve nuclei important for speech production. The trigeminal and facial nerves have their nuclei located within the pons.

Medulla. The most inferior portion of the brain stem is called the **medulla,** sometimes termed **medulla oblongata.** Through visual inspection, this structure has a cone-shaped appearance. It is extremely important for speech production since it contains numerous descending fibers that carry motor information to several cranial nerve nuclei. It also contains the motor fibers that descend to the spinal cord for innervation of the spinal nerves. The cranial nerves that have their nuclei housed within the medulla are the vestibuloacoustic, glossopharyngeal, vagus, accessory, and hypoglossal nerves. The vestibuloacoustic, a purely sensory nerve, is extremely important for the neural integration of hearing.

Connecting Fibers in the Central Nervous System

Thus far, we have described the structures of the brain as separate entities for the sake of discussion. However, these structures are by no means isolated in function. Although most of the structures of the brain do have some specialized function, we know that complex interconnections must be made for the actual communication of neural impulses. For example, if the primary motor cortex were not connected to the spinal cord somehow, the motor movements initiated there would not reach the periphery (e.g., arms, legs, toes).

In this section, we will address the connecting fibers of the central nervous system that permit interhemispheric (between the hemispheres) and intrahemispheric (within each hemisphere) communication. These interconnecting nerve fibers are made up primarily of white matter or myelinated axonal fibers. They form the **medullary** center of the brain (Barr & Kiernan, 1988; Bhatnagar & Andy, 1995). The nerve fibers of the medullary center are typically categorized as projection, association, or commissural fibers, depending on the nature of their connections.

Projection Fibers. The projection fibers run in a vertical direction, and they establish connections between the cortex and subcortical structures such as the basal ganglia, the cerebellum, the brain stem, and the spinal cord. Some of these fibers carry sensory information, while others carry motor information. The motor projection fibers primarily originate in the primary motor and premotor areas in the frontal lobe. They form the upper motor neuron system of the pyramidal tract. The pyramidal tract is the direct activation pathway for voluntary motor movements. We will discuss the pyramidal system with greater detail in a later section. The sensory projection fibers transmit **cutaneous** and **proprioceptive** information from the skin and joints and project them to various primary sensory areas in the cortex.

Association Fibers. Association fibers interconnect various areas of the cortex within each hemisphere. Some association fibers are short; others are relatively long. The shorter association fibers connect gyri that are adjacent to each other (within the same lobe), and the long fibers connect distant cortical areas (between lobes).

Although there are many specialized association fibers, one of the most important for speech is the **arcuate fasciculus.** This long bundle of nerve fibers connects Wernicke's area in the temporal lobe with Broca's area in the frontal lobe. Theoretically, a lesion to the arcuate fasciculus disconnects these important cortical areas for speech and language and may lead to a language disorder known as **conduction aphasia.** Other short association fibers help connect the auditory cortex to Wernicke's area within the temporal lobe and the primary motor cortex to Broca's area within the frontal lobe.

Commissural Fibers. The commissural fibers in the brain run horizontally and help interconnect the two hemispheres. Although there are several commissural pathways that interconnect the cortical areas in both hemispheres, the major bundle of fibers is known as the **corpus callosum.**

Peripheral Nervous System

The **peripheral nervous system** is the second major division of the human nervous system. It is made up three types of nerves that are located outside the skull or spinal column: the cranial nerves, the spinal nerves, and the peripheral autonomic nerves. Peripheral nerves carry sensory information originating in various peripheral organs to the brain, while motor nerves transmit motor nerve impulses originating in the brain to the muscles, glands, and organs in the body. The autonomic nerves help control many involuntary functions of the body. The spinal nerves and cranial nerves are more directly implicated with speech production, and thus our discussion will be limited to these.

Cranial Nerves

The cranial nerves originate from the brain stem and exit the base of the skull through small apertures called **foramina.** They **innervate** various muscles including those of the head, neck, face, larynx, pharynx, tongue, and some glands. The cranial nerves are part of the lower motor neuron system of the corticobulbar tract of the pyramidal system (to be discussed with greater detail later on). Several of the cranial nerves are essential for speech production, while others serve special senses such as vision, audition, smell, and taste. The cranial nerves can be sensory, motor, or both sensory and motor (mixed). There are 12 pairs of cranial nerves that are named according to function and numbered in the sequence by which they exit the brain, in relation to the height in the brain at their point of exit (Perkins & Kent, 1986). Table 1.2 outlines the 12 cranial nerves according to their name, Roman numeral, and basic function.

The first two cranial nerves, *olfactory* (I) and *optic* (II), are sensory and originate in the nasal cavity and the retina of the eye, respectively. The remaining 10 originate in and exit at various parts of the brain stem. Cranial nerves III (*oculomotor*) and IV (*trochlear*) are motor in function. They both originate in the midbrain

Table 1.2. The Cranial Nerves and Their Functions

Roman Numeral	Name	CNS Level	General Function
I	Olfactory	Telencephalon	Sensory: Sense of smell
II	Optic	Diencephalon	Sensory: Sense of vision
III	Oculomotor	Midbrain	Motor: Eye movements, pupillary constriction
IV	Trochlear	Midbrain	Motor: Eye movements
V	Trigeminal	Mid pons	Sensory: Ophthalmic & maxillary areas of the face Motor: Mandibular musculature
VI	Abducens	Inferior pons	Motor: Eye movement
VII	Facial	Pons-medulla junction	Motor: Facial expression, stapedial reflex, elevation of hyoid bone Other efferent: Lacrimation, salivation
VIII	Vestibulocochlear (auditory)	Pons-medulla junction	Sensory: Balance and hearing
IX	Glossopharyngeal	Medulla	Sensory: Tongue, pharynx, tonsils Motor: Pharyngeal musculature
X	Vagus	Medulla	Sensory: Viscera of neck, thorax, abdomen Motor: Larynx, pharynx, soft palate
XI	Spinal accessory (accessory)	Medulla	Motor: Strap muscles of neck
XII	Hypoglossal	Medulla	Motor: Tongue

Mnemonic device for names of cranial nerves: <u>O</u>n <u>O</u>ld <u>O</u>lympus <u>T</u>owering <u>T</u>ops <u>A</u> <u>F</u>inn <u>A</u>nd <u>G</u>erman <u>V</u>ended <u>A</u>t <u>H</u>ops

and innervate muscles responsible for eye movement. With the exception of cranial nerve VI (*abducens*)—also important for eye movement—the remaining cranial nerves are intricately related to speech or hearing. Cranial nerves V, VI, VII, and VIII originate in the pons, and cranial nerves IX, X, XI, and XII exit from the medulla oblongata.

Cranial Nerves for Speech

Trigeminal Nerve. The *trigeminal nerve* (V) is both a sensory and a motor nerve. The motor fibers of the trigeminal nerve innervate various muscles of the jaw including the masseter, temporalis, lateral and medial pterygoids, tensor tympani, tensor veli palatini, mylohyoid, and the anterior belly of the digastric muscle. The sensory fibers are made up of three branches: mandibular, maxillary, and ophthalmic. The mandibular branch is sensory to the tongue, mandible, lower teeth, lower lip, part of the cheek, and part of the external ear. The maxillary branch is sensory to the upper lip, maxilla, upper teeth, upper cheek area, palate, and maxillary sinus. The ophthalmic nerve is sensory to the forehead, eyes, and nose. Perhaps you have experienced the effect of temporary anesthetization of the trigeminal nerve during a visit to the dentist.

Facial Nerve. The *facial nerve* (VII) is also a mixed nerve, meaning that it has both a sensory and a motor function. The facial nerve is a relatively complex nerve in terms of its anatomy. The motor fibers innervate various muscles important for speech production (articulation) and facial expression including orbicularis oris, zygomatic, buccinator, orbicularis oculi, platysma, stylohyoid, stapedius, the posterior belly of the digastric, and various labial muscles. The sensory component of the facial nerve is partly responsible for taste (in the anterior two thirds of the tongue).

Vestibuloacoustic Nerve. The *vestibuloacoustic nerve (vestibulocochlear)* is made up of two branches, the *vestibular* and the *auditory*. It is a sensory nerve for hearing and balance. The auditory branch carries sensory information from the cochlea in the inner ear to the brain (the primary auditory cortex). The vestibular branch is primarily responsible for the maintenance of balance or equilibrium.

The auditory division of the vestibuloacoustic nerve has many endings in the cochlea (discussed in the Basic Unit of this chapter). These nerve endings are in contact with the hair cells to pick up the sound vibrations that were transformed from mechanical energy into neural impulses. Some 30,000 nerve fibers of the auditory nerve can be found in the cochlea.

The auditory nerve exits the inner ear through the **internal auditory meatus.** The nerve impulses carried by the left and the right auditory pathways then enter the brain stem. At the brain stem, many auditory nerve fibers that come from one ear cross over (**decussate**) to the opposite side, forming **contralateral** pathways. Some continue on the same side, forming **ipsilateral** pathways. Because of this crossover of signals, the brain can compare sounds sent to it from each of the two ears. It helps the brain localize and integrate the sounds. The two sides of the temporal cortex are interconnected, so additional integration of sounds is possible.

Glossopharyngeal Nerve. The *glossopharyngeal nerve* (IX) is another mixed nerve. It contains sensory and motor fibers. The motor fibers innervate the stylopharyngeus, a pharyngeal muscle that contributes to the elevation of the pharynx and the larynx. The movements generated by the innervation of the stylopharyngeus muscle are very important for swallowing. The sensory component of the glossopharyngeal nerve helps in processing taste information from the posterior one third of the tongue. It also provides general sensation to the pharynx, soft palate, faucial pillars, tonsils, ear canal, and tympanic cavity.

Vagus Nerve. The *vagus nerve* (X) is a very complex nerve that has both a sensory and a motor function. It is the largest cranial nerve and has a wide distribution. Because of this wide distribution, it is sometimes termed the wandering nerve.

The vagus nerve conveys sensory information from the larynx, pharynx, trachea, heart, and digestive system. Its motor fibers supply the heart, lungs, and digestive system.

In addition to these important organs, some of the motor fibers of the vagus innervate the muscles of the pharynx, the soft palate, and the intrinsic muscles of the larynx, making it an extremely important nerve for speech production. The **pharyngeal branch** of the vagus nerve supplies the pharyngeal constrictors and all of the muscles of the soft palate, with the exception of the tensor tympani, which is innervated by the trigeminal nerve. Motor innervation of the muscles of the soft palate contributes to appropriate resonance changes during speech production. The left and right branches of the **recurrent laryngeal branch** innervate the intrinsic muscles of the larynx; an exception is the cricothyroid, which is supplied by the **superior laryngeal nerve branch.** Appropriate phonation is highly dependent on adequate innervation of the intrinsic laryngeal muscles by the vagus nerve through its recurrent laryngeal and superior laryngeal branches.

Accessory Nerve. The *accessory nerve* (XI) is a motor nerve. Unlike any other of the cranial nerves, the accessory is actually a cranial and a spinal nerve; some of its fibers originate in the brain stem, while others originate in the spinal cord. Along with the vagus nerve, its cranial fibers innervate the uvula and levator veli palatini (muscles of the soft palate). The spinal root supplies the sternocleidomastoid and trapezius muscles, which assist in turning, tilting, and thrusting the head forward and shrugging the shoulders.

Hypoglossal Nerve. The *hypoglossal nerve* (XII) is a motor nerve that primarily innervates the muscles of the tongue. It supplies all the intrinsic muscles of the tongue and three extrinsic tongue muscles: the genioglossus, hyoglossus, and styloglossus. Together, the intrinsic and extrinsic muscles of the tongue are responsible for various tongue movements important for speech production, particularly for the articulation of specific sounds. Innervation of the tongue is also important for effective bolus formation and swallowing.

Spinal Nerves

In addition to the cranial nerves, the peripheral nervous system is made up of 31 pairs of spinal nerves. The spinal nerves emerge from the spinal cord through an afferent (sensory) and efferent (motor) root. The afferent root is on the dorsal surface of the spinal cord (the part of the spinal cord that faces the back). The efferent root is on the spinal cord's ventral surface (the portion facing the abdomen). The 31 pairs of spinal nerves are divided into the following segments: cervical, thoracic, lumbar, sacral, and coccygeal. They are named after the region of the spinal cord to which they are attached and are numbered in sequence. This results in:

- 8 pairs of cervical spinal nerves, numbered C1–C8
- 12 pairs of thoracic spinal nerves, numbered T1–T12
- 5 pairs of lumbar spinal nerves, numbered L1–L5
- 5 pairs of sacral spinal nerves, numbered S1–S5
- 1 pair of coccygeal spinal nerves, numbered C1 (not to be confused with cervical 1 spinal nerve)

Spinal nerves are both sensory and motor and, thus, mixed in function. They carry sensory information from peripheral receptors to the central nervous system and transmit motor information from the CNS to the muscles. Although not all spinal nerves are directly implicated in speech production, some contribute to it greatly through innervation of the respiratory musculature. For example, the diaphragm, which is considered the chief muscle of inhalation, is innervated by the motor branches of the C3–C5 spinal nerves (phrenic nerves). Several other respiratory muscles are innervated by the thoracic spinal nerves (e.g., the internal and external intercostals).

The reader may refer to Appendix A for a detailed review of the musculature associated with the production of all English consonants and their cranial or spinal nerve supply.

Integrating the Systems: Neuromotor Control of Speech

Up to this point, we have described the various anatomical parts of the human nervous system by grouping them into a *central nervous system* and a *peripheral nervous system*. Again, it is emphasized that this division helped to highlight the important structures of the brain that have some effect on speech, language, and hearing. However, how do all these structures interconnect to initiate, regulate, coordinate, and synthesize speech and language? In this section we will attempt to integrate the function of these various structures so that the dynamic neuromotor control of speech can be addressed. Love and Webb (1996) indicate that the production of speech requires the action of various systems or mechanisms at five major levels: (1) cerebral cortex, (2) subcortical nuclei, (3) brain stem, (4) cerebellum, and (5) spinal cord (p. 106). For clinical purposes, the integration of these systems is more commonly divided into the pyramidal system, the extrapyramidal system, and the cerebellar system.

Cerebral Initiation

To set up the upcoming sections on the pyramidal, extrapyramidal, and cerebellar systems, we will begin by assuming that a person is having a conversation with someone and that he or she has just received some auditory information in the form of a question. Obviously, in a dyadic (two-person) conversation, a person who is asked a question is expected to respond. So what must this person experience to perform a task that he or she does without thinking throughout the course of a normal day?

Assuming that this person received the question in the auditory modality, this sensory information is transmitted from the cochlea in the inner ear to the primary auditory cortex in the temporal lobe via the vestibuloacoustic nerve (cranial nerve VIII). Recall that the auditory cortex perceives spoken information. The information perceived by the auditory cortex is then transmitted to the auditory language association area (Wernicke's area), where the meaning of the words is actually understood. As the information is understood, the person may opt to respond to the question. If the person decides to speak, his or her choice of words is formulated in Wernicke's area and transmitted to Broca's area through a long bundle of association fibers, theoretically the arcuate fasciculus in this case.

Broca's area, located in the inferior frontal gyrus of the frontal lobe, receives the information and then plans the patterns of skilled movements necessary for speech production. The supplementary motor cortex is also believed to have some effect on motor planning.

The motor movements planned in Broca's area and the supplementary motor cortex are then transmitted to the primary motor cortex, specifically the lower one third of the precentral gyrus in the frontal lobe, through short association fibers. The parts of the motor cortex that mediate the movements of the speech muscles (i.e., tongue, lips, soft palate, face, and larynx) then send out neural impulses through long projection fibers. The projection nerve fibers continue their vertical path through the **internal capsule,** an area of concentrated and compact projection fibers near the brain stem, and communicate with the cranial nerve nuclei for cranial nerves V, VII, IX, X, XI, and XII located in the brain stem.

The cranial nerves then exit the skull through the small holes called foramina and actually innervate the muscles of the face, tongue, soft palate, pharynx, and larynx for the movements necessary for speech. Remember that the respiratory muscles involved in speech production are innervated by the spinal nerves in the spinal cord, not the cranial nerves. It is also important to note that the movements initiated at a cortical level are further regulated, integrated, fine tuned, and coordinated through subcortical structures such as the basal ganglia and the cerebellum. This seemingly long process actually occurs with such great speed that many of us never think about talking, unless our system becomes damaged at some level.

With this illustration in mind, we can now begin our discussion of the neuromotor control of speech with greater detail. This information will be reviewed according to three important clinical divisions: the pyramidal system, the extrapyramidal system, and the cerebellar system.

Pyramidal System

The pyramidal system has been described as the direct motor activation pathway (Duffy, 1995). It is primarily responsible for facilitating voluntary movement of the muscles, including those for speech. Thus, the pyramidal system is thought to be excitatory in function. The nerve fiber tract of the pyramidal system courses from the cerebral cortex to the spinal cord and brain stem to eventually supply the muscles of the head, neck, and limbs (e.g., legs, arms, toes, fingers). The voluntary movements necessary for speech production are initiated at the primary motor cortex in the lower one third of the precentral gyrus.

The pyramidal system consists of the **corticospinal** and the **corticobulbar tracts.** Keep in mind that the word *tract* refers to a bundle of nerve fibers running through the central nervous system. It is important to visualize the pyramidal system and its two tracts as a group of myelinated nerve fibers carrying important neural impulses. Although the corticospinal and corticobulbar tracts are part of one system, they are addressed separately for ease of discussion. The *projection fibers* of both tracts originate in the cerebral cortex; however, the point of termination for their neural messages influences their classification.

The nerve fibers of the **corticospinal tract** descend from the motor cortex of each hemisphere through the internal capsule. They continue to travel vertically through the midbrain and pons, and at the level of the medulla approximately 85 to 90% of the fibers cross over or **decussate.** The decussated fibers then enter the spinal cord to communicate with the spinal nerves at various levels. Finally, the spinal nerves exit the **neuraxis** through the **vertebrae foramina** along the spinal column to innervate the muscles of the trunk and limbs.

Because of the high level of crossover at the medulla, the left side of the body is typically controlled by nerve fibers that originate in the right cerebral cortex, and vice versa. A person who has a stroke in the left cerebral hemisphere and has right-sided hemiparesis best illustrates the concept of contralateral motor control.

The **corticobulbar tract** is extremely important for speech production. These fibers control all voluntary movements of the speech muscles, with the exception of the respiratory muscles. Like the fibers of the corticospinal tract, the fibers of the corticobulbar tract originate in the cerebral cortex, the motor cortex primarily. They also descend in a vertical fashion through the internal capsule and run along with the fibers of the corticospinal tract. However, the fibers of the corticobulbar tract terminate at the motor nuclei of the cranial nerves (III–XII) in the brain stem. Their point of decussation is at the level of the brain stem where they terminate. For example, the fibers that terminate at the motor nuclei of the facial nerve (VII) decussate in the medulla, whereas fibers that terminate at the motor nuclei of the trigeminal decussate in the pons. The cranial nerves for speech then exit the skull through small foramina and innervate the muscles of the face, lips, tongue, soft palate, pharynx, and larynx for the formation of sounds and words.

For clinical purposes, the corticospinal and corticobulbar tracts have been further subdivided into **lower** and **upper motor neurons.** This division is of clinical significance because of the varying symptoms associated with lower versus upper motor neuron damage.

The nerve fibers that originate in the cerebral cortex and descend to the spinal cord and those that terminate at the cranial nerve nuclei in the brain stem are all considered upper motor neurons. Love and Webb (1996) indicate that upper motor neurons do not exit the neuraxis (brain or spinal cord), meaning that they stay within the central nervous system. Technically, upper motor neurons include the pathways of both the pyramidal and extrapyramidal systems. However, the term is most frequently used in reference to the motor neurons of the pyramidal system.

The lower motor neurons include nerve fibers that in fact exit the neuraxis and communicate with the cranial and spinal nerves—peripheral nerves—for innervation of the muscles. By definition, the lower motor neurons are part of the peripheral nervous system. The lower motor neurons are considered the final route by which centrally mediated neural impulses are actually communicated to the peripheral muscles. Lower motor neuron activity results in muscular movement.

Extrapyramidal System

Another motor system that plays an important role in speech production is the **extrapyramidal system.** The prefix *extra-* makes reference to motor tracts that are not part of the pyramidal system. The extrapyramidal system is made up various *subcortical* nuclei including the basal ganglia, subthalamus, substantia nigra, and red nucleus and the various pathways that connect them. The extrapyramidal system is considered an indirect activation system, as opposed to the pyramidal system, which has a more direct connection with the lower motor neurons. It interacts with various motor systems in the nervous system before exerting an influence on the lower motor neurons.

The neuronal activity of this motor system, like that of the pyramidal system, begins in the cerebral cortex and ultimately exerts an influence on the lower motor neurons. Remember that the final result of lower motor neuron activity is voluntary muscular movement. The extrapyramidal system helps regulate this movement and assists in the maintenance of posture and tone.

As indicated earlier, the pathways of the extrapyramidal system are indirect, in contrast to the direct pathway of the pyramidal tract. The long axons of the corticospinal tract make only one synapse with the spinal nerves via the motor nuclei in the spinal cord. In the case of the corticobulbar tract, the synapse is with the cranial nerves via the cranial nerve nuclei at different levels of the brain stem. This is referred to as **monosynaptic** connections.

The extrapyramidal tract, on the other hand, is **polysynaptic.** It makes many synaptic connections before impulses reach the lower motor neurons to effect regulated and coordinated muscular movement. The effect of the extrapyramidal system on muscular movement is primarily **inhibitory,** rather than **facilitatory** as in the pyramidal (or direct) system.

It is important to keep in mind that functionally the two systems are difficult to distinguish. This distinction is more clinical in nature because of the effect that each has on muscular movement. Damage to the pyramidal system results in different clinical symptoms than those that result from damage to the extrapyramidal system.

Because of the emergence of involuntary movements when a person incurs extrapyramidal damage, it is assumed that this system (in normal condition) regulates muscle tone, suppresses unnecessary movements, and reduces extraneous motor activity associated with automatic movements. It is also thought to be concerned with the regulation of some coarse and stereotyped movements.

Motor Movement Disorders Resulting from Extrapyramidal Damage

The motor disturbances of the extrapyramidal system are usually classified as "involuntary movement disorders." The most commonly used technical term for these movement disorders is "dyskinesia" (*dys* = disorder, and *kinesia* = movement). *Hyperkinesia* is a term used to describe dyskinesias that have too much or excessive movement. The excessive movement may be of a slow or fast type. *Hypokinesia* is the term used to describe too little movement or a limited range of movement. *Bradykinesia* refers to slow movement.

These disorders encompass a full range of bizarre postures and unusual movement patterns. Often, the unusual movements that dominate the trunk and limbs of the dyskinetic patient are reflected in the face and the speech mechanism. The result is dysarthria. In general, the dysarthria reflects the specific symptoms of each specific type of dyskinesia. The characteristics of the various dysarthrias will be addressed in the Advanced Unit of Chapter 6.

It is important to note that medical professionals do not use the term *hypokinesia* to refer to the limitation in movement resulting from lesions of the pyramidal tract (upper and lower motor neuron system). The terms *hemiplegia, quadriplegia,* and *paraplegia* are used instead. This is an important clinical distinction that also applies to speech–language pathology.

Several specific types of dyskinesias have been identified (Love & Webb, 1996, adapted from p. 126–130):

• *Tremors*—purposeless hyperkinetic movements that are rhythmic, oscillatory, and involuntary. Tremors are pathologic if they occur in a disease and are characteristic of that disease. **Rest tremor** describes a type of tremor that occurs while the muscles are at rest. Its presence has been associated with **Parkinson's disease.** This tremor temporarily suppresses when the limb is moved, and sometimes it can be inhibited by conscious effort. Tremor may affect the voice, giving it a tremulous quality.

• *Chorea*—quick, random, hyperkinetic movements. It is a fast type of hyperkinesia. The speech, facial, and respiratory movements, as well as movements of the extremities, are affected by this type of movement disorder. Hyperkinetic chorea is a symptom of **Huntington's disease.**

• *Athetosis*—slow, irregular, coarse, writhing, or squirming movements. Even though they are slow movements, they occur in excess, and thus are classified as a hyperkinetic movement disorder. Athetosis usually involves the extremities as well as the face, neck, and trunk. Its movements interfere with the fine and controlled movements of the tongue, larynx, soft palate, pharynx, and respiratory mechanism. Athetotic movements may disappear in sleep. The site of lesion in pure athetosis is often in the putamen and caudate nucleus portion of the basal ganglia. Hypoxia, or lack of oxygen at birth, is a common cause of damage.

• *Dystonia*—distorted static postures of the limbs resulting from excess tone in *selected* parts of the body. Dyskinetic postures are slow, bizarre, and often grotesque. Movements may be writhing, twisting, and turning. Dysarthria may result if the speech musculature is affected, in which case, this disorder primarily affects the larynx, though the face, tongue, lips, palate, and jaw may also be involved. Some neurologists believe that dystonias contribute to spastic or **spasmodic dysphonia,** a voice disorder characterized by aphonia along with a strained, labored whisper. However, to date, etiology of spasmodic dysphonia is not very clear.

• *Myoclonus*—abrupt, brief, almost lightning-like muscular contractions. This movement disorder is most common in the limbs and trunk, but it may also occur in the facial, mandibular, lingual, and pharyngeal muscles. Several causes for this disorder have been described, including stroke in the brain stem. An example of a normal physiologic myoclonic reaction occurs when we are drifting off to sleep and are suddenly awakened by a rapid muscle jerk.

• *Orofacial dyskinesia or tardive dyskinesia*—bizarre movements limited to the mouth, face, jaw, and tongue. There is grimacing, pursing of the mouth and lips, and writhing of the tongue. These movements may affect articulation of speech. They may develop after the prolonged use of powerful tranquilizing drugs (e.g., phenothiazines).

Cerebellar System

The cerebellum is a neurological mechanism that functions as an error control device. It constantly monitors all motor outputs to muscles by receiving projections from the motor cortex and sensory signals from joint receptors and muscle spindles (Bhatnagar & Andy, 1995).

The cerebellum monitors intended movements by comparing the efferent (outgoing) commands with the sensory information it receives. It considers the targeted movement or movements in relation to (a) body position, (b) muscle preparedness, (c) muscle tone, (d) body equilibrium, (e) distance, and (f) movement over time. It functions as a conductor, modifier, adjuster, and regulator of movement. If any sensorimotor discrepancy is detected during the comparison between body position and motor impulse, the cerebellum sends the necessary corrective adjustments to the motor cortex via the deep cerebellar nuclei and the brain stem.

The cerebellum (cerebellar system) is vital to the control of very rapid muscular movement and activities such as *speaking,* running, typing, playing the piano, dancing, *writing, eating,* dressing, and so forth. These activities require the highest level of constantly changing muscle synergy and velocity.

Muscle tone regulation involves maintaining constant tension in healthy muscles and ensuring that muscles are prepared. Appropriate equilibrium is necessary to ensure a stable posture in space for the execution of motor movements. Voluntary movement, without assistance from the cerebellum, is clumsy, uncoordinated, and disorganized. The motor defect of the cerebellar system has been called **asynergia** or **dyssynergia.**

The cerebellum is connected with the rest of the central nervous system via the superior, middle, and inferior peduncles at the level of the brain stem. All afferent (incoming) and efferent fibers traveling to and from the cerebellum pass through these three fiber bundles. Fibers that travel through the inferior and middle cerebellar peduncles are afferent (receptive of sensorimotor information); they mediate almost all sensorimotor information to the cerebellum. Afferent fibers originate from the spinal cord, the brain stem, cranial nerve VIII, the temporal lobes, and the motor cortex.

Fibers of the superior cerebellar peduncle are largely efferent (conveying regulated outgoing information); they transmit cerebellar outputs to the brain stem and from there to the thalamus, motor cortex, and spinal cord. Motor, auditory, tactile, and visual regulation areas exist in the cerebellum and project to similar areas in the cerebrum, which in turn project back to corresponding cerebellar areas.

The cerebellum, therefore, is not completely vestibular, proprioceptive, or motor in function. It actually serves to reinforce or diminish sensory and motor impulses, acting as a "modulator" of neuronal activity. Through its afferent and efferent feedback circuits (loops), it ensures a desired level of neural activity in the motor parts of the nervous system.

Summary of the Advanced Unit

• The human brain is a relatively small structure weighing only 2½ to 3 pounds; however, it is amazingly powerful and controls all body functions.

• The nervous system is divided into two major subsystems: the central nervous system and the peripheral nervous system

• Nerve cells are the most basic building blocks in the central nervous system. They are responsible for receiving, transmitting, and synthesizing neural information.

• Each nerve cell consists of three major parts: the cell body, several dendrites, and a single axon.

• Dendrites transmit information toward the cell body of their own neuron, while the axon transmits neural information away from its cell body.

• Nerve cells communicate with one another at the synaptic junction.

• The information from one neuron travels to another neuron by the release of neurotransmitters at the synaptic junction.

• The brain is subdivided anatomically into five major components: cerebrum, basal ganglia, thalamus, cerebellum, and brain stem.

• The cerebrum is made up of two cerebral hemispheres, four primary lobes, and the cerebral cortex.

• The cerebral cortex houses several structures important for speech production, including the primary motor cortex, the supplementary motor cortex, Broca's area, Wernicke's area, and the primary auditory cortex.

• The basal ganglia are deep subcortical structures that play an important role in regulating the skilled motor movements necessary for speech.

• The cerebellum does not initiate motor movements; however, it helps monitor, regulate, and coordinate the speed, range, force, and strength of skilled motor movements including speech.

• The brain stem houses the cranial nerve nuclei for the cranial nerves involved in speech production.

• The brain stem is divided into the midbrain, pons, and medulla.

• There are 12 pairs of cranial nerves, and 7 are directly implicated in speech production: trigeminal, facial, vestibuloacoustic, glossopharyngeal, accessory, vagus, and hypoglossal.

• The spinal nerves play an indirect role in speech production by supplying several of the respiratory muscles, including the diaphragm, abdominals, and internal and external intercostals.

• Clinically, the central nervous system is often divided into the pyramidal, extrapyramidal, and cerebellar systems.

• The pyramidal system is considered a direct motor activation pathway, while the extrapyramidal system is considered a more indirect motor pathway. The cerebellar system does not initiate motor movements but does help in their coordination.

Chapter 2

◆ ◆ ◆ ◆ ◆ ◆ ◆ ◆ ◆ ◆ ◆ ◆ ◆ ◆ ◆ ◆ ◆

Perspectives in Articulation and Phonology

Basic Unit

♦ ♦ ♦ ♦ ♦ ♦ ♦ ♦ ♦ ♦ ♦ ♦ ♦ ♦ ♦ ♦ ♦ ♦ ♦

Basic Perspectives in Articulation and Phonology

An educated Southerner has no use for an r *except at the beginning of a word.*

—MARK TWAIN
Life on the Mississippi

Speech is a widely used vehicle for communication. Through a complex combination of sounds, speakers of a language produce words and sentences to verbally express their thoughts, feelings, and desires. Language appears to be rule-governed behavior, although the rules often are extracted from regularities in observed behaviors. Phonological rules are derived from patterns of phonological productions. Phonological rules refer to the systematic organization of sounds in forming words for communication. The study of these rules is known as **phonology.** More specifically, phonology refers to the study of speech sounds, speech sound production, and the rules for combining sounds in meaningful words and sentences.

Because most people acquire speech naturally, without formal instruction, few ever stop to think about the complexity of sound production. Most individuals intuitively follow the systematic rules of speech without difficulty, but if asked to do so could not explain those rules. However, those of us who specialize in speech–language pathology or are in any way involved in the remediation of articulation or phonological disorders* have a vested interest in studying sound production with great detail.

In this Basic Unit, we will address various aspects of sound production. For some readers, part of the information will be review from previous study, while other components may be completely new. For those who do not have a background in the subject matter, we believe that the information is presented in such a fashion that

---

*Although the terms *phonology disorder* and *disordered phonology* are often used in the literature, we prefer the terms *phonological disorder* or *disordered phonological skills* when referring to the inappropriate or delayed acquisition of the sound system and the rules that govern it. If we break down the word *phonology,* it becomes evident that the suffix *-ology* refers to the "study of," while the base word *phono* refers to "sound." Therefore, the term *disordered phonology* would literally mean the disordered study of sound and *phonology disorder* would mean the study of sound disorder. It is doubtful that these are the intended meanings. It may become easier to see the inappropriate use of the terms if we substitute the word *phonology* with *biology* or *geology.* Most of us would never say *disordered biology* or *disordered geology,* and we would definitely not say *biology disorder* or *geology disorder.*

it is easy to follow and simple to integrate. The specific perspectives addressed in this Basic Unit are an overview of (a) phonetics and phonetic transcription, (b) the speech production mechanism, (c) phoneme classification systems, (d) coarticulation and the dynamics of speech production, (e) phonological rules, (f) phonological processes, and (g) the clinical distinction between articulation and phonology.

To preserve the simplicity of the Basic Unit, more technical and theoretical information will be addressed in the Advanced Unit of this chapter. Such perspectives as aerodynamic, acoustic, suprasegmental, and perceptual aspects of speech production will be reviewed in detail in the Advanced Unit. Also, varied phonological theories will be introduced, and the clinical implications of these will be carefully evaluated. The clinician's role in applying and testing theories advanced by linguists and theoretical phonologists will be considered.

Phonetics

Phonetics is the study of speech sounds, their production and acoustic properties, and the written symbols that represent them. Because different professionals are interested in answering different questions about sound production, several branches have evolved within this field of study. Edwards (1997) identified the five major branches of phonetics as experimental, articulatory or physiological, acoustic, perceptual, and applied.

Experimental phonetics focuses on the development of scientific methods for the study of speech sounds. A method that has been developed by experimental phoneticians is speech synthesis or the generation of speechlike sounds by a computer. **Articulatory** or **physiological phonetics** concentrates on how a speaker of a language produces speech sounds. The vocal tract and related anatomical structures are studied extensively to describe what happens when speech sounds are produced. **Acoustic phonetics** is the study of the properties of the sound waves as they travel from the vocal tract of a speaker to the ear of a listener. The sound waves are studied according to their patterns of tone and noise. In **perceptual phonetics** the perception of sounds by the listener is studied in great detail. This study ranges from sound awareness to sound interpretation. Finally, as the name implies, **applied phonetics** is the branch dedicated to the practical application of the knowledge derived from experimental, articulatory, acoustic, and perceptual phonetics. According to Edwards (1997), this branch is dedicated to answering such questions as, "How does a dialect affect the sounds of American English?" "When do children acquire the sounds of English?" and "What phonetic symbols should be used to record sound production?" (p. 5).

It is beyond the scope of this Basic Unit to expand on the very detailed information offered by the many branches of phonetic study. Rather, because students at this level would be expected to have gained this information in a phonetics course, our review will be limited to the aspects of phonetics essential to understanding the study of articulation and phonological development and its disorders.

Several Important Terms

To establish a common base before we proceed, it is important to tackle the specialized vocabulary of phonetics. The term *phonetics* is derived from the word *phone.* Technically, the word **phone** is a generic term for any sound that can be produced by the vocal tract; a phone may or may not be a speech sound (Edwards, 1997). However, in the study of speech production, a phone is typically considered a single speech sound.

A **phoneme** is a family of phones or sounds perceived to belong to the same category by the listener. It is considered to be a group of sounds rather than a single sound because it consists of many productions that vary slightly when made in the context of words and or sentences. These slight variations, when they occur, do not change the meaning of the word containing the phoneme. For example, in the word *tea,* the *t* sound can be produced with lingual (tongue) contact against the alveolar ridge in one sentence, whereas in another sentence it can be produced with a more forward contact against the upper front teeth. Such variations in the production of *t* may occur because of the sounds that precede or follow it. If you say the word **tea** alternating from alveolar to dental contact, you will see that the meaning of the word does not change. You have simply produced two different phones that belong to the same phoneme group. In short, a phone is the actual speech sound uttered at a given moment, while a phoneme is a group of phones *perceived* to fall within the same sound family.

Phonemes have the linguistic function of distinguishing morphemes, or making a contrast in the meaning of words. A **morpheme** is the minimal unit of meaning, or the smallest unit of language carrying semantic interpretation. A **free morpheme** is a whole word that cannot be linguistically broken down into smaller units. **Bound morphemes** are word endings (suffixes) or beginnings (prefixes) that attach to a word (a free morpheme) to alter the meaning of that word. Although phonemes do not have any meaning in and of themselves, they can make a distinction between words such as **bit, sit, hit,** and **fit.** These words are all free morphemes that are contrasted only by one phoneme. Morphemes that are similar except for one phoneme are called **minimal pairs.** Using such minimal pairs, it can be determined whether a sound is a phoneme in a given language. For example, we know that *t* and *d* are two distinct phonemes in American English because they contrast word pairs such as *tie–die* and *ten–den.* The study of these sound differences in a language is called **phonemics** (Shriberg & Kent, 1995).

A variant or alternate form of a phoneme within a language is technically called an **allophone.** An allophone may be thought of as a member of the phoneme family. Allophones do not change the meaning of a word and, thus by definition, are not distinct phonemes. In our previous example of the word *tea,* the alveolar and the dental production of the /t/ sound are considered **allophonic variations** of the same phoneme because they do not change the meaning of the word. The occurrence of allophones is the direct result of the phonetic contexts that surround a phoneme. Continuing with our example of *tea,* the /t/ sound may be produced with lingual-alveolar contact in the sentence "He has tea," because the sound preceding the *t,* or the /z/, is also produced with lingual-alveolar contact. However, in the sentence "I loathe tea," the /t/ sound is produced with a more lingual-dental contact because the preceding sound /ð/ is produced **interdentally.** Try producing the two sentences interchangeably and you will notice (feel) the subtle difference. The effects of phonetic context on phoneme articulation will be described further in upcoming sections of this chapter.

✎ Activity

DIRECTIONS: Define the following terms in your own words.

Allophone: _____

Morpheme: _____

Bound morpheme: _____

Free morpheme: _____

Minimal pairs: _____

Phone: _____

Phoneme: _____

Phonetic Transcription

Recall that the definition of phonetics offered earlier included the phrase *"the written symbols* that represent [sounds]." In the study of sound production, our profession has adopted the symbols of the **International Phonetic Alphabet** (IPA) to represent the many phonemes of the English language.

The IPA was created in 1888 and was most recently revised in 1989. It was developed because orthographic spelling does not always represent how a sound is pronounced, thus creating confusion among professionals. For example the *f* sound in mainstream American English may be represented by the orthographic symbols "f" (*f*at), "ff" (pu*ff*iness), "ph" (*ph*ysician), or "gh" (lau*gh*ter). The different letters and letter combinations that can be used to represent the same phonemes are known as **allographs** (Shriberg & Kent, 1995).

To further complicate matters, any one allograph can represent different sounds, and it can also be silent. For example, the letter combination "gh" represents the *f* sound in the word *laughter* and the *g* sound in the word *ghost,* and in the word *sight* it is silent. No wonder people learning English as a second language have difficulty mastering written English.

Speech–language pathologists generally use the symbols of the IPA to transcribe sound production. This allows for a consistent and mutually agreed upon system that decreases the confusion created by allographic variations. All students in speech–language pathology should be proficient in the use of the sound-symbol association of the IPA. A copy of the International Phonetic Alphabet is found in Appendix B. (Not all of the symbols given in Appendix B are discussed in this text.)

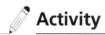 **Activity**

DIRECTIONS: Transcribe the following othographically written words using the phonetic symbols of the International Phonetic Alphabet.

computer _____	medicine _____
exercise _____	international _____
jogging _____	phonetics _____
vase _____	laughter _____
nose _____	program _____

The idealized or abstract description of a sound is transcribed according to the IPA and enclosed between slash marks or **virgules,** as in /t/. This is called **phonemic transcription** because the variations in actual phoneme production are not depicted. The sounds that are actually produced by an individual are transcribed and placed between brackets as in [t]; this is known as **phonetic transcription.**

Brackets alone, however, fail to indicate exactly how a sound has been produced. Therefore, the phonetic symbols enclosed by brackets may sometimes be further modified by special symbols called **diacritic markers.** For example, a dentalized production of /t/ would be transcribed as [t̪]. The mark placed under the [t] is the IPA symbol indicating the dentalized production of a phoneme. This detailed form of transcription is called **narrow phonetic transcription,** as opposed to **broad phonetic transcription.**

Table 2.1 lists the phonetic symbols for the 24 American English consonants, 14 American English vowels, and 6 American English diphthongs and several orthographically written key words. Table 2.2 lists several diacritic markers believed to be important for our discussion as we proceed.

Quick Review of the Speech Production Mechanism

In Chapter 1 we described the anatomical structures and organs that are important in speech production. We also addressed the neural integration of these. As a simple overview: The process of respiration supplies the air necessary for speech production. This air is then phonated at the level of the vocal cords for voiced consonants and vowels; for unvoiced consonants it continues past the level of the vocal cords unmodified. As the vibrated or unvibrated air continues to travel, it enters various cavities (e.g., pharyngeal, oral, and nasal) for further modification. This process is called resonation. The resonated sound is ultimately shaped into specific speech sounds through the various structures in the mouth, in a process described as articulation.

Recall that these oral structures are typically divided into movable articulators (tongue, lips, velum, and mandible) and immovable articulators (hard palate, teeth, and alveolar ridge). The immovable articulators serve as a point of contact for the mobile articulators for the modification of the airstream (voiced or

Table 2.1. Phonetic Symbols for English Consonants, Vowels, and Diphthongs

Phonetic Symbol	Sample Allographic Representations
Consonants	
/b/	**b**a**b**y, ra**bb**it
/p/	**p**an, pe**pp**er, hiccou**gh**
/d/	**d**o, la**dd**er, begg**ed**, shoul**d**
/t/	**t**op, a**tt**ack, talk**ed**, dou**bt**, recei**pt**, **Th**omas
/g/	**g**et, e**gg**, **gu**est, **gh**ost, va**gue**
/k/	**k**it**ch**en, a**c**tor, a**cc**ustom, **ch**emistry, bouti**que**
/m/	**m**oon, ha**mm**er, to**mb**, ple**ghm**, hy**mn**, psal**m**
/n/	**n**ot, di**nn**er, **kn**ow, **gn**at, **pn**eumonia, **mn**emonic
/ŋ/	bri**ng**, i**nk**, to**ngue**, a**nx**ious
/z/	**z**oo, bu**zz**er, **x**yloghone, hi**s**, a**s**thma
/s/	**s**ay, a**ss**a**ss**in, **ps**y**ch**iatrist, li**s**ten, **c**ent
/v/	**v**alentine, sa**vv**y, wife'**s**, Ste**ph**en
/f/	**f**an, a**ff**air, tou**gh**, tele**ph**one, hal**f**
/ð/	**th**at, ba**the**
/θ/	too**th**, **th**in
/ʒ/	mea**s**ure, a**z**ure, gara**ge**
/ʃ/	**sh**ip, **s**ugar, **ch**ef, mi**ss**ion, loca**ti**on
/h/	**h**op, **wh**o
/dʒ/	**j**ob, **j**u**dge**, marria**ge**, **g**em, exa**gg**erate
/tʃ/	**ch**ur**ch**, ki**tch**en, na**t**ure, **c**ello
/w/	**wh**en, **w**in, **o**ne, **qu**est, **ch**oir
/ʍ/	**wh**ich, **wh**ite (dialectical variations)
/j/	**y**ellow, halle**l**ujah, opin**io**n
/r/	**r**abbit, ma**rr**y, **wr**ite, **rh**yme, Peace Co**rps**
/l/	**l**adder, ba**ll**, is**l**and, funn**el**
Vowels	
/ɑ/	f**a**ther, b**ou**ght, m**o**cking
/æ/	c**a**t, bl**a**st, j**a**ck, f**a**mily
/e/	m**a**te, l**a**ke, vac**a**tion, rel**ay**
/ɛ/	b**e**tter, **e**lephant, **e**xit, **e**xplain
/o/	b**oa**t, m**o**st, t**oa**st, t**o**te
/ɔ/	p**oo**r, f**ou**r, m**o**re, sh**o**re
/u/	m**oo**n, s**ui**tcase, tr**ue**
/i/	h**ea**t, p**ie**ce, m**ee**k
/ɪ/	p**i**g, m**i**tt, j**i**ngle, **i**gloo
/ʊ/	c**oo**k, p**u**t, r**oo**kie
/ɚ/	batt**er**, jok**er**, col**or**, mak**er**
/ɝ/	p**ur**ple, b**ir**d, d**ir**ty
/ə/	**u**ntie, **e**xtra
/ʌ/	c**u**p, **u**nder, **u**p, b**u**tter
Diphthongs	
/aɪ/	p**i**pe, m**y**, m**igh**t, r**i**te
/au/	c**ow**, h**ou**se, t**ow**n, p**ou**t
/ɔi/	t**oi**l, b**oy**, m**oi**st, l**oi**ter
/ju/	**u**nited, **u**sed, f**ew**, b**eau**tiful
/eɪ/	vac**a**tion, t**a**ke, f**a**ce
/ou/	l**oa**n, thr**o**ne, ph**o**ne

Table 2.2. Diacritic Markers and Phonetic Symbols for Selected Non-English Sounds

Diacritic Markers		Phonetic Symbols for Non-English Sounds	
[ˌ]	syllabic consonant	[ř]	voiced alveolar trill
[˳]	partially devoiced	[χ]	voiceless velar fricative
[ˬ]	partially voiced	[ɣ]	voiced velar fricative
[¨]	breathy	[ɸ]	voiceless bilabial fricative
[ʰ]	aspirated	[β]	voiced bilabial fricative
[=]	unaspirated	[ɲ]	palatal nasal
[˥]	unreleased	[λ]	palatal lateral approximant
[̪]	dentalized	[ʕ]	voiced pharyngeal stop
[ˏ]	lateralized	[ʕ]	unvoiced pharyngeal stop
[˜]	nasalized	[Δ]	posterior nasal fricative
[≈]	nasal emission	[ʑ]	voiced mid-dorsum palatal stop
[̷]	denasalized	[ʒ]	voiceless mid-dorsum palatal stop
[ʾ]	rounded vowel		
[ʿ]	unrounded vowel		
[̫]	labialized consonant		
[̪]	nonlabialized consonant		
[:]	lengthened		
[>]	shortened		
[˄]	whistled		

unvoiced) into specific speech sounds. Figure 2.1 illustrates all the articulators involved in the production of English phonemes. It is important to keep these structures in mind as we proceed to phoneme classification. Refer to the Basic Unit in Chapter 1 for more detailed information.

Phoneme Classification

English phonemes are divided into two main categories: consonants and vowels. **Consonants** are phonemes produced by some narrowing or closing of the vocal tract. The closure may be complete, as in the production of /b/ and /k/, or partial, as in the formation of sounds like /f/ and /l/. Consonant sounds produced in side-by-side combination are termed **clusters.** American English has a large set of **prevocalic** (before a vowel) and **postvocalic** (after a vowel) consonant clusters. The words *tree, break,* and *street* all contain prevocalic clusters, while *park, best,* and *help* have postvocalic clusters.

Unlike consonants, **vowels** are produced with a relatively open vocal tract configuration. In the production of vowels, the tongue does not make contact with any specific articulator for closure as it does with consonants. Vowels are further subdivided into simple or pure vowels and diphthongs. Pure vowels are also termed **monophthongs,** and they constitute most of the vowel system of American English (Lowe, 1996). The terms *pure vowels* and *monophthongs* connote that these sounds have a single or unchanging quality as they are produced. **Diphthongs** are made by the quick gliding of two simple vowels so that they cannot be perceptually separated, as in the words *toy* and *bye.* Compared to pure vowels, diphthongs make up a much smaller set of sounds in American English.

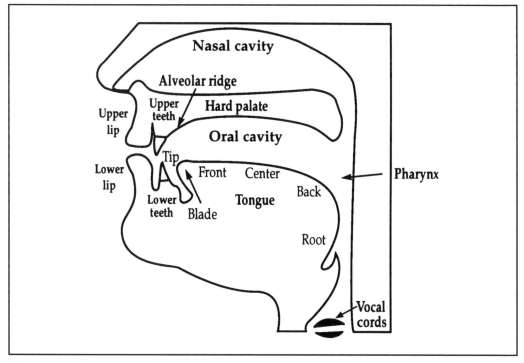

Figure 2.1. The articulators and the resonating cavities. *Note.* From *Applied Phonetics: The Sounds of American English* (2nd ed., Figure 3.2, p. 21), by H. T. Edwards, 1997, San Diego, CA: Singular Publishing Group. Copyright 1997 by Singular Publishing Group, Inc. Reprinted with permission.

Linguistically, vowels and diphthongs are the carriers of syllables, while consonants and consonant clusters attach to vowels to form various syllable shapes. Because of their syllable-forming status, vowels are also termed **syllabics.** In addition to vowels, a few English consonants can take on a syllabic nature, meaning that they can also form the nucleus for a syllable. These consonant syllabics include /m/, /n/, /l/, and /r/. The special diacritic marker /ˌ/ is used to differentiate the consonantal versus syllabic property of these sounds. Below are examples of words containing these sounds as consonants and syllabics.

Sound	Consonant Property	Syllabic Property
/m/	/mæn/, /ləmɛnt/	/prizm̩/
/n/	/nɛkst/, /æntik/	/bʌtn̩/
/l/	/lamp/, /əlon/	/æpl̩/
/r/	/red/, /əraund/	/æftr̩/

Whereas vowels actually form a syllable or syllables in a word, consonants serve to initiate a syllable, terminate a syllable, or both. A syllable that ends in a vowel or diphthong is **open,** while one that ends in a consonant is **closed.** Such words as *my, key,* and *blue* are examples of open syllables; *stop, make,* and *took* are closed syllables.

Depending on how consonants attach to vowels, various syllable shapes can be formed. Languages across the world have different sequencing rules dictating how consonants and vowels can attach to each other to form syllable shapes. The following are one- and two-syllable words representing some of the many possible syllable shapes in English. For simplicity, V refers to vowel and C refers to consonant.

One-Syllable Words (Shriberg & Kent, 1995)		**Two-Syllable Words** (Ohde & Sharf, 1992)	
V	I	VCV	away
VC	up	CVCV	buddy
CV	bye	VCVC	along
CCV	brew	CVCVC	buddy's
CVC	hat	VCCV	also
VCC	its	VCCVC	applies
CCCV	straw	VCCCV	astray
VCCC	asks	VCCCVC	astride
CVCC	hard	CVCCV	toaster
CCVC	break	CVCCVC	replies
CCCVC	streak	CCVCV	story
CVCCC	palms	CCVCVC	prefers
CCVCC	stork	CCVCCV	prosper
CVCCCC	sixths	CCVCCVC	prospers
CCCVCC	streets	CVCCCV	sixty
CCVCCCC	glimpsed	CVCCCVC	describe
CCCVCCC	sprints	CCVCVCC	prevent
CCCVCCCC	strengths	CCVCVCCC	protests

Consonants that precede a vowel are **prevocalic;** those that occur between vowels are **intervocalic;** and those that follow a vowel are **postvocalic.** Other terms used to describe the position of a sound are **initial, medial,** and **final.** *Initial* refers to a sound that is located at the beginning of a word, and *medial* and *final* denote sounds that are made in the middle and at the end of a word, respectively. These terms are more commonly used in clinical practice.

The terms *initial* and *final* can be used to denote the position of sounds in both words and syllables. A sound may be in the initial position of a syllable but not in the initial position of the word. For example, in the word *de-tec-tive,* the first *t* is in the medial position of the word but the initial position of the second syllable. The same is true for sounds in the final position. Sounds in syllable-initial and syllable-final positions are also termed syllable-**releasing** and **-arresting** sounds, respectively. Sounds that initiate a syllable are said to release the syllable, while those that terminate a syllable are said to arrest the syllable (Shriberg & Kent, 1995).

We have made reference to a **syllable** on various occasions, but what exactly is a syllable? Many of us can probably remember as children having to identify the number of syllables in words, a skill known as **syllabification.** The literature has shown that most first graders can correctly identify the number of syllables in words (Owens, 1996), but despite the fact that we can identify the number of syllables in words with a high level of accuracy at a very young age, the majority of us cannot define the term *syllable.*

Yavas (1998) provides us with a simple, yet thorough description of the components of a syllable. He defines a syllable as a small unit of speech that has three essential components: **onset, nucleus,** and **coda.** Nucleus and coda are collectively known as **rhyme.**

The onset component of a syllable is the consonant or consonant cluster that initiates it, while the rhyme is the remaining part. Within the rhyme, the vowel or diphthong that follows the initial consonant or cluster is the nucleus. The consonant or consonant cluster that follows the nucleus makes up the coda. For example, in the word *break,* the cluster *br* is the onset, the diphthong *ea* is the nucleus, and the *k* is the coda. Together, the diphthong *ea* and the final *k* make up the rhyme. In American English, neither the onset nor the coda components are obligatory; many words start or end with a vowel (e.g., *egg, in, act, see, you,* and *blue*).

Multisyllable words may have more than one onset, nucleus, and coda. Some may have more than one coda, while others may not contain a coda at all. The first syllable in a multisyllable word may or may not have an onset. To illustrate this point we will use the words *backpack, tomorrow,* and *entire.* The word *backpack* consists of two syllables: *back* and *pack.* Each of these syllables contains an onset, a nucleus, and a coda. The word *tomorrow* consists of three syllables: *to, mo,* and *rrow.* Each of its syllables has an onset and a nucleus. There are no codas in the word *tomorrow* since neither of its syllables ends in a consonant or consonant cluster. It should be noted that *w* in the syllable *rrow* is only an orthographic consonant. Phonetically, the syllable ends in the vowel /o/. The word *entire* has two syllables: *en* and *tire.* The syllable *en* begins with the nucleus *e* and ends with the coda *n.* The syllable *tire* has an onset, a nucleus, and a coda.

As we indicated earlier, syllables that end in a vowel or diphthong are termed *open syllables,* while those ending in a consonant or consonant cluster are called *closed syllables.* For an excellent and more detailed examination of what exactly constitutes a syllable, the reader may consult Shriberg and Kent (1995, pp. 11–12 and pp. 102–104).

Activity

DIRECTIONS: Identify the onset, nucleus, and rhyme for each syllable in the following words.

	Onset	**Nucleus**	**Coda**
Joke (1 syll)	_____	_____	_____
Today (2 syll)	_____	_____	_____
Fun (1 syll)	_____	_____	_____
Glasses (2 syll)	_____	_____	_____
Art (1 syll)	_____	_____	_____

In the upcoming sections the sounds of the English language will be described in detail according to the traditional and more current classification systems. By the end of this chapter, the reader should be able to answer such questions as "What is the voiceless bilabial stop?" and "What is the high-front, tense, and unrounded vowel?"

Consonant Production

Manner, Place, and Voicing Features

Consonants have been traditionally described according to place, manner, and voicing dimensions. **Place of articulation** indicates *where* along the vocal tract the consonant is formed; **manner of articulation** indicates *how* it is formed; and **voice** indicates *whether* the vocal folds are vibrating during its production.

English consonants are typically defined according to their place of production as follows:

- *bilabial:* mutual contact of the upper and lower lips
- *labiodental:* placement of the upper front teeth over the lower lip
- *linguadental or interdental:* placement of the tongue tip between the upper and lower front teeth
- *lingua-alveolar or alveolar:* contact of the tongue tip against the alveolar ridge
- *linguapalatal or palatal:* contact of the tongue blade against the hard palate
- *linguavelar or velar:* contact of the tongue dorsum against the velum
- *glottal:* vibration of air at the level of the vocal cords

The manner of production refers to the nature or amount of articulatory constriction. If the vocal tract is completely closed off for a short period of time, the sound is a **stop.** This name indicates the temporary stoppage of sound production at its place of constriction. Because the release from the stoppage may be forceful in nature, these sounds are also frequently referred to as **plosives.** The name **stop-plosive** depicts both the temporary stoppage and the forceful release of the airstream in the production of these sounds. **Fricatives** are sounds produced by an incomplete and narrow constriction that results in a friction, or hissing type of noise. **Affricates** are formed by a combination of stopping and fricative characteristics. These sounds are formed initially as stops followed by a fricative release.

Sounds formed from a coupling of the oral and nasal cavities are called **nasals** because of the nasal quality that results from the resonation of sound in the nasal cavity. **Glides** are vowel-like sounds produced by a transitional movement of the tongue from one area of the mouth to another. **Liquids** also are vowel-like sounds that are produced with a relatively open vocal tract configuration. A narrowed tongue permitting air to pass around its sides produces a **lateral** sound.

If the vocal folds are vibrating during sound production, the consonants are referred to as **voiced.** If the consonants are activated by the airstream only, they are labeled **voiceless** or **unvoiced.** Many sounds of the English language vary only in the voicing dimension. Such sound pairs as /p-b/, /t-d/, and /s-z/ share the same place and manner of production; however, they differ in the voicing feature. These sound pairs are called **cognates.** Table 2.3 represents the English consonants by place, manner of production, and voicing.

Manner of Articulation

Stops. As the name implies, stop consonants are formed by complete closure of the vocal tract at some point so that the airflow ceases, or stops, and air pressure

Table 2.3. Manner, Place, and Voicing Features of English Consonants

Phoneme	Voicing	Manner	Place
/b/	voiced	stop	bilabial
/p/	voiceless	stop	bilabial
/d/	voiced	stop	alveolar
/t/	voiceless	stop	alveolar
/g/	voiced	stop	velar
/k/	voiceless	stop	velar
/m/	voiced	nasal	bilabial
/n/	voiced	nasal	alveolar
/ŋ/	voiced	nasal	velar
/z/	voiced	fricative	alveolar
/s/	voiceless	fricative	alveolar
/v/	voiced	fricative	labiodental
/f/	voiceless	fricative	labiodental
/ð/	voiced	fricative	linguadental
/θ/	voiceless	fricative	linguadental
/ʒ/	voiced	fricative	palatal
/ʃ/	voiceless	fricative	palatal
/h/	voiceless	fricative	glottal
/dʒ/	voiced	affricate	palatal
/tʃ/	voiceless	affricate	palatal
/w/	voiced	glide	velar/bilabial
/ʍ/	voiceless	fricative	glottal/bilabial
/j/	voiced	glide	palatal
/r/	voiced	liquid, rhotic*	palatal
/l/	voiced	liquid, lateral*	alveolar

*Distinctive feature term

builds up behind the point of closure (Shriberg & Kent, 1995). As stated earlier, this buildup of air pressure eventually is released and may produce a short burst of noise. Because of this audible burst of noise, stop consonants are also referred to as stop-plosives (*plosive* referring to the explosion of air upon its release). Shriberg and Kent (1995) emphasize that the plosive phase does not occur in the production of all stop sounds or in all word positions. For example, many stop sounds in word-final position are unreleased and, thus, are not plosive in nature.

The stop consonants that are part of the English language include /p/, /b/, /t/, /d/, /k/, and /g/. Although these sounds all share the same manner of production, they are produced in different places along the vocal tract.

Articulatory Summary for Stops
(Shriberg & Kent, 1995, p. 64)

1. The oral cavity is completely closed off at some point for a brief interval.
2. The velopharynx is closed (otherwise, the air within the oral pressure chamber would escape through the nose).
3. Upon release of the stop closure, a burst of noise is typically heard.
4. The closing and opening movements for stops tend to be quite fast, usually the fastest movements in speech.

Fricatives. Fricative sounds are so termed because of the hissing-like or turbulent quality that results from the continuous forcing of air through a narrow constriction. Although all fricatives are noisy, the intensity of the noise depends on the sound's place of articulation (Shriberg & Kent, 1995). The fricatives are /s/, /z/, /f/, /v/, /θ/, /ð/, /ʃ/, /ʒ/, /tʃ/, and /dʒ/.

Articulatory Summary for Fricatives
(Shriberg & Kent, 1995, p. 65)

1. The articulators form a narrow constriction through which airflow is channeled. Air pressure increases in the chamber behind constriction.
2. As the air flows through the narrow opening, a continuous friction noise is generated.
3. Because effective noise production demands that all escaping air be directed through the oral constriction, fricatives are produced with a closed velopharynx.

Affricates. Affricate sounds actually have a stop and a fricative component. Although these sounds begin as stops, they are released as fricatives. Because of this, Shriberg and Kent (1995) term them *combination* sounds (p. 67). There are only two affricates in the English language: /tʃ/ and /dʒ/.

Articulatory Summary for Affricates
(Shriberg & Kent, 1995, p. 67)

1. Affricates are a combination of a stop closure and a fricative segment, with the frication noise closely following the stop portion.
2. Affricates are made with complete closure of the velopharynx.

Nasals. Nasals are produced by lowering the velum so that the velopharyngeal port is opened. Opening of the velopharyngeal port allows air vibrated by the vocal cords to enter the nasal cavity; this adds a nasal resonance to some consonants. Only three consonants in English are produced with nasal resonance, /m/, /n/, and /ŋ/. However, in connected speech, oral sounds may become nasalized when they are surrounded by nasal sounds. For example, the vowel /æ/ in the word *cat* is fully resonated in the oral cavity, but in the word *man* it is nasalized because of the preceding and following nasal sounds. If you alternate between producing *cat* and *man,* paying close attention to the vowel in the two words, you will notice the subtle difference.

Articulatory Summary for Nasals
(Shriberg & Kent, 1995, p. 65)

1. The oral tract is completely closed, as it is for a stop.
2. The velopharyngeal port is open to permit sound energy to radiate outward through the nasal cavities.
3. Even if the oral closure is broken, sound may continue to travel through the nose as long as the velopharynx remains open.

Glides. Glides, also known as **semivowels,** are produced by a quick transitioning of the articulators as they move from a partly constricted state to a more open state for the vowel that follows the glide. Edwards (1997) uses the term *onglide* to describe this movement. Glides are formed by a relatively unrestricted and transitory point of constriction in comparison to other consonants, particularly stops, fricatives, and affricates. Only two English sounds are glides, /w/ and /j/. Try saying the words <u>w</u>ent and <u>y</u>am, and you will notice the gradual gliding property as you progress from the glide consonant to the following vowel. You may also notice the more open point of constriction. Although some phoneticians consider /l/ and /r/ as glides, these are more commonly termed liquids. For our purposes, only /w/ and /j/ will be considered glides.

Articulatory Summary for Glides
(Shriberg & Kent, 1995, p. 67)

1. The constricted state for the glide is narrower than that for a vowel but wider than that for stops and fricatives.
2. The articulators make a gradual gliding motion from the constricted segment to the more open configuration for the following vowel.
3. The velopharynx is generally, if not always, closed.
4. The sound energy from the vocal folds passes through the mouth in a fashion similar to that for vowels.

Liquids. The terms used to classify sounds up to this point tend to make logical sense. Stops are actually stopped at some point in their production, fricatives make friction noise, and glides are made with a gliding motion. However, the term **liquid** tends to be a standard that on the surface does not very well explain the manner of production for these sounds. Nevertheless, two sounds generally fall under this category, /l/ and /r/. Although their individual productions vary, /l/ and /r/ are both made with a vocal tract that is obstructed only slightly more than for vowels. Thus, these sounds are sometimes considered vowel-like consonants. The /l/ is also called a **lateral** because during its production the lateral, midsection part of the tongue is open, and thus air is directed through the sides of the tongue. The /r/, also termed **rhotic,** may be produced in various ways. However, two of the most common ways of making this sound are by (1) curling the tongue tip back slightly so that it approximates but does not touch the alveolar ridge or palatal area, and (2) bunching or humping the tongue in the palatal area. An /r/ made by curling the tongue tip back is called a **retroflex** /r/, while one made by bunching and elevating the blade portion of the tongue is known as a **bunched** or **humped** /r/. The terms *lateral* and *rhotic* will be explained further under the section on distinctive features.

Articulatory Summary for Liquids
(Shriberg & Kent, 1995, p. 65)

1. Sound energy from the vocal folds is directed through a distinctively shaped oral passage, a configuration that can be maintained indefinitely for sustained production of the sound, if required.
2. The velopharynx is always (or at least almost always) closed.
3. The oral passageway is narrower than that for vowels but wider than that for stops, fricatives, and nasals.

Place of Articulation

We previously discussed the manner of articulation associated with all English sounds. However, manner of production is not sufficient for the identification of specific sounds. To help differentiate one sound from another, it is useful to consider their place of articulation. Place of articulation refers to the location in the vocal tract of the point of constriction for specific sounds. For example, although /p/, /t/, and /k/ all share the same manner of production, they are made with different points of constriction. This classification system considers the relationship between the primary articulators that help shape the sounds. What follows is a description of English sounds according to their place of articulation, progressing from front to back.

Bilabials. These sounds are produced by pressing the two lips together, thus the term **bilabial.** The stops /b/ and /p/ and the nasal /m/ make up the bilabial sound class. The glide /w/ is also considered a bilabial, but it is not made by pressing the two lips together as with /b/, /p/, and /m/. Rather, /w/ is made by rounding the lips while the tongue dorsum elevates toward the velum. Thus, /w/ is frequently categorized under two places of articulation, bilabial and **velar** (we will discuss this later).

Labiodentals. Labiodental sounds are formed by placing the lower edge of the upper incisors (teeth) on the upper portion of the lower lip. The contact between the upper incisors and the lower lip is very light, forming a narrow point of constriction. Only two English consonants, /f/ and /v/ are made with labiodental contact; they are both fricatives.

Linguadentals. Linguadental sounds, also termed **interdental,** are made by protruding the tip of the tongue slightly between the cutting edge of the upper and lower front teeth. This forms a narrow constriction from which airflow is directed. For obvious reasons, the point of contact between the tongue and the teeth is light. Only two fricative consonants are linguadentals, /θ/and /ð/.

Lingua-alveolars (alveolars). By definition, lingua-alveolar sounds are produced by articulation of the tongue and the alveolar ridge. Several sounds make up this sound class: /t/, /d/, /s/, /z/, /l/, and /n/. Although the tip of the tongue is raised so that it makes contact with the alveolar ridge for all of these sounds, the type of contact varies according to the sound's manner of articulation.

For the stops /t/ and /d/, the tip of the tongue is placed firmly against the alveolar ridge so that it completely impedes the flow of air for a short period of time. Contact for the fricatives /s/ and /z/ is characterized by placement of the tip of the tongue against the alveolar ridge so that a narrow constriction is formed. This narrow constriction is actually shaped by a midline groove of the tongue that serves as a passageway for the escaping air.

The liquid lateral /l/ is formed by light contact of the tongue tip against the alveolar ridge for midline closure and lateral opening at both sides of the mouth. The air escapes through this lateral opening. Finally, /n/is formed similarly to /t/ and /d/ in terms of place of articulation, with firm contact of the tongue tip against the alveolar ridge. The important distinction between the stops /t/ and /d/ and the nasal /n/ is their resonance. While /t/ and /d/ are fully resonated in the oral cavity, /n/ is produced with an open velopharyngeal port for nasal resonance.

Linguapalatals (palatals). Placement of the tongue blade against the hard palate forms the point of constriction for **linguapalatal** sounds. The actual point of contact on the hard palate is typically just posterior to the alveolar ridge. The fricatives /ʃ/ and /ʒ/, the affricates /ʤ/ and /ʧ/, the liquid /r/, and the glide /j/ make up the palatal class according to place of articulation. The difference between these sounds is their manner of articulation. The consonants /ʃ/ and /ʒ/ are fricatives made with an intense noise, while /ʤ/ and /ʧ/ are affricates made with a stop and fricative component. The /r/ is a liquid, and /j/ is a glide.

Velars. Velar sounds are made by elevation of the tongue dorsum against the soft palate (velum). The /k/, /g/, and /ŋ/ sounds form the velar class. Some definitions of velars include /w/ in this sound class because as it is produced, the tongue elevates toward the soft palate. While /k/, /g/, and /ŋ/ are made with firm contact of the tongue against the velum, in the production of /w/ the tongue merely approximates the soft palate. The manner of production for these sounds varies: /k/ and /g/ are stops; /ŋ/ is a nasal; and /w/ is a glide.

Glottals. As the name implies, glottal sounds are made at the level of the glottis. In mainstream American English, /h/ is the only glottal consonant that has a phonemic property. However, although the glottal stop [ʔ] is not a distinct phoneme of American English, it may occur as an allophonic variation of some stops in connected speech (Edwards, 1997). Words such as *button* [bʌʔn] and *cotton* [kaʔn] demonstrate the use of [ʔ] as an allophone of /t/. In this case, [ʔ] is an allophone and not a phoneme because it does not create a contrast in meaning. In other words, the meaning of *button* remains constant whether it is pronounced as [bʌʔn] or [bʌtn]. The same is true for *cotton*. The glottal stop /ʔ/ is phonemic in some languages, such as Danish and Arabic (Edwards, 1997). Children with cleft palate speech often replace a glottal stop for many **pressure consonants,** which include stops and fricatives.

Voicing

Consonant production is also classified according to the voicing feature. **Voicing** refers to the movement of the vocal folds in the production of sounds. Sounds that are made while the vocal folds are vibrating are termed **voiced sounds.** Sounds made in the absence of vocal fold vibration are known as **unvoiced** or **voiceless sounds.** The voiced consonants of American English are /b/, /d/, /g/, /z/, /v/, /ð/, /ʒ/, /ʤ/, /m/, /n/, /ŋ/, /l/, /r/, /w/, /j/. The voiceless sounds are /p/, /t/, /k/, /z/, /f/, /θ/, /ʃ/, /ʧ/, and /h/. Some sounds are identical in their manner of production and place of articulation but differ in the voicing feature. These are known as **cognate pairs.** The cognate pairs of American English are /p–b/, /t–d/, /k–g/, /s–z/, /f–v/, /θ–ð/, /ʃ–ʒ/, and /ʧ–ʤ/.

Distinctive Features

An alternative way of describing phonemes is by their distinctive features (Chomsky & Halle, 1968; Jakobson, Fant & Halle, 1952; Jakobson & Halle, 1956). A distinctive feature is an articulatory or acoustic parameter that according to its presence or absence helps define a phoneme. Using this classification system, each phoneme is examined according to a cluster of features that is either present or absent in that phoneme.

Chomsky and Halle (1968) developed what is now a classic **binary** system, by which a phoneme (consonant or vowel) is given a plus (+) value if a feature is present or a minus (−) value if the feature is absent. An example of a distinctive feature offered by Chomsky and Halle's definitions is the **vocalic** feature, which refers to sounds that are not produced with a marked constriction of the vocal tract; all vowels and the liquid consonants have this feature, while the remaining consonants do not. Phonemes may share certain features, but each phoneme has a unique set of features that distinguishes it from all other phonemes. While some phonemes vary by a large number of features, some may differ only by one or two. For example, /s/ and /z/ share all the same distinctive features with the exception of voicing; /s/ has a (−) voice feature, and /z/ has a (+) voice feature.

The 16 sets of binary features and their definitions as described by Chomsky and Halle are reviewed below.

1. **Vocalic.** Sounds that do not have a marked constriction in the vocal tract. The level of constriction is no more than is necessary for the production of /i/ and /u/ or the liquids /l/ and /r/ (Edwards, 1997). Vocalic sounds are associated with spontaneous voicing. All vowels are vocalic, but only the /l/ and /r/ consonants have this feature.

2. **Consonantal.** Sounds that have a marked constriction along the midline region of the vocal tract. Although traditionally all sounds apart from vowels are considered consonants, Chomsky and Halle do not consider /h/, /w/, and /j/ as consonantal. The remaining consonants have a (+) consonantal feature: /f/, /v/, /θ/, /ð/, /t/, /d/, /s/, /z/, /n/, /l/, /ʃ/, /ʒ/, /r/, /ʧ/, /ʤ/, /k/, /g/, /ŋ/, /p/, /b/, /m/.

3. **High.** Sounds that are made with the tongue elevated above the neutral position required for the production of /ə/. The (+) high consonants are: /ʃ/, /ʒ/, /j/, /ʧ/, /ʤ/, /k/, /g/, /ŋ/.

4. **Back.** Sounds that are made with the tongue retracted from the neutral position required for the production of /ə/. The consonants with the (+) back feature are: /k/, /g/, and /ŋ/.

5. **Low.** Sounds made with the tongue lowered for the neutral position of /ə/. Of all English consonants, only the /h/ has a (+) low feature.

6. **Anterior.** Sounds that are made with a point of constriction located farther forward than that of the palatal /ʃ/. The place of production for /ʃ/ creates the boundary between anterior and nonanterior sounds. The consonants that have this feature are: /w/, /f/, /v/, /θ/, /ð/, /t/, /d/, /s/, /z/, /n/, /l/, /p/, /b/, /m/.

7. **Coronal.** Sounds made with the tongue blade raised above the neutral position required for the production of /ə/. The (+) coronal consonants are: /θ/, /ð/, /t/, /d/, /s/, /z/, /n/, /l/, /ʃ/, /ʒ/, /r/, /ʧ/, /ʤ/.

8. **Round.** Sounds made with the lips rounded or protruded. Only two consonants are rounded: /r/ and /w/.

9. **Tense.** Sounds made with a relatively greater degree of muscle tension or contraction at the root of the tongue. The (+) tense consonants are: /p/, /t/, /k/, /ʧ/, /ʤ/, /f/, /θ/, /s/, /ʃ/, /l/. You will notice that all of these are (−) voice consonants with the exception of /ʤ/ and /l/.

10. **Continuant.** Sounds made with an incomplete point of constriction. The flow of air is not entirely stopped at any point. Because of this, many continuant sounds can be maintained in a steady state until the person runs out of the necessary supply of air to make the sound. How long can you sustain an /f/ before turning blue? The continuant consonants are: /w/, /f/, /v/, /θ/, /ð/, /s/, /z/, /l/, /ʃ/, /ʒ/, /j/, /r/, /h/.

11. **Nasal.** Sounds that are resonated in the nasal cavity. The velum is lowered so that the nasal and oral cavities become coupled. Only three sounds of English are nasal: /m/, /n/, and /ŋ/.

12. **Strident.** Sounds made by forcing the airstream through a small opening, resulting in the production of intense noise. These sounds typically include the fricatives /f/, /v/, /s/, /z/, /ʃ/, /ʒ/, and the affricates /ʧ/, /ʤ/.

13. **Sonorant.** Sounds that allow the airstream to pass relatively unimpeded through the oral or nasal cavity. The sonorant consonants are the glides /w/, /j/, the liquids /l/, /r/, and the nasals /n/, /m/, /ŋ/.

14. **Interrupted.** Sounds that are produced by complete blockage of the airstream at their point of constriction. The stops /t/, /d/, /k/, /g/, /p/, /b/ and affricates /ʧ/, /ʤ/ are (+) interrupted.

15. **Lateral.** Sound made by placing the front of the tongue against the alveolar ridge (midline closure) and lowering the midsection of the tongue on both sides (lateral opening). Only the /l/ sound in English is (+) lateral.

16. **Voice.** Sound produced with vibration of the vocal folds. The (+) voice consonants are: /w/, /v/, /ð/, /d/, /z/, /n/, /l/, /ʒ/, /j/, /ʤ/, /r/, /g/, /ŋ/, /b/, /m/. Sounds that are identical in every respect except the voice feature are commonly known as **cognates.** These cognate pairs are /s–z/, /p–b/, /k–g/, /t–d/, /θ–ð/, /ʃ–ʒ/, and /ʧ–ʤ/.

The following are examples of how these features can be used to analyze and describe individual phonemes:

/p/	**/v/**	**/n/**
−vocalic	−vocalic	−vocalic
+consonantal	+consonantal	+consonantal
−high	−high	−high
−back	−back	−back
−low	−low	−low
+anterior	+anterior	+anterior
−coronal	−coronal	+coronal
−voice	+voice	+voice
−continuant	+continuant	−continuant
−nasal	−nasal	+nasal
−strident	+strident	−strident

Table 2.4 describes the distinctive features of all English consonants according to Chomsky and Halle's (1968) binary system. It should be noted that although this system initially appears very different from the more traditional analysis of manner, place, and voicing (M-P-V), the two systems do share various similarities. Although the vocabulary may be somewhat different, most distinctive features have M-P-V counterparts. For example, the distinctive features *strident* and *continuant* can be equated with the traditional phonetic term *fricative,* and the distinctive feature *interrupted* is comparable to the more traditional term *stop.*

Other distinctive features that may be clinically useful include obstruent, sibilant, approximant, rhotic, and syllabic. Consonants that are made with a complete closure or narrow constriction in the oral cavity so that the airstream is stopped or friction noise is produced are collectively termed **obstruents;** these include the

Table 2.4. Distinctive Features for Consonants of American English (Chomsky & Halle, 1968)

Features	p	b	t	d	k	g	f	v	s	z	ʃ	ʒ	tʃ	dʒ	θ	ð	h	m	n	ŋ	l	r	w	j
																								Consonants
Vocalic	−	−	−	−	−	−	−	−	−	−	−	−	−	−	−	−	−	−	−	−	+	+	−	−
Consonantal	+	+	+	+	+	+	+	+	+	+	+	+	+	+	+	+	−	+	+	+	+	+	−	−
High	−	−	−	−	+	+	−	−	−	−	+	+	+	+	−	−	−	−	−	+	+	−	−	+
Back	−	−	−	−	+	+	−	−	−	−	−	−	−	−	−	−	−	−	−	+	−	−	−	−
Low	−	−	−	−	−	−	−	−	−	−	−	−	−	−	−	−	+	−	−	−	−	−	−	−
Anterior	+	+	+	+	−	−	+	+	+	+	−	−	−	−	+	+	−	+	+	−	+	−	+	−
Coronal	−	−	+	+	−	−	−	−	+	+	+	+	+	+	+	+	−	−	+	−	+	+	−	−
Round	−	−	−	−	−	−	−	−	−	−	−	−	−	−	−	−	−	−	−	−	−	+	+	−
Tense	+	−	+	−	+	−	+	−	+	−	+	−	+	+	+	−	−	−	−	−	−	−	−	−
Continuant	−	−	−	−	−	−	+	+	+	+	+	+	−	−	+	+	+	−	−	−	+	+	+	+
Nasal	−	−	−	−	−	−	−	−	−	−	−	−	−	−	−	−	−	+	+	+	−	−	−	−
Strident	−	−	−	−	−	−	+	+	+	+	+	+	+	+	−	−	−	−	−	−	−	−	−	−
Sonorant	−	−	−	−	−	−	−	−	−	−	−	−	−	−	−	−	−	+	+	+	+	+	+	+
Interrupted	+	+	+	+	+	+	−	−	−	−	−	−	+	+	−	−	−	−	−	−	−	−	−	−
Lateral	−	−	−	−	−	−	−	−	−	−	−	−	−	−	−	−	−	−	−	−	+	−	−	−
Voiced	−	+	−	+	−	+	−	+	−	+	−	+	−	+	−	+	−	+	+	+	+	+	+	+
	p	b	t	d	k	g	f	v	s	z	ʃ	ʒ	tʃ	dʒ	θ	ð	h	m	n	ŋ	l	r	w	j

stops, fricatives, and affricates (Ohde & Sharf, 1992). **Sibilant** sounds are high-frequency sounds that have a more strident quality and longer duration than most other consonants (Ohde & Shard, 1992). It is generally agreed that the sibilants include the fricatives and affricates /s/, /z/, /ʃ/, /ʒ/, /tʃ/, and /dʒ/ (Bleile, 1996). Glides and liquids are sometimes called **approximants** because of the approximating nature of the contact between the two articulators that help form them. Although they are certainly produced by the approximation of two articulators, the degree of contact is not nearly as closed as with stops, fricatives, and affricates (Ohde & Sharf, 1992). A sound with /r/ coloring is sometimes termed **rhotic.** This term may be used for the /r/ consonant and its various allophonic variations (Shriberg & Kent, 1995). Finally, **syllabics** are sounds that serve as a nucleus for a syllable; all vowels are syllabics, while most consonants are not (Shriberg & Kent, 1995). The consonants that can take on a syllabic property include the nasals /m/ and /n/ and the liquids /l/ and /r/.

Easy Reference of the English Consonants According to Commonly Used Distinctive Feature Terms

- **Consonantal:** f, v, θ, ð, t, d, s, z, n, l, ʃ, ʒ, r, tʃ, dʒ, k, g, ŋ, p, b, m
- **Vocalic:** l, r
- **Anterior:** w, f, v, θ, ð, t, d, s, z, n, l, p, b, m

(continues)

- **Back:** k, g, ŋ
- **Voice:** w, v, ð, d, z, n, l, ʒ, j, ʤ, r, l, g, ŋ, b, m
- **Continuant:** w, f, v, θ, ð, s, z, l, ʃ, ʒ, j, r, h
- **Interrupted:** t, d, k, g, p, b, ʧ, ʤ
- **Strident:** f, v, s, z, ʃ, ʒ, ʧ, ʤ
- **Obstruent:** f, v, θ, ð, t, d, s, z, ʃ, ʒ, ʧ, ʤ, k, g
- **Sonorant:** w, l, r, j, n, m, ŋ
- **Approximant:** w, l, r, j
- **Sibilant:** s, z, ʃ, ʒ, ʧ, ʤ
- **Nasal:** m, n, ŋ
- **Rhotic:** r

Singh and Polen (1972) developed a relatively more simplistic distinctive feature program. As opposed to Chomsky and Halle's (1968) system, this system focuses only on consonant motor production. Consonants are identified into seven paired feature classes using a binary system of "1" and "0." The classes are arranged according to opposing features (e.g., front/back, nonlabial/labial, and voiceless/voiced). The features given a "0" value are front, nonlabial, nonsonorant, nonnasal, stop, nonsibiliant, and voiceless. Their respective contrastive features are given an "1" value: back, labial, sonorant, nasal, continuant, sibilant, and voiced.

1. **Front/Back:** Front (0) consonants are those that are articulated on or in front of the alveolar ridge. These are /p/, /b/, /t/, /d/, /f/, /v/, /θ/, /ð/, /s/, /z/, /l/, /m/, and /n/. Back (1) consonants are produced posterior to the alveolar ridge. These consonants are /ʃ/, /ʒ/, /ʧ/, /ʤ/, /k/, /g/, /h/, /j/, /w/, and /r/.

2. **Nonlabial/Labial:** Nonlabial (0) consonants are produced without the lips. These are /t/, /d/, /k/, /g/, /θ/, /ð/, /s/, /z/, /ʃ/, /ʒ/, /ʧ/, /ʤ/, /j/, /r/, /l/, /n/, and /h/. Labial (1) consonants are produced with the lips as the main place of articulation. These are /p/, /b/, /m/, /f/, /v/, and /w/.

3. **Nonsonorant/Sonorant:** Sonorant (0) consonants are produced with an unobstructed airflow and spontaneous voicing. This distinctive feature sound class is made up voiced stops, fricatives, and affricates. Sonorant (1) sounds are those made with an obstruction along the vocal tract. These are /l/, /r/, /w/, /j/, /m/, /n/, and /ŋ/.

4. **Nonnasal/Nasal:** As the term implies, nonnasal (0) consonants are produced without nasal resonance. This class includes all sounds except /m/, /n/, and /ŋ/. Sounds that are part of the nasal class (1) are produced with nasal resonance. There are only three nasal sounds in English: /m/, /n/, and /ŋ/.

5. **Stop/Continuant:** Stop (0) consonants include all of those sounds produced with a rather abrupt termination of airflow. These include /p/, /b/, /t/, /d/, /k/, and /g/. Continuants (1), on the other hand, are not produced with a continuous airflow that can be sustained. The continuants are /θ/, /ð/, /s/, /z/, /ʃ/, /ʒ/, /r/, /l/, /j/, /w/, /m/, /n/, and /ŋ/.

6. **Nonsibilant/Sibilant:** Sibilant sounds have been previously described under the more traditional definition of distinctive features. Singh and Polen (1972) used the term in a similar light. Their category of sibilant (1) sounds included /s/, /z/, /ʃ/, /ʒ/, /ʧ/, /ʤ/. All other sounds were considered nonsibilants (0).

7. **Voiceless/Voiced:** This feature was previously described under Chomsky and Halle's (1968) binary distinctive feature system. The voiceless (0) sounds are

/p/, /t/, /k/, /s/, /f/, /ʃ/, /tʃ/, and /h/. The voiced cognates for these sounds, /m/, /n/, /ŋ/, /r/, /l/, /j/, and /w/, make up the voiced (1) class.

Consonant Clusters

Consonants can be produced as singletons (alone) or in side-by-side combination with other consonants to form clusters. Consonant clusters occur in prevocalic and postvocalic word positions. American English contains many two- and three-member clusters, and a few four-member clusters in the final position of words. Although the definition for clusters is not consistent from one source to another, we will use the term in reference to the contiguous combination of consonant sounds that precede or follow a vowel within the same syllable. Consonant clusters are also known as **blends.** As with singleton consonants, clusters attach to vowels to create various syllable shapes. Table 2.5 shows examples of several clusters that occur in American English; several key words have been provided for each.

Vowel Production

Tongue Position, Lip Rounding, and Tenseness Features

Vowel articulation has been traditionally described according to (a) the position of the tongue, (b) the shape of the pharynx, (c) the shape of the lips, and (d) the muscular tension associated with production. Unlike consonants, the voicing feature is not typically used to characterize vowels since all of the English vowels are voiced unless a person produces whispered speech, which can result in devoiced vowel productions.

These features help distinguish all English vowels. It is amazing to think that even a slight difference — in tongue height, for example — can create an important linguistic distinction between two sounds (e.g., /ɪ/ and /i/). Word pairs like *bit–beat, mitt–meat,* and *fit–feet* vary by only one sound: their vowel. However, this vowel distinction can make the difference between a sentence that is logical — "I used my new mitt during last night's baseball game" — and one that does not make much sense — "I used my new meat during last night's baseball game."

Tongue position. As stated earlier, one way of classifying vowels is according to the position of the tongue along two major dimensions: tongue height (*high, mid,* or *low*) and tongue advancement (*front, central,* or *back*). High vowels are produced in the highest position possible, with the tongue close to the roof of the mouth. Low vowels, on the other hand, are produced with the tongue depressed in the mouth. Vowels in between the high and low dimensions are categorized as mid vowels. Tongue advancement or retraction for vowels is determined by comparing their production with the highest-front vowel /i/, the lowest-front vowel /æ/, the highest-back vowel /u/, and the lowest-back vowel /ɑ/. A **vowel quadrilateral** defines the four extreme points of vowel production: *high, low, front,* and *back.* This four-sided figure, with /i/, /u/, /æ/, and /ɑ/ at its extreme corners, has been used to categorize the production of all vowels according to tongue position into seven general categories: high-front, mid-front, low-front, mid-central, high-back, mid-back, and low-back.

The *front-to-back* dimension of the position of the tongue has a direct effect on the shape of the pharynx. As the tongue is carried in a more forward position, the

Table 2.5. Several Syllable-Initiating and Syllable-Terminating Clusters of American English and Allographic Representations

Consonant Cluster	Sample Allographic Representations	Consonant Cluster	Sample Allographic Representations
Syllable-Initiating		**Syllable-Terminating**	
kw-	quick, queen, quack, quantity	-mp	ramp, lamp, stomp
tw-	tweezers, twist, twang, twenty	-nt	ant, pleasant, count, plant
sw-	swim, sweat, swap, sweeten	-nd	hand, bend, fond, blind
pl-	play, plan, plastic, place	-ns	prince, cleanse
kl-	clown, clock, clap, clean	-rd	hard, weird, guard, chard
fl-	flag, flick, flounder, flack	-nz	lens, plans, buns
bl-	black, blast, blink, Blake	-ks	parks, lacks, plaques
gl-	glasses, gloat, glimpse, glad	-st	past, best, post, nest
sl-	slide, slap, slender, sleep	-kt	act, fact, deduct, induct
pr-	prize, present, practical, prepare	-ld	held, mold, peeled
br-	brown, brag, brain, bring	-rt	art, fort, mart, sort
tr-	truck, tree, train, trap	-ts	bets, mats, ports
dr-	drive, drink, drastic, dramatic	-rn	barn, burn, fern, churn
fr-	front, frog, frost, French	-rm	arm, farm, alarm, charm
θr-	through, threat, thrive	-lb	bulb
kr-	crown, crop, create, creep	-lp	pulp, help, gulp
gr-	green, gray, grass, gripe	-lt	halt, malt, fault
st-	stop, steel, steak, stork	-lf	half, calf
sp-	spot, sport, speak, Spanish	-lk	bulk, stalk, walk
sk-	school, scar, score, Scott	-rst	burst, first
sn-	snake, snow, sniff, snack	-zd	buzzed, blazed
sm-	small, smile, smack, smudge	-rk	park, mark, fork
nj-	news, newsworthy, newcomer	-mz	arms, aims, stems
fj-	few, fugitive, fumes, future	-lz	balls, malls, steals
kj-	cute, coupon, accused	-gz	bugs, pegs
mj-	music, amused, musician	-pt	opt, stopped, dropped
ʃr-	shrink, shriek, shrine	-ft	left, stuffed, lift
str-	stray, street, strong, strange	-rf	scarf
skw-	squander, squat, squint	-rv	starve, carve, swerve
spl-	splash, splendor, splint	-mpt	stomped, stamped
spr-	spray, sprint, sprinkle	-mps	lamps, cramps, blimps
skr-	scram, scream, screech	-nts	ants, pants, prints
		-ngz	strings
		-ngk	thank, bank, frank
		-ndz	hands, grounds

pharynx is enlarged, while a posterior placement of the tongue narrows the pharyngeal cavity. The different pharyngeal dimensions that result from varying tongue placement create the unique resonance characteristics of each vowel.

HIGH-FRONT VOWELS: /i/ AND /ɪ/. The /i/ vowel is produced with the tongue in the highest and most forward position compared to other English vowels. It can be made in the initial, medial, and final positions of words. Although /ɪ/ is also categorized as a high-front vowel, it is produced with the tongue in a slightly lower and more posterior position than /i/. This vowel also occurs in all positions, with the exception of the final position in monosyllabic words (Ohde & Sharf, 1992).

MID-FRONT VOWELS: /e/ AND /ɛ/. The /e/ vowel is produced lower than the position required for the high vowels and slightly back from the position required for /ɪ/. It can occur in all positions of monosyllabic and polysyllabic words. Although it is produced lower than the position for /e/, the /ɛ/ vowel can still be categorized under the mid vowels. Some phoneticians call /ɛ/ a low-mid-front vowel (Ohde & Sharf, 1992). This vowel occurs only in word-initial and -medial positions.

LOW-FRONT VOWELS: /æ/. Only the /æ/ vowel falls under this category. It represents one of the lowest vowels in English. It is produced with the tongue lower and more posterior from the position required for /ɛ/. Key words include *hat, at,* and *stamp.*

MID-CENTRAL VOWELS: /ɝ/, /ɚ/, /ə/, AND /ʌ/. Although these four vowels are generally categorized as mid-central vowels, their place of production varies from one to the other. The /ɝ/ is typically produced with the blade of the tongue bunched and raised toward the hard palate. The tongue height is about equal to that of /e/ and /ɪ/, and it is retracted toward /o/. It occurs in the initial, medial, and final positions of monosyllabic and polysyllabic words. The /ɚ/ vowel, sometimes called **schwar,** has the same point of production in the oral cavity as /ɝ/; however, in transcription it is used to represent the production of /ɝ/ in unstressed syllables in words like *barber* and *color* (Ohde & Sharf, 1992). The third mid-central vowel, /ə/, is made with the tongue lowered in relation to /ɝ/. It occurs in all positions in polysyllabic words, but in monosyllabic words it does not occur in the final position. This vowel is also known as the unstressed schwa since it occurs in unstressed syllables. The stressed counterpart of **schwa** is the /ʌ/ vowel. It is produced in a position close to /ə/, but the tongue is slightly more retracted toward /ɑ/.

HIGH-BACK VOWELS: /u/ AND /ʊ/. The /u/ vowel is produced in the highest and most retracted position compared to all other English vowels, as in the words *soon, moon,* and *blue.* The other high-back vowel, /ʊ/, is produced slightly lower and more forward than /u/. The /u/ vowel occurs in all positions of monosyllabic and polysyllabic words, while /ʊ/ occurs only in word-medial positions (Ohde & Sharf, 1992).

MID-BACK VOWELS: /o/ AND /ɔ/. The /o/ vowel is produced slightly lower in the oral cavity in comparison to /u/. It occurs in the initial, medial, and final positions of monosyllabic and polysyllabic words. In relation to /o/, the /ɔ/ vowel has a slightly lower point of production. Like /o/, this vowel also occurs in all positions of monosyllabic and polysyllabic words.

LOW-BACK VOWELS: /ɑ/. The /ɑ/ vowel has the lowest and most retracted point of production of all vowels. It occurs in all word positions in monosyllabic and polysyllabic words. Ohde and Sharf (1992) indicate that although it occurs in final-word position in monosyllabic words, this happens only occasionally.

Lip Rounding

The shape of the lips during the production of vowels may be considered according to the amount of rounding. Vowels that are produced with the lips somewhat protruded, as in the words *who, cook,* and *boat,* are categorized as **rounded.** Vowels that are produced with the lips in a more neutral or retracted position, as in the words *bet, hat, hot,* and *hey,* are called **unrounded.** Sometimes more descriptive terms are used in reference to lip configuration, including *rounding, protrusion, retraction, spreading, eversion,* and *narrowing* (Shriberg & Kent, 1995). However, the terms *rounded* and *unrounded* are by far the most common.

Rounded Vowels	**Unrounded Vowels**
/u/ — *moon*	/i/ — *meet*
/ʊ/ — *cook*	/ɪ/ — *bit*
/o/ — *boat*	/e/ — *bake*
/ɔ/ — *caught*	/ɛ/ — *met*
/ɝ/ — *bird*	/æ/ — *hat*
	/ɑ/ — *pot*
	/ɚ/ — *butter*
	/ə/ — *untie*
	/ʌ/ — *up*

You will notice by the examples provided above that only the back vowels and the central vowel /ɝ/ are rounded, while all the front vowels and the central vowels /ɚ/, /ə/, and /ʌ/ are unrounded. Some phoneticians also categorize /ɝ/ as unrounded (Ohde & Sharf, 1992).

Tenseness. Although the exact level of muscular tension associated with vowels has not been experimentally confirmed (Shriberg & Kent, 1995, p. 28), the terms **tense** and **lax** are often used to describe their production. Theoretically, the tense vowels are longer in duration and have a higher degree of muscular tension associated with their production, while the lax vowels are shorter and require less muscular effort. Shriberg and Kent indicate that the distinction *long–short* might be more appropriate, as some vowels are almost always short and others are almost always long. They also indicate that this dimension can be identified more easily under experimental conditions.

The vowels traditionally described as tense are: /i/, /e/, /u/, /o/, /ɔ/, and /ɝ/. The lax vowels are: /ɪ/, /ɛ/, /æ/, /ʊ/, /ɑ/, /ɚ/, /ə/, and /ʌ/. Linguistically, tense or long vowels can occur in open syllables — *he, bay, Sue, toe* — and closed syllables — *heat, bait, boot, bird.* Lax or short vowels can appear in stressed closed syllables — *bit, bet, bat, book, pot, cup* — but not stressed open syllables.

Distinctive Features

As with consonants, a more recent way of describing vowels is according to their distinctive features. Chomsky and Halle's (1968) binary +/− system discussed under consonant production has also been applied to vowels. The following distinctive features have been specifically used to describe vowels:

- **Vocalic**—Sounds that are made without a marked constriction in the vocal tract. The level of constriction is no more than that necessary for the production of /i/ and /u/. All vowels are vocalic.

- **Consonantal**—Sounds that are made with a marked constriction along the midline region of the vocal tract. No vowels are consonantal.

- **Sonorant**—Sounds that are produced as the airstream passes relatively unimpeded through the oral or nasal cavity. All vowels are sonorant.

- **Rhotic**—Sounds made with an /r/ coloring. The mid-central vowels /ɚ/ and /ɝ/ are the only two vowels sharing the +rhotic feature.

- **High**—Sounds made with the tongue elevated above the neutral position required for the production of /ə/. The /i/, /ɪ/, /u/, and /ʊ/ are all high vowels.

- **Low**—Sounds made with the tongue lowered for the neutral position of /ə/. Only /æ/ and /ɑ/ share this distinctive feature.

- **Front**—Sounds made with the tongue in a more forward position than that required for the production of /ə/. The vowels /i/, /ɪ/, /e/, /ɛ/, and /æ/ are all considered +front vowels.

- **Back**—Sounds made with the tongue retracted from the neutral position required for the production of /ə/. Five American English vowels are +back vowels: /ɑ/, /ɔ/, /o/, /u/, and /ʊ/.

- **Rounded**—Sounds made with the lips rounded or protruded. The /ɚ/, /ɝ/, /ɔ/, /o/, /ʊ/, and /u/ vowels are classified as rounded.

- **Tense**—Sounds made with a relatively greater degree of muscle tension or contraction at the root of the tongue. The +tense vowels are /i/, /e/, /ʌ/, /ɝ/, /o/, and /u/.

- **Voiced**—Sounds produced with vibration of the vocal folds. All American English vowels are voiced.

Table 2.6 shows the English vowels according to various distinctive features.

Diphthongs

Diphthongs can be defined as vowel-like sounds resulting from a gradually changing place of articulation (Shriberg & Kent, 1995). Diphthongs contain two segments: an initial segment and a final segment. The initial and final segments are also known as onglide and offglide segments, respectively. The onglide is the vowel that initiates the diphthong, and the offglide is the vowel to which it changes (Lowe, 1996). Diphthongs are represented phonetically by digraph symbols that highlight the initial and final elements. A phonetic mark known as a *ligature* is sometimes placed underneath the diphthong to highlight the unity of the onglide and offglide portions. Table 2.1 shows the phonetic symbols used for the diphthongs of American English and various key words.

Linguistically, diphthongs serve the same function as pure vowels, in that they form the nucleus for a syllable (e.g., *boy* [bɔi], *bite* [bait], and *train* [trein]). In American English, diphthongs can be **phonemic** or **nonphonemic.** Diphthongs that cannot be reduced to pure vowels or monophthongs without changing the meaning of the words in which they occur are categorized as phonemic. The American

Table 2.6. Distinctive Features for Vowels of American English (Chomsky & Halle, 1968)

Features	Vowels													
	i	ɪ	e	ɛ	æ	ɑ	ɔ	o	ə	ʌ	ɝ	ɚ	ʊ	u
Vocalic	+	+	+	+	+	+	+	+	+	+	+	+	+	+
Consonantal	−	−	−	−	−	−	−	−	−	−	−	−	−	−
Sonorant	+	+	+	+	+	+	+	+	+	+	+	+	+	+
Rhotic	−	−	−	−	−	−	−	−	−	−	+	+	−	−
Advanced	−	−	−	−	−	−	−	−	−	−	−	−	−	−
Front	+	+	+	+	+	−	−	−	−	−	−	−	−	−
High	+	+	−	−	−	−	−	−	−	−	−	−	+	+
Low	−	−	−	−	+	+	−	−	−	−	−	−	−	−
Back	−	−	−	−	−	+	+	+	−	−	−	−	+	+
Rounded	−	−	−	−	−	−	+	+	−	−	+	+	+	+
Tense	+	−	+	−	−	−	+	−	+	+	−	−	−	+
Voiced	+	+	+	+	+	+	+	+	+	+	+	+	+	+
	i	ɪ	e	ɛ	æ	ɑ	ɔ	o	ə	ʌ	ɝ	ɚ	ʊ	u

English diphthongs that fall under this category are /ai/, /au/, /ɔi/, and /ju/. Although /j/ was previously described as a consonant glide, recall that this sound also has a vowel-like quality. Therefore, when it occurs side by side with /u/, as in the words *cue* [kju̲], *few* [fj̲u̲], and *pew* [pj̲u̲], it is also considered the onglide component of the /ju/ diphthong. The phonemic nature of /ai/, /au/, /ɔi/, and /ju/ can best be highlighted by contrasting words containing the onglide component of the diphthong as a pure vowel and words that contain the actual diphthong.

Contrast	**Pure Vowel**	**Diphthong**
/a–ai/	*pop* /p̲a̲p/	*pipe* /p̲a̲ip/
/a–au/	*pot* /p̲a̲t/	*pout* /p̲a̲ut/
/ɔ–ɔi/	*tall* /t̲ɔ̲l/	*toil* /t̲ɔ̲il/
/u–ju/	*coo* /k̲u̲/	*cue* /kj̲u̲/

Only two American English diphthongs, /ei/ and /ou/, are nonphonemic since they do not create a change in word meaning when they are replaced by their pure vowel counterparts /e/ and /o/. Whether a person says *take* as [teik] or [tek], it is perceived as the same word by the listener. Although /ju/ was described as a phonemic diphthong, in some instances it can also be nonphonemic, meaning that it does not create a contrast in words made with the diphthong or its pure vowel counterpart. Examples of this are the words *coupon* and *news*. The meaning of these words does not change if they are produced as [kjupɑn] or [kupɑn] and [njuz] or [nuz].

Diphthongs in which one of the stressed vowels combines with schwar /ɚ/ are sometimes described as **rhotic** or **centering diphthongs** (Secord, 1981a). This class of diphthongs includes /ɪɚ/ as in *fear*, /ɛɚ/ as in *bear*, /ɑɚ/ as in *far*, and /ɔɚ/

as in *poor*. It should be noted, however, that these terms are not used consistently in the field of speech–language pathology.

Speech Production: A Dynamic Human Behavior

Although sounds are traditionally categorized according to place, manner, and voicing features, this classification system has several limitations. One of the major limitations is that it gives the impression that sounds are produced in isolated units and thus always articulated "perfectly." However, in connected speech, sounds do not occur in isolation and typically stray from their textbook-defined production. Kent (1998) indicates that "when sounds are put together to form syllables, words, phrases, and sentences, they interact in complex ways and sometimes appear to lose their separate identity" (p. 36). And since most of us do not talk in "ooos" and "eees" unless we have not surpassed the coo and goo stage, it is important to consider the interactions of sounds in contextual speech.

Coarticulation refers to the influence that sounds have on one another when they are linked to make words, phrases, and sentences. All sounds are affected by their neighboring sounds, especially by those sounds that immediately precede or follow them. We have all become cognizant at some point of the effects of coarticulation in our own speech when we actually catch ourselves making an error such as "I bought a new pomputer [computer]." As effective language users, we frequently identify our errors, correct them, and get a good laugh from them. The average layperson would probably not stop to analyze why such an error occurred. However, as presented here, it may have become clear that the initial /k/ in "computer" more than likely became a /p/ because of the following /p/ sound in the word. Coarticulation may be subclassified as adaptation or assimilation, depending on the degree of perceptual changes that it effects on a sound (Creaghead, Newman, & Secord, 1989).

Creaghead et al. (1989) describe phonetic **adaptations** as articulatory movement variations and changes in the configuration of the vocal tract in the production of a sound according to the sounds that precede or follow it. Because speech is a dynamic process, sounds are not usually made the same way twice. Simply stated, a sound that undergoes adaptation takes on the properties of a surrounding sound or sounds. This is best illustrated by the /t/ sound in the words *tin* and *took*. The word *tin* is followed by a front vowel and consonant, while *took* is followed by two back sounds. When producing *tin,* the /t/ is made at the alveolar ridge, which is the textbook-defined point of constriction for that sound. However, the /t/ in *took* is produced with a slightly more retracted tongue position because of the back vowel and consonant that follow it. It should be noted that although /t/ adapted, this change did not create a perceptual change. In other words, the /t/ in *tin* and the /t/ in *took* are perceived as the same sound by the listener, despite their varying points of constriction.

In **assimilation,** however, the modification may be extensive enough that a perceptual change is detected. The affected sound may take on some audible characteristics of the sound effecting the change. In some instances, the sound that is affected becomes completely like its neighboring sound, as in our previous example of *pomputer* for *computer*. In other cases, the modification, although perceptible, may not be as dramatic. An example of this is the devoicing of /z/ in the sentence, "Yeah, it's a fat zebra" because of the preceding voiceless consonant /t/. Assimilation will be discussed further in this Basic Unit under the section on phonological processes.

Phonological Rules of a Language

Every language of the planet appears to have certain phonological rules that govern the production of sounds by its users. While some phonological rules are language specific, others are universal across languages. As rule-governed behavior, the sound system of any language can be analyzed according to the following four parameters: (1) the sound inventory of the language (contrastive phonemes), (2) the allowable combinations of sounds, (3) the acceptable allophonic variations of sounds, and (4) the morphophonemic alterations in sound combinations (Stoel-Gammon & Dunn, 1985).

Inventory of Sounds

Phoneme refers to the smallest linguistic unit of language that can signal a difference in meaning. Although a phoneme produced in isolation does not carry meaning, when it is combined with other phonemes it can help create words. By definition, phonemes also create meaningful contrasts in word pairs like *pop–mop, bat–fat,* and *shake–take* (**minimal pairs**). Therefore, phonemic contrasts are linguistic contrasts that have the potential to produce different morphemes and words (Shriberg & Kent, 1995, p. 7). Each language has an inventory of sounds that is part of the phonological system of that language.

While some phonemes are shared across languages, others are unique to a particular language. Shriberg and Kent (1995) indicate that there are about 100 total phonemes used in the many languages of the world. However, some languages, such as English, have a large number of sounds that make up their phonetic inventory, while other languages have a more limited repertoire.

The sound inventory of American English includes 24 consonants, 14 vowels, and 6 diphthongs. Several allophonic variations result from this large phonemic inventory, which help create the many **dialects** of American English. Ethnocultural and dialectical variations will be addressed in detail in Chapter 5.

You will recall from previous sections in this Basic Unit that a phoneme is actually a family of phones, or sounds, that are perceived by the listener to belong to the same category. However, as we have said, the idealized production of a sound rarely occurs in connected speech. Due to the effects of coarticulation, adaptation, and assimilation, phonemes may vary from one moment to another. Subtle phonetic modifications that are not extensive enough to create a difference in meaning in the words that contain them are known as **allophonic variations.**

Allophonic Variations

We previously defined an allophone as a variant or alternate form of a phoneme within a language. While *phoneme* refers to an abstract concept of sound production, *allophone* refers to the actual sound uttered at a given moment in time.

Allophonic variations typically are a result of phonetic environment in coarticulated speech. The words *kit* and *coop* exemplify this. The /k/ in *kit* is articulated with the tongue in a more forward position in comparison to the /k/ in *coop*. Although not a perceptible change, this subtle variation in the sound's point of constriction is an effect of the vowel that follows it; *kit* contains a front vowel, while *coop* has a back vowel. Shriberg and Kent (1995) summarize the concept of allophones nicely by stating that two allophones of the same phoneme never contrast to produce two different morphemes. Only phonemes have that linguistic function.

Allophonic variations of a single phoneme may occur in free variation or complementary distribution. Allophones occur in **free variation** when they *can* be exchanged for one another in a certain phonetic context without affecting the word. In American English, for example, allophones of /t/ can occur in free variation in word-final position. For example, in the word *bat,* the /t/ may be released with a small burst of air, or it may be unreleased if the tongue remains in position for a few seconds. The released production is transcribed [bætʰ], while the unreleased production of the same word is transcribed [bæt ̚]. The diacritical markers [ʰ] and [̚] symbolize the aspirated versus the unreleased production of a sound, respectively.

Some allophonic variants occur in specific places but not in others (Edwards, 1997). Such allophones are said to be in **complementary distribution** because they *cannot* be exchanged for one another in specific phonetic contexts. For example, in American English, /t/ has various allophonic variations that are context specific. In word-initial positions, /t/ is made with an aspirated release. However, when it is part of an /s/ cluster, it is unaspirated. Words such as *top* and *stop* would be transcribed [tʰap ̚] and [st ̚ap ̚] if using **narrow phonetic transcription.** The use of narrow phonetic transcription helps to highlight the aspirated and unreleased allophonic variations of /t/ in the two words. That allophonic variants are in complementary distribution does not mean that if exchanged in certain phonetic contexts the meaning of words would be affected. For example, if we choose to produce *top* as [t ̚ap ̚] instead of [tʰap ̚], the word may sound nonstandard, but the meaning remains unaffected. Such allophonic exchanges are not uncommon in people learning English as a second language or in children and adults using a nonmainstream dialect of American English.

Phonotactics

Edwards and Shriberg (1983) define *phonotactics* as the rules for how sounds can be combined to form syllables and how these sounds can be distributed. Although all languages have phonotactic rules, the exact rules are not equivalent across languages. For example, in English, words cannot be initiated with /ɛs + stop/ clusters, whereas Spanish has many words that begin with such clusters in words like *escuela* [ɛskwɛla] and *estoy* [ɛstoi].

As already indicated, phonotactic rules dictate the possible combination or sequencing of sounds in syllables and the permissible distribution of sounds according to initial, medial, and final positions. Weiss, Gordon, and Lillywhite (1987) indicate that in a specific language, there are restrictions about:

- where certain sounds can appear;
- the possible combinations of sounds;

- the number of consonants that can be combined in the initial and final positions of words; and

- the possible order of the occurrence of the sounds.

If some of these restrictions are applied to American English, the following can serve as examples of phonotactic rules within this language:

Where certain sounds can appear

- The /p/ sound can occur in the initial, medial, and final positions of words.

- The /h/ sound can occur in the initial and medial positions of words but not in the final position.

- The /ŋ/ sound can occur in the final and medial positions of words but not in the initial position.

The possible combinations of sounds

- The /t/ and /r/ consonants can be combined in the initial position to create words like *train, truck,* and *try.*

- The /k/ and /l/ consonants can be combined in the initial position of words to create words like *clown, clap,* and *clean.*

- The /b/ and /g/ sounds cannot be combined to initiate or terminate words.

- The consonant /r/ and a nasal consonant can be combined in the final position to create words like *farm, born,* and *barn.*

The number of consonants that can be combined in the initial and final positions of words

- Two-consonant combinations are permissible (e.g., /pl-/, /br-/, /st-/, and /-rm/, /-rk/, and /-ld/).

- Three-consonant combinations are permissible (e.g., /str-/, /spr-/, /skr-/, and /-rst/, /-kst/, and /-nts/).

- Four-consonant combinations are permissible, though rare, only in the final position (e.g, /-ŋθs/ in *strengths* and /-mpst/ in *glimpsed*).

Morphophonemics

Morphophonemics refers to the sound alternations that result from the modification of free morphemes. Morphophonemic rules specify how sounds are produced in combination in morphemes. For example, in American English there are identifiable and predictable voicing morphophonemic rules regarding the attachment of certain bound morphemes to the end of a free morpheme.

- **Plural -s.** When a free morpheme (noun) is modified for plurality, the following morphophonemic rules apply:

  1. If a noun ends in a voiceless sound, the **allomorph** /-s/ is attached at the end to create a plural form. Examples:

     [hæts]   [plets]   [bʊks]   [bæskɪts]

2. If a noun ends in a voiced sound, the allomorph /-z/ is attached at the end to create a plural form. Examples:

   [dɑgz]   [ʃuz]   [bɑlz]   [pɛnz]

3. If a noun already ends in /s/ or /z/ or any other sibilant, the allomorph /-ɪz/ or /-ɛz/ is attached to the end to create a plural form. Examples:

   [bʌsɪz]   [glæsɪz]   [mætʃɪz]   [ʤʌʤɪz]

• **Past Tense.** When a free morpheme (verb) is modified to indicate past tense, the following morphophonemic rules apply:

1. If a verb ends in a voiceless sound, the **allomorph** /-t/ is attached at the end to create a past-tense form. Examples:

   [tɑkt]   [wɑkt]   [kʊkt]   [pɑpt]

2. If a verb ends in a voiced sound, the allomorph /-d/ is attached at the end to create a plural form. Examples:

   [pled]   [tʃenʤd]   [græbd]   [lɪvd]

3. If a verb already ends in /t/ or /d/, the allomorph /-ɪd/ or /-ɛd/ is attached to the end to create a plural form.

   [wantɪd]   [blɛndɪd]   [ɛkspɛktɪd]   [rɪtaird]

The voicing morphophonemic rules discussed for the plural grammatical marker also apply for the possession-bound morpheme and the regular third-person present tense.

Phonological Processes

In the last two to three decades a new way of describing sound production errors has become increasingly popular. Rather than focusing on individual phonemes, many recent researchers have shifted their attention to analyzing sound production according to **phonological processes.** Lowe (1996) describes a phonological process as "a systematic sound change that affects classes of sounds or sound sequences and results in a simplification of production" (p. x).

The term *phonological process* is most frequently used to describe the patterned modifications of the adult model by normally developing children. For example, a three-year-old child who has not yet acquired many fricative sounds may often substitute stops for those sounds, a phonological process known as **stopping.** In other words, the child simplifies the complex adult model by substituting sounds that are within his or her phonetic repertoire for those sounds that he or she has not yet acquired. Clinically, this term is also used to describe the sound error patterns used by children diagnosed with a phonological disorder.

It is important to realize that the use of a phonological process to "simplify" the adult model is probably not a psychological reality for the young child. It is improbable that the child consciously and cognitively selects certain sounds within one sound class to substitute for sounds within another sound class. However, the fact remains that very often children's production errors can be reliably classified according to various phonological processes. Grunwell (1997b) summarizes this notion nicely in stating that "the concept of phonological process in the clinical assessment of child speech is applied primarily as a **descriptive device** that identifies or analyzes systematic patterns in children's pronunciations by comparison with the target adult pronunciations" (p. 47, emphasis added).

Varying Definitions

Varying definitions of individual phonological processes inundate the literature (Dean, Howell, Hill, & Waters, 1990; Grunwell, 1985; Hodson, 1980; Ingram, 1981; Lowe 1994, 1996; Shriberg & Kwiatkowski, 1980; Stoel-Gammon & Dunn, 1985; Vihman, 1998; Weiner, 1979). This can be confusing and extremely frustrating for the student who does not have the foundational knowledge for understanding the concept of phonological processes, much less their inconsistent definitions. To simplify our presentation of various phonological processes, we will consider all of these sources but primarily draw from the work of Stoel-Gammon and Dunn (1985) and Lowe (1994, 1996). In our opinion, their presentation covers the most naturally occurring and clinically relevant phonological processes in a relatively simplistic manner. We also believe that upon review of these major phonological processes, the reader who is not well versed with them will gain an adequate foundation for future learning. It is important to note that Lowe follows Ingram's (1981) system of syllable structure, substitution, and assimilation processes. Appendix C defines and provides examples of processes that are less commonly observed in either normal or disordered phonological development.

Syllable Structure Processes

Syllable structure processes describe the sound changes that modify the syllabic structure of words as the child attempts to produce the adult target. These processes include unstressed-syllable deletion, reduplication, final-consonant deletion, initial-consonant deletion, cluster deletion, cluster substitution, and epenthesis. In syllable deletion, reduplication, and epenthesis, the number of syllables in a word is affected; while in initial- and final-consonant deletion, cluster deletion, and cluster substitution, it is the syllable shape of the word that is altered.

Unstressed-Syllable Deletion (USD)

Unstressed-syllable deletion describes the omission of one or more syllables from a polysyllabic word. As the name implies, the syllable with the least stress is typically the one deleted. However, deletion of stressed syllables can also occur. This process is also called weak-syllable deletion and syllable deletion. Lowe (1996) prefers the term *syllable deletion* because, in his opinion, in connected speech "it is often difficult to determine the stress being placed on a particular syllable" (p. 13). **Examples include:**

[medo] for **to**mato	[ɛfənt] for **elephant**	[məs] for **Chris**tmas
[tɛfon] for te**le**phone	[nænə] for **ba**nana	[said] for **out**side

Activity

DIRECTIONS: Provide an example of the effects of syllable deletion on the following words:

1. popsicle _____
2. pencil _____
3. hamburger _____
4. computer _____
5. wagon _____

Reduplication (Redup)

Reduplication is the repetition of a syllable of a target word; this repetition results in the creation of a multisyllabic word form. Because of the duplicating nature of this process, it is sometimes called **doubling.** Reduplication may be total or partial. Total reduplication occurs when the entire syllable is repeated (e.g., /baba/ for *bottle*). Partial reduplication occurs when only part of the syllable is repeated (e.g., [babi] for *bottle*). Stoel-Gammon and Dunn (1985) indicate that reduplication is often accompanied by final-consonant deletion in productions such as [kækæ] for *cat,* in which the final /t/ is deleted first and then the syllable /kæ/is totally reduplicated (p. 37). **Examples include:**

[baba] for *bottle* (total)　　　　[bada] for *bottle* (partial)
[dada] for *dog* (total)　　　　　[dadi] for *dog* (partial)
[tata] for *television* (total)　　[tatu] for *television* (partial)

Activity

DIRECTIONS: Provide an example of the effects of reduplication on the following words:

	Total Reduplication	Partial Reduplication
1. hat	_____	_____
2. doll	_____	_____
3. shoe	_____	_____
4. book	_____	_____
5. hamburger	_____	_____

Diminutization (Dim)

Diminutization is the addition of /i/, or sometimes [Ci] (C = consonant), to the target word. Lowe (1996) describes diminutization as a special form of partial reduplication (p. 13). **Examples include:**

[kʌpi] for *cup*   [dali] for *doll*   [hæti] for *hat*
[buki] for *book*   [papi] for *pencil*   [fofi] for *finger*

✏️ Activity

DIRECTIONS: Provide an example of the effects of diminutization on the following words:

1. egg   _____
2. coat   _____
3. toe   _____
4. food   _____
5. cake   _____

Epenthesis

Epenthesis can be characterized by the insertion of an unstressed vowel, usually the schwa /ə/, between two consonants. Typically the vowel is inserted between two contiguous consonants that make up an initial cluster as in [bəlu] for *blue* (Stoel-Gammon & Dunn, 1985). Stoel-Gammon and Dunn indicate that epenthesis can also occur when an unstressed vowel is added after a final voiced stop. **Examples include:**

[səpun] for *spoon*   [pəlet] for *plate*   [kəraun] for *crown*
[kʌpə] for *cup*   [bækə] for *back*   [lʊkə] for *look*

✏️ Activity

DIRECTIONS: Provide an example of the effects of epenthesis on the following words:

1. clean   _____
2. please   _____
3. tree   _____
4. leg   _____
5. lamp   _____

Final-Consonant Deletion (FCD)

Final-consonant deletion is characterized by the omission of a final singleton consonant in a word. Stoel-Gammon and Dunn (1985) and Khan and Lewis (1986) also consider the deletion of all members of a final-consonant cluster as part of FCD. It is important to note that the entire cluster must be deleted for this type of error to fall under the category of FCD. Considering this, [bɛ] for *best* would be considered

FCD because the entire final cluster is deleted, but the production [bɛs] for the same target word would not since only one member of the cluster is omitted. In essence, the deletion of a final consonant or final-consonant cluster alters the syllable shape of the word so that a word that should be closed is produced as an open-syllable word. A **closed-syllable word** is one that ends in a consonant or consonant cluster, whereas an **open-syllable word** ends in a vowel. It is also important to keep in mind that a production error such as [glæt] for [glæsɪz] is not considered FCD since the word still ends in a final consonant. This error pattern is best described by stopping (to be discussed later) and syllable deletion. **Examples of FCD include:**

[bu] for *book**s***	[da] for *do**g***	[hæ] for *ha**nd***
[ma] for *mo**m***	[karpɪ] for *carpet*	[wægɪ] *for wagon*

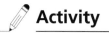 **Activity**

DIRECTIONS: Provide an example of the effects of final-consonant deletion on the following words:

1. jump   _____
2. basket   _____
3. keep   _____
4. leg   _____
5. stamp   _____

Initial-Consonant Deletion (ICD)

Initial-consonant deletion or the omission of singleton consonants in the initial-word position is not a naturally occurring process, meaning that it is rare in normal phonological development. However, it may be observed in some children (especially those who have a severe phonological disorder) and, thus, be worth discussion. Khan and Lewis (1986) also consider omission of the *entire* initial cluster as an exemplar of ICD. Thus, [ek] for *break* would be considered an example of both total cluster reduction and initial-consonant deletion since all members of the cluster are deleted. However, the production [bek] for the same target would be considered partial cluster reduction since only one member of the two-member cluster is deleted. If the word is analyzed according to its syllable shape, it still begins with a consonant and thus cannot be considered an instance of ICD. This concept is easily understood if it is remembered that as in final-consonant deletion, this process alters the syllable shape of a word; a word that should begin with a singleton consonant or consonant cluster now starts with a vowel. **Examples of ICD include:**

[on] for *phone*	[u] for *shoe*	[ap] for *stop*
[azɪt] for *closet*	[ɪndou] for *window*	[it] for *seat*

✎ Activity

DIRECTIONS: Provide an example of the effects of initial-consonant deletion on the following words:

1. lake   _____
2. please   _____
3. fat   _____
4. table   _____
5. brown   _____

Cluster Reduction (CR)

Cluster reduction may be defined as the deletion or substitution of some or all members of a cluster. Although cluster deletion and cluster substitution are often categorized under the same phonological process of cluster reduction, we agree with Lowe (1996) that they should be discussed separately to better highlight some of their important distinctions. Hodson and Paden (1991) use the term **consonant-sequence reduction** to describe the "omission of one or more sound segments from two or more contiguous consonants" (p. 39). Although cluster reduction can occur in both initial and final clusters, Dean, Howell, Hill, and Waters (1990) consider deletion of final clusters as a rare or atypical process. A more inclusive term is **cluster simplification,** which highlights omissions or substitutions that in essence simplify or make the cluster easier to produce.

Cluster Deletion. Cluster deletion is the deletion of one or all members of a cluster. When all members of a cluster are deleted, it is considered total-cluster reduction (TCR), whereas omission of only some of the members of a cluster is regarded as partial-cluster reduction (PCR). In partial-cluster reduction, sound deletion often follows a general developmental pattern, in that the sound that is more difficult to produce or later developing is typically the one deleted. The sound that is most difficult to produce within a cluster is often called the **marked member** and the sound that is theoretically easier to make is considered the **unmarked member.** Stoel-Gammon and Dunn (1985, p. 38) describe some of the most common reduction patterns as follows:

- Children attempting to produce a /stop + liquid/ cluster will typically delete the liquid (e.g., [gin] for **green**, [bed] for **bread**).

- Children attempting to produce a /liquid + stop/ or /liquid + nasal/ postvocalic cluster usually delete the liquid (e.g., [pak] for *park*, [bon] for *born*).

- Children attempting an /s + stop/ or /s + nasal/ cluster will typically delete the /s/ (e.g., [tov] for *stove*, [niz] for *sneeze*).

Further examples of cluster deletion include:

Total-Cluster Reduction	**Partial-Cluster Reduction**
[æg] for *flag*	[fæg] for *flag*
[ap] for *stop*	[tap] for *stop*
[et] for *straight*	[tet] for *straight*
[da] for *dark*	[dak] for *dark*
[pa] for *palm*	[pam] for *palm*

✎ Activity

DIRECTIONS: Provide an example of the effects of cluster deletion on the following words:

	TCR	PCR
1. drop	_____	_____
2. glue	_____	_____
3. strike	_____	_____
4. lamp	_____	_____
5. past	_____	_____

Cluster Substitution. As children mature in their phonological development, they often progress from cluster reduction to cluster substitution. As reviewed earlier, cluster reduction is the deletion of some or all members of a cluster. Cluster substitution, on the other hand, is the substitution of one or all members of a cluster by another sound. Like cluster reduction, cluster substitution tends to follow a general developmental pattern, in that the sound that is more difficult to produce or later developing is typically the one substituted (e.g., [bwed] for *bread* and [pwes] for *place*). Cluster substitution most often affects clusters that contain a liquid (Lowe, 1996). Stoel-Gammon and Dunn (1985) describe a pattern by which all the members of the cluster are replaced by a sound that was not a member of the *target* cluster (e.g., [pag] for *frog*, [bov] for *stove*, [dit] for *street*).

✎ Activity

DIRECTIONS: Provide an example of the effects of cluster substitution on the following words:

1. drop	_____
2. glue	_____
3. strike	_____
4. tree	_____
5. grow	_____

Substitution Processes

Substitution processes are those processes in which one class of sounds is substituted for another class of sounds. To fully understand the various substitution processes that will be discussed, it is important to understand the concept of sound-class substitution.

In the traditional sense, the term *substitution* is used to indicate the replacement of one sound with another, as in the production of an /f/ for /v/ or /p/ for /s/. However, some children's substitution errors affect not only one or two sounds but several phonemes within one sound class. An example of this would be the child who substitutes alveolar sounds (one sound class) for velar sounds (another sound class), a phonological process known as **velar fronting.**

Although many substitution processes have been reviewed in the existing literature, we will primarily focus on the following seven processes:

1. stopping

2. deaffrication

3. velar fronting

4. depalatalization

5. backing

6. liquid gliding

7. vocalization

Stopping (Stop)

Stopping is most frequently defined as the substitution of stops for fricatives and affricates. Some definitions are very inclusive, stating that stopping can affect fricatives, affricates, liquids, and glides (Lowe, 1996). Some researchers, however, question the categorization of stops for affricates as stopping, since an affricate by definition already has a stop component (Hodson, 1986a). Whether the definition is liberal or conservative, this process can affect many sounds, especially considering the high number of fricatives in American English. Stopping of fricatives is a common process in normal phonological development. Although stopping can occur in all word positions, it is most often observed in word-initial position. **Examples (limited to fricatives and affricates) include:**

[pæt] for *fat*	[tek] for *shake*
[pain] for *vine*	[top] for *sop*
[tɛr] for *chair*	[pu] for *zoo*
[dɑb] for *job*	[pʌm] for *thumb*

Activity

DIRECTIONS: Provide an example of the effects of stopping on the following words:

1. suit   _____
2. zipper   _____
3. bus   _____
4. cough   _____
5. shoe   _____

Deaffrication

Deaffrication refers to the replacement of an affricate with a stop or fricative. In other words, the intended affricate is changed to a stop or a fricative. Lowe (1996) is quite liberal in his definition; he considers any sound change that results in a nonaffricate as deaffrication. Other definitions, however, are narrower and consider deaffrication as the substitution of a fricative for an affricate. Since the affricate class includes only /tʃ/ and /dʒ/, this phonological process can affect only two sounds. **Examples of deaffrication include:**

[ter] for *chair*	[dɑb] for *job*
[sɑp] for *chop*	[dɪm] for *gym*
[karm] for *charm*	[zæn] for *Jan*

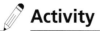 **Activity**

DIRECTIONS: Provide an example of the effects of deaffrication on the following words:

1. chip   _____
2. John   _____
3. couch   _____
4. page   _____
5. chin   _____

Velar Fronting (VF)

Velar fronting is the replacement of the velars /k/, /g/, /ŋ/ with sounds that are made in a more anterior position, typically an alveolar stop. This process affects place of articulation. The more common substitutions are [t/k], [d/g], and [n/ŋ]; however, other substitutions can occur (e.g., [d/k], [k/ŋ]). Stoel-Gammon and Dunn (1985) indicate that velar fronting occurs more commonly in word-initial than word-final position. **Examples of VF include:**

[tɑp] for *cop*	[tʌp] for *cup*	[pæt] for *pack*
[dʌn] for *gun*	[do] for *go*	[bɛd] for *beg*
[rin] for *ring*	[tʌm] for *gum*	[dɪs] for *kiss*

✎ Activity

DIRECTIONS: Provide an example of the effects of velar fronting on the following words:

1. get   _____
2. sing   _____
3. kite   _____
4. seek   _____
5. fog   _____

Depalatalization (Dep)

Depalatalization is characterized by the substitution of an alveolar fricative for a palatal fricative. Stoel-Gammon and Dunn (1985) also categorize the substitution of an alveolar affricate for a palatal affricate as depalatalization. In this type of substitution, /dz/ typically replaces /ʤ/, and /ts/ replaces /ʧ/. Although /dz/ and /ts/ are not considered American English phonemes, in our experience it is not unusual for children to replace the English affricates with these non-English sounds if they have /s/ and /z/ in their repertoire. Lowe (1996) considers any sound change that replaces a palatal with a nonpalatal sound as an instance of depalatalization. **Examples include:**

[tɛk] for *check*	[dʌdz] for *judge*
[mætsiz] for *matches*	[den] for *Jane*

✎ Activity

DIRECTIONS: Provide an example of the effects of depalatalization on the following words:

1. chew   _____
2. edge   _____
3. John   _____
4. chop   _____
5. chicken   _____

Backing

Although backing is not a commonly occurring phonological process in normal development, it may be observed in children with severe phonological disorders. This process, in essence, is the opposite of velar fronting. That is, sounds with an anterior point of constriction are replaced by posterior sounds. This process typically affects alveolar and palatal consonants. The most typical substitutions are [k/t], [g/d], and [ŋ/n], although others are possible. Some children may also substitute [h/s] in addition to the more typical sound replacements already described. **Examples include:**

    [kɑp] for *top*   [gaɪm] for *dime*

    [hop] for *soap*   [baɪk] for *bite*

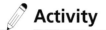 **Activity**

DIRECTIONS: Provide an example of the effects of backing on the following words:

1. chew   _____

2. doll   _____

3. shop   _____

4. ten   _____

5. so   _____

Liquid Gliding (LG)

Liquid gliding is defined as the substitution of a glide for a prevocalic liquid. This process affects manner of articulation. The liquids /r/ and /l/ are typically replaced by the glides /w/ and /j/, respectively. Stoel-Gammon and Dunn (1985) indicate that the substitution pattern for /l/ is at times determined by the vowel following, so that /l/ is replaced by /j/ before front vowels and by /w/ elsewhere. **Examples of LG include:**

    [wæbit] for *rabbit*   [wing] for *ring*

    [wuk] for *look*   [jif] for *leaf*

Liquid gliding can also occur in consonant clusters that contain a liquid:

    [bwɛd] for *bread*   [bwæk] for *black*

    [gwin] for *green*   [gwæs] for *glass*

✎ Activity

DIRECTIONS: Provide an example of the effects of liquid gliding on the following:

1. let _____
2. red _____
3. right _____
4. brake _____
5. laugh _____

Lowe (1996) describes another form of gliding, called fricative gliding. In fricative gliding, a fricative is replaced by a liquid or a glide. Examples include [ju] for *shoe,* [lʌ] for *the,* [jup] for *soup,* and [lop] for *soap.* Fricative gliding does not occur as frequently as liquid gliding.

Vocalization (Voc)

Vocalization, also called vowelization, is the substitution of a vowel for a syllabic liquid (Stoel-Gammon & Dunn, 1985). Lowe (1996) indicates that this process can also affect syllabic nasals. When the mid-central vowels /ɚ/ and /ɝ/ are replaced by /ə/ or any other vowel, this is also considered vocalization. This may seem a bit contradictory since the sound affected and the resulting sound are both vowels. However, in reviewing the literature on phonological processes, this is a common way of categorizing such error patterns. The most common replacements are [o] or [u] for a syllabic liquid. **Examples of vocalization include:**

[sɪmpo] for *simple*	[kwækə] for *cracker*
[abu] for *able*	[pepo] for *paper*
[tabo] for *table*	[boθde] for *birthday*

Stoel-Gammon and Dunn (1985) and Hodson and Paden (1983) indicate that vocalization can also affect postvocalic liquids (liquids that occur after a vowel). Postvocalic liquids are considered consonants rather than syllabics. Typically, the postvocalic liquid is deleted so that the syllable or word ends in a vowel. For words that end in postvocalic liquids, this pattern can technically also fall under the category of final-consonant deletion. However, when children demonstrate a pattern of vocalization of syllabics, the substitution of a vowel for postvocalic liquids is most often categorized under vocalization rather than final-consonant deletion. In our experience, it is not unusual for children to demonstrate vocalization of postvocalic liquids in the absence of true final-consonant deletion. **Examples of vocalization of postvocalic liquids include:**

[kɑ] for *car*	[bo] for *bowl*
[bɑni] for *Barney*	[teu] for *tell*

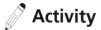 **Activity**

DIRECTIONS: Provide an example of the effects of vocalization on the following words:

1. hair _____
2. together _____
3. able _____
4. ball _____
5. car _____

Assimilation Processes

We previously discussed **assimilation** under the section on speech dynamics. Recall that *assimilation* refers to the phenomenon by which one sound changes to become more like another sound, particularly its neighboring sound. A sound can become more like sounds that come before it or sounds that follow it. When discussing assimilation as a phonological process, this term also refers to the effects of one sound or sounds on the production of another. Lowe (1996) wisely advises that to understand this process, a person must keep in mind that for assimilation to occur there has to be a sound that changes and a sound that causes or effects the change.

The process of assimilation can affect a sound's manner of production, place of articulation, and voicing features. With this in mind, several specific types of assimilation have been advanced in the literature. You will quickly realize by the name given to a process whether it is place of articulation, manner of production, or voicing that is affected. The most widely recognized types of assimilation include labial assimilation, velar assimilation, nasal assimilation, alveolar assimilation, prevocalic voicing, and postvocalic devoicing.

Labial Assimilation

Labial assimilation is the process by which a nonlabial consonant becomes a labial because of the influence of another labial sound in a word. Stoel-Gammon and Dunn (1985) indicate that in most cases labial assimilation affects alveolar and palatal sounds; however, any nonlabial sound can be affected. For purposes of labial assimilation, the labial consonants that can affect other sounds include /b/, /p/, /m/, and /w/. **Examples include:**

[bʊb] for *book*   [pɛb] for *pen*
[wæp] for *wax*   [mob] for *moss*

Velar Assimilation

Velar assimilation is characterized by assimilation of a nonvelar sound to a velar sound. In other words, a nonvelar sound becomes a velar because of the influence of another velar in the word. Velar assimilation typically affects alveolar and palatal consonants. The velars that can influence the change are /k/, /g/, and /ŋ/.

[kʌg] for *cup*   [gog] for *goat*

[kik] for *keep*   [wɪŋ] for *win*

Nasal Assimilation

Nasal assimilation is the process by which a nonnasal sound assimilates to become a nasal because of the influence of another nasal in the word. The nasals that can influence this type of change are /m/, /n/, and /ŋ/. We previously included /m/ under a sound that could influence labial assimilation and /ŋ/ as a sound that could create velar assimilation. Remember that in this case the sound that changes becomes a nasal, not merely a labial or a back sound. In other words, the nasal affects a sound's manner of production. **Examples include:**

[mɑm] for *mop*   [non] for *nose*

[nɑŋ] for *long*   [maim] for *Mike*

Alveolar Assimilation

Alveolar assimilation is characterized by assimilation of a nonalveolar sound to an alveolar sound. A nonalveolar sound becomes an alveolar because of the influence of another alveolar in a word. **Examples include:**

[tɑt] for *toss*   [dod] for *door*

[sut] for *soup*   [lɪd] for *lip*

Prevocalic Voicing

Prevocalic voicing is the process by which a voiceless sound preceding a vowel (prevocalic) becomes voiced. The prevocalic sound that should be voiceless is likely taking on the voicing feature of the vowel that follows it. Stoel-Gammon and Dunn (1985) indicate that prevocalic voicing can affect all obstruents, but of these the most commonly affected are stops. **Examples include:**

[dɛn] for *ten*   [vait] for *fight*

[zut] for *suit*   [bai] for *pie*

Postvocalic Devoicing

In postvocalic devoicing a voiced obstruent following a vowel (postvocalic) becomes voiceless or devoiced. Lowe (1996) indicates that the assimilation may be to the "voiceless feature of the following word boundary" (p. 37). This would explain why productions like [nos] for *nose* and [bait] for *bike* would be considered postvocalic devoicing despite the fact that the target word does not contain any voiceless consonants that can influence this type of change. **Examples of postvocalic devoicing include:**

[pɪk] for *pig*   [sæt] for *sad*

[tʌk] for *tug*   [bis] for *bees*

The term **consonant harmony** is sometimes used in reference to assimilation processes that affect manner of production or place of articulation (i.e., labial assimilation, velar assimilation, nasal assimilation, and alveolar assimilation).

Assimilation can also be classified as progressive and regressive depending where the sound that changes is located in relation to the sound that causes the change. If the sound that changes *precedes* the sound that causes the change, the modification is categorized as **regressive** or **anticipatory assimilation.** Along the same lines, if the sound that changes *follows* the sound that influences the change, the modification is considered **progressive assimilation.** In regressive assimilation, the characteristics of the sound influencing the change "regress" on to the sound that actually changed. An example of regressive assimilation is the production [tot] for *coat;* the sound that changed, /k/, preceded the sound that influenced the change, /t/. In progressive assimilation, the characteristics of the sound causing the change "progress" on to the changed sound. The production [bib] for *bean* is an example of progressive assimilation because the sound that changed, /n/, followed the sound that created the change, /b/.

Assimilation can be total or partial. In **total assimilation,** a sound that changes becomes identical to the sound that causes the change, while in **partial assimilation** the changed sound takes on only some of the characteristics of the sound effecting the change. **Examples of total and partial assimilation include:**

	Total Assimilation	**Partial Assimilation**
• Velar assimilation	[kʌk] for *cup*	[kʌg] for *cup*
• Nasal assimilation	[mɑm] for *mop*	[mɑn] for *mop*
• Labial assimilation	[bʌb] for *bug*	[bʌp] for *bug*
• Alveolar assimilation	[tɑt] for *top*	[tɑd] for *top*

To complicate matters more, assimilation has also been described as **contiguous** or **noncontiguous.** If the sound that changes and the sound that influences the change are adjacent to each other, with no interfering sound between them, this is *contiguous assimilation.* However, if the changed sound and the sound that effects the change are separated by an intervening sound, the term *noncontiguous assimilation* applies.

Clinical Distinction Between Articulation and Phonology

Although a distinction between **articulation** and **phonology** has not always been made, most researchers and clinicians today emphasize that indeed there is an important difference between the two terms. This distinction is thought to have important clinical implications, in that a child with an articulation disorder may present with different characteristics than a child with a phonological disorder. Although the theoretical distinction is increasingly emphasized, in clinical practice, speech–language pathologists do not always distinguish between articulation and phonological disorders. However, as a profession grows, it is important to keep abreast of developments and incorporate the use of new and more specific terminology when appropriate.

Articulation

In anatomy, the term *articulation* is used to depict the point of junction of two or more structures, particularly bones (Zemlin, 1998). For example, the mandible and the temporal bones have a point of articulation at the **temporomandibular joint.** However in the description of human communication, articulation is most often used to refer to the physical movements and placement of the articulators and the motor abilities necessary for the production of speech sounds. Lowe (1996) refers to articulation as the *overt level* of speech production. Articulation describes the motor components of the sounds that can be seen, heard, and produced. Stoel-Gammon and Dunn (1985) indicate that the phonetic or articulatory component of the sound system encompasses (a) the way sounds are formed by the speech mechanism, (b) their acoustic or physical components, and (c) their perception by the listener.

Phonology

Phonology is a broader and more abstract term, defined as the system of rules underlying sound production and sound combinations in the formation of words. Edwards and Shriberg (1983) define phonology as the study of the sound component of language. In his comparison of phonetics (articulatory production) and phonology, Lowe (1994) indicated that "phonology is much more concerned with the system of contrastive sounds and how they are used in conveying meaning" (p. 2). Articulation or the physiological formation of sounds, therefore, is a part of phonology. That is, individual sounds are articulated, but when they are combined to make words for communication, a system of linguistic rules is followed.

To produce the word *bed* [bɛd], for example, the individual phonemes must be articulated according to their physical properties; however, they must also be sequenced and combined appropriately so that the phonological rules of the language are followed. The arbitrary word [bɛd] is permissible in the English language for several reasons: (1) /b/, /ɛ/, and /d/ are all part of the English phonemic system; (2) /b/ and /d/ can occur in the initial and final positions of words, respectively; and (3) /b/ can precede /ɛ/, and /d/ can follow it. If the sounds were rearranged to form the sequence [dbɛ], the articulation of these sounds might remain intact, while the linguistic rules would be violated since /d/ and /b/ cannot occur contiguously in word-initial position and /ɛ/ cannot occur in the final position of words.

Lowe (1996) further described phonology as having a *covert* level, or a level of phonological knowledge. The specific components of this level as outlined by Edwards and Shriberg (1983) are: (1) an inventory of contrastive sounds, (2) morpheme structure rules and sequential constraints that determine permissible word and syllable formations, (3) morphophonemic rules for correctly producing combinations of morphemes, and (4) allophonic rules for correctly producing allophones of phonemes (cited in Lowe, 1996).

Articulation Disorder Versus Phonological Disorder

Articulation errors, also termed *phonetic errors,* are sound productions resulting in nonstandard speech sounds. However, as emphasized by Lowe (1994), these productions usually do not affect the contrastiveness of the sound system. A mild distortion of /r/ highlights an articulation error that results in nonstandard English productions that do not typically affect the meaning of words. A lateralized production of /s/ that is mild in nature also demonstrates a sound production error that does not necessarily create a difference in meaning in the words that contain it.

Unlike articulation errors, phonological errors result in a neutralization of sound contrast (Lowe, 1994). If in an attempt to say *fun,* a child says *gun,* the phonemic contrast between the words is lost. In other words, due to the sound production error, the meaning of the word *fun* is affected.

If adhering to this fine distinction between articulation and phonological errors, the term *articulation disorder* could be used only to diagnose sound production errors that do not affect the meaning of words or neutralize the phonemic contrast in the language. Therefore, by definition, this narrow category could apply only to mild or moderate sound distortions that affect the phonetic properties of the sound but do not generally affect meaning. A *phonological disorder,* on the other hand, is reserved to diagnose sound production errors that result in the collapse of phonemic contrasts and indeed affect meaning.

As logical as this distinction is, in practice most clinicians do not make such a discrimination. Articulation disorder is the diagnostic category most often used in the following cases:

- in reference to sound production errors associated with an organic, structural, or neurological origin (whether they are phonetic, phonological, or both);
- in reference to sound production errors limited to only a few sounds; and
- in reference to sound production errors for which an identifiable pattern could not be found.

Clinicians most often reserve the diagnosis of phonological disorder to describe the patterned sound production errors for which some underlying rule can be identified. Phonological processes that persist in children's speech beyond an expected age would probably lead to the diagnosis of a phonological disorder. A child with very poor intelligibility and a limited phonetic inventory may also be diagnosed with a phonological disorder.

Grunwell (1997b) identified five characteristics of disordered phonological development that could be identified through a phonological process analysis:

1. persisting normal processes
2. chronological mismatch
3. unusual processes
4. systematic sound preference
5. variable use of processes

Grunwell describes *persisting normal processes* as normal phonological processes that continue in a child's production error patterns "long after the age at which they would be expected to have been suppressed" (p. 69). *Chronological mismatch* is described as the production of some earliest normal simplifying processes in co-occurrence with sound production patterns characteristic of later stages in phonological development. Some children may exhibit some *unusual patterns,* which Grunwell defines as "patterns that have been rarely attested in normal phonological development or that appear to be different from normal developmental processes and may, therefore, be idiosyncratic" (p. 69). Other children may show a *systematic sound preference,* in that they use one type of consonant for a large range of different targets. This results in the significant loss of phonemic contrasts and may have severe effects on intelligibility. The last indicator offered by Grunwell is the *variable use of processes* by a child. This is observed when a child uses more than one phonological process with the same target type of structure. This results in variable and unpredictable productions. Grunwell offers the following examples:

rake [leik]	*rabbit* [abɪt]
ring [wing]	*red* [oɛd]

One can quickly identify the varied simplification processes affecting the same target sound, /r/. On one occasion it is replaced by an /l/ and on another by a /w/, both instances of liquid gliding. Furthermore, the sound is deleted in the word *rabbit* (initial-consonant deletion) and is vowelized in the word *red*. It is interesting to note that in a traditional description, these errors would have been classified as inconsistent articulation errors.

Summary of the Basic Unit

• Speech is a widely used vehicle for communication.

• Speakers convey their thoughts, feelings, and desires by a complex combination of sounds into words and sentences.

• Language appears to be rule-governed behavior.

• **Phonological rules** are extracted from patterns of phonological productions.

• The study of phonological rules is called **phonology.**

• **Phonetics** is the study of speech sound production and the special symbols that represent speech sounds.

• There are five main branches of phonetic study: experimental, articulatory, acoustic, perceptual, and applied.

• A **phoneme** is a family of sounds that are perceived to belong to the same category.

• Phonemes have the linguistic function of distinguishing morphemes, or making a contrast in the meaning of words.

• Phonemes do not carry meaning in and of themselves.

• An **allophone** is a variant or alternate form of a phoneme within a specific language.

• Speech–language pathologists use the symbols of the **International Phonetic Alphabet** when transcribing sounds.

• **Diacritical markers** are special symbols that help identify the precise production of a sound.

• The four main processes of speech production are: respiration, phonation, resonation, and articulation.

• **Consonants** are sounds that are produced by a narrowing or closing of the vocal tract at some point.

• Consonants can be **prevocalic, intervocalic,** or **postvocalic.** The terms **initial, medial,** and **final** are often used to refer to the position of a consonant within a word.

• **Vowels** are sounds produced with a relatively open vocal tract configuration.

• **Diphthongs** are a combination of two pure vowels made by a quick gliding of the articulators so that perceptually the two vowels cannot be separated.

• A **syllable** is a small speech unit that has three essential components: **onset, nucleus,** and **coda.** The nucleus and the coda of the syllable are collectively known as a **rhyme.**

• Consonants have traditionally been categorized according to **place, manner,** and **voicing features.**

• A relatively newer way of describing consonants is by their **distinctive features.** Distinctive features are articulatory or acoustic parameters that are either present ($+$) or absent ($-$) in a particular phoneme.

• Consonants that occur in side-by-side combination within the same syllable are called **consonant clusters** or **blends.**

• Vowels are often categorized according to **tongue position, lip rounding,** and **tenseness.**

• Distinctive features have also been used to categorize vowels.

• Connected speech is often influenced by the effects of **coarticulation, adaptation,** and **assimilation.**

• Every language of the planet has an **inventory of sounds, allophonic variations,** and **phonotactic** and **morphophonemic rules.**

• **Phonological processes** refer to systematic sound changes that affect classes of sounds or sound sequences. The application of these processes by children results in simplification of the adult model.

• The many phonological processes that have been reviewed in the literature can be categorized into **syllable structure, substitution,** and **assimilation processes.**

• The term **articulation** describes the motor components of sounds that can be seen, heard, and produced.

• **Phonology** is a more inclusive term that refers to the system of rules underlying sound production and sound combinations in the formation of words.

• Theoretical and clinical distinctions have been made between **articulation** and **phonological disorders.**

Advanced Unit

◆ ◆ ◆ ◆ ◆ ◆ ◆ ◆ ◆ ◆ ◆ ◆ ◆ ◆ ◆ ◆ ◆ ◆

Advanced Perspectives in Articulation and Phonology

The Basic Unit summarized some fundamental concepts relative to speech sounds: their classification, analysis in terms of place-manner-voice features, distinctive features, and phonological processes. In this Advanced Unit, we will discuss certain additional parameters of speech sound production. These parameters include aerodynamic, acoustic, suprasegmental, and perceptual aspects of speech sounds and their production. In addition, we will summarize some newer phonological theories and offer a critical evaluation of such theories in light of clinical empiricism. We will raise the issue of scientific progress in the study of articulation by asking whether multiple phonological theories and concepts represent serial or parallel analyses of articulatory and phonological phenomena. We will conclude this section with a brief discussion of the varied roles of the theoretician and the clinician.

Aerodynamic Aspects of Speech

Recall from Chapter 1 that air supply from the lungs is essential for normal speech production. Breathing, being a biological function necessary to sustain life, provides energy for speech as well. The amount of air needed to produce and sustain speech is not much different from the amount used in normal, quiet breathing except in cases where special emphasis or loudness is required.

The air supplied by the lungs is valved and modified in various ways to produce different kinds of speech sounds as well as to create different resonatory effects. The valving and modification function includes a variety of changes in the air as it leaves the lungs and flows over the laryngeal structures. Changes in the rate of airflow, its volume, and its pressure result in the necessary modifications to produce different speech sounds. Such changes are rapid and constant and follow certain physical rules.

A system of physiological valves is involved in effecting changes in the airflow, its volume, and pressure as a person begins to speak. The vocal folds are the first level of valves that open and close to change the flow of air and its pressure. Closed vocal folds stop the flow of air from the lungs. The velopharyngeal mechanism provides a valve at the next level. Opening and closing of this mechanism respectively couples and uncouples the oral and nasal cavities. The airflow is directed through the nasal cavity when it is open. The flow is directed through the oral cavity when the nasal cavity is closed and the oral cavity is open. The different degrees of constriction of the oral cavity and the complete closing of the lips provide the next and final valve that maximizes, minimizes, or completely eliminates the airflow through the oral cavity.

Activity

DIRECTIONS: Describe the three primary levels of valving of airflow for speech production.

Level 1: _____

_____

Level 2: _____

_____

Level 3: _____

_____

It is common knowledge that the direction of airflow necessary to sustain normal speech production is from the lungs to the outside world. This direction of airflow is called *regressive* (from the inside out). The airflow mechanism used in producing most speech sounds of the languages of the world is called the *pulmonic egressive airstream mechanism* (Yavas, 1998).

Physically, air flows only in one direction. The direction is determined by the relative pressure in surrounding regions. Air is forced to move from a region of greater pressure to a region of lower pressure. If the flow is stopped at any point, air pressure then builds up. In the case of speech sound production, the air that flows from the lungs to the outside world may be stopped at the level of the glottis. This creates an increase in the air pressure below the glottis. Such a pressure is called the *subglottic air pressure*. As described in Chapter 1, increased subglottic air pressure is a significant phenomenon in speech production. Because of the increased subglottic air pressure, the vocal folds are blown apart and the air begins to flow from the lungs to the outside world.

Air pressure may be built up in the oral cavity as well. This happens when the lips are closed or the oral cavity is constricted as the air flows out of the lungs. Such a buildup of air pressure in the mouth is necessary to produce various consonants, especially the *pressure consonants,* which include voiceless stops and fricatives. In producing various pressure consonants, the laryngeal valve is open so the air flows freely into the oral cavity. The velopharyngeal mechanism is closed to prevent the flow of air from the lungs into the nasal cavity. The air flowing from the lungs reaches the severely constricted or even closed oral cavity. Because of the built-up pressure in the oral cavity, a puff of air is forced out of the mouth. This puff of air may be articulated into such speech sounds as voiceless stops (e.g., /p/, /t/, or /k/). In producing such voiceless fricatives as /s/ and /sh/, the oral cavity is severely constricted and the built-up air pressure is released to produce such sounds. Incidentally, intraoral air pressure is greater in children than in adults.

Vocal fold vibration is necessary to produce voiced stops and fricatives. Therefore, the vocal folds are not completely closed during the production of voiced sounds. Instead, they only approximate and vibrate to produce voice sounds. Because of this lack of complete laryngeal closure, a certain amount of air pressure is lost. Consequently, the voiced sounds are produced with less intraoral air pressure than the voiceless sounds.

Minimal intraoral air pressure is associated with the production of nasal sounds. As in the production of all voiced sounds, the vocal folds vibrate and only approximate, resulting in minimal subglottic air pressure. The velopharyngeal port is open to let the vibrating sound pass through the nasal cavity. The oral cavity is constricted as in the production of voiced stops. The addition of nasal resonation results in the characteristic perceptual quality of nasal sounds.

Intraoral air pressure also is minimal for vowel productions, as the oral cavity is more open so that the laryngeally generated tone freely passes through it. English vowels, unless they are preceded or succeeded by a nasal consonant, do not require nasal resonation. Therefore, the air passes only through the oral cavity in the production of English vowels. A similar air pressure and oral cavity features are associated with the production of liquids and glides.

Studies of different languages of the world have revealed that the pulmonic egressive airstream mechanism, although it is the most frequently used airstream management mechanism across all languages, is not the only one used in speech sound production. Varied airstream management mechanisms are employed in speech sound production. For example, in certain Native American and African languages, the *glottic airstream mechanism* is used to produce certain sounds. In that mechanism, the air above the larynx is used to initiate speech sounds. This is accomplished (a) by raising the larynx and closing the vocal folds, (b) by raising the velum to close the velopharyngeal port, and (c) by closing an oral valve. This creates a supralaryngeal chamber in which air pressure is increased. The vocal tract closure is then suddenly released to produce a kind of stop known as an *ejective* (Yavas, 1998).

Another airstream mechanism used in speech sound production is known as the *glottic ingressive airstream mechanism.* Contrary to the glottic airstream mechanism, the glottic ingressive airstream mechanism involves a *lowered* larynx and partially *open* vocal folds. As the larynx is lowered, it sucks the air inward. The sucking action sets the partially open folds into vibration. The speech sounds thus produced are known as implosives and are observed in certain African languages. Ejective and implosive speech sounds are also called *glottalized* or *laryngealized* sounds (Yavas, 1998).

Yet another airstream mechanism used in speech sound production is called the *velaric airstream mechanism.* Observed in speakers of southern African languages, the velaric airstream mechanism involves trapping the air in the oral cavity. To accomplish that, a closure at the back of the oral cavity is created by drawing the back of the tongue against the velum and by achieving another closure forward in the oral cavity. The more frontal closure may be achieved at the level of the lips or the alveolar ridge. The trapped air is made to rush inward by a downward and backward movement of the tongue and by releasing the closure at the front. The sound thus produced is called a *click* (Yavas, 1998).

🖉 Activity

DIRECTIONS: From the information offered in the text, describe the following terms.

Pulmonic egressive airstream mechanism: _____

_____

Glottic airstream mechanism: _____

_____

Glottic ingressive airstream mechanism: _____

_____

Velaric airstream mechanism: _____

_____

Several neural and physiological pathologies affect the flow and pressure of air used to produce speech. Such pathological conditions negatively affect speech production. For example, various neural pathologies that affect the normal functioning of the vocal folds may result in an inefficient use of the airflow in producing speech. Paralyzed vocal folds cannot approximate to build sufficient subglottic air pressure. This may result in excessive air leakage, resulting in breathy voice. Similarly, clefts of the soft palate may cause an inadequate velopharyngeal mechanism that cannot adequately close the velopharyngeal port. This will result in undesirable nasal resonance in the production of oral sounds. Also, any kind of respiratory disorder may reduce the air supply needed to sustain speech at sufficient loudness.

Acoustic Aspects of Speech

Acoustics is the scientific study of sound as a physical phenomenon. It is a branch of physics. Oral speech is a form of sound, and as such it can be analyzed in terms of its physical properties. A more comprehensive understanding of speech requires that we study not only the physiological aspects of speech sound production, but also the physical aspects of the signal thus produced. An analysis of speech as a physical signal is the domain of acoustics.

To create sound, which is a physical force, an object that can vibrate and a medium are needed. To perceive sound, one needs a biological (hearing) mechanism that is sensitive to sound vibrations. A physical force sets an object into vibration. The vibrations create waves of disturbance in the molecules of gas, liquid, or a solid object. An elastic medium such as gas, liquid, or a solid object transmits the vibrations. In the case of speech sounds, the elastic vocal folds provide the physical mechanism that vibrates. The air supply from the lungs and other aerodynamic mechanisms described in the previous section provide the physical force that sets the folds into vibration. The air molecules in the laryngeal, pharyngeal, nasal, and oral cavities transmit the sound as it is also modified and articulated into speech sounds.

All sounds may be described as acoustic signals. Oral communication begins as speech sound production, and, therefore, speech is an acoustic signal. All acoustic signals have certain physical properties, including frequency, amplitude, and duration. Therefore, speech sounds, too, have those physical properties.

Frequency, the first physical property of sound, is the rate at which an object vibrates. Frequency is measured in terms of the number of vibrations per unit of time, typically per second. A sound may be of a single frequency or a combination of frequencies. A tuning fork, for example, is designed to vibrate at a single frequency. The sound of a single frequency that repeats itself is called a **pure tone.** However, very few naturally occurring sounds, including speech sounds, are of a single frequency. Most naturally occurring sounds, including speech, are described as **complex tones** because they consist of different frequencies. The vibrations that constitute a complex tone may be **periodic,** in that they have a pattern that repeats itself, or **aperiodic,** in that they have no such pattern. Thus, sounds differ in the pattern of physical energy across different frequencies. The **spectrum** of a sound describes a pattern of physical energy across a frequency range. Different speech sounds have different *spectra*. It is these spectral differences that help us distinguish one sound from the other.

Differences in frequency are perceived as differences in the **pitch** of a sound. Therefore, whether a sound is a nonspeech sound or a speech sound, its perceived pitch is a direct function of the frequency with which the source of the sound vibrates. In the case of speech sounds, the frequency of vocal fold vibrations determines the pitch. English vowels, liquids, and glides are produced within a range of low to mid frequencies. Hence, their pitch is within the low to mid range. Nasals are produced with vocal fold vibrations at low frequency; strident fricatives and affricates (e.g., /s/, /z/, /ʃ/, and /ʧ/) are produced with vocal fold vibrations at high frequency. Stops as a class are produced with vocal fold vibrations within a wide range of frequency. Alveolars are produced with vocal fold vibrations at mid to high frequencies; velars are produced within a mid-frequency range; and bilabials are produced within a low-frequency range.

Amplitude or **intensity,** the second characteristic of a sound signal, refers to the magnitude of the vibration of a sound source. The greater the magnitude of vibration, the higher the amplitude of the sound. The higher the amplitude, the greater the loudness of the sound. While amplitude or intensity refers to physical measurements, loudness refers to an auditory (perceptual) experience. Sounds of greater intensity (or amplitude) are perceived as louder than those of lower intensity. Speech sounds, too, have characteristic amplitude profiles. Therefore, the loudness of different sounds varies. Vowels are the most intense speech sounds. Low vowels are more intense than high vowels. Glides and liquids, though not as intense as vowels, are more intense than other classes of sounds. Strident fricatives, affricates, and nasals are of moderate intensity, whereas stops and nonstrident fricatives are among the weakest.

Duration, the third important property of sound, is the measure of time during which vibrations are sustained. Speech sounds are sustained for relatively brief durations. As a class, vowels have the longest duration of all speech sounds. Individual vowels, however, vary significantly in their duration. Some vowels may be as long as one half of a second, whereas others do not exceed 50 msec. Glides and liquids are of short to moderate duration. However, the glides /w/ and /j/ are generally longer than the liquids /l and /r/. Strident fricatives and affricates have a moderate duration, whereas nonstrident fricatives have a short to moderate duration. Compared to other consonants, stridents generally are longer in duration. As a class, fricatives are longer than affricates. Nasal sounds have short to moderate duration, whereas the stop sounds have the shortest duration of all speech sounds.

Certain physiological variables affect the acoustic properties of speech produced by different speakers. Age and gender are two significant physiological variables to be considered. The speech (and voice) of males generally is of lower frequency (hence, lower pitch) than that of females. Children's speech is of highest frequency. Men have longer and more massive vocal tracts than women or children. Longer and more massive folds vibrate at a lower rate. Therefore, adult males tend to have lower vocal pitch than females or children. Furthermore, normative acoustic data on women and children are limited. Also limited are the normative acoustic data on speakers of different ethnocultural backgrounds. Because the readily available acoustic data pertain mostly to white men, caution must be exercised in extrapolating such data to women, children, and speakers of different ethnocultural backgrounds.

🖊 Activity

DIRECTIONS: Briefly define the following terms.

Acoustics: _____

Frequency: _____

Period: _____

Aperiodic: _____

Spectrum: _____

Pitch: _____

Amplitude: _____

Duration: _____

Suprasegmental Aspects of Speech

Consonants and vowels, described and classified in the section on phonetics, are typically considered *segmentals*. Segmental units in a speech analysis correspond to phonemes or phonetic units. Properties of speech that become evident when such larger units as words, phrases, sentences, and continuous speech are produced are described as **suprasegmentals.** In essence, when phonemes are produced in sequence, additional characteristics emerge. These are suprasegmentals, also known as prosodic features. We will briefly consider pitch, stress, rate of speech, and juncture as suprasegmentals.

Pitch

Pitch, as defined earlier, is the sensory experience related to the frequency of vibration. Also as noted earlier, pitch of speech (or, more appropriately, the voice) is determined by the frequency with which the vocal folds vibrate. Of particular interest in this section on suprasegmentals is the observation that pitch variations suggest differences in meaning. Speakers of all languages vary the pitch of their voice in conversational speech.

Pitch may fall or rise in conversational speech. Such falls and rises signify different meanings. An utterance such as "She ate ten hamburgers," produced with a falling intonation means that it is a statement of observation. However, the same utterance produced with a rising pitch is understood as a question, not a statement of fact. Thus, the same words, produced in the same syntactic arrangement, may mean different things depending on the pitch contour of the utterance produced. A mere analysis of the meaning of the words and the syntactic structure will not reveal this fact. Pitch falls and rises in conversational speech give the speech its melodious quality. Therefore, pitch rises and falls are sometimes described as the melody of a phrase. Systematic changes in pitch contours are known as **intonation.**

Variables that affect intonation or the pitch contour of an utterance include the emotional state of the speaker, the stress pattern employed, and the tongue position used in producing vowels. Generally, high vowels have a higher fundamental frequency (higher pitch).

Pitch variations may be involved in signaling new information in a conversational exchange. To draw listener attention to it, speakers may raise the pitch of words and phrases that contain new information. For instance, the speaker who has been talking for a while may say, "What I am saying now is something very important," and may raise the pitch on *now* and *very important.*

In some languages of the world, differences in meaning may be signaled by pitch variations applied even to single or monosyllabic words. Such languages are called tonal languages (Yavas, 1998). In a **tonal language,** a single word produced with different pitches means different things. Yavas gives the example of Mandarin Chinese, in which the word [ma] may be produced with a high-level, high rising, falling rising, or low falling tone, to mean "mother," "hemp," "horse," or "scold," respectively. In a nontonal language like English, such a word as *mother* will mean the same thing regardless of the pitch with which it is produced. In a few tonal languages, even such grammatical distinctions as tense shift and possession may be indicated by pitch variations (Yavas, 1998).

Stress

Linguistic **stress** is defined as a device that gives prominence to certain syllables within a sequence of syllables. Stress is an important suprasegmental feature that works at the level of syllables. Within a syllable, it is the vowel segment that is primarily stressed. Stressed syllables stand out in a sequence of unstressed syllables.

Three acoustic features distinguish stressed syllables from unstressed syllables. First, stressed syllables are produced with greater vocal intensity. Louder syllables in a sequence of syllables stand out. In producing stressed (louder) syllables, the speaker must expend more air from the lungs. Second, the duration of stressed syllables is longer than that of unstressed syllables. Third, stressed syllables are produced with higher pitch. Thus, a combination of increased intensity, longer duration, and higher frequency characterizes stressed syllables in speech. Research on stress patterns in spoken English has shown that higher pitch, longer vowel duration, and increased intensity, in that order, are important in producing stressed syllables (Fry, 1965).

Stress, while emphasizing certain parts of an utterance, also may be used to distinguish noun/verb forms of the same word. English contains many such words in which two forms share identical phonemes. For example, the noun *convict* and the verb *convict* are produced with different stress patterns to distinguish the two forms in conversational speech. The noun form is produced with primary stress on the first syllable, the verb form with stress on the second. Other examples of words whose noun/verb forms are distinguished by differential stress patterns include *import, insult,* and *permit.* Also, words that are spelled the same but have different meanings are distinguished by different syllabic stress. For example, the word *object* may mean "protest" or "thing," depending on which syllable is stressed.

A form of stress that helps contrast two or more possibilities while emphasizing one of them is known as **contrastive stress.** A speaker who says, "Give me that *blue* pen," with emphasis on the italicized word, uses this type of contrastive stress. Sometimes contrastive stress may be used to negate an implied or previously made statement. A speaker who says, "No, I didn't buy a Saturn, I bought a *Toyota,*" with emphasis on the italicized word, uses this type of stress.

When stress patterns change, an additional linguistic parameter that also may change is the vowel quality. In the word *object,* for example, when the stress shifts to the second syllable to indicate a verb, the first syllable is reduced to a schwa [ə]. Therefore, it is important to consider stress as a phenomenon in which the importance of certain syllables is enhanced while that of others is decreased.

Interlanguage phonological studies, as summarized by Yavas (1998), have shown that in English and other Germanic languages, the position of stress is variable, whereas in many other languages of the world, the stress position is fixed. In many languages, the fixed position that is stressed is that of the first syllable in a word (Yavas, 1998).

Stress patterns have an effect on the spoken rhythm of a language. Different stress patterns create characteristic rhythms that are unique to their languages. Based on the stress-based rhythms, languages are sometimes classified into one of two categories: stress-timed or syllable-timed. In **stress-timed languages,** which include English, German, Russian, and Arabic, stressed syllables tend to be produced at regular intervals. In **syllable-timed languages,** which include French, Italian, Greek, Spanish, Turkish, and Hindi, syllables, not necessarily stress syllables, tend to be produced at regular intervals. Most languages, however, are difficult to classify unambiguously into one of these categories. On stress-related variables, languages vary on a continuum (Yavas, 1998).

Rate of Speech

Variations in the rate of speech are a significant aspect of speech suprasegmentals. Relatively faster or slower rates affect prosodic features of speech. Alternate measures of the rate of speech consist of the number of words, syllables, or phonemes produced per second.

Individuals differ in their rates of speech. Some speak noticeably slower than others. At faster rates, some speakers can maintain intelligibility better than others. By and large, when speakers increase their rate, some loss of intelligibility occurs. As the speaker increases speech rate, sound productions are often negatively affected. Increased speech rate may not involve faster articulatory movements; instead, a faster overall rate is achieved by eliminating pauses and decreasing the duration of vowels and such longer consonants as fricatives. Reduction in vowel duration is particularly striking in faster speech. For instance, the vowels /i/ and /e/ are reduced to /ɪ/, which may be further reduced to /ə/. Many other vowels also tend to be reduced to the schwa. In addition, some articulatory positions that can be sustained at a normal or slower rate are missed at faster rates. Omitting certain articulatory positions while speaking faster than the normal is called *undershooting*.

The rate of articulation has clinical implications. A slower rate is necessary in treating most speech disorders. The speech rate may be slowed in treatment to show different articulatory positions or certain segmental features (e.g., the duration of different vowels). Treatment for the disorders of stuttering and cluttering often involves a slower rate.

Speech rate is a major aspect of prosody. A rate that is slower than the norm negatively affects prosody, as seen in articulation therapy and perhaps even more dramatically in stuttering and cluttering therapy. Speech at slower rates tends to be monotonous, softer, more deliberate, and less spontaneous. Listeners tend to perceive the prosody of slow speech as unnatural. Clinical observations suggest that as the rate of speech is allowed to approximate the norm, natural prosody also becomes evident. Teaching each client to sustain what may be a normal rate for him or her is a necessary procedure to induce normal prosody.

Juncture

Juncture is a suprasegmental device that helps make semantic or grammatical distinctions in speech. It includes brief pauses in speech to signal what might be punctuations in written language. Among other things, punctuations in written languages and pauses in spoken language help keep different grammatical clauses separate so that the meaning of an utterance is not confused. For instance, "John, let us do it" is a request to John, whereas "John let us do it" is a statement of fact. This distinction becomes clear to the listener when the speaker pauses after "John" in one case and not in the other.

Pauses also may be used to make lexical distinctions and, hence, semantic distinctions in speech. The same sequence of syllables uttered with or without a pause may mean something different because the pause, when injected, will mean two words rather than one. For instance, *cocktail* is clearly different from *cock tail* because of the pause that splits the compound word into two separate words, signaling different meanings.

Junctures may also involve pitch variations, which may be combined with brief pauses in speech. For instance, the pitch contour for "John" in "John, let us do it" may be different (higher) than that in "John let us do it."

Pauses, along with pitch variations described earlier, may help signal new or important information about to be offered in discourse and formal lectures. A brief pause in speech may help draw the attention of listeners and hence may precede utterances that contain new or important information.

Activity

DIRECTIONS: Describe the effects that the following suprasegmental devices have on speech production.

Intonation: _____

_____

Stress: _____

_____

Rate of speech: _____

_____

Juncture: _____

_____

Varied Phonological Theories

The study of speech sound production has undergone many changes, and the field continues to evolve. Articulation was once the primary field of speech sound production. Classical developmental research on articulation was concerned with the production and acquisition of individual phonemes. Classical description of articulation disorders also was primarily concerned with the correctness of individual phoneme productions. Treatment of articulation disorders, in turn, emphasized techniques designed to remediate the production of individual phonemes.

Newer perspectives in the study of speech sound production emerged because of the influence of linguistic theories. Linguistic theories, propelled especially by the generative grammar theories, had asserted that language is governed by a system of organized principles. Such a perspective began to look at speech sound production within the framework of an organized system of language. These theories, including those of distinctive features and phonological processes, began to emphasize that it is inefficient and perhaps incorrect to consider each speech sound as an independent behavior. Instead, the theories suggested that there are principles of organization that govern both correct and incorrect productions of speech sounds. Speech sound production was considered within the larger framework of language that helps create an organized system of communication. In sections of the Basic

Unit in this chapter, linguistically based distinctive feature and phonological process perspectives have been described. In this Advanced Unit, a few newer phonological theories will be briefly summarized.

Theory of Naturalness and Markedness

Often described as natural phonology (which is a misnomer), the theory of naturalness and markedness is thought to make an important distinction in phonological patterns found within and across languages. All segments and segmental sequences are not equally distributed in languages. Some are more frequently observed than others. For example, stops are found in almost 100% of languages. Among the stops, voiceless stops are more common than voiced. The voiced-voiceless distinction also is a common feature of languages. Among the fricatives, voiceless are more common than voiced. Among the voiceless fricatives, the dental alveolar /s/ is found most frequently across the languages of the world. Most languages have at least two or three nasals; a language with a single nasal is unusual. Front unrounded vowels (e.g., /e/) are found in more languages of the world than are front rounded vowels (e.g., /y/). At the level of syllables, CV is the most common structure.

The theory of naturalness and markedness states that certain segments, segment combinations, and phonological processes are more natural than others. A **natural** segment or process is one that is more common among the languages of the world. A natural segment or process also is called **unmarked.** The theory further states that processes that are less common across languages and those that are unique to certain languages are less natural. Less natural features of languages are called **marked.** In essence, unmarked or more natural aspects of languages are observed more frequently, whereas marked and less natural aspects of languages are observed less frequently (Yavas, 1998).

It should be noted that naturalness and markedness are not strictly categorical across languages. Features of languages vary on a continuum of naturalness. Therefore, it is appropriate to think of naturalness and markedness as *relative,* not absolute, concepts.

Developmental studies have suggested that more natural (unmarked) features are learned more easily or earlier than those that are less natural (marked). For example, unmarked unrounded vowels are acquired sooner than marked rounded vowels. More natural stops are acquired earlier than less natural sounds. Naturalness and markedness are reflected also in children's speech error patterns. For example, unrounding of rounded vowels is more common than the reverse. Children with articulation disorders tend to make fewer mistakes on more natural stops than on less natural sounds. Children also master a more natural syllable structure (CV) earlier than less natural syllable structures (e.g., CVC, CCV).

The presence and frequency of certain phonological processes, too, may be influenced by naturalness and markedness (Yavas, 1998). Some of the more common phonological processes tend to move toward naturalness. For example, final-consonant deletion, a common phonological process, creates open syllables or the CV type, which is the most unmarked syllable type. Another phonological process, the stopping of fricatives and affricates, also indicates that the tendency in such error patterns is to move from the less natural or marked (fricatives and affricates) to the more natural (stops). In essence, many instances of articulatory error patterns tend to eliminate or diminish marked features and thus create more natural segments.

Linear Versus Nonlinear Phonological Theories

Classical theories of phonology, especially those of distinctive features, assumed that segmental properties or features of a phoneme (e.g., vocalic, sonorant, low, nasal, voiced) are independent of each other. The standard or classical theories (e.g., Chomsky and Halle's 1968 theory of distinctive features) implied that phoneme segments may act independently of each other and may combine with any other segment. There was no implication in the standard theories that features of a phoneme may be hierarchically organized. In the more recent literature (see Ball & Kent, 1998; Yavas, 1998, for details), the standard theories that assumed that segments are a bundle of independent features or characteristics of a phoneme with no hierarchical organization are referred to as **linear phonological theories.** In essence, linear theories presumed that phonological properties are linear strings of segments (Clements & Keyser, 1983; Stevens & Keyser, 1989).

Several newer theories challenge the assumption that segmental aspects of a phoneme are simply a bundle of independent and unorganized features that may freely combine with each other. Such theories are known as **nonlinear phonological theories.*** Nonlinear phonological theories also were needed because linear theories do not adequately account for the effect of prosody on speech production. Linear theories did not handle such phenomena as stress, tone, and intonation, which influence speech beyond the segmental levels. Standard linear theories even ignored the syllable, as they presumed the morpheme to be the basic phonological unit (Yavas, 1998). In essence, suprasegmentals were not effectively handled in linear theories.

A common feature of nonlinear theories is some sort of a hierarchy that helps organize segmental and suprasegmental phonological properties (units). There are several theories or variations of theories that propose somewhat different, nonlinear hierarchies to organize phonological units. We will briefly describe selected theories to indicate the emergence of new directions in phonology.

Metric Theory

One of the nonlinear phonological theories, known as the **metric theory,** suggests a hierarchy based on feet, syllables, and segments (Goldsmith, 1990; Hayes, 1988). Metric theory pays particular attention to the syllable structure and stress patterns. As described in this chapter's Basic Unit, the syllable is described in terms of an onset and rhyme. The rhyme, in turn, is described in terms of the nucleus and the coda. Thus, the onset, and nucleus and coda (the rhyme) constitute the basic structure of a syllable.

The initial consonant or consonant cluster is the onset of a syllable, as it launches a syllable. For instance, /fl/ launches the word *flute,* and /f/ launches the

---

*In most textbooks, a new phonological theory is described as a *phonology,* and multiple theories are described as *phonologies,* a practice not followed here. A new theory within a field of study does not create a new discipline.

word *fan.* The onset, however, may be absent when the syllable starts with a vowel, as many words in English do. The rhyme includes everything except the onset of a syllable. The nucleus is the vowel or the diphthong that follows the consonant, and the coda is the final consonant. For example, in the word *tap,* the /t/ is the onset, the middle vowel is the nucleus, and the final /p/ is the coda. The onset and the coda may both contain more than one sound. For example, in the word *strict,* /str/ is the onset, and /ct/ is the coda.

In a metric theory, rhythm involves alternating patterns of stress. When weak and strong syllables are produced in alternating positions, a rhyme is created. A rhyme may also be thought of as a timing unit called a **foot,** which consists of a stressed syllable and one or more unstressed syllables. While monosyllabic words have a single foot, some (but not all) disyllabic and polysyllabic words may have multiple feet. Multiple syllables that are stressed in a word may receive relatively more or less stress. That is, stress is a relative concept; of two stressed syllables, one may be relatively stronger. Thus, syllables in a foot and feet in a word vary in strength. Such strength variations create the typical rhythm of speech. In the metric theory, then, the syllable with its expanded structure is the main vehicle of prosodic features (the rhythm of speech).

In essence, according to the metric theory, before reaching the segmental level, a word consists of such hierarchies (or tiers) as the foot, the syllable, the onset rhyme, and the CV. These different tiers account for prosodic effects in speech. As we shall see in the next section, other phonological theories have extended this type of hierarchical analysis to the segmental level as well.

Feature Geometry

Another nonlinear phonological theory, feature geometry extends the concept of hierarchies to the segmental level. The **feature geometry** theory proposes that feature combinations of a segment also are hierarchically organized. As noted earlier, the standard or classical phonological theory, such as the well-known theory proposed by Chomsky and Halle (1968), viewed features as unorganized and thus free to combine with one another. However, features do not freely combine with each other. Certain feature combinations are more commonly observed than certain other feature combinations. For instance, it is known that [high], [back], and [low] vowels show the assimilation process, whereas [high], [nasal], and [ATR] show no or infrequent assimilation. (ATR refers to *advanced tongue root,* which is a feature in which sounds are produced with the tongue root pushed forward.) Feature geometry was proposed to solve these and other problems that are inherent to standard phonological theory (Yavas, 1998).

In organizing the segmental features and their combinations, the theory of feature geometry employs the anatomical structures used in speech production. The six articulators that create feature differences are the glottis, soft palate, lips, tongue blade, tongue body, and tongue root. Some feature specification is entirely due to the action of an articulator. For instance, the feature [labial] is due to lip action, and the feature [nasal] is due to the velopharyngeal action (opening). Other features are a function of several articulators. For instance, the features [consonantal] and [sonorant] are not limited to any one articulator and thus specify a category with no particular articulator. Therefore, features that are entirely due to the action of a single articulator are called **articulator-bound,** and those that are produced with multiple articulators are called **articulator-free.**

The articulator-free features are classified into two categories: the major class features and the stricture (manner) features. The major class features include [consonantal] and [sonorant], and the stricture features include [continuant], [strident], and [lateral]. Among these, the [consonantal] and [sonorant] are considered root features, which give rise to major classes of sounds. The stricture or manner features are derived from the root features. Thus, a hierarchy of features is created instead of a bundle of unrelated features. Features trees based on feature geometry show all related features in an organized manner. For instance, the specification of a terminal feature implies a particular articulator and all other higher features. For instance, consonants may be specified as *supralaryngeal,* which branch out into tongue root and soft palate on the one hand and oral place on the other. The oral place branches out into labial, coronal, and dorsal, each of which branches out into specific nodes. For instance, the dorsal branches out into [high], [low], and [back]. Thus, an articulator and its branching feature mechanisms are hierarchically organized (Halle, 1992; Yavas, 1998).

Summary of Newer Phonological Theories

Several newer phonological theories have been proposed to overcome the limitations of the standard or classical phonological theories of the kind proposed by Chomsky and Halle (1968). The standard theories are now considered linear in their assumptions, whereas the newer theories are considered *nonlinear.* Nonlinear theories suggest ways in which segmental and suprasegmental features are related and organized in a hierarchical fashion. It is believed that these theories more effectively account for stress and other aspects of prosody. The metric theory and the feature geometry are among the more prominent newer nonlinear theories. The metric theory proposes a hierarchy of features based on feet, syllables, and segments and pays particular attention to the syllable structure and stress patterns (suprasegmental features). The feature geometry proposes that feature combinations of a segment also are hierarchically organized. In specifying the features and their permissible combinations, this theory uses the six anatomical structures used in speech production: the glottis, soft palate, lips, tongue blade, tongue body, and tongue root. Each terminal node in the feature tree implies an articulator and all higher features associated with it.

There are several other theories and variations of better-known nonlinear theories. The reader is referred to other sources for details of theories summarized here and for additional theories (Ball & Kent, 1998; Yavas, 1998).

Evaluation and Clinical Implications of Phonological Theories

As described in the two units of this chapter, the study of speech sound production contains varied perspectives. Standard, newer, and varied phonological theories create an ever changing scene in the study and analysis of speech sounds, their patterns, and their acquisition. Old and new theories claim to have important developmental and clinical implications, thus suggesting a need for clinicians to master them.

Clinicians should understand phonological theories as well as critically evaluate them. Most clinicians find the current perspectives in phonology excessively theoretical. Before the developmental and clinical implications of one approach are fully explored and explained to clinicians, a newer approach emerges, which devalues the older approaches. Clinicians need to develop critical standards by which to judge the usefulness or relevance of newer theories. It is suggested here that among other possibilities, the nature of development in the field and the empirical status of theoretical concepts provide two such standards. The nature of development may be parallel (hence not cumulative) or serial (hence cumulative), and the theoretical concepts may be empirical (hence clinically useful) or merely formal (hence only theoretical). These two standards are further explored in the next two sections.

Parallel or Serial Concepts in Articulation and Phonology

Classically, phonetics has been the study of speech sound production, its physiological mechanisms, and its acoustic properties. In the 1950s and 1960s, a newer perspective called *distinctive features* emerged. This view was hailed as revolutionary in that it helped organize patterns of feature combinations that distinguish one phoneme from the other. It was claimed that the traditional phonetic analyses did not help identify such patterns. Over the years, some limited clinical application of distinctive features in treatment of articulation disorders has yielded somewhat conflicting results, as summarized in the Basic Unit.

Before the distinctive feature approach could be fully clinically tested, a newer approach, called the *phonological approach,* emerged. Early phonological theories claimed that the traditional phonetic analyses did not classify sounds based on certain patterns and that the sounds were described individually, as isolated phonetic events. Although this criticism was widely accepted, it is not entirely true that only the distinctive feature approach helps organize phoneme features while the traditional phonetic approach only describes sounds individually. Phonetics has always classified sounds into groups. The physiological parameters involved in the production of speech sounds (e.g., vowel classification based on tongue position and consonant classification based on manner, place, and voicing) provide a well-known classification system. The revolutionary distinctive feature method, while adding the binary method of feature specification, retains many of the traditional aspects of phoneme classification. For instance, its *cavity features* [high], [low], [back], [rounded], and [nasal] are nothing new. What is new in the distinctive feature approach is the binary coding system, which says that a consonant is not a vowel (−vowel) or a low vowel is not a high vowel (−high) or an unvoiced sound is not a voiced sound (−voiced). However, the theoretical power and clinical usefulness of such a binary system are debatable.

The phonological approach, which overshadowed the distinctive feature approach, was considered another revolutionary view in the study of speech sounds. Phonology, being the study of speech sounds and their patterns in languages, is concerned with speech sounds, their arrangement to form words, and rules by which sounds are manipulated (e.g., added, deleted, or changed). Clinicians learned much about phonological processes, which are simplifications or changes in the production of speech sounds. Various phonological theories, as sampled in this chapter, have been proposed in fairly quick succession. Each new theory is considered a significant advancement over the previous theories.

One gains the impression that changing perspectives indicate significant scientific progress in the study of speech sounds and their patterns across languages. However, it is possible that different perspectives are parallel notions, not scientifically cumulative, forming a more comprehensive view of speech sounds used in different languages. Many varied, conflicting, and competing theoretical models of speech sounds and their production indicate only that observations are still inadequate and theories mostly premature. For example, the once widely accepted standard phonological feature theory did not account even for prosody, a basic feature of speech. Most phonological theories have alternate forms and significant limitations, and none is universally accepted. Nonlinear phonological theories propose different hierarchies to organize segmental and suprasegmental features of speech, and there is no agreement on any hierarchical system. If the history of phonology is indicative of its future, most of these theories will be modified or replaced before their clinical applications are tried.

Empirical Status of Phonological Concepts

The most relevant and perhaps the most troubling issue for clinicians is the empirical status of phonological concepts, especially phonological rules and processes. Phonological rules and processes are theoretical assumptions. A phonological theoretical assumption may be **empirical** in the sense that what is stated is realized in the experience of child and adult speakers. In other words, a phonological rule is empirical if it relates to the speaker's experience. A phonological theoretical assumption may be only **formal,** on the other hand, in that it is only an expression of certain observations, which means that what is stated may or may not be the personal experience of speakers. In other words, strictly formal rules do not refer to personal experience. As defined, empirical observations have a much greater relevance to a clinical science such as speech–language pathology than do formal theoretical deductions.

Phonological rules and processes often are stated in empirical terms; that is, a stated rule is implied to capture a child's linguistic or verbal experience. For example, formal theorists often suggest that a child who does not produce consonants in word-final positions *follows the rule* of final-consonant deletion. More strongly empirically oriented scientists, however, wonder in what sense a child *follows* such a phonological rule. Whether a speaker follows a rule or behavioral regularities simply give that impression is an important empirical issue. We will soon return to this issue.

Nonlinear phonological theories do not emphasize rules or processes. Instead, they emphasize *representations*. Most of these theories assume that there are underlying, abstract phonological representations for different phonemes, phonemic features, and their permissible combinations. Presumably, children keep these underlying phonological representations somewhere in their head. This is similar to transformational generative linguists' well-known assertion that children *have* the universal syntactic rules of languages. Children who learn to produce the phonemes and their combinations correctly are supposed to have correctly *realized* their underlying phonological representations. On the contrary, however, children who make phonological errors are presumed to have failed to realize the underlying (accurate) phonological representation. Unfortunately, convincing empirical evidence about the underlying, abstract representation of phonological systems in children is lacking. It may be clear that a child is making phonological or articulatory errors, but it is not equally clear that the child has an underlying representation that has not been correctly realized. For the formal theorist, a presumed, underlying, unobserved, unmeasured entity is essential to explain observed behavioral regularities.

An understanding of how the phonological rules are formed gives us an insight into their empirical or formal status. Phonological rules are statements that describe observed patterns of phonological behaviors. To give a simple example, when children do not produce certain phonemes in word-final positions, the observer captures this behavior by stating the rule of final-consonant deletion. Does this mean that the children somehow have discovered the rule of final-consonant deletion and are following it? Or does it mean that someone has taught the children to follow the rule of final-consonant deletion? Neither is likely.

There is an important distinction between *rule following* and *rule extraction*. **Rule following** is evident when a person's behavior meets the requirements of an explicitly stated rule, a rule that has been formally taught and that the person can state. To give a simple example from everyday life, children who do not touch hot surfaces because they have been told that it is dangerous to do so are following a rule. A behavior is **rule-governed** only when it explicitly follows a rule. There is no empirical evidence to show that children normally and typically follow phonological rules or that phonological productions are rule-governed. It is not because they are following a rule that English-speaking children do not produce /mb/ sequence in initial-word positions. It is because they have not heard it in their language. Similarly, their production of all acceptable sound sequences is not a function of phonological rules; they produce them because they have heard them.

While rule following is a behavioral phenomenon, **rule extraction** is a scientific-analytic activity. Phonologists *extract* rules from regularities in the phonological production of children. Extracted rules economically describe patterns of behaviors. The rules do not explain those patterned behaviors, nor are they part of the skill, knowledge, or ability of the behaving persons. Therefore, there is no compelling reason to drive the rules extracted from children's patterned speech–language productions back into their minds.

Linguistic rules, whether syntactic or phonologic, may be explicitly taught to speakers. Typically, students learn syntactic or phonologic rules only through explicit instruction. Speakers of foreign languages, whose speaking may evidence overgeneralization of their native language patterns, may learn rules and follow them. Therefore, there may be instances in which linguistic behaviors follow rules, but that is generally not the case with children who acquire their native language.

The Clinician and the Theoretician

The clinical research on the application of phonological theories has always lagged behind theoretical advances. The distinctive feature approach, which has a history of several decades now, can still boast only a few treatment studies in which its clinical assumptions have been tested (see Chapter 8 for details). Currently popular phonological approaches, too, need many more controlled treatment studies, in which treatment is compared with no treatment and with other forms of treatment, to establish their absolute and relative efficacy. Many treatment studies use the case study method and thus lack experimental controls.

The newer phonological theories (e.g., the metric theory and the feature geometry) may have encouraging clinical implications, but clinicians need applications. Generally, clinical implications of newer theories are justified on logical grounds, and, while such justifications are necessary, they are not sufficient. There is a need for controlled treatment studies in which the presumed power, usefulness, or application of phonological theories is tested. Most linguists and theoretical phonologists who suggest clinical implications of their new theories often cannot conduct controlled treatment studies to evaluate their assumptions. Therefore, it will be the responsibility of speech–language pathologists who accept such theories to test their clinical application possibilities. Practicing clinicians who remain skeptical of newer theories until such tests are conducted and the results support theoretical deductions may save their time and energy. Because of ever shifting theoretical grounds in phonology, Yavas stated that "any application of the hierarchy [such as those suggested by feature geometry] for remediation [is] tentative at best" (1998, p. 278).

Summary of the Advanced Unit

- Certain additional parameters of speech include aerodynamic, acoustic, suprasegmental, and perceptual factors.

- Air supply from the lungs is essential for normal speech production.

- A system of physiological valves, including the vocal folds, the velopharyngeal mechanism, constriction of the oral cavity, and the lips are involved in effecting changes in the airflow, its volume, and its pressure as a person begins to speak.

- As a branch of physics, **acoustics** is the scientific study of sound as a physical phenomenon.

- **Frequency** is the rate at which an object vibrates; variations in frequency create variations in the perceived pitch of a sound.

- **Amplitude** or **intensity** is the magnitude of vibration of a sound source; the greater the magnitude of vibration, the higher the amplitude.

- **Duration** is a measure of time during which vibrations are sustained.

- Consonants and vowels are typically considered *segmentals*. Properties of speech that become evident when such larger units as words, phrases, sentences, and continuous speech are produced are **suprasegmentals.**

- A suprasegmental feature of speech, **pitch** is the sensory experience related to the frequency of vibration; pitch variations can affect meaning and give speech its melodic quality.

- Linguistic **stress** is a device that gives prominence to certain syllables within a sequence of syllables; the vowel segment is typically stressed; stressed syllables are higher in intensity and pitch and longer in duration.

- A form of stress that helps contrast two or more possibilities while emphasizing one of them is known as **contrastive stress.**

• In **stress-timed languages,** stressed syllables tend to be produced at regular intervals, whereas in **syllable-timed languages,** syllables, not necessarily stress syllables, tend to be produced at regular intervals.

• Variations in the **rate of speech** are a significant aspect of speech suprasegmentals; the rate is increased by decreasing pauses and the durations of vowels and longer consonants.

• **Juncture** is a suprasegmental device used to make semantic or grammatical distinctions in speech and includes brief pauses in speech.

• According to the theory of naturalness and markedness, a **natural** segment or process, also called **unmarked,** is more common among the languages of the world. Less natural or unique features of languages are called **marked.** Unmarked elements are generally acquired earlier than marked elements, and a greater number and pattern of errors are associated with marked elements than unmarked elements.

• Several newer phonological theories have been proposed to overcome the shortcomings of the **linear** standard phonological theories of the kind proposed by Chomsky and Halle (1968).

• Newer **nonlinear** theories suggest ways in which segmental and suprasegmental features are related and organized in a hierarchical fashion and thus more effectively account for stress and other aspects of prosody.

• The nonlinear **metric theory** proposes a hierarchy of features based on feet, syllables, and segments and pays particular attention to syllable structure and stress patterns (suprasegmental features).

• The **feature geometry** proposes that feature combinations of a segment also are hierarchically organized and that combinations are based on the six anatomical structures used in speech production: the glottis, soft palate, lips, tongue blade, tongue body, and tongue root.

• Developments in the basic and clinical study of speech sounds and their patterns, including such new approaches as the distinctive feature theory, phonological process theory, and newer phonological theories may be more parallel than serial; frequent shifts in theories are an indication of the prematurity of suggested theories.

• Phonological concepts and processes are theoretical and formal and may not be empirical; that is, they may not reflect the actual experience of children learning phonological systems or speakers who exhibit patterned phonological behaviors.

• Though typically asserted as such, phonological productions normally may not be rule-governed. Experts extract phonological behaviors from patterned behaviors; this does not mean that the speakers follow those rules.

• The clinical implications of newer phonological theories need to be experimentally verified in treatment research studies.

Chapter 3

◆ ◆ ◆ ◆ ◆ ◆ ◆ ◆ ◆ ◆ ◆ ◆ ◆ ◆ ◆ ◆ ◆ ◆

Development of Articulation and Phonological Skills

Basic Unit

♦ ♦ ♦ ♦ ♦ ♦ ♦ ♦ ♦ ♦ ♦ ♦ ♦ ♦ ♦ ♦ ♦ ♦

Normal Development of Articulation and Phonological Skills from Infancy Through the Early School Years

Communication is the name of the game.
—ANDY ROONEY

Children continually fascinate adults with their incredible daily developments. One of the most impressive accomplishments is the child's ability to produce speech sounds and the ability to combine those sounds to form words. Parents and significant others view the development of the first word as a major achievement that is remembered always. This event typically earns a spot in the child's "milestones" scrapbook.

As fascinating as the development of speech is, many times it is taken for granted and viewed as something that just happens in human beings. However, the acquisition of speech sounds and the phonological skills that allow a child to verbalize his or her first words is a complex motor and linguistic process that begins in infancy and proceeds through the early school years. Many experts in the fields of child development, developmental linguistics, and speech–language pathology have studied this acquisition process.

Such intensive study is extremely important for the speech–language pathologist (SLP) since one of the primary responsibilities of the SLP is to distinguish normal from disordered phonological development in a particular child and to base treatment on that distinction. However, to completely understand abnormal development, it is essential to also understand general developmental trends across children. This Basic Unit will focus on the development of articulation and phonological skills from infancy through the early school years. Approximate ages for the various stages of articulation and phonological development will be provided.

Although a developmental approach will be taken, individual variability in the development of speech sounds and phonological skills will be considered. In recent years, the existence of individual differences in communicative development has been increasingly documented (Davis & MacNeilage, 1995; Stoel-Gammon, 1985; Stoel-Gammon & Cooper, 1981; Vihman, 1998).

In defense of the developmental approach, however, it is necessary to provide students and practicing professionals with basic guidelines that will help them separate normal from abnormal development. Although individual variability certainly exists, general trends in the acquisition of articulation and phonological skills can be established. The reader should carefully view such trends as a general framework from which diagnostic and therapeutic decisions may be initiated, not completed.

In the Advanced Unit of this chapter, we will consider methodological and theoretical issues in speech perception and discrimination research. Theories of articulation and phonological development and a comparative evaluation of linguistic and behavioral explanations of phonological development will also be addressed.

Prelinguistic Development

In recent years there has been an increasing legal and professional emphasis on the provision of speech–language pathology services to the 0- to 3-year-old population. Professionals working with infants and toddlers are continually faced with many tough assessment and management decisions. The difficulty in making appropriate diagnostic and therapeutic conclusions is more pronounced with the infant population (birth to 1 year) due to a historical lack of research with respect to the communication development in that age group.

The professional working with this population must be able to determine whether an infant judged to be at risk for a communication disorder is on the proper course of speech and language development. However, to make such a determination the speech–language pathologist must have a basic understanding of what is normally expected in an infant at varying stages of communication development. Fortunately, with a growing acknowledgment that the infant population must be served and that important communication milestones indeed occur in infancy, an increased knowledge base of early speech development has emerged in recent years.

Before reviewing this information, we would like to note the common use of the term *prelinguistic* in reference to infant vocalizations. This term implies that sound productions at this level are not entirely linguistic since they are not used meaningfully by the child. In essence, these sounds or sound combinations often lack a specific referent and communicative intent, especially in the very early stages. However, you will notice the preference of the term *prelinguistic* over *nonlinguistic*. As a prefix, *pre-* means "before," whereas *non-* means "not" or "absent." Therefore, vocalizations during the infant stage are considered "before" true language rather than "not" language altogether. This important distinction is highlighted because recent research has supported the notion that there is some relationship between early infant vocalizations and the later development of adult-based words (Locke, 1983; Oller, 1980; Oller, Wieman, Doyle, & Ross, 1975; Stark, 1978, 1979, 1980; Stoel-Gammon & Cooper, 1981; Vihman, 1998; Vihman, Macken, Miller, Simmons, & Miller, 1985).

Infant Speech Perception

It is logical to assume that the natural development of articulation and phonological skills involves the perception as well as the production of speech sounds. But what exactly does the word *perception* refer to? **Perception** has been defined as the process "by which a person selects, organizes, integrates, and interprets sensory stimuli he is receiving (Hulitt & Howard, 1997, p. 89). *Stedman's Concise Medical Dictionary* defines perception in the following manner: "the mental process of becoming aware of or recognizing an object or idea; primarily cognitive, rather than **affective** or **conative,** although all three aspects are manifested" (Dirckx, 1997, p. 661, emphasis added). Since perception is an internal cognitive state that cannot be directly observed, a person's ability to select, organize, integrate, and interpret sensory stimuli is typically inferred by the presence or absence of an outward behavior. For example, an audiologist testing a person's hearing assumes that the individual did or did not hear specific pure tones based on some observable behavior (e.g., hand raising, button pushing, or verbalization).

More specific to our discussion, **speech perception** refers to "the identification of speech sounds, mainly from acoustic cues" (Dirckx, 1997, p. 661). If we extrapolate from these definitions, then *infant speech perception* pertains to the infant's inferred ability to identify and perceive speech stimuli. The question emerges then, Can an infant perceive speech stimuli, or is that a skill that develops later? Most of us would probably agree that older children and adults possess the skills to distinguish speech sound contrasts such as *p* and *t* or *u* and *i*. But does an infant also have this skill, and if he or she does, at what age can this be expected to develop? Several researchers sought to answer such questions, and thus, the study of infant speech perception broadened in the early 1970s. Since that time, a vast number of investigations have been conducted, resulting in an abundant amount of information in this realm of infant development.

Sound Localization and Auditory Discrimination

Research has shown that one of the most basic perceptual skills of an infant is sound localization. That an infant localizes a source of sound is inferred from observable behaviors, notably an eye movement or a head turn toward the source of sound. In 1979, Muir and Field sought to gain some information about infants' sound localization skills. Their criterion for sound localization was a head-turn response. The authors found that infants as young as 2 to 7 days turned in the direction of a rattling noise 75% of the time. Muir and Field's data support the notion that infants can determine the direction of incoming noise from a very early age. This is not as astonishing as it may seem because infants' hearing abilities are well developed by about the 20th week of gestation (Birnholz & Benacerraf, 1983; Elliot & Elliot, 1964; Johansson, Wedenberg, & Westin, 1964; Kuczwara, Birnholz, & Klodd, 1984). These data suggest that the newborn infant has been hearing sounds for approximately 4 months prior to his or her birth.

Other studies have shown that newborn infants can discriminate between varied pure-tone frequencies (Bridger, 1961) and pure-tone loudness levels (Bartoshuk, 1964). Bench (1969) also demonstrated that the newborn could discriminate differing white noise levels. Spring and Dale (1975) offered further support that infants between 1 and 4 months of age can discriminate sound location, fundamental frequency, intensity, and duration.

Infants have also been found to show a greater interest in human speech than other noises (Eisenberg, 1976; Jensen, Williams, & Bzoch, 1975). There is some evidence that a child as young as 3 days can recognize his or her mother's voice and discriminate it from the voices of other women (DeCasper & Fifer, 1980). Furthermore, DeCasper and Spence (1986) documented that an infant may prefer a speech passage that his or her mother read while she was pregnant over speech passages that she did not read.

Speech Perception

The infant's tendency to localize sound, discriminate frequency and loudness levels, and prefer human voice to nonhuman noises are all quite remarkable skills. However, a relatively more complex perceptual skill may be the infant's ability to discriminate among classes of speech sounds.

But since infants do not use true words to communicate, how do we know when they have perceived the difference between speech sounds? Two major methods have been used to find an answer to this question: high-amplitude sucking and visually reinforced head turn. The high-amplitude sucking method is used with very young infants (from birth to about 5 months of age) because of its conditionability in such infants. With older infants, the visually reinforced head-turn method is used.

In the **high-amplitude sucking method,** two groups of infants, one experimental and the other control, are allowed to suck on a pacifier attached to a pressure transducer. By varying the rate of sucking, the infant can control the presentation of speech stimuli. Initially, a baseline sucking rate is established. When the sucking rate is stabilized, the experimenter presents a repeating speech stimulus (e.g., *pa pa pa*). There may be an increase in the infant's sucking rate as a result of this reinforcing sound stimulus presentation. However, with repeated presentation of the sound stimulus, the sucking rate levels off and begins to decrease because of adaptation to the sound stimulus. Following such adaptation, the infants in the experimental group are presented with a different sound stimulus (e.g., *ba ba ba*), while those in the control group continue to hear the original sound stimulus. An increase in the sucking rate of the infants in the experimental group while a stabilized or decreasing rate of sucking occurs in the control group is taken to mean that the infants in the experimental group discriminated the new speech stimulus from the old stimulus.

The **visually reinforced head-turn method** exploits the tendency to turn toward a source of sound and reinforces this behavior visually. A reliable head-turn response is evident in infants as young as 5–6 months of age. During the experiment, an infant's attention is held by manipulating a toy in his or her visual field. The experimenter then presents a repeated speech stimulus (e.g., *va va va*) through a loud speaker. The infant gets adapted to this auditory syllable stimulus and keeps looking at the toy being manipulated. The experimenter then presents a different speech sound stimulus (e.g., *sa sa sa*). If the infant promptly turns his or her head toward the speaker when the stimulus is changed from *va va va* to *sa sa sa,* this head turn is immediately reinforced by an animated toy that is lighted. The Plexiglas box housing the toy is placed in front of the speaker. *Control trials* (e.g., the continued and repeated presentation of *va*) and *change trials* (e.g., the new stimulus *sa sa*) are alternated a few times to see if the infant reliably turns his or her head toward the reinforcing box when the change trials are presented but not when the control trials are presented. If this is the outcome of the experiment, it is then concluded that the infant perceived and discriminated the two sets of syllables (Eilers, 1980; Kuhl, 1987).

Speech sound discrimination experiments have been conducted with animals as well. The most frequently used animal is the chinchilla, a rodent (Kuhl & Miller, 1978). The other animal used in speech perception experiments is the dog (Baru, 1975). With animal subjects, the method used is instrumental (operant) avoidance conditioning, in which the animal is exposed to shock if a particular response is not made when a speech (or other sound) stimulus is presented. In speech discrimination experiments, the method allows conditioning an avoidance response to speech stimuli (Burdick & Miller, 1973; Kuhl & Miller, 1978).

Using the methods described, many studies have been conducted on infant speech perception (see Eimas, Siqueland, Jusczyk, & Vigorito, 1971; Morse, 1972; Eilers & Minifie, 1975; Eilers, Wilson, & Moore, 1977; see Miller, Kent, & Atal, 1991, for a collection of papers; and see also Eilers, 1980; Kuhl, 1987, for reviews of studies, results, and theories). Additional studies with varied methods have been concerned with infant's perception and discrimination of pitch contours (Morse, 1972), syllable stress levels (Spring & Dale, 1975), sounds produced at different places of articulation (Eimas, 1974), voice onset times (Eimas et al., 1971), and utterances in their own language from those in other languages (Mehler, Jusczyk, Lambertz, Halsted, Bertoncini, & Amiel-Tison, 1988).

There is a good deal of consistency among findings, although some discrepant findings are reported in certain areas. Generally speaking, the studies have shown that infants can be conditioned to respond differently to different sounds and syllables at a very young age; in fact, infants that are only 4 days old have been conditioned. It should be noted that while most investigators and textbook writers report that infants can discriminate among speech sounds, we prefer to report that *infants can be trained, taught, or conditioned to discriminate among speech sounds*, as the methods used in the studies are of learning and conditioning, mostly operant conditioning. This generally ignored methodological issue is addressed in the Advanced Unit of this chapter.

The many studies on infant speech perception, taken as a whole, have generally shown that:

• Very young infants can be taught to make fine distinctions among speech sounds.

• Infants 6 months old can be taught to discriminate distinctions in pitch contours.

• Infants can be taught to discriminate among syllable stress levels.

• Infants can be conditioned to discriminate sounds produced at different places of articulation.

• Infants can be taught to discriminate varied voice onset times.

• Infants as young as 1 month can be conditioned to discriminate between /pa/ and /ba/.

• Infants as young as 2 months can be conditioned to discriminate between /ba/ and /ga/.

• Infants between 2 and 3 months can be conditioned to discriminate between /ra/ and /la/.

• Infants between 1 and 4 months can be conditioned to discriminate between /sa/ and /va/ and /sa/ and /ʃa/.

• Infants between 1 and 4 months can be conditioned to discriminate the vowel contrasts /u/ and /i/ and /a/ and /ɪ/.

• Infants between 5 and 6 months can be conditioned to discriminate between /a/ and /i/.

• Infants between 6 and 8 months can be conditioned to discriminate between /sa/ and /za/.

• Infants between 14 and 18 weeks can be conditioned to discriminate between phonetically similar pairs (e.g., /pi/ and /pu/) more readily than between phonetically dissimilar pairs (e.g., /pi/ and /ka/).

• Infants can transfer (generalize) their learned discrimination to syllables or sounds produced by different speakers (e.g., if conditioned to discriminate syllables produced by a male speaker, the infants could discriminate the same syllables produced by a female speaker or a child speaker).

• Infants between 6 and 8 months can be conditioned to discriminate speech sounds that are not used in their native language.

• As the infant becomes older (reaching 12 months of age or so), it becomes increasingly difficult to condition infants to discriminate sounds not used in their native language.

• Infants as young as 4 days can discriminate utterances (not specific speech sounds) from their own language from those of an unfamiliar language.

Studies also have shown that:

• Infants as old as 12 to 14 months *cannot* be easily conditioned to discriminate between /θa/ and /fa/.

• Infants between 1 and 4 months *cannot* be easily conditioned to discriminate between /sa/ and /za/.

• Young infants *cannot* be easily conditioned to discriminate between /fi/ and /θi/.

• Young infants *cannot* be easily conditioned to discriminate between stops used in multisyllabic productions with relatively short syllable durations (e.g., /ataba/ vs. /atapa/).

✎ Activity

DIRECTIONS: As discussed in the text, briefly describe the two main procedures used to study infant speech perception and discrimination.

1. **High-amplitude sucking method:** _____
   _____
   _____
   _____
   _____
   _____

2. **Visually reinforced head-turn method:** _____
   _____
   _____
   _____
   _____
   _____

Infant Speech Perception: Innate or Learned Skill?

That infants could be conditioned to make fine distinctions between speech sound contrasts has triggered the question of whether infants have an innate ability to discriminate speech sounds or learn those skills after some initial exposure to language. In an attempt to answer that question, Trehub (1976) conducted a study in which a group of Canadian infants was presented with native (English) and nonnative (Czech) sound contrasts. The infants were all part of English-speaking homes and had never been exposed to any Eastern European language. This eliminated exposure to the language as a variable in the speech discrimination skills of the infants, since they had not been previously exposed to the Czech language. The logical assumption would be that the infants would do better in discriminating English sound contrasts than Czech sound contrasts since English was their native language and they had been exposed to it since birth. The results of the study did not support that assumption, however.

Contrary to logical expectation, Trehub found that the infants in her study discriminated between the syllables containing the Czech sounds (i.e., [ʒa] and [řa]) just as well as they discriminated between those containing the English sounds (i.e., [pa] and [ba]). The results of this and other studies on infant speech perception and discrimination were originally interpreted to mean that infants have an innate ability to make fine discriminations between speech sounds (native and nonnative). The strong version of this interpretation meant that infants have a special, linguistic-specific speech decoder innately built into their speech processing mechanism.

Results of subsequent studies have questioned the earlier interpretation of a specific speech decoder mechanism innately available to infants. Some studies also revealed that infants could not be conditioned to make certain kinds of speech discriminations. For example, Eilers and Minifie (1975) found that infants aged 1 to 4 months could not distinguish [sa] from [za], and Eilers et al. (1977) reported that infants as old as 12 to 14 months could not perceive the difference between [fa] and [θa]. Other studies have shown that discrimination between /f/ and /θ/ continues to be difficult even in children 3 to 4 years of age (e.g., Locke, 1980a, 1980b). These findings support the assumption that children may require at least some learning or experience for discrimination of specific sound contrasts.

A second portion of Trehub's just cited study lends further support to the idea that the environment does have a role in speech perception. In addition to presenting native and nonnative sound contrasts to young infants, Trehub tested adult monolingual English-speaking subjects for their ability to discriminate between the two Czech sounds presented to the infant group. Although the infants could discriminate the two pairs of sound syllables equally well, the adult subjects had a high degree of difficulty in discriminating the Czech sounds. The adults' linguistic knowledge of English may have interfered with their ability to discriminate sound contrasts that were not functional or relevant in their native language.

The idea that a person's primary language can interfere with the ability to discriminate sound contrasts that are not part of the native language is further supported by Werker and Tees's (1984) study. They presented non-English sound pairs to infants between 6 and 8 months, 8 and 10 months, and 10 and 12 months of age. Werker and Tees found that the youngest age group had little difficulty perceiving the difference between Hindi and Thompson (a Salish language spoken in Canada) sound contrasts. They further found that the 8- to 10-month-old group performed more poorly than the 6- to 8-month-old group, and the 10- to 12-month-old group performed worse than the two younger groups. This indicated that the infants' ability to discriminate nonnative sound contrasts deteriorated as they got older. As infants grow older and begin to pay increasing attention to the surrounding language, their ability to discriminate speech sounds in other languages tends to deteriorate.

The hypothesis that humans have an innately given linguistic decoder that helps discriminate speech sounds early in infancy also meant that subhuman animals, lacking language, also lack a linguistic decoder, and hence, are incapable of speech perception (Liberman, 1970). However, evidence of speech perception and discrimination in animals, especially in the chinchilla and the dog, as summarized in the Basic Unit, mounts an even more serious challenge to the hypothesis of innate, speech-specific skill in infants. Research evidence now clearly shows that learning to discriminate between speech sounds is not an exclusively human skill (Baru, 1975; Burdick & Miller, 1975; Kuhl & Miller, 1975; Miller & Kuhl, 1976). These studies also include evidence that once trained with a set of speech stimuli, the animals show generalized responding when presented with similar stimuli or stimuli generated from different speakers, including male, female, and child speakers.

Thus, the well-documented evidence on animal discrimination of speech sounds suggests that a mammal with an auditory system similar to that of humans can be taught to make certain phonemic distinctions. The evidence does not support the theory of a special speech-specific mechanism responsible for phonemic discriminations. Sensitivity to sound differences may be a general characteristic of the auditory system of many organisms. This is supported by the results of a study that has shown that 2-month-olds can perceive differences in nonspeech sounds as well (Jusczyk, Rosner, Cutting, Foard, & Smith, 1977). Possibly, the auditory mechanism's general sensitivity and conditionability may have had certain adaptive or survival values in the evolutionary scale.

An appropriate interpretation of the results of infant speech perception and discrimination experiments requires a due consideration of the experimental methods used. The methods are essentially those of operant conditioning, and hence the results most forcefully show that infants can be taught to make speech discriminations. The methods used in the studies do not allow for a direct test of some innate ability. We will return to this methodological issue in the Advanced Unit of this chapter.

Infant Speech Production

In the not so distant past, true articulation and phonological development was thought to begin with the production of the child's first meaningful words. The production of the "first word" was viewed as the child's initial step toward the acquisition of adultlike speech. Therefore, most of the pioneering articulation developmental studies included children between 2 and 8 years of age in their investigations.

However, the study of the speech skills that an infant must acquire before he or she can actually produce his or her first words began to flourish in the late 1970s and early 1980s (e.g., Oller, 1980; Oller et al., 1975; Stark, 1978, 1979, 1980). Research since that time has done away with the notion that vocal behaviors prior to the one-word stage are unimportant productions bearing no relationship to the development of meaningful speech. Roman Jakobson's (1941/1968) "discontinuity" hypothesis, stating that infant babbling is a random series of vocalizations with no apparent order or consistency, has come under severe scrutiny. Jakobson's notion that a child typically undergoes a period of silence between the end of the babbling period and development of the first real words is no longer accepted as fact.

In actuality, recent research focusing on infant speech development has repeatedly documented that babbling is not random behavior, all possible sounds are not produced during the babbling stage, and the transition between babbling and the first words is not abrupt but continuous (Bauman-Waengler, 1994).

Infant Developmental Stages

An infant's primary method of communication with the adult world is through crying and fussing. A few months after birth, the infant also begins to produce sequences of consonant-vowel and vowel-consonant combinations with adultlike intonations. These distinct vocal productions are typically divided into two general categories: **reflexive vocalizations,** which are automatic responses reflecting the physical state of the infant, including crying, coughing, burping, and hiccuping; and **nonreflexive vocalizations,** which are voluntary productions, including cooing, babbling, and playful screaming and yelling (Oller, 1980; Stark, 1980).

In 1980 Oller advanced several specific stages that mark the acquisition of articulation and phonological skills during the first year of speech development. Oller's stages are widely accepted and frequently used in reference to prelinguistic vocalizations. Some overlap in vocalizations exists from one stage to another; however, each new stage is characterized by vocal behaviors not observed in the previous stage. The stages must be viewed only as approximate ages of infant speech production that may differ from one infant to another.

Stage 1: Phonation Stage. This stage progresses from birth to 1 month.

• Reflexive vocalizations such as crying, fussing, coughing, sneezing, and burping predominate. Speechlike sounds are rare.

• Some nonreflexive vocalizations resembling syllabic nasals occur.

• Vocalizations resembling vowels occur. However, these are termed *quasi-resonant nuclei* since they occur with normal phonation but limited oral resonance.

Stage 2: Coo and Goo Stage. This stage characterizes infant vocalizations from 2 months to about 3 months.

• Sounds are produced that are acoustically similar to back vowels and consonant-vowel (CV) and vowel-consonant (VC) syllables containing back vowels and back consonants (velars, uvulars).

• The syllable sequences produced at this stage are considered *primitive* because of the irregular timing in the opening and closure of the consonantal and vocalic segments (as compared to those of adults).

Stage 3: Exploration-Expansion Stage. This stage typically progresses from about 4 months to 6 months.

• This stage is characterized as a period of vocal play in which the child gains better control of the laryngeal and articulatory mechanisms.

• Squeals, growls, yells, **raspberries** (bilabial or lingualabial trills), vowel-like elements, and friction noises may be observed in this stage. These vocalizations attest to the better laryngeal and articulatory functions in the infant.

• The infant's predominant vocalizations may vary daily and weekly.

• Vowels have better oral resonance and are more adultlike. Thus, at this point they are termed *fully resonant nuclei.*

• **Marginal babbling** appears. Productions labeled as such are characterized by CV and VC syllable sequences. However, the timing of opening and closure is still difficult at this point. The distinction between the syllable sequences at this stage and those at the previous stage is the increased resonance for vowel-like sounds and better constriction for consonant-like sounds.

Stage 4: Canonical Babbling Stage. This stage progresses from 7 months to 9 months. It is also known as the **reduplicated babbling stage.**

• CV syllables continue and now have more adultlike timing for closure and opening. The sounds are more constricted and resonated so that they now resemble true consonants and vowels.

• The CV syllables become longer at this point and may be *reduplicated* so that syllable sequences such as [baba], [kaka], and [tata] result. For parents, CV reduplicated syllables that resemble [mama] and [dada] are of prime importance (for obvious reasons).

• Although some reduplicated syllable sequences resemble real words, particularly [mama] and [dada], these are not used with true intention by the infant (to every parent's dismay). That is, the infant may use these productions when alone, when looking at the family dog (as reported by one of our colleagues in reference to her own son's production of [mama] at 7 months), when looking at a toy, or when looking at Mom.

• The infant's phonetic repertoire, although limited, may consist of stops, nasals, glides, and the lax vowels /ɛ/, /ɪ/, /ʌ/.

• The production of back sounds (velars) declines sharply, while the production of front sounds (alveolars and bilabials) increases.

Stage 5: Variegated Babbling Stage. The last infant vocalization stage advanced by Oller (1980) progresses from 10 months to about the first year.

• CV syllable sequences continue but are no longer simply reduplicative in nature.

• The infant in the variegated babbling stage combines a variety of CV sequences resulting in productions like [madaga], [putika], and [tikadi].

• The infant's vowel and consonant repertoire increases significantly at this point (this will be discussed in detail in an upcoming section).

• The infant's intonation patterns take on a more adultlike quality, especially as the first year approximates.

- The infant's connected strings of variegated syllable sequences may resemble real statements, questions, and exclamations prosodically; however, these strings do not contain real words.

Babbling Revisited

As previously discussed, infant babbling was once believed to be random behavior bearing little or no relationship to the development of meaningful speech. This belief was primarily nourished by Jakobson's (1941/1968) discontinuity theory. This theory postulated that babbling is random in the sense that infants produce the full range of possible human speech sounds (sounds in and out of the child's ambient language) instead of systematically producing only those sounds that are part of the native language.

Jakobson further claimed that infants typically undergo a period of silence between the end of the babbling stage and the beginning of the true speech stage. According to the discontinuity viewpoint, this period of silence, in addition to marked differences in the phonetic repertoires of the two stages, depicts the lack of relationship between babbling and meaningful speech in a child's phonological development.

More recent investigations have provided little support for Jakobson's discontinuity hypothesis. Recent investigations have shown that although there are individual differences, most children continue to babble for approximately 3 to 4 months after the appearance of the first "true" word (Stoel-Gammon & Dunn, 1985). In addition, studies have shown that the phonological patterns of babbling and meaningful speech are very similar in relation to syllable types and phonetic repertoires (Stoel-Gammon & Cooper, 1981, 1984; Stoel-Gammon, 1985; Vihman, Macken, Miller, Simmons, & Miller, 1985).

Locke (1983) reviewed a large number of studies of infants from English-speaking environments, infants from other linguistic environments, and deaf and Down syndrome infants. He found very little support for the assumption that infants babble all of the sounds of English or that they babble all of the possible speech sounds. Rather, he found that infants babble a fairly small or preferred set of sounds. Considering these more recent findings in our discussion, infant babbling behavior will be viewed as an important developmental milestone leading the way to the development of later articulation and phonological skills.

Forms of Babbling. Babbling begins at approximately 6–7 months of age and extends until the child's first words appear at age 10–13 months. As previously discussed, most infants continue to babble a few months after production of their first words. Despite recent controversies regarding the sequential nature of babbling (Holmgren, Lindblom, Aurelius, Jalling, & Zetterstrom, 1986; Smith, Brown-Sweeney, & Stoel-Gammon, 1989; Mitchell & Kent, 1990), babbling continues to be divided into two distinct stages. The initial portion of babbling is known as **reduplicated babbling,** usually starting at about 7 months of age. This form of babbling is characterized by the reduplication of similar consonant-vowel syllable strings such as [mama], [papa], and [baba]. A variation in the vowel sounds may occur from syllable to syllable; however, the consonant tends to remain constant (e.g., [mamu]).

Nonreduplicated or **variegated babbling** is marked as the second portion of babbling. This period usually begins at approximately 9–10 months of age and is characterized by varying consonant and vowel productions from one syllable string to another (e.g., [mabi], [pamu], and [banu]). Reduplicated and variegated babbling have frequently been included in a single stage of development called **canonical babbling** because of the difficulty that often arises in distinguishing the two (Smith et al., 1989; Mitchell & Kent, 1990).

A form of babbling that frequently overlaps with the early period of meaning-ful speech is characterized by strings of sounds and syllables produced with a variety of stress and intonational patterns. This form of babbling has been called **conversational babble, modulated babble,** and **jargon** (Berko Gleason, 1993). Oller (1980) referred to this infant vocal behavior as "gibberish." For ease in dis-cussion and comparison with other textbooks, we perfer the term *jargon*.

Jargon usually begins once the variegated babbling stage has been reached, at approximately 10 months of age. The primary difference between variegated bab-bling and jargon is the infant's increasingly varied and consistent use of intona-tion, rhythm, and pausing in the latter. Jargon may be thought of as variegated babbling with intonation patterns superimposed on the sound productions. Because of the varied use of intonation patterns, adults are often left with the impression that the infant is producing whole sentences to make statements, make commands, and ask questions. Although the child sounds as if he is saying some-thing meaningful, his or her productions cannot be understood based solely on the articulated sounds. The adult's ability to infer some meaning from the older infant's jargon may be related more to the accompanying gestures and pointing and the communicative context than the actual articulated sounds.

Sounds and Syllable Shapes of Babbling. The sounds and syllable shapes used by infants during the babbling stage have been investigated by various researchers (Davis & MacNeilage, 1995; Irwin, 1947a, 1947b, 1948, 1952; Irwin & Chen, 1946; Fisichelli, 1950; Locke, 1983; Oller, Wieman, Doyle, & Ross, 1975; Pierce & Hanna, 1974; Stoel-Gammon & Cooper, 1981, 1984; Vihman et al., 1985). As can be identi-fied by the dates of the various studies, infant speech development has been inves-tigated over the past 50 years.

VOWELS. To determine the vowel-like sounds used most often by children at the end of the variegated babbling stage, Bauman-Waengler (1994) compared Irwin's (1948) data with a more current study conducted by Kent and Bauer (1985). Some differences and similarities were noted in the data. The rank order of the six most prevalent vowels according to Irwin's study was /ɛ/, /ɪ/, /ʌ/, /ʊ/, /ɑ/, /u/. Kent and Bauer reported a different rank order: /ʌ/, /ɛ/, /æ/, /ɑ/, /ʊ/. Although the rank order varied slightly, at least four sounds remained constant across the two studies as the most prevalent: /ɛ/, /ʌ/, /ɑ/, and /ʊ/.

A recent longitudinal study by Davis and MacNeilage (1995) with 6 infants (3 males, 3 females) from monolingual English-speaking homes revealed much indi-vidual variability in the use of vowels. However, some trends were identified. Davis and MacNeilage analyzed the vowel data according to tongue height and tongue advancement dimensions. In relation to tongue height, the vowels were grouped into *high* (i, ɪ, u, ʊ), *mid* (e, ɛ, ʌ, ə, ɔ, o), and *low* (æ, a). For tongue advancement, the vowels were categorized as *front* (i, ɪ, e, ɛ, æ), *mid* (a, ʌ, ə), and *back* (u, ʊ, ɔ, o).

According to the tongue height dimension, mid vowels, particularly [ʌ, ə, and ɛ], predominated in 3 subjects, while high vowels, particularly [u, ʊ, and ɪ], predominated in the remaining 3 subjects. In relation to tongue advancement, front vowels, particularly [ɛ, æ, and ɪ], predominated in 4 subjects, and the mid vowels [a, ʌ, ə] predominated in the remaining 2 subjects. If the vowels used by this infant group are analyzed according to tongue height and advancement combined, the most commonly used vowels in the canonical babbling period are identified as [ʌ, ə, ɛ, u, ʊ, ɪ, æ]. Overall, these data are in close agreement with both Irwin's (1948) and Kent and Bauer's (1985) studies.

CONSONANTS. What consonant-like sounds have been documented to be the most frequent in the late babbling period? Locke (1983) provides an overview of three major studies, Irwin (1947b), Fisichelli (1950), and Pierce and Hanna (1974), in an attempt to answer this question. In his overview of these three studies, Locke noted that /h/, /d/, /b/, /m/, /t/, /w/, and /j/ were reported as the most frequently occurring consonant-like sounds. Furthermore, 12 sounds were found to make up between 92 and 97% of the total sounds used by 11- to 12-month-old infants across the three studies. These included /h/, /d/, /b/, /m/, /t/, /g/, /s/, /w/, /n/, /k/, /j/, and /p/. The less frequently occurring consonant-like sounds were transcribed as /v/, /ʒ/, /ʃ/, /z/, /f/, /θ/, /ð/, /l/, /ŋ/, /r/, /tʃ/, and /dʒ/, which occurred approximately 3–6% of the time across the three studies.

Davis and MacNeilage's (1995) study also offered some information on the use of consonants during the canonical babbling period. Again, their study showed much individual variation among the subjects; however, some overall trends were identified. The most frequently produced consonants according to place of articulation were labials /b/, /m/, /w/, alveolars /d/, /n/, and velars /g/, /ŋ/. However, labials and alveolars occurred with a higher frequency than velars. In regard to manner of production, oral stops occurred with the highest level of frequency, followed by nasals and glides. Although Davis and MacNeilage did not report their data in relation to voicing dimensions, an analysis of their information reveals that voiced consonants occurred most frequently. This more current study lends some support to Locke's (1983) overview of the consonant sounds used most frequently during the late babbling period.

SYLLABLE SHAPES. In our discussion of Oller's stages of infant development, the combination of consonant- and vowel-like sounds was said to begin during the Exploration Stage at about 4 to 6 months. During the later babbling period, open syllables or syllables ending in a vowel are the most frequently occurring syllable shapes (Bauman-Waengler, 1994). Kent and Bauer (1985) found that V, CV, VCV, and CVCV syllable structures accounted for approximately 94% of all the syllables produced at the end of the babbling period. They also emphasized that while closed syllables (syllables ending in a consonant) occurred, they were found to be very limited in the repertoire of the infant at this stage of development.

🖉 Activity

DIRECTIONS: Provide the name given to each of Oller's five prelinguistic stages. List at least two major characteristics for each stage.

Stage I: _____

_____

(continues)

🖉 (Continued)

Stage II: _____

Stage III: _____

Stage IV: _____

Stage V: _____

Individual differences aside, what are the most frequently occurring consonants, vowels, and syllable shapes during the late babbling period?

☐ Consonants: _____

☐ Vowels: _____

☐ Syllable shapes: _____

From Babbling to Meaningful Speech: The Transition Period

The transition from babbling to meaningful speech is a very important milestone in the development of articulation and phonological skills. It is at this point that the child moves from prelinguistic to linguistic phonological development. Although the infant has made an amazing transition from vegetative crying and fussing to the use of jargon in a very short period of time, the development of articulation and phonological skills has really just begun.

Contrary to what was previously thought, children do not merely stop babbling, undergo a period of silence, and then begin using meaningful speech. There is typically an overlap of a few weeks to several months in the use of babbled and meaningful productions (Stoel-Gammon & Dunn, 1985). Children may even use a combination of babbling and meaningful speech in a single utterance (Branigan, 1977).

A child's first meaningful productions have frequently been labeled proto-words (Menn, 1975). **Protowords,** also known as *vocables* (Ferguson, 1978), *phonetically consistent forms* (Dore, Franklin, Miller, & Ramer, 1976), *invented words* (Locke, 1983), *sensori-motor morphemes* (Carter, 1974, 1979) and *quasi-words* (Stoel-Gammon & Cooper, 1984) are vocalizations absent of a recognizable adult model that are used consistently by the infant.

These sounds or sound combinations function as words for the infant, even though they are not based on the adult model. Because they are not based on adult words, these vocalizations do not qualify as "true words." However, they cannot be considered babbling either because they have some phonetic and semantic consistency (Stoel-Gammon & Dunn, 1985). Ferguson (1978) described protowords as "babbling-like sounds used meaningfully" (p. 281).

Protowords are frequently tied to a specific context and are often accompanied by a consistent gesture. These vocal productions have frequently been considered the link between babbling and adultlike speech. Researchers have reported four phonetic forms that are frequently used in protowords: (1) single or repeated vowels, (2) syllabic nasals, (3) syllabic fricatives, and (4) single or repeated consonant-vowel syllables in which the consonant is a nasal or a stop (Ferguson, 1978; Halliday, 1975; Lewis, 1951).

Carter (1974, 1979) studied the progression from protowords to real words in a single subject named David. She termed his productions "sensori-motor morphemes." Carter reported that between the ages of 1 year, 1 month, and 1 year, 2 months, David produced vocalizations that differed from babbling in that they had some phonetic consistency and were frequently accompanied by a gesture. The specific patterns identified by Carter are as follows:

- David used [mm], [ma], [may], or [mə] when reaching for an object;
- David used [la], [læ], [da], [dæ], or [də] when pointing to an object; and
- David used [hɪ], [hɪy], [he], [hə], or [hm] when giving or receiving an object.

Carter further speculated that the use of these sound combinations accompanied by a gesture served as a foundation for the development of conventional (adult-based) words. For example, she believed that:

- the /m + vowel/ vocable accompanied by a reaching gesture led to the acquisition of the words *more, my,* and *mine;*

- the /l + vowel/ or /d + vowel/ vocable accompanied by a pointing gesture led to the acquisition of words such as *look, these,* and *this;* and

- the /h + vowel/ vocable accompanied by a giving or receiving gesture led to the acquisition of words such as *here, where,* and *have.*

It should be emphasized that Carter's speculations are theoretical assumptions that may or may not be factual, as logical or probable as they may seem.

Ferguson (1978) stated that children develop about 12 vocables as they transition from babbling to the use of adult-based words. However, Stoel-Gammon and Cooper's (1984) study failed to support Ferguson's claim. Rather, their study with 3 subjects showed a wider variation among children. Stoel-Gammon and Cooper found that 1 subject used 13 vocables during the acquisition of 50 conventional words, while the other 2 subjects used only one vocable each during the same period. Their data also offered no support for Carter's (1974, 1979) claim that vocables may develop into adult-based words, as with her subject David. In their study none of the children showed such a pattern.

Development of Meaningful Speech: The First Real Words

The use of protowords marks the development of meaningful verbal productions in the speech of young children. However, as indicated earlier, these productions cannot be considered true words because they are not based on an adult model. As the child is making use of protowords for meaningful communication efforts, however, he or she is also attempting to produce words based on an adult model.

So what exactly constitutes a "true" word? Although an indisputable answer does not exist for this question, a general definition has been developed over the years. Many authors and researchers define a **true word** as a stable phonetic form that is used consistently by the child in a particular context. How does this differentiate it from protowords, however? The second part of the definition is usually the determining factor. To qualify as a true word, the child's production, in addition to being stable and consistent, must be phonetically similar to the adult-word form in a particular language.

While a protoword by definition is used consistently in a particular situation, the production often does not resemble the adult word. For example, a child may use the phonetic form [lala] consistently when requesting a toy car; however, that production does not resemble the adult name for the object (i.e., *toy* or *car*). On the other hand, if a child says [ka] consistently when requesting a toy car, the production would qualify as a true word because the child's production and the adult target are phonetically similar, although not identical. Obviously, the use of true words can be identified only if the adult target is known, so that a comparison can be made between the child's production and the target production. This may create some inherent problems with the definition of true words. Is a word only a true word if adults know exactly what the child is saying?

Studies of the phonetic configuration of early adultlike words have revealed common patterns in their overall form and in the sounds that occur (Jakobson, 1968; Stoel-Gammon, 1984, 1985; Stoel-Gammon & Cooper, 1981; Winitz & Irwin, 1958). During this early stage of true-word production, children typically use single syllables or fully or partially reduplicated words. Closed syllables occur but are less common. This pattern of syllable shapes was also noted during the latter stages of the babbling period. Speech sound production is generally characterized by the use of stops, nasals, and/or glides. Fricatives occur much less frequently. Stops, nasals, and glides are speech sounds that are also characteristic of the late babbling period. From these data, it appears that the production of a child's first true words is influenced by the phonetic repertoire and syllable structure of the productions in the late babbling period. Recent studies have documented a continuity between babbling and early word forms (Stoel-Gammon, 1984, 1985; Vihman, Ferguson, & Elbert, 1986; Vihman, Macken, Miller, Simmons, & Miller, 1985).

An interesting occurrence that has been identified in the phonological system of young children is the presence of *progressive idioms* and *regressive idioms* (Moskowitz, 1973; Ferguson & Farwell, 1975). Stoel-Gammon and Dunn (1985) refer to these as *advanced forms* and *frozen forms,* respectively. **Progressive idioms** or **advanced forms** are words that have an advanced pronunciation in comparison to the child's current phonological system or production of other words. Leopold (1947) offers one of the earliest examples of progressive idioms. He noted that his daughter Hildegarde produced the word *pretty* as [prəti] at 10 months of age, a point at which she did not produce any other words with the initial cluster /pr/. He also noted that several months later, as Hildegarde's phonological system matured, she produced *pretty* as [pɪti] or [bɪdi]. These forms more closely matched Hildegarde's other word forms.

Regressive idioms or **frozen forms** are the child's static or unchanging pronunciations despite his or her progression into a more advanced phonological system. That is, words that are less advanced in comparison to the adult target remain that way even as the child's phonological system becomes more sophisticated. Creaghead (1989) indicates that these word forms likely develop from names of familiar people or pets that are used often. The first author's nickname probably developed as a regressive idiom. Although her name is Adriana [e·dri·a·na], some of her immediate family members still call her Nani [na·ni]. When she asked how such a nickname developed, her mother indicated that when Adriana was very young one of her young cousins called her Nana [na·na] because she could not pronounce Adriana's long name. Because the cousin continued to call her that even as they got older, others picked it up, modified it a little, and followed suit.

The cousin's production of [na·na] for [e·dri·a·na] probably resulted from the use of the phonological processes of *syllable deletion* and *total reduplication*. Something that began as a developmentally appropriate simplification process continued even as her phonological system matured because Nana more than likely became her name for Adriana.

✎ Activity

DIRECTIONS: Define the following terms in your own words. Give an example for each.

> **Marginal babbling:** _____
>
> **Reduplicated babbling:** _____
>
> **Variegated babbling:** _____
>
> **Canonical babbling:** _____
>
> **Protoword:** _____
>
> **True word:** _____
>
> **Progressive idiom:** _____
>
> **Regressive idiom:** _____

Development of the Sound System

Around their second birthday, children are more consistent in their use of words and begin to combine words to make simple phrases. They have progressed from the use of early infant vocalizations such as cooing and babbling to the use of protowords, to their first meaningful productions. However, this progression is not linear, as children often use a combination of variegated babbling, jargon, protowords, and true words in their communicative attempts during the first 50-word stage.

By the time children are 2 years of age, their phonetic and lexical inventories have increased dramatically as they continue their route to acquiring an adultlike phonological system. At this point the use of early forms such as variegated babbling, jargon, and protowords is virtually eliminated, while the production of true words increases daily. Their words become phonetically more systematic, and as a result the adult targets are more identifiable.

Several studies have been conducted to investigate the acquisition process during the preschool and early school years. Earlier studies focused on the sequence in which children acquire single speech sounds and the chronological ages at which they master their production. More recent research has focused on the acquisition of distinctive features and the systematic use and disappearance of phonological processes.

Single Phonemes

The acquisition of individual speech sounds in preschool- and early school-age children has been extensively studied since the late 1930s. Several large-scale investigations have been conducted to gain a better understanding of the ages at which children can be expected to master certain speech sounds. Many of these now classic studies set out to develop group norms of articulation using the cross-sectional research method. Other studies have used the longitudinal method to assess the phonological development of individual children.

Cross-Sectional Studies

In the **cross-sectional method,** researchers select a certain number of children from each of the age groups targeted in the study. An effort is made to obtain a group of children that reflects the socioeconomic distribution of the population as a whole. Because hearing and language problems have been associated with articulation and phonological delays, researchers also attempt to exclude children with a reported or documented history of hearing loss or a language disorder.

Once the group has been selected, each child's speech production is sampled by using various test stimuli. Typically, the child is asked to name a picture or an object representing the target sound in a single word. If the child cannot identify the target word upon picture or object presentation, the examiner may provide a model of the target production. The child is then asked to imitate. The degree of imitation permitted may vary from one study to another.

At each age level the specific sounds mastered by a majority of children are determined. A criterion is established that represents the *age of acquisition* or *age of mastery* for each sound. For example, a sound may be considered mastered when 90% of the children tested in a particular age group produced the sound correctly in the initial, medial, and final positions of words. The selected mastery criterion is consistently applied to all sounds tested.

Cross-sectional normative studies yield group data. Individual performance is not considered, and specific error types are not identified. The results provide information on the ages at which children may be expected to produce a sound correctly according to the adult standard. At least five major cross-sectional studies on the acquisition of individual phonemes have been conducted over the last 65 years (Arlt & Goodban, 1976; Poole, 1934; Prather, Hedrick, & Kern, 1975; Templin, 1957; Wellman, Case, Mengert, & Bradbury, 1931).

In her review of these now classic studies Smit (1986) noted some similarities in the research methodology used, particularly the subjects' ages and the sound evoking procedures (see Smit, 1986, for details). However, because of methodological differences in the data collection and analysis, the studies do not always agree on the age at which children master production of specific consonant sounds. One of the primary methodological issues that may account for the difference in age of mastery is the use of differing criteria. For example, some studies considered a consonant mastered when 90% of the study population produced it correctly, whereas other studies considered it mastered when 75% of the population produced it correctly. Another issue that may contribute to some differences is the word positions in which the phoneme was tested. Some studies tested the phoneme only in the initial and final positions, while others tested it in initial, medial, and final positions.

Shipley and McAfee (1998) state that normative data from similar studies can vary because of many factors, including when and where the study was conducted, the size and characteristics of the sample, and the design followed. These factors in addition to the mastery criteria used and the sound positions tested pose an inherent problem in comparing phoneme development data presented by different researchers.

Table 3.1 outlines the exact ages of sound mastery as reported by various classic studies. Despite the differences previously emphasized, the information offered by each of the studies clearly reveals that the acquisition of speech sounds is a relatively lengthy process. Some sounds are mastered quite early, while others continue to be misarticulated until the early elementary school years.

In addition to the studies cited in Table 3.1, Fudala and Reynolds (1986) and Smit, Hand, Freilinger, Bernthal, and Bird (1990) offer more recent information on the acquisition of sounds. Unlike many of the earlier large-scale studies, Fudala

Table 3.1. Ages of Consonant Development

Consonant	Wellman et al. (1931)	Poole (1934)	Templin (1957)	Prather et al. (1975)	Arlt & Goodban (1976)
	Age of Acquisition				
m	3	3½	3	2	3
n	3	4½	3	2	3
h	3	3½	3	2	3
p	4	3½	3	2	3
f	3	5½	3	2-4	3
w	3	3½	3	2-8	3
b	3	3½		2-8	3
ŋ		4½	3	2-8	3
j	4	4½	3½	2-4	
k	4	4½	4	2-4	3
g	4	4½	4	2-4	3
l	4	6½	6	3-4	4
d	5	4½	4	2-4	3
t	5	4½	6	2-8	3
s	5	7½	4½	3	4
r	5	7½	4	3	5
ʧ	5	4½		3-8	4
v	5	6½	6	4	3½
z	5	7½	7	4	4
ʒ	6	6½	7	4	4
θ		7½	6	4	5
ʤ		7	4	4	
ʃ		6½	4½	3-8	4½
ð		6½	7	4	5

and Reynolds extend data on consonants, some consonant clusters, and vowels. The Smit et al. study is also somewhat unique by offering information on word-initial consonant clusters in addition to singleton consonants.

Fudala and Reynolds's (1986) developmental information is based on the data they collected for standardization of the second edition of the *Arizona Articulation Proficiency Scale*. Their normative data are based on a sample of 5,122 children drawn from four states in the western United States. The study population used for the development of their standardized articulation test ranged in age from 1 year, 6 months, to 13 years, 11 months. They analyzed sound production in the initial and medial positions of words and considered a sound mastered when 90% of the children in a given age group produced the sound correctly in a specific position. The information in the following table was reported (a slash mark indicates that the sound does not occur or was not tested in that position).

Sound	Age of Mastery	
	Initial Position	**Final Position**
h	1½	—
w	1½	—
m	2½	1½
f	2½	3
k	2½	3
b	2	3
n	2	2
g	2½	3
j	3	—
d	2½	2½
p	2	3
ŋ	—	3
t	3	4
l	5	5
ʤ	5	—
v	5½	5½
r	5½	—
ð	5½	—
hw	6	—
ʧ	5½	5½
θ	6	6
ʃ	5½	5½
z	11	11
s	11	11

It is interesting to note the ages of acquisition for /s/ and /z/ offered by Fudala and Reynolds. In comparison to other studies, their age of mastery for these sounds appears to be quite late. A careful analysis of their actual data revealed an interesting pattern. The 90% mastery criterion was originally reached for initial [z-] and [s-] by the 6-0 to 6-5 age group. The actual percentage of children producing the sound correctly at that age was 93.3% for both sounds. However, as the groups got older the percentage of children who produced the sound correctly decreased to less than 90% (as low as 62% for the 7-0 to 7-11 age group). These data seem to indicate that the production of those sounds could be expected to decline as children get older. The percentage began to gradually increase again at 8-0 to 8-11 years until 98.4% of the 11-0 to 11-11 group produced the sound correctly. Similar results were obtained for final [-z] and [-s].

Fudala and Reynolds concluded that those sounds show "two cycles of development." The first cycle ends at approximately age 6, and the second cycle ends at about age 11. The authors concluded that "the developmental cycle stops with the loss of the central incisors" (p. 19). Our own clinical experience with young children would seem to support Fudala and Reynolds's conclusion that as children get older and lose their deciduous central incisors (a process that usually begins at about 6 years), their production of /s/ and /z/ may be compromised. This is an important diagnostic variable that should be considered in the evaluation process.

Smit et al. (1990) provided some normative information on the acquisition of speech sounds in children residing in Iowa and Nebraska. Their study population ranged in age from 3 to 9 years. They developed and used an assessment instrument that tested all word-initial and word-final consonant singletons with the exception of /ʒ/ and word-final /ð/. They also assessed production of intervocalic /r/ and /l/, syllabic /l/, postvocalic /ɚ/, and several word-initial consonant clusters. Because they found a statistically significant difference on sound acquisition according to gender in the preschool age groups, their data were presented in two groups: male and female. Smit et al. provided information on sound acquisition at a 75% level primarily for comparison with Templin's (1957) data. However, their recommended clinical age of mastery was based on 90% levels of acquisition. If the 90% acquisition criterion is applied to Smit et al.'s original data, the information in the following table can be drawn.

Sound	Age of Mastery	
	Male Group	**Female Group**
h-	≤3-0	≤3-0
w-	≤3-0	≤3-0
j-	3-6	4-0
m-	3-6	≤3-0
-m	≤3-0	≤3-0
n-	≤3-0	3-6
-n	≤3-0	3-6
-ŋ	>9-0*	>9-0*
b-	≤3-0	≤3-0
-b	≤3-0	≤3-0
p-	3-6	≤3-0
-p	≤3-0	≤3-0
g-	4-0	≤3-0
-g	≤3-0	4-0
t-	3-6	≤3-0
-t	4-0	4-0
d-	≤3-0	≤3-0
-d	3-6	≤3-0
k-	4-0	≤3-0
-k	≤3-0	≤3-0
f-	4-0	3-6
-f	5-6	5-6

(continues)

Sound	Age of Mastery	
	Male Group	**Female Group**
v-	5-6	4-6
-v	5-6	4-6
θ-	7-0*	6-0
-θ	7-0*	6-0
ð-	7-0*	4-6
s-	9-0*	9-0*
-s	9-0*	9-0*
z-	9-0*	9-0*
-z	>9-0*	>9-0*
ʃ-	7-0*	6-0
-ʃ	7-0*	6-0
ʧ-	7-0*	5-6
-ʧ	7-0*	6-0
ʤ-	6-0	4-6
-ʤ	7-0*	6-0
l-	6-0	5-0
-l	7-0*	6-0
-l-	6-0	5-6
r-	8-0*	8-0*
-ɚ	8-0*	8-0*
-r	8-0*	8-0*

Note. x- = prevocalic
-x = postvocalic
-x- = intervocalic

*Beginning with the 7-0 age group, the data represent the average of males and females. The authors did not separate the data according to male and female performance. We presumed this to be the age of acquisition.

When they are examined closely, it is noted that with a few exceptions the earlier studies of the 1930s and 1950s report later ages of sound acquisition when compared to more recent studies. Again, this is probably due to methodological differences. As good clinical practice, we recommend that the more recent and updated information be used during the diagnostic and therapeutic decision-making process. It should be emphasized, though, that despite the differences in the reported ages of acquisition for specific phonemes from one study to another, the order of acquisition of sounds and sound classes was significantly similar: stops, nasals, and glides are mastered earlier, followed by liquids, fricatives, and affricates.

When the various studies are considered, several generalizations can be made:

• **By age 3-0,** consistent production of the following sounds can be expected: /h/, /w/, /m/, /n/, /b/, /p/, and /f/.

• **By age 4-0,** consistent production of the above sounds plus the following can be expected: /d/, /t/, /j/, /k/, /g/, and /ŋ/.

• **By age 6-0,** consistent production of the following sounds in addition to those already given can be expected: /l/, /ʤ/, /ʧ/, /ʃ/, and /v/. Errors on /r/, /s/, /z/, /θ/, /ð/, and /ʒ/ may persist.

- **By age 8-0 through 9-0,** a child can be expected to closely match the adult standard for the production of all consonant sounds.

Range of Development

Because norms are based on statistical averages that apply to large groups of children, articulation studies using this research method provide specific ages of sound acquisition. However, individual performance is not very predictable based on normative data. Individual children may vary in the development of articulatory skills. Some children may begin using a sound at a given age but not master that sound until a few months or a few years later. Sander (1972) tried to counteract some of these problems by reanalyzing the Wellman et al. (1931) and Templin (1957) normative data to provide an age range rather than a specific age of development.

Sander suggested that the findings of the early developmental studies would be more useful if they were presented according to the **age of customary production** (the age at which 50% of the children tested produced the sound correctly in at least two positions) and the **age of mastery** (the age at which 90% of the children produced the sound correctly in all three positions). Sander's reinterpretation of the Wellman et al. and Templin data is presented in Table 3.2.

Sander's data are clinically significant in that they provide a range of sound acquisition. The presentation of age ranges allows a clinician to see development as a gradual process that may differ from one child to another. If strictly adhering to a criterion based on correct production by nearly all children (e.g., 90%), some children with potential speech delays may be missed; a specific age of mastery could obscure the fact that 50% of children achieve mastery at an earlier age. In other cases, children who simply demonstrate developmentally appropriate errors may be diagnosed with an articulation disorder.

Table 3.2. Age of Customary Production and Age of Mastery for English Consonants According to Sander (1972)

Age	Consonants Customarily Produced (at least 50% correct production)	Consonants Mastered (at least 90% correct production)
Under 2-0	p, b, m, n, w, h[a]	
2-0	t, d, k, g, ŋ	
3-0	f, s, r, l, j	p, m, n, w, h
4-0	v, z, ʃ, ʧ, ʤ	b, d, k, g, f, j
5-0	θ, ð	
6-0	ʒ[b]	t, ŋ, r, l
7-0		θ, ʃ, ʧ, ʤ
8-0		v, ð, s

Note. Adapted from *Normal and Disordered Phonology in Children* (Table 2.3, p. 31), by C. Stoel-Gammon and C. Dunn, 1985, Austin, TX: PRO-ED. Copyright 1985 by PRO-ED, Inc. Reprinted with permission.

[a]These consonants exceeded 70% correct production at 2-0, the youngest level tested.

[b]This consonant was not "mastered" by 8-0 and therefore does not appear in the right-hand column.

If we select one sound in particular from Sander's data, /r/ for example, it becomes evident that the range of acquisition may extend over several years. Whereas only 50% of children can be expected to produce /r/ correctly at age 3, by 6 years of age nearly 90% of children produce this sound correctly. In general, the time span between the age of customary production and the age of mastery is greater for fricatives and affricates, especially for /s/ (Stoel-Gammon & Dunn, 1985). Again, this highlights the fact that sound acquisition is a gradual process, and children cannot be expected to adhere to a specific mastery criterion.

A reanalysis of Fudala and Reynolds's (1986) information according to an age range of acquisition was performed for comparison with Sander's data. We chose to use an age of development, age of routine production, and age of mastery criterion. *Age of development* reflects the age at which 50% of the children produced the sound correctly in initial and final positions. *Age of routine production* and *age of mastery* are considered the ages at which 75% and 90% of the children produced the sound correctly in the initial and final positions, respectively. Refer to Table 3.3 for this information.

Table 3.3. Age of Development, Age of Routine Production, and Age of Mastery of English Consonants

Age	Consonants Developed (at least 50% correct production)	Consonants Routinely Produced (at least 75% correct production)	Consonants Mastered (at least 90% correct production)
Under 1-6 to 1-11	f, k, g, j, d, ŋ, t[a]	m, b, n, p[b]	h, w[c]
2-0 to 2-5	l, ʤ, ð	f, k, b, g, j, d, ŋ, t	m, b, n, p
2-6 to 2-11			f, g, d
3-0 to 3-5	v, r		k, j, ŋ, t
3-6 to 4-0	ʧ, ʃ, s		
4-0 to 4-5	z	θ[d], ʤ, v, ʧ	l[e]
4-6 to 4-11	hw	r	ð[e]
5-0 to 5-5		ʃ	ʤ
5-6 to 5-11		hw	v, r, ʧ, ʃ
6-0 to 6-5			θ, z,[f] s,[f] hw
6-6 to 6-11			
7-0 to 7-11			
8-0 to 8-11		z, s	
9-0 to 9-11			
10-0 to 10-11			
11-0 to 11-11			z,[f] s[f]

Note. The data for this table were obtained from Fudala and Reynolds (1986).

[a]These phonemes ranged from 58 to 88% correct production at 1-6, the youngest age group tested.

[b]These phonemes exceeded 78% correct production at 1-6, the youngest age group tested.

[c]These phonemes exceeded 90% correct production at 1-6, the youngest age group tested.

[d]This phoneme never reached 50% correct production prior to reaching 75% correct production. The highest production level prior to 75% correct production was 47%.

[e]These phonemes advanced from 50% correct production to 90% correct production. The 75% correct production criterion was not reached prior to 90% correct production.

[f]The phonemes /s/ and /z/ appeared to have undergone two cycles of acquisition. The initial mastery criterion was reached by 6-0, but the percentage of children producing the sounds correctly decreased to below 65% at 7-0 and then gradually increased until 90% correct production was again reached at 11-0.

As in Sander's study, application of a range of development to Fudala and Reynolds's original data revealed that the age of development and the age of mastery for fricatives and affricates may span a long period of time, up to 3 years for sounds like /v/, /ʤ/, /ð/, /s/, and /z/. Also the data were similar for both studies, with a few exceptions, in that two major groups of mastery could be identified:

- earlier mastered sounds: j, w, m, n, ŋ, p, b, k, g, d, t, f, h
- later mastered sounds: l, r, ð, θ, ʧ, ʤ, ʃ, ʒ, s, z, v

Longitudinal Studies

Another method that has been used to study the development of speech sounds has been the **longitudinal method.** Using this research method, investigators set out to study the acquisition process by following a few children for an extended period of time. Unlike cross-sectional studies, in longitudinal studies spontaneous speech samples from the same child are recorded frequently to trace the development of speech sounds. Although longitudinal studies cannot provide norms, they do provide more specific information regarding the individual acquisition process of speech sounds.

Stoel-Gammon performed such a study in 1985. She investigated the phonetic inventories of 34 children (19 boys and 15 girls) between the ages of 15 and 24 months. Using spontaneous speech samples, she investigated the range and type of consonantal phones in the inventory of children using meaningful speech. All children were 9 months of age at the beginning of data collection. The samples were collected every 3 months, at ages 9, 12, 15, 18, 21, and 24 months.

Although Stoel-Gammon collected data for both prelinguistic vocalizations and meaningful speech, she limited her analysis to the meaningful speech productions. Her criterion for meaningful speech was the spontaneous production of at least 10 identifiable words during a 1-hour recording session. Because children reached this criterion at different age levels, the number of children in the 15-, 18-, 21-, and 24-month age groups varied. At 15 months, only 7 children had reached the criterion, while at 18 and 21 months, respectively, 19 children and 32 children had reached the criterion. At 24 months, only 1 child had not reached the meaningful speech criterion. This clearly highlights the reality of individual variability in the acquisition of speech and language skills.

Stoel-Gammon analyzed the data according to each child's phonetic inventory in word-initial and word-final positions. Singleton phones were considered part of the child's inventory when they occurred in a given position in at least two different words. Although individual variability was recorded, Stoel-Gammon reported that the early phonetic inventories in the initial position of words were primarily voiced anterior stops, nasals, and glides. By 24 months, voiceless stops, velars, and a few fricatives were included in the initial position. In the final position, the children's phonetic inventories were made up primarily of voiceless stops and alveolar consonants. Voiced stops tended to appear first in the initial position, while /t/ and /r/ appeared first in the final position. The following specific patterns were identified in the study:

- At 15 months of age /b/, /d/, and /h/ were in the inventories of 50% of the subjects in the initial position. In the final position, no sounds met the criterion.

• At 18 months of age /b/, d/, /m/, /n/, /h/, and /w/ were in the inventories of 50% of the subjects in the initial position. In the final position, /t/ was the only phone in the inventory of 50% of the subjects.

• At 21 months of age /b/, /t/, /d/, /m/, /n/, and /h/ were in the inventories of 50% of the subjects in the initial position. In the final position, only /t/ and /n/ were in the inventories of 50% of the subjects.

• At 24 months of age /b/, /t/, /d/, /k/, /g/, /m/, /n/, /h/, /w/, /f/, and /s/ were in the inventories of 50% of the subjects. In the final position, /p/, /t/, /k/, /n/, /r/, and /s/ were in the inventories of 50% of the subjects.

As can be determined from the above information, the subjects' phonetic inventory was significantly larger in the initial position of words. This is not surprising since children at this age tend to use open-syllable words more often than closed-syllable words, where final consonants would be expected to occur. Also, the subjects' phonetic inventories increased from means of 3.4 and 0.6, respectively, in word-initial and word-final positions at 15 months to means of 9.5 and 5.7 at 24 months.

Although Stoel-Gammon's data demonstrated much individual variability, the results are somewhat comparable with some of the large-scale cross-sectional studies in that they substantiated the early development of stops, nasals, and glides. In regard to the ages at which 50% of the subjects produced particular phones, this study is most comparable to Sander's (1972) and Fudala and Reynolds's (1986) information on phoneme mastery for children at 2 years of age.

Consonant Clusters

A review of the existing literature revealed very little information on the development of consonant clusters. Most cross-sectional studies provided information on the development of singleton consonant phonemes. Templin's (1957) study did include norms on the mastery of initial- and final-consonant clusters as well as single consonants. As in single phonemes, consonant clusters were considered mastered when 75% of the subjects produced them correctly. The ages of mastery of clusters are presented in Table 3.4. Templin's findings revealed that by the age of 4-0, 75% of subjects correctly produced /s + stop/, /s + nasal/, /stop + liquid/ (except /gr/), and /stop + w/ initial clusters. Fewer final clusters had been mastered by the same age group, and the acquisition in terms of sound classes was less predictable. Mastery for 3-member clusters and clusters containing a fricative member continues through the age of 8.

Smit et al.'s (1990) previously described study also included data on the development of word-initial consonant clusters. Again, their study population ranged in age from 3 to 9 years. Because they found a statistically significant difference in sound acquisition according to gender in the preschool age groups, their data were presented in two groups: male and female. Although Smit et al. provided information on sound acquisition at a 75% level for comparison with Templin's (1957) data, their recommended clinical age of mastery was based on 90% levels of acquisition. If the 90% acquisition criterion is applied to Smit et al.'s original data, the following information can be drawn for prevocalic or word-initial clusters:

Consonant Cluster	Age of Mastery	
	Male Group	**Female Group**
tw-	3-6	4-0
kw-	5-6	4-0
sp-	9-0*	9-0*
st-	9-0*	9-0*
sk-	>9-0*	>9-0*
sm-	>9-0*	>9-0*
sn-	>9-0*	>9-0*
sw-	>9-0*	>9-0*
sl-	9-0	9-0
pl-	6-0	5-6
bl-	6-0	6-0
kl-	6-0	5-0
gl-	6-0	6-0
fl-	7-0*	5-6
pr-	8-0*	8-0*
br-	8-0*	8-0*
tr-	8-0*	8-0*
dr-	8-0*	8-0*
kr-	8-0*	8-0*
gr-	8-0*	8-0*

Consonant Cluster	Age of Mastery	
	Male Group	**Female Group**
fr-	8-0*	8-0*
θr-	>9-0*	>9-0*
skw-	9-0*	9-0*
spl-	9-0*	9-0*
spr-	>9-0*	>9-0*
str-	>9-0*	>9-0*
skr-	>9-0*	>9-0*

*Beginning with the 7-0 age group, the data represent the average of males and females. The authors did not separate the data according to male and female performance. We assumed this to be the age of acquisition.

As in the development of single phonemes, longitudinal studies (e.g., Greenlee, 1974; Moskowitz, 1973) have revealed individual differences in the rate and order of consonant cluster acquisition. As evidenced by the scant data, further research is needed before any conclusive statements can be made on the acquisition of consonant clusters. Thus, the data offered by Templin (1957) and Smit et al. (1990) should be used with caution.

Table 3.4. Age of Mastery of Consonant Clusters According to Templin (1957)

Age	Initial Clusters	Final Clusters
4-0	pl, bl, kl, gl pr, br, tr, dr, kr tw, kw sm, sn, sp, st, sk	mp, mpt, mps, ngk lp, lt, rm, rt, rk pt, ks ft
5-0	gr, fl, fr, str	lb, lf rd, rf, rn
6-0	skw	lk rb, rg, rθ, rdʒ, rst, rtʃ nt, nd, nθ
7-0	spl, spr, skr sl, sw ʃr, θr	sk, st, kst lθ, lz dʒd
8-0		kt, sp

Note. A cluster is "mastered" when produced by 75% of the subjects. The clusters are listed cumulatively; only newly mastered clusters are listed for each age. Adapted from *Normal and Disordered Phonology in Children* (Table 2.5, p. 33), by C. Stoel-Gammon and C. Dunn, 1985, Austin, TX: PRO-ED. Copyright 1985 by PRO-ED, Inc. Reprinted with permission.

Vowels

The acquisition of vowels is another area of phonemic development that has been historically neglected (Bauman-Waengler, 1994). This area of development has been primarily discounted due to reports by many researchers that children acquire all of the English vowels by the age of 3 (e.g., Templin, 1957). Little information is available on the order and rate of vowel acquisition before the age of 3, a time in which children appear to be undergoing major development.

In 1983 Irwin and Wong edited a textbook that contains a series of studies. Those studies focused on the phonological development of children between the ages of 18 and 72 months. A total of 100 children participated in the study, with 10 males and 10 females in each of the following age groups: 18 months, 2 years, 3 years, 4 years, and 6 years. A total of five investigators collected the data, one per age group. However, the same data collection and analysis procedures were used for all groups. In regard to the development of vowels and diphthongs, the studies lend support to the common notion that vowels develop quite early. By the age of 3, individual children and the total group of 20 produced all of the vowels and diphthongs with 99–100% accuracy. At 2 years of age, all vowels and diphthongs were produced with at least 80% accuracy with the exception of /ɚ/ and /ɝ/. At 18 months of age only /ɑ/, /u/, /i/, and /ʌ/ were produced with at least 70% accuracy.

Fudala and Reynolds (1986), in the second edition of the *Arizona Articulation Proficiency Scale,* also offer some developmental information on the acquisition of vowels. Their normative data are based on a sample of 5,122 children drawn from four states in the western United States. The study population used for the development of their standardized articulation test ranged in age from 1 year, 6 months, to 13 years, 11 months.

When applying a 90% mastery criterion to their data— 90% of the subjects in a given age group produced the sound correctly—all of the target vowels and diphthongs developed quite early. An exception to this was the mid-central vowels /ɝ/ and /ɚ/ and the rhotic diphthongs /ɪr/, /ɛr/, /or/, and /ar/. The following vowels and diphthongs all reached the 90% mastery criterion by the youngest age group of 1-6 to 1-11: /ə/, /ʌ/, /ɛ/, /a/, /æ/, /ɔ/, /ɪ/, /i/, /ʊ/, /u/, /ou/, /ai/, /ei/, and /au/. The actual percentage of children producing each of these vowels correctly in the youngest age group ranged from 97.7 to 100.

The mid-central vowels /ɝ/ and /ɚ/ did not reach the mastery criterion of 90% until the 5-6 to 5-11 age group. The rhotic diphthongs also reached the mastery criterion at the 5-6 to 5-11 age group, with the exception of /ɛr/, which reached the 90% acquisition level at the 4-6 to 4-11 group. In summary, from this information it can be gathered that most vowels and diphthongs develop very early in a child's phonological system with the exception of rhotic vowels and diphthongs. This helps explain why the vowelization phonological process, or the substitution of /a/, /u/, and /ou/ for /ɝ/ and /ɚ/, persists for several years.

Despite the apparent evidence that all vowels are mastered early in development, further research is needed in this area. A more specific order and rate of development are needed. Patterns in vowel substitutions may also be clinically relevant, especially with phonologically delayed children, who often show a disordered vowel system.

Common Error Types

What types of errors can be expected to occur on specific sounds or particular sound classes? Experienced clinicians' own interactions with children probably help them answer that question. Students, however, may have a more difficult time. Smit (1993a, 1993b) attempted to provide some of this information by reanalyzing the data offered by Smit et al. in their 1990 Iowa-Nebraska articulation study. The most common error patterns outlined by Smit are summarized below; others have reported similar error patterns (e.g., Bassi, 1983; Dyson, 1986; Hare, 1983; Irwin & Wong, 1983; Macken & Barton, 1980; Olmsted, 1971; Singh & Frank, 1972).

Nasals

• Denasalization of /m/ and /n/ (the replacement of a nasal consonant by a non-nasal sound made in the same place of articulation such as [doz] for *nose*).

• Final /n/ replaced by [m] and [ŋ].

• Final /ŋ/ replaced by [n].

Glides

• Deletion of /w/, /j/, and /hw/.

• Substitution of [w], [d], [h], and [l] for /j/.

Stops

• Deaspiration of initial voiceless stops. This is also known as initial-consonant voicing, or the replacement of a voiced for a voiceless consonant.

- Fronting of initial velars to alveolars common. Fronting affects initial stops more commonly than final stops.

- Deletion of final stops. Deletions are less common for velars than for labial or alveolar stops.

Liquids

- Substitution of [w] for initial /l/ and /r/.

- Deletion of initial liquids.

- Substitution of a rounded vowel and schwa for final /l/ and /r/.

- Deletion of final /l/ and /r/.

Labial and Dental Fricatives

- Substitution of stops for fricatives, primarily initial fricatives.

- Substitution of [f] for /θ/.

- Substitution of [b] for initial and final /v/.

- Substitution of fricatives for other fricatives (e.g., [f] for /v/ and [f] for /θ/).

- Substitution of a fricative [s, f] for initial /θ/ and substitution of a stop [d] for its voiced cognate /ð/.

Alveolar and Palatal Fricatives and Affricates

- Deletion of final fricatives /s/, /z/, /ʃ/.

- Stopping of fricatives and affricates in the youngest age groups, primarily in the initial position.

- Devoicing of final /z/ and /dʒ/. Can also affect initial /z/.

- Depalatalization of initial and final palatals /ʃ/, /tʃ/, /dʒ/. Manner of production is preserved.

- Deaffrication of initial and final /tʃ/.

- Stopping of initial /s/.

- Dental distortions of /s/ (dental and interdental variants, including /θ/ and /ð/).

Consonant Clusters

- A tendency for obstruent + /w/ clusters to be reduced to the obstruent.

- A tendency for obstruent + /l/ clusters to be reduced to the obstruent. An exception to this is the /fl/ cluster, which tends to be reduced to an approximant [w].

- A tendency for obstruent + /r/ clusters to be reduced to the obstruent (sometimes the remaining obstruent is a substitute for the clustered obstruent).

- A tendency for clusters made up of /s/ + consonant to be reduced to the [w], nasal, or stop component of the cluster.

- Three major error patterns expected on three-member clusters:

  1. When children reduce the cluster to a single element, they usually retain the stop or a stop substitute.

  2. When children reduce the cluster to two elements, a wide variety of errors can be expected, but the most common is the preservation of a stop at the appropriate place of articulation together with the **approximant** (or its substitute).

  3. When all three members are preserved, the /s/ and the approximant (especially /r/) become vulnerable to errors that are typical for that consonant, such as dentalized [s] and [w] for /r/.

Patterns of Development

The information previously discussed addressed speech sound acquisition in an isolated manner by delineating specific ages of acquisition for individual phonemes. In that method of analysis, patterns of development are not well represented. Patterns of correct and incorrect productions have received increasing attention in the past few years. Researchers have looked at patterns of sound production in terms of sound classes, distinctive features, and phonological processes.

Development of Sound Classes

Despite some differences in ages of sound mastery in many of the cross-sectional studies, a pattern of sound class acquisition was noted. Nasal, stops, and glides are mastered early. Liquids, fricatives, and affricates generally develop later.

Nasal consonants are among the earliest to develop. Within the sound class, /m/ and /n/ are mastered quite early, at about 3 years of age, while /ŋ/ is mastered a bit later, at about 3 to 4 years. *Stops* are also acquired very early, with /p/ and /b/ being the earliest mastered within the sound class, at about 2 to 3 years. There is no specific order of acquisition for the alveolar stops /t/, /d/ or velar stops /k/, /g/. Great individual variation has been noted in the acquisition of the alveolar and velar stops; children develop /t/ and /d/ prior to /k/ and /g/ and vice versa. In her study on the acquisition of velars by 2-year-old children, Dyson (1986) found that final velars are acquired before initial velars. In addition to nasals and stops, *glides* are early-developing sounds. The /w/ consonant is mastered by about 2 years, while /j/ is mastered at about 3 years of age.

Fricatives, affricates, and liquids are the later-developing sound classes, although there is much variation in the acquisition of individual sounds within each class. The *fricative* sound class is quite large, containing nine consonants /h/, /s/, /z/, /f/, /v/, /ʃ/, /ʒ/, /θ/ /ð/. The affricate /tʃ/, /dʒ/ and liquid /l/, /r/ sound classes have only two sounds each. Among the fricatives, /h/ and /f/ are among the earliest mastered, at about 3 and 4 years, respectively. The remaining fricatives develop somewhat later, between the ages of 4 and 6. The fricatives /ʒ/, /θ/, and /ð/ tend to be mastered the latest by most children. The *affricates* /tʃ/ and /dʒ/ are both mastered at about 6 years of age. The *liquids* /l/ and /r/ are also mastered quite late, at approximately 6 years of age. Errors of /l/ and /r/ are not uncommon among preschool and early school-age children (Irwin & Wong, 1983; Kenney & Prather, 1986; Olmsted, 1971).

Development of Distinctive Features

A child's articulation and phonological development has also been described according to the acquisition of distinctive features (Menyuk, 1968; Prather, Hedrick, & Kern, 1975; Singh, 1976; Blache, 1982). In Chapter 2 we defined distinctive features as articulatory or acoustic characteristics that are present or absent in a particular phoneme or group of phonemes. Research on the development of various distinctive features has focused on the ages at which children can be expected to use specific features in their sound system.

Menyuk (1968) conducted one of the earliest studies on the acquisition of distinctive features. Using Jakobson, Fant, and Halle's (1952) distinctive feature system, she analyzed the use of several distinctive features by American preschool children between the ages of 2½ and 5 years. After collecting spontaneous speech samples, Menyuk analyzed those samples for the presence of the following features: gravity, diffuseness, voicing, continuancy, stridency, and nasality. She determined the percentage of sounds containing each feature that were used by the children at varying ages. After her analysis, Menyuk advanced the following rank order of distinctive feature mastery, from earliest to latest development:

1. **+nasal**—sounds resonated in the nasal cavity
2. **+grave**—sounds produced at the very front
3. **+voice**—sounds produced with vibration of the vocal folds
4. **+diffuse**—sounds made at the very back
5. **+strident**—sounds made by forcing the airstream through a small opening, resulting in the production of intense noise
6. **+continuant**—sounds that are made with an incomplete point of constriction, thus not entirely stopping the flow of air at any point

After collecting information on the acquisition of consonant segments in children aged 2 to 4, Prather, Hedrick, and Kern (1975) analyzed their data according to the presence of distinctive features. They applied the same feature analysis system used by Menyuk (1968). Prather et al. found a similar rank order of acquisition, with the exception of the continuant and strident features. Their order of acquisition was as follows: +nasal, +grave, +diffuse, +voice, +continuant, and +strident.

Blache (1982) advanced various stages of distinctive feature acquisition based on the information of early psychoacoustic research, Jakobson's phonological acquisition model, and Wellman, Case, Mengert, and Bradbury's (1931), Poole's (1934), and Templin's (1957) developmental studies. He developed the following six stages of systematic growth in children's phonemic acquisition: (1) primitive, (2) vocalic, (3) stop-nasal, (4) semivowel, (5) continuant, and (6) sibilant.

Primitive System

The primitive stage progresses between the prelinguistic period and 2 years of age. During this stage the child develops control of the nasal-nonnasal and labial-lingual features. The child typically produces four utterance types:

1. a nasal, labial utterance, which is usually an [m];
2. a nasal, lingual utterance, which is usually an [n];

3. a nonnasal, labial utterance, which is usually a [p]; and
4. a nonnasal, lingual utterance, which is usually a [t].

Vocalic System

The vocalic system is typically completed by the end of year 3. During this stage, the development of the vowel system is completed. The child initially learns distinctions between high-front, low-front, high-back, and low-back vowel utterances, with finer distinctions learned later. Many vowels are still confused with each other; but high vowels are typically not confused with low vowels, and front vowels are not confused with back vowels.

Stop-Nasal System

The stop-nasal system is usually learned by 4 years of age. This stage results in finer distinctions of the nasal-nonnasal and the labial-lingual features. Stops and nasals are now distinguished by a three-point place of articulation scheme: lip, front of the tongue, and back of the tongue. Stops are further distinguished by an additional manner of production feature: voiced versus voiceless. The result of this distinction is a nine-category consonantal system. The development of such distinctive features constitutes the use of the following phonemes: [m], [n], [ŋ], [p], [b], [k], [g], [d], and [t].

Semivowel System

The semivowel system is learned near the end of year 4. At this stage, the child will establish production of consonants with vowel-like characteristics. Semivowels are organized into a three-point place of articulation scheme similar to that of stops and nasals. The development of this distinctive feature adds the semivowels [w], [j], [l], and [r] to the sound system used by the end of the stop-nasal system.

Continuant System

The child begins controlling the continuant system by the end of year 5. This stage marks the introduction of the continuant feature, which greatly expands the child's sound system. The development of the continuant feature increases the child's phonetic system by about 50% to include [f], [v], [s], [z], [ʃ], [ʒ], [tʃ], and [dʒ]. At the end of this stage, the layperson perceives few articulatory errors. The professional may note a developmental "lisp" and general difficulty with sibilants.

Sibilant System

The sibilant system is established after the age of 6 years. It is developed when the child learns the strident–mellow feature; it is a refinement of the continuancy feature. Strident sounds are continuants that are made with an unobstructed airflow striking the teeth; these include [f], [v], [s], [z], [ʃ], [ʒ], [tʃ], and [dʒ]. Mellow sounds are made with a slightly obstructed airflow against the teeth; these are /θ/ and /ð/. At this stage, the child separates the sounds with voiced–voiceless and front–back tongue contrasts. Failure to develop the front–back tongue contrast may result in a "lateral lisp." Failure to develop the stridency feature may result in an interdental lisp.

Phonological Processes in Normal Development

Since Stampe (1969) pioneered the notion of phonological processes, more recent developmental research has focused on gathering information about the productive duration and elimination (or suppression) of such processes. We defined several phonological processes in the Basic Unit of Chapter 2. Less common processes are examined in Appendix C. The reader is referred to that information for a review of the definitions offered for individual simplification processes.

Several investigators have attempted to describe the phonological processes that characterize children's speech in the normal course of development. In Chapter 2 we defined phonological processes as systematic sound changes that affect classes of sounds and the syllable structure of words. The processes that have been found to occur in the speech of children with normally developing phonological skills and those with phonological disorders have been categorized according to syllable structure processes, substitution processes, and assimilation processes (Ingram, 1976; Stoel-Gammon & Dunn, 1985; Lowe, 1994). Processes that have been reported to occur in young children have been outlined as follows:

Syllable Structure Processes

- final-consonant deletion
- cluster reduction
- unstressed-syllable deletion
- reduplication
- epenthesis

Substitution Processes

- stopping
- liquid gliding
- vocalization
- depalatalization
- velar fronting
- deaffrication
- stridency deletion

Assimilation Processes

- labial assimilation
- velar assimilation
- nasal assimilation
- voicing assimilation

The most widespread processes in the normal development of phonological skills include final-consonant deletion, cluster reduction, unstressed-syllable deletion, stopping, fronting, and liquid gliding (Stoel-Gammon & Dunn, 1985; Grunwell, 1987; Ingram, 1976). These processes are present in the speech of nearly all children.

Although certain processes have been noted to occur more frequently in normally developing children, limited and often contradictory information currently exists on the developmental appearance, productive duration, and suppression of phonological processes. The different age levels at which the processes appear and are eventually eliminated are not clearly identified. The information advanced by several researchers poses the problem of not being directly comparable since differing criteria have been used to identify when a process is occurring. Also, the establishment of varying terminology and definitions to refer to similar processes from one study to another creates problems for a direct comparison. With this in mind, we will provide a chronological review of the information available on the use of phonological processes in normally developing children.

Ingram (1976) gathered information on the phonological skills of English- and non-English-speaking children from various sources. He identified several phonological processes that characterize the speech of children from 1 year, 6 months, to 4 years. He provided ages at which children are likely to use the phonological processes; however, this was not consistently done for each of the processes. Some of the developmental information offered was also vague, with statements such as "may occur late in development" and "may persist over several years." This is likely due to a lack of specific data in this area of development, especially at the time that Ingram collected such information.

Grunwell (1982) offered a chronology highlighting the gradual disappearance of the phonological processes common in the normal development of young children. She outlined these "simplifying processes" as: weak-syllable deletion, final-consonant deletion, reduplication, consonant harmony, cluster reduction, stopping, fronting, gliding, and context-sensitive voicing. A summary of this information is found in Figure 3.1. If we follow one of the phonological processes depicted by Grunwell, weak-syllable deletion, the figure would read in the following manner:

• The solid black line progressing across the age band of 2-0 to 2-6 and 3-0 to 3-6 indicates that weak-syllable deletion can be expected to occur at this age.

• The broken line between the ages of 3-6 and 4-0 indicates that weak-syllable deletion begins to disappear at this age level and is probably eliminated after 4 years of age.

It should be noted that Grunwell (1982) provides developmental information on the use, productive duration, and eventual suppression of stopping for each specific fricative and affricate that can be affected by the process. This highlights the fact that although stopping is usually categorized as an individual process, its eventual elimination is gradual since the sounds affected are acquired at different ages. For example, we know from the classic sound segment studies that /f/ is one of the earliest developing fricatives, whereas /ð/ tends to develop somewhat later. Therefore, the suppression of stopping would be expected sooner on /f/ than on /ð/.

Hodson and Paden (1981) noted that the phonological processes known to affect intelligibility the most in young children were rarely used by the 60 "normally developing" intelligible children between the ages of 4 and 5 years in their study. Hodson and Paden indicated that by that age the "articulation" performance of the children in the study sample closely approximated the adult model (p. 371). They did note devoicing of final obstruents, production of anterior strident phonemes to replace nonstrident interdentals, liquid deviations, tongue protrusions, depalatalization, nasal assimilation, labial assimilation, velar assimilation, and metathesis in varying numbers of children. However, these deviations were judged not to greatly affect the children's intelligibility. Unfortunately, Hodson and Paden did not report their data according to the total number of instances in which a process was used by each group or by each child or the actual percentage of occurrences for each process.

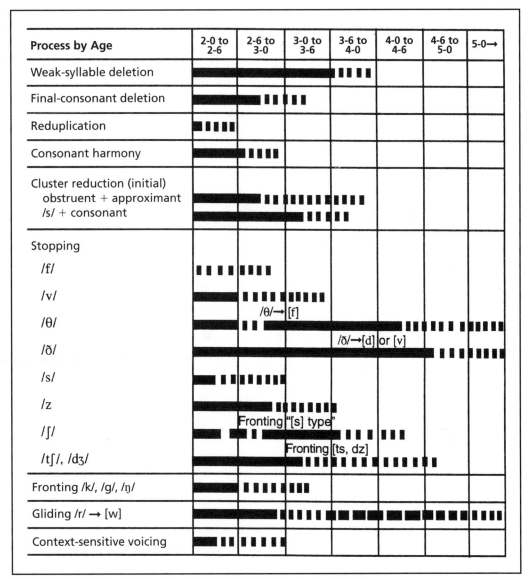

Figure 3.1. Chronology of the active duration and eventual suppression of various phonological processes. *Note.* From "Natural Phonology" (Table 3.3, p. 68), by P. Grunwell. In *The New Phonologies: Developments in Clinical Linguistics* edited by M. J. Ball and R. D. Kent, 1997, San Diego, CA: Singular Publishing Group. Copyright 1997 by Singular Publishing Group, Inc. Reprinted with permission.

Dyson and Paden (1983) investigated the elimination of the following five phonological processes by 40 2-year-old children: gliding, cluster reduction, fronting, stopping, and final-consonant deletion. Using 36 words to provide the opportunity for the occurrence of these five processes, they tested the children at 3-week intervals beginning at 2 years and ending 7 months later. Throughout the study, the processes were ordered from the most frequently occurring to the least frequently occurring. During the initial testing, the order for the frequency of occurrence was as follows: gliding, cluster reduction, fronting, stopping, and final-consonant deletion. During the last testing, at the age of 2 years, 7 months, the order remained the same. However, at that point Dyson and Paden found that final-consonant deletion was almost completely eliminated, fronting and stopping were infrequent, and gliding and cluster reduction were still common.

Lowe, Knutson, and Monson (1985) studied the incidence of fronting in 1,048 preschool children between the ages of 2 years, 7 months, and 4 years, 6 months. They observed fronting in 6% of the study participants and noted that velar fronting was more common than palatal fronting. They also noted that palatal fronting did not occur in the absence of velar fronting. They stated that fronting infrequently occurred after the age of 3 years, 6 months.

Haelsig and Madison (1986) investigated the occurrence of 16 phonological processes in 3-, 4-, and 5-year-old children. Fifty children were divided into five 6-month age groupings, resulting in the participation of 10 children in each of the following age groups: 3-0, 3-6, 4-0, 4-6, 5-0. Using the *Phonological Process Analysis* (Weiner, 1979), the investigators obtained the frequency of occurrence for the following phonological processes: weak-syllable deletion, cluster reduction, glottal replacement, deletion of final consonants, gliding of fricatives, labial assimilation, alveolar assimilation, vocalizations, fronting, velar assimilation, prevocalic voicing, final-consonant devoicing, stopping, affrication, denasalization, and gliding of liquids. McReynolds and Elbert (1981a) suggested that to qualify as a process, a specific phonological process must have a possibility of occurring four times and be used at least 20% of the time. If these criteria are applied to Haelsig and Madison's group performance across the various age groups, the following patterns can be identified:

• The 3-0 age group used final-consonant deletion, weak-syllable deletion, glottal replacement, cluster reduction, labial assimilation, vocalizations, and gliding of liquids in at least 20% of possible occurrences.

• The 3-6 age group used weak-syllable deletion, glottal replacement, cluster reduction, alveolar assimilation, stopping, vocalizations, and gliding of liquids in at least 20% of possible occurrences.

• The number of processes used at least 20% of the time significantly decreased in the 4-0 age group. The processes that met the criteria in this age group were weak-syllable deletion, vocalizations, and gliding of liquids.

• The 4-6 age group used only one process at least 20% of the time: weak-syllable deletion.

• The 5-0 age group did not use any processes in at least 20% of possible occurrences.

• Several processes were rarely used by any of the age groups, including fronting, final-consonant devoicing, velar assimilation, prevocalic voicing, gliding of fricatives, affrication, and denasalization.

Table 3.5 represents a reanalysis of Haelsig and Madison's data according to the average percentage of occurrence for each of the phonological processes that occurred at least 20% of the time in at least one of the five age groups. In this study, "the greatest reduction in use of the phonological processes occurred between 3 and 4 years" (p. 114). The investigators did note individual variation across the subjects and the five age groups, and they acknowledged that the sample size in this study was limited.

Table 3.5. Percentage of Occurrence of Phonological Processes in Children 3-0 to 5-0

Chronological Age Group	3-0	3-6	4-0	4-6	5-0
Phonological Process	**Mean Percentage of Occurrence**				
Deletion of final consonants	22	15	6	10	5
Weak-syllable deletion	38	31	26	28	13
Stopping	14	21	8	6	0
Glottal replacement	38	31	7	8	8
Liquid gliding	48	55	23	13	0
Vocalization	21	41	28	6	1
Alveolar assimilation	8	25	8	2	2
Labial assimilation	30	14	14	4	2

Note. From "A study of phonological processes exhibited by 3-, 4-, and 5-year-old children," by P. C. Haelsig and C. L. Madison, 1986, *Language, Speech, and Hearing Services in the Schools, 17,* pp. 107–114.

Preisser, Hodson, and Paden (1988) reported percentage-of-occurrence averages for eight phonological processes in 60 normally developing children. The subjects were divided into three age groups at 3-month age intervals as follows: 1-6 to 1-9, 1-10 to 2-1, and 2-2 to 2-5. Preisser et al. classified the phonological processes according to omissions and class deficiencies. Omissions included cluster reduction, postvocalic and prevocalic obstruent omission, and syllable reduction. Class deficiencies were categorized as liquid deviation, stridency deletion, velar deviation, and nasal-glide deviation. Table 3.6 outlines the data provided by Preisser et al. Using McReynolds and Elbert's (1981a) 20% criterion, the youngest age group of

Table 3.6. Percentage of Occurrence of Phonological Processes for Three Chronological Age Groups

	Chronological Ages (Number of Subjects)		
	1-6 to 1-9 (20)	1-10 to 2-1 (20)	2-2 to 2-5 (20)
Phonological Processes	**Percentage of Occurrence**		
Omissions			
Cluster reduction	93	76	51
Postvocalic obstruent	45	13	4
Syllable reduction	43	10	3
Prevocalic obstruent	14	12	3
Class Deficiencies			
Liquid deviation	91	75	64
Stridency deletion	56	41	23
Velar deviation	45	23	14
Nasal/glide deviation	49	23	11
Average	55	34	22

Note. Adapted from *Targeting Intelligible Speech: A Phonological Approach to Remediation* (2nd ed., Table 3, p. 66), by B. W. Hodson and E. P. Paden, 1991, Austin, TX: PRO-ED. Copyright 1991 by PRO-ED, Inc. Used with permission.

1-6 to 1-9 used all of the processes at a significant level, with the exception of prevocalic obstruent omission, which occurred at an average of 14%. By the oldest age group of 2-2 to 2-5, only liquid deviation, stridency deletion, and cluster reduction occurred at a significant level.

Roberts, Burchinal, and Foote (1990) conducted a more recent study. They investigated the phonological skills of children between 2 years, 5 months, and 8 years by testing them at varying times throughout the course of their study. As they followed the children's development, they noted a noticeable decline in the use of phonological processes between the ages of 2 years, 5 months, and 4 years. They reported that by age 4 only cluster reduction, liquid gliding, and deaffrication had an occurrence level of at least 20%.

In an attempt to provide some guidelines regarding the productive use and suppression of phonological processes, Stoel-Gammon and Dunn (1985) developed two major categories. Their now classic information divides phonological processes according to those that are likely to disappear by 3 years and those that would be expected to persist beyond the age of 3. The data previously reviewed would seem to support Stoel-Gammon and Dunn's primary divisions.

Processes Disappearing by 3 Years	**Processes Persisting After 3 Years**
• unstressed-syllable deletion	• cluster reduction
• final-consonant deletion	• epenthesis
• doubling	• gliding
• diminutization	• vocalization
• velar fronting	• stopping
• consonant assimilation	• depalatalization
• reduplication	• final devoicing
• prevocalic voicing	

Speech Intelligibility

The use of phonological processes to simplify the adult form along with the incorrect use of individual phonemes will undoubtedly affect a child's intelligibility level. As the child begins to master individual phonemes and suppress the use of various phonological processes, speech intelligibility is likely to improve. Therefore, how understandable a child is seems to be directly affected by the development of articulation and phonological skills.

So how intelligible can we expect children to be in the normal course of development? Shipley and McAfee (1998) offer some cursory percentages of speech intelligibility for different age levels. According to them, a child at 19 to 24 months would be 25–50% intelligible to strangers, at 2 to 3 years would be 50–75% intelligible, at 3 to 4 years would be 80% intelligible, and at 4 to 5 years would be 90–100% intelligible. Vihman and Greenlee' s (1987) study with 10 3-year-old children revealed an average level of intelligibility of 73% for that age group. It should be noted, however, that the range was quite broad, from 54% to 80%. Gordon-Brannan (1994) reported a level of intelligibility for 4-year-old children. She found a mean percentage of intelligibility of 93% for that age group, with a range of 73% to 100%. The range of intelligibility reported by these studies highlights the prevalence of individual variability among children.

Anecdotal data, clinical experience, and parental reports support the notion that by 5 years of age, normally developing children are nearly 100% understandable. However, that a child is understood 90–100% of the time by the age of 5 years does not suggest that the child has "perfect" speech. It simply means that the child is understood most of the time despite the possible presence of some developmentally appropriate misarticulations. Speech intelligibility is likely to vary from child to child according to his or her articulation and phonological development.

Easy Reference for Speech Intelligibility Expectations

Age	Intelligibility Level
19–24 months	25–50%
2–3 years	50–75%
4–5 years	75–90%
5+ years	90–100% (a few articulation errors may persist)

Development in the School Years: Phonological Awareness and the Acquisition of Reading

The mastery of some individual speech sounds and the suppression of some phonological processes may continue into the early elementary school years. A few fricatives, the affricates, and the liquids, in particular, are not mastered by all children until about age 7 or 8. Children at that age level may also display difficulties with some consonant clusters and multisyllabic words. In general, however, the majority of children by first grade will have a well-developed phonological system. Their production of most sounds will closely match the adult model, and their speech intelligibility will be approximately 90–100% in connected speech.

A more significant development during the early elementary school years, which has received much attention in recent years, is phonological or phonemic awareness (Goswami & Bryant, 1990; Stackhouse, 1997). **Phonological awareness** refers to a child's underlying knowledge that words are created from sounds and sound combinations. A child with good phonological awareness, for example, could identify that the first sound in the word *bat* is *b* and the last sound in the word *stop* is *p*. In essence, the child can break down the word and analyze its individual components. Robertson and Salter (1997) describe phonological awareness as "the knowledge of meaningful sounds, or phonemes, in our language and how those sounds blend together to form syllables, words, phrases, and sentences" (p. 5). Among some of the skills believed to indicate the development of phonological awareness are the following:

• *rhyming*—the ability to identify words that sound alike or rhyme; the ability to provide a word that rhymes with a presented word; the ability to sort rhyming from nonrhyming words

• *alliteration*—the ability to identify words that begin or end with a certain sound

• *phoneme isolation*—the ability to identify whether a specific sound occurs in the beginning, end, or middle of a word

• *sound blending*—the ability to blend two or more sounds that are temporally separated by a few seconds into a word

- *syllable identification* — the ability to identify the number of syllables in a word through clapping, finger tapping, or verbally stating the number of syllables

- *sound segmentation* — the ability to break down a word into its individual sound components (identification of the number of phonemes in the word)

- *invented spellings* — the ability to spell words phonetically. Such spellings would indicate that the child is aware of the phoneme-grapheme association between spoken and written words. These spellings are phonetic in nature (e.g., "kat" for *cat*, "fon" for *phone*, and "sin" for *sign*).

The emergence of phonological awareness seems to parallel the child's development of metalinguistic skills. **Metalinguistics** refers to an individual's ability to analyze, think about, and talk about language; it is the inherent capacity to use language to analyze language. Phonological skills are one aspect of language. The term **metaphonological** would be more specific to the metalinguistics of phonology.

A child's ability to analyze words and break them down into their phonological components has been correlated with the acquisition of early reading skills (Robertson & Salter, 1997; Stackhouse, 1997; Swank, 1994; van Kleeck, 1995). Robertson and Salter indicate that "since English uses a sound-based representational system, the beginning reader needs to learn to decode printed letters (graphemes), store their associated sounds in short-term memory, and then blend these stored sounds to form words" (p. 5). Because speech–language pathologists, especially those employed in the public school setting, are becoming more and more involved in the intervention of children's reading and writing problems through either direct methods or consultation, we will address the assessment and intervention of phonological awareness skills in the Basic Unit of Chapter 7.

Bilingual and Ethnocultural Variables in the Development of Articulation and Phonological Skills

The United States has developed a culturally and linguistically diverse population through welcoming people of various origins within its borders. In a single community across the United States it is not uncommon to find people who speak various languages or use different dialects of American English. Many pleasures and benefits can be derived from this cultural pluralism.

Our profession has embraced the view that cultural and linguistic diversity is an important consideration in the study of normal and disordered communication development. Understanding the speech patterns of children who speak languages other than English or speak dialects other than mainstream American English is extremely important for today's speech–language pathologist. This understanding (or lack thereof) may determine whether phonological variations produced by linguistically and culturally diverse children are diagnosed as "different" or "disordered."

The view that cultural and linguistic differences must be considered in the diagnostic and therapeutic decision-making process has posed some inherent difficulties for both monolingual English-speaking and bilingual speech–language pathologists. It is not sufficient to inform professionals that differences exist in the phonological development of culturally and linguistically diverse children and expect them to make appropriate diagnostic and therapeutic decisions. With this in mind, we have chosen to devote an entire chapter to the many issues surrounding bilingual phonological development, dialectical variations, ethnocultural variations, and the assessment and treatment implications. The reader can find this information in the Basic and Advanced Units of Chapter 5.

Summary of the Basic Unit

• For assessment and treatment purposes, it is critical that speech–language pathologists understand normal development of articulation and phonological skills in children.

• Infants' sound productions are commonly referred to as **prelinguistic** vocalizations.

• **Infant speech perception** has been extensively studied since the early 1970s primarily through conditioning procedures.

• Studies have shown that infants can reliably localize sound soon after birth. Other studies have documented infant discriminations between varied pure-tone frequencies, pure-tone loudness levels, and differing white noise levels.

• Infants have been found to show a greater interest in human speech than in other noises.

• Some studies suggest that infants as young as 3 days can recognize their mother's voice from various other female voices.

• Two methods have been used to study infant speech perception: the **high-amplitude sucking method** and the **visually reinforced head-turn method.**

• Infants as young as 2 months have been conditioned to discriminate various syllable contrasts (e.g., /pa/ and /ba/).

• Infants cannot be conditioned to discriminate all syllable contrasts (e.g., /fa/ and /θ/).

• Conditioning studies have documented that animals (e.g., chinchillas, dogs) can also be taught to discriminate speech sounds, suggesting that such skills are not unique to human infants.

• Infant vocalizations have been divided into two major categories: **reflexive vocalizations** and **nonreflexive vocalizations.**

• Oller (1980) advanced five specific stages describing infant vocalizations: **phonation stage (Stage I), coo and goo stage (Stage II), exploration-expansion stage (Stage III), canonical babbling stage (Stage IV),** and **variegated babbling stage (Stage V).**

• **Babbling** has been divided into two portions: **reduplicated babbling** and **nonreduplicated babbling.**

• Studies have shown that infants babble some sounds more frequently than others toward the end of the babbling stage and use a select type of syllable structure.

• **Protowords** are vocalizations used consistently by the infant that are absent of a recognizable adult model. These vocalizations are believed to be the link between babbling and adultlike speech.

• Production of the child's first **true words** appears to be influenced by the phonetic repertoire and syllable structure of productions of the late babbling period.

• **Progressive idioms** are words that have an advanced pronunciation in comparison to the child's current phonological system and production of other words.

• **Regressive idioms** are the child's static or unchanging pronunciation of certain words despite his or her progression into a more advanced phonological system.

• The acquisition of speech sounds in the preschool and early school years has been extensively documented since the 1930s.

• Several **cross-sectional studies** have documented the age of mastery of English consonants. The specific information offered by each study varies somewhat, but some similarities have been identified. Nasals, stops, and glides tend to develop early, while fricatives, affricates, and liquids develop much later.

• Studies using the **longitudinal method** have shown individual differences in the acquisition of articulation and phonological skills.

• More recently, studies have assessed children's phonological development according to sound classes, **distinctive features,** and **phonological processes.**

• A child's **speech intelligibility** seems to be directly affected by the misarticulation of sounds and the use of phonological processes. As the child's articulation and phonological skills increase, his or her speech intelligibility can also be expected to improve.

• Recently, the development of a child's **phonological awareness** skills and their relationship to the acquisition of reading have received much attention.

• **Bilingual** and **ethnocultural variables** in the development of articulation and phonologial skills must be considered.

Advanced Unit

♦　♦　♦　♦　♦　♦　♦　♦　♦　♦　♦　♦　♦　♦　♦　♦　♦

Theories of Articulation and Phonological Development

The Basic Unit of this chapter has summarized the information on articulation and phonological development. In this Advanced Unit, we will address theoretical issues related to speech perception and discrimination, theories of normal development of articulation and phonological skills, and the clinical implications of developmental research.

Methodological and Theoretical Issues in Speech Perception and Discrimination Research

As noted in the Basic Unit, a considerable amount of research on the early (prelinguistic) stages of speech sound development has been concerned with speech perception in infants. Perception is a sensory experience, and, as such, it is a private event. It is measured only through some action on the part of the perceiver. Perception is measured by presenting a certain external stimulus and noting an overt response. However, investigators of perception tend to make inferences regarding what goes on in the person who reacts to a stimulus. In this sense, perception is a presumed process that begins *within* an organism soon after a stimulus has been presented and perhaps ends when an overt response has been initiated.

Researchers of early speech perception depend on a discriminated response from an infant. While the concept of *perception* comes from the classical sensory psychology, the concept of *discrimination* comes from the behavioral science of classical and operant conditioning. A discriminated response is a changed or different response when stimuli are changed. As a behavioral process, discrimination is an observable and measurable change in responses when stimuli are systematically changed under well-controlled experimental arrangements. As a psychological process, perception is a directly unobservable and, hence, unmeasurable mental activity inferred from observable behaviors. A point not well appreciated is that speech perception researchers have combined the concepts and methods of behavioral science with those of sensory psychology. Consequently, some methodological and theoretical issues arise in research on infant speech perception and discrimination.

The two major methods commonly used to study infant speech perception and discrimination—high-amplitude sucking and visually reinforced head turn—were described in the Basic Unit of this chapter (Eilers, 1980; Kuhl, 1987). Both are essentially operant conditioning methods in which some overt response to changes in speech stimuli is positively reinforced. In the high-amplitude sucking method, a new speech stimulus positively reinforces increased sucking response. In the other method, a head-turn response toward the loud speaker that presents a new stimulus is positively reinforced by a lighted and animated toy.

It is important to note the methodological difference between the two methods. In both methods, a new speech sound stimulus is a reinforcer. In the high-amplitude sucking method, the new speech sound stimulus increases the sucking response rate. In the other method, the new sound stimulus evokes a head-turn response, which is reinforced (increased) by an animated and lighted toy.

Some of the major results and conclusions of infant speech perception and discrimination experiments are summarized in the Basic Unit. Essentially, the investigators have come to the conclusion that infants have an ability to perceive certain speech sounds and to discriminate between certain classes of sounds. The results often are summarized by stating that infants can perceive and discriminate speech sounds and categories of sounds. Investigators have debated whether this ability is innate, learned, or a combination of both. Some strongly believe that humans have a specific phonetic processing mechanism that is innately given (Liberman, 1970) and is distinguished from the general auditory processing mechanisms. Others believe that speech perception skill in the infant may be a function of the general sensitivity of the auditory system to discontinuities in the sound stream. This controversy also is briefly summarized in the Basic Unit; therefore, here we will concentrate mostly on the methodological issue involved in infant speech perception and discrimination experiments.

That the experimental methods used in infant speech perception and discrimination are operant conditioning procedures is rarely recognized in the literature on infant speech perception and discrimination. Lack of this recognition has led to claims regarding data that are incongruent with the methods by which those data are gathered. The results of high-amplitude sucking and head-turn experiments *do not* forcefully demonstrate that infants can perceive and discriminate speech sounds and their categories without conditioning or some form of experimental manipulation. The results of high-amplitude sucking and head-turn experiments most forcefully show that infants *could be conditioned* to respond differently to different speech stimuli. The studies are experiments in learning. In these experiments, infants have *learned* to reliably respond to speech stimuli. If the experiments are a test of an innate ability, they are so only in a trivial sense: that *infants have an ability to learn* to respond to speech sounds and respond differently to different speech sounds. Any kind of learning, in persons of all ages and members of all species, presupposes such a general ability to learn, and, hence, it is not a powerful explanation of anything.

Theories of Articulation and Phonological Development

We know more about *what* children learn in acquiring speech and language than *how* and *why* they accomplish that task. Theoreticians of various backgrounds, notably psychologists and linguists, have speculated on how children acquire speech sounds as a part of language acquisition. We will sample a few representative hypotheses followed by a critical evaluation of theories of speech acquisition.

A theory explains a phenomenon. To explain a phenomenon, a theorist should find its cause or causes. In technical terms, researchers need to identify the independent variables (causal factors) that are associated with the dependent variables (speech sound perception and production) in a systematic and organized manner. Such independent variables need to be isolated in experimental research. In the present context, theorists of articulation and phonological development need to find out why that development takes place.

Explanations of speech sound acquisition in children fall into two main groups: linguistic and behavioral. Linguistic explanations are offered by both linguists and psycholinguists (psychologists who specialize in linguistic studies), with occasional contributions from speech–language pathologists. Linguistic explanations are plenty, popular, and ever changing. Behavioral explanations of speech acquisition are scarce, underappreciated, and underdeveloped. We will soon find out why this is the case and what it means for an evaluation of contrasting positions.

Questions asked about the nature of a phenomenon often determine the form of the explanation offered and the methods of research used to gather evidence to support that explanation. In phonological research, certain basic questions identify what needs to be explained. First, researchers often ask what is meant by speech sound acquisition. What exactly is mastered? Second, researchers ask what internal mechanisms help promote the acquisition of whatever is acquired. What external variables assist in the acquisition process? Theories differ in their answers to these and related questions. Even linguistic theories differ in their emphasis on certain kinds of assumptions, but linguistic and behavioral theories differ the most.

Linguistic Explanations

Linguistic explanations of acquisition of a speech sound system are influenced by linguistic views of language. With some variations, linguists view language as a mental system of representations, processes, and rules. These experts believe that internal representations, processes, and rules dictate speech and language production. Therefore, a good explanation of speech (and language) acquisition or production should contain a clear view of what these internal representations, processes, and rules are.

Classic research on speech development was concerned mostly with the mastery of individual speech sounds. In explaining the acquisition of individual speech sounds, researchers investigated potential independent variables that might promote or impede the acquisition of individual sounds. This line of investigation was not heavily influenced by linguistic theories. As reviewed in Chapter 4, such variables as oral anatomical structures, intelligence, and socioeconomic status were correlated with speech development. By and large, this line of investigation to find out the potential independent variables of speech sound acquisition has been discouraging. No variables have been isolated in such a way as to explain speech sound acquisition. In recent years, this line of investigation has not been pursued to any significant extent.

Subsequent explanations of articulation and phonological development have been more significantly influenced by linguistic theories. Unfortunately, linguistic theories on the nature of speech and language and inferred internal mechanisms of their production have been an ever changing scene. Therefore, at any one point, only a few historically significant theories may be sampled.

While the classical researchers were concerned with the acquisition of speech sounds, the more recent, linguistically oriented researchers, on the other hand, consider speech sound acquisition a part of the acquisition of the larger system called language. Also, unlike the classical researchers, linguistic researchers have been concerned with the acquisition of a phonological system rather than individual sounds.

There are significant parallels between the linguistic theories of language acquisition and those of speech sound system acquisition. Both sets of theories emphasize that the infant and the child face a formidable task of mastering an abstract system of rules and processes while getting relatively little or no help from the environment. Theorists point out that the child accomplishes this difficult task at an amazing speed. Both sets of theories seek to explain not just observable productions (speech sounds or language) but also underlying, inferred, abstract systems of one kind or the other.

Jakobson's (1968) study produced one of the early linguistic explanations of speech sound acquisition. His views, described as the **hypothesis of discontinuity** between babbling and later speech acquisition, have been summarized in the Basic Unit of this chapter. Essentially, Jakobson proposed that speech sounds are not shaped out of early vocalizations found in the babbling stage. This view contrasted with the behavioral view that early vocalizations, including babbling, provide a foundation for later speech development. Instead, Jakobson thought that the speech sound acquisition process was distinct from the early stages of vocalization and babbling, which he considered random activity. He believed that speech sound acquisition followed a universal and innate pattern in which the distinctive features were acquired in a hierarchical manner. Just as the generative grammarians proposed that language unfolds within a predetermined, innate sequence, Jakobson proposed that the acquisition of distinctive features is an unfolding process.

For Jakobson, acquiring the sound system meant differentiating sounds with contrasting features. Initially, the sounds that are acquired are those that contrast the most. For instance, the child might first learn the bilabial stop /p/ and the vowel /a/; those two phonemes contrast maximally. Jakobson believed that the child continues to differentiate different classes of sounds that share certain distinctive features. For instance, the child will continue to learn such contrasts as the nasal and oral consonants, labial and dental consonants, and so forth. He suggested that the child acquires the features of stops, nasals, bilabials, and dentals before acquiring the features of fricatives, affricates, and liquids. In essence, Jakobson proposed that the child's mastery of distinctive features follows feature contrasts, starting with simpler contrasts and moving toward more complex or difficult contrasts. He considered the order of phonological acquisition to be universal and attributed the process of phonological mastery to presumed innate mechanisms.

Another influential explanation of articulatory and phonological development was proposed by Stampe (1969), whose theoretical views are a part of natural phonology. **Natural phonology** (Donegan & Stampe, 1979; Stampe, 1969) describes universal phonological processes evident in children's speech and considers those processes as innate mechanisms of simplifying adult productions. Natural phonological processes (e.g., cluster reduction or final-consonant deletion) reflect the limitations of the human speech production mechanism. They also reflect universal patterns in phonological productions in all languages of the world.

The most controversial aspect of the theory of natural phonology is that the phonological processes are real mental operations going on in the mind of the child. This is known as the *hypothesis of psychological reality of phonological processes.* In other words, phonological processes are empirical; they are a part of the child's active understanding and processing of phonological input. In simple terms, children know that they are using a phonological process and as they become more mature, they actively suppress those processes.

The natural phonology presumes that because of the innate phonological processes, children accurately perceive speech sounds from the very beginning. They do not have unique phonological strategies; their strategies are both universal and accurate. Children's speech errors are only production problems, not perceptual problems. Children's task in phonological acquisition is to suppress natural tendencies to simplify adult models and thus achieve the adult phonological skills. This process is guided mostly by innate mechanisms. According to Stampe (1969), children's erroneous patterns of production are *explained* on the basis of the innate, psychologically real phonological processes. This is known as the *hypothesis of the explanatory power of phonological processes*. Thus, in essence, the natural phonological theory proposes that phonological processes are psychologically real, are innate, and explain production errors (Yavas, 1998).

Some of the newer phonological theories, especially **nonlinear phonological theories** (see the Advanced Unit of Chapter 2 for a description) also make strong nativist assumptions about phonological acquisition that are similar to Chomsky's (1981) on language acquisition. Phonological acquisition is made possible because the child is born with a set of universal phonological principles (Bernhardt, 1994). These innate principles provide a framework, like templates, that help the child acquire a phonological system. Phonological input is decoded and encoded according to the innate templates. Universal principles or templates help categorize certain common features of language. For example, the environmental input fits the template that states that CV structure is common to all languages or that all languages have vowels. When certain phonological aspects of a child's language differ from the universal templates, the input of that language helps set up new parameters. For example, a particular input from a specific language might help set up the parameter that the language has few or no final consonants or that the syllable stress pattern is unique (different from what is specified in the template).

A different set of theories emphasize children's cognitive functions in acquiring their phonological systems. Known as the **cognitive model,** theories taking this approach propose that children actively test hypotheses regarding phonological constraints and systems (Menn, 1983; Macken & Ferguson, 1983; Ferguson, 1978, 1986). Children's eventual acquisition of the adult phonological skills depends on accepting certain assumptions they make about their language and discarding certain others.

Cognitive theorists believe that children test hypotheses about phonological patterns they hear against what they know about those patterns. That belief is supported by several kinds of observational data, including the following. First, the child's identifiable initial words are different for different children. It seems that each child has a preference for certain early words; for example, a child might prefer only two-syllable words starting with a particular consonant such as a stop or a nasal. Cognitive theorists interpret this to mean that children select certain unique strategies to master phonological skills. Second, children seem to have unique ways of simplifying complex or polysyllabic adult forms. Cognitive theorists find this to be a tendency to explore different ways of producing a difficult word. Third, children may show a tendency to *initially* use a correct word form with adult phonemic sequence and *later* revert to a more simplified form. The typical example given is that of a child who first produced the word *pretty* correctly and later incorrectly produced the same word as [bɪdi]. Researchers have observed that the initial correct productions do not match the child's overall phonological skills, but the subsequent incorrect productions do. This phenomenon is known as *phonological regression* and is interpreted as evidence that the child is testing certain hypotheses about adult phonological forms.

Theorists disagree as to whether children initially learn phonemic sequences or whole words. While most theorists pay attention to the acquisition of *segments* (speech sounds with defined features) that children master, at least one view, known as the **prosodic view,** pays attention to *words* as the initial learning units (Waterson, 1981). In fact, the prosodic view of phonologic acquisition is that children's acquisition of phonological skills begins with the mastery of certain initial words. In that theory, the early words are schemata of adult forms that include such common features as intonation and syllable structure. The theory proposes that children do not have a complete and accurate phonological system to begin with; instead, they have an imperfect perceptual production mechanism that is progressively refined to match the adult phonological system.

A distinction between **underlying phonological representations** and actual **realization in production** is common to many linguistic views of phonological development. Recent linguistic theories of phonological development propose that children have underlying phonological representations that change through development. Underlying phonological representations may be similar to the innate systems of linguistic knowledge that generative linguists have attributed to children. When a nativist bias is not included, underlying representations mean remembered and cognitively stored forms of what the child hears in the adult speech.

Different phonological theories propose different sorts of underlying phonological representations. Some theories presume that children's underlying representations are complete, in that all phonemes of language, their entire inventory of features, and their permissible combinations are already available. This is similar to transformational generative linguists' assertion that children have an innate knowledge of universal syntactic rules. When children with a complete or universal phonological representation begin to experience a given language, they delete what is redundant or irrelevant to their specific language. This means that a complete phonological underlying representation leads to a sequence of phonological development that proceeds from a general knowledge of the universal phonological system to that of a particular language (Yavas, 1998).

An alternative view of phonological representation is that it contains only a universally specified, minimal set of contrastive features. These contrasts include [consonantal], [sonorant], and [continuant]. With this basic phonological equipment, children begin to receive linguistic input from their environment. Because of this input, children begin to add what is missing in their universally specified minimal sets of feature contrasts. Children's underlying, minimal, and universal representation is thus expanded to include all the relevant features of their particular language. In that view, children progress from a set of simpler, minimal feature specifications to a more complex, comprehensive system (Yavas, 1998).

Behavioral Explanations

The behavioral view, as traditionally conceived, is the view of behavioral scientists with the Skinnerian outlook. Nonbehavioral psychologists often are in agreement with linguists and in fact have carved out a specialty called psycholinguistics. The behavioral view, therefore, is an extension of the tenets of behaviorism to the study of speech and language.

A comprehensive description of the behavioral view of speech–language development is currently problematic for three main reasons. First, behavioral scientists use an entirely different paradigm of speech–language behaviors. They do not see speech and language as a mental system with cognitive representations that underlie productions. Unlike linguists, they see speech–language as verbal behavior that is similar to nonverbal behaviors. Although verbal behavior has certain unique properties, it does not have a special status. Certain generative linguists of the Chomskyan orientation attribute special status to language by stating that it is the creation of a unique mental apparatus at the human level. Therefore, the differences between the behavioral and linguistic views are based on fundamental paradigmatic differences and are not just due to differences in certain assumptions and explanatory concepts.

Second, behavioral scientists are less inclined to explain a phenomenon based on data obtained from nonexperimental methods. Much of phonological developmental data (as well as language developmental data) are merely observational. Observational data do not rule out alternative hypotheses and, hence, when used exclusively, are inadequate to support any kind of theory. Some strong theoretical statements often are based on observations of a single subject, usually the child of the observer. The questionable reliability of such observations and potential investigator biases in recording them are problems in such investigations. Behavioral explanations often are based on experimental research in which some variable is systematically manipulated under controlled conditions and the effects of such manipulations are carefully noted. Typically, there are no such data available on phonological development.

Third, in the absence of experimental data, certain extrapolations of behavioral and developmental data are possible, but behavioral scientists generally have not made much systematic effort to advance a contemporary behavioral view of speech–language development. Behavioral scientists have been more interested in the experimental and clinical methods of modifying speech–language problems than in explaining their normal development. Consequently, textbooks and research articles typically provide some dated references to an inadequately formulated behavioral view and then summarily dismiss it.

Traditionally, the behavioral view described in various sources is that of Mowrer's 1960 theory, supplemented by Olmsted's 1971 theory. The basic idea in this view is that speech sounds are shaped out of babbling by environmental contingencies of positive reinforcement. During the course of the day, the infant receives much care from the caretaker, often the mother, in the form of feeding and changing. During such activities, the mother also produces many vocalizations and even clearly articulated sequences of speech sounds (syllables and words). Such maternal productions are associated with activities that provide for the infant primary positive reinforcement (e.g., food) and negative reinforcement (e.g., elimination of discomfort when changed). In due course, maternal vocalizations and speech productions signal primary reinforcement for the infant. The infant's own babbling and other vocalizations acquire secondary reinforcement because of their similarity to the maternal vocalizations that are associated with primary reinforcement. The infant's babbling and other vocalizations, even if they begin as vocal play or random behaviors, are highly sensitive to environmental contingencies. For example, experimental studies on infant vocalizations have shown that babbling can be increased by contingent positive reinforcement and decreased by extinction (McLaughlin, 1998). In essence, the essential feature of the classical behavioral view formulated by Mowrer (1960) is that interaction between the infant's initial vocal behaviors and environmental events helps shape speech sounds.

This behavioral account is certainly incomplete, in that it does not address phonological development in any detail. The patterns of later acquisition and phonological disorders are not addressed in the theory. Nonetheless, the fundamental assumption that babbling provides a basis for shaping speech sounds has received much recent research support. As noted previously, Jakobson's (1968) view that babbling is not systematically related to later speech sound acquisition has been rejected in light of more recent developmental data. Most theorists now believe that later speech sound productions are significantly related to earlier babbling. Therefore, the fundamentally behavioral hypothesis that speech sounds are shaped out of babbling remains credible.

Linguistic theories of both phonological and language development have generally rejected the behavioral view that environmental contingencies are important in learning speech and language skills. The debate is old in the language acquisition literature and is only newly reflected in phonological theories. The role of environmental contingencies is typically reduced to *input* in linguistic theories. The child is supposed to use this input to construct a phonological and language system mostly with the help of innate or cognitive mechanisms. However, such mechanisms remain highly speculative, and they are different across ever changing theories.

Research on language acquisition has shown that environment provides more than just input. Moerk's (1992) reanalysis of Brown's classic data on language acquisition, along with research on motherese (Newport, Gleitman, & Gleitman, 1977; Snow, 1977; Stern, 1977), has clearly shown that adults do use certain strategies that promote speech–language learning in infants. More relevant to the present context, these strategies include the use of slower and more clearly articulated speech sounds when adults speak to young children.

Comparative Evaluation of Linguistic and Behavioral Explanations

There are notable differences among the varied linguistic theories of phonological development. Collectively, however, some features are shared to varying degrees by linguistic theories that contrast with the behavioral view of speech–language acquisition. Several features of linguistic theories as summarized in various sources contrast with the behavioral view. See, among other sources, Ball and Kent, 1997; Ferguson, Menn, and Stoel-Gammon, 1992; and Yavas, 1998, for a description of various linguistic theories.

First, most linguistic theories propose innate phonological mechanisms that cause an unfolding of universal and invariable stages of development. Some theorists believe that common patterns of phonological acquisition and production observed in children and across children speaking a variety of languages support the notion of an innate mechanism that controls and guides phonological development.

Second, linguistic theories generally minimize the influence of environmental events on the speech–language acquisition process. Theorists do not believe that environmental reinforcement contingencies can effectively account for such patterning within and across languages. They do not think that reinforcement contingencies can effectively shape speech sounds from babbling and other infant vocalizations. Linguists generally think that speech and language acquisition involves mastery of a system of rules or knowledge. Linguists further assert that this system is both too abstract and too complex to be learned and that the input is not specific enough to teach infants and children how to acquire such a system.

Third, linguistic theories make a distinction between internal phonological representations and external realizations of those representations. While theorists differ on whether underlying representations are complete, partial, fully correct, or partially correct, they do propose the existence of underlying representations of phonemes that are realized in actual productions. Linguists assert that articulatory mistakes children make in producing a word are better understood in terms of an underlying representation of that word, which is often assumed to be the correct adult form, and the rules that change an accurate representation into an inaccurate production (realization). For instance, Smith (1973), who made a detailed analysis of his son's phonological development, gave the example of [gɪk], which was his son's production of the word *zinc*. Assuming that there is a correct underlying representation of *zinc*, Smith proposed a series of rules that operated on this representation to convert it into a phonetic realization in the form of [gɪk]. According to Smith, one rule deleted the nasal consonant in the underlying representation. Another rule assimilated the coronal fricative with the final velar consonant. Yet another rule converted the fricative into a stop. It is because of these rules that the child wrongly realized a correct underlying representation. Linguists propose that a distinction between the underlying representations and the phonetic realizations and rules that operate on the representations help us understand both the correct and incorrect productions.

Fourth, several linguistic theories attribute complex cognitive processes to children in terms of hypothesis testing and evaluation of phonological input. Cognitive theorists propose that children need to analyze linguistic input and match that input with certain innate phonological templates, that children need to make certain hypotheses about the nature of the input and test them against the templates to arrive at a correct phonological system. Children are described as active learners, who analyze linguistic data, accept or reject the hypotheses they make about the data, and thus actively pursue a system of phonological knowledge. Theorists sometimes contrast this view with the behavioral view, which, in their opinion, reduces children to passive roles in the learning process.

Fifth, although now controversial, some of the linguistic theories assert that phonological processes are empirical. This means that rules of phonological processes are psychologically real for the child. Theorists believe that errors are rule generated and that phonological rules are an excellent means of understanding how and why children wrongly realize their correct phonological representations. Psychological reality implies that children actively use phonological processes to simplify complex adult productions.

The behavioral view of phonological acquisition, though underdeveloped, contains certain features that contrast with the linguistic views. First, the behavioral view assigns an active role for the environmental contingencies that shape behaviors. Behavioral scientists think that early infant vocal conditioning studies, the continuity of babbling and speech sound acquisition, operant conditioning studies on teaching infants to discriminate speech sounds (the so-called infant speech perception studies), and widely used reinforcement techniques in teaching speech (and language) skills to clinical populations provide ample evidence that speech and language behaviors are as sensitive to reinforcement contingencies as are non-verbal behaviors. Recent research on language acquisition (especially the mater-nal adaptation of speech addressed to children) and Moerk's (1992) reanalysis of Brown's classic data suggest the influence of environmental variables, especially teaching strategies that caretakers use, that may facilitate speech and language learning in children. Behavioral scientists do not believe that learning within the operant (Skinnerian) model reduces the child to a passive learner. Operant learn-ing is purposeful, active learning based on contingent interactions between the learner and those surrounding that learner.

Second, the behavioral view would not support a distinction between underly-ing phonological representations and phonetic realizations. Linguists have only the observable phonetic productions, and underlying representations are inferred entities. There is no independent evidence of such representations. In the behav-ioral view, such inferred entities do not explain observable phonetic productions. According to the behavioral view, when a child makes errors, it is not clear that dif-ferent rules convert correct underlying representations into erroneous phonetic realizations.

Third, the behavioral view questions the power and explanatory usefulness of language-specific innate mechanisms that are supposed to create invariable, uni-versal stages of acquisition. The experimental evidence on speech sound discrimi-nation in chinchillas and dogs, reviewed in a previous section, clearly indicates that subhuman animals, too, can learn to discriminate between speech sounds. Therefore, even among the linguistic theorists, the concept of a language-specific innate mechanism is now controversial.

Fourth, the behavioral view is skeptical about the assumption of hypothesis testing by children in speech–language acquisition. That children compare input with innate templates of phonological patterns is too rich an assumption about what children do and, presumably, what they are capable of. When there is little or no evidence of such conscious hypothesis testing of speech and language input in the case of adult speakers, the assumption of such cognitive activity in children as young as 12 months (when the first words and acceptable phonemic sequences are observed) seems to be excessive theorizing.

Fifth, the behavioral view questions the empirical status (psychological real-ity) of phonological processes. Psychological reality, though rarely precisely defined in the linguistic literature, may mean that children actively use phonological rules to simplify adult productions. As with the cognitive hypothesis testing, the behav-ioral science view finds the psychological reality of phonological processes an unproven assumption about what goes on in the minds of young children learning to speak their language. That this may also be excessive theorizing is indicated by disagreement among linguistic theorists themselves. Several linguistic and clini-cal experts believe that phonological processes are only descriptive devices (Grun-well, 1985; Ingram, 1981; Stoel-Gammon & Dunn, 1985; Yavas, 1998). Behavioral scientists would agree.

A fundamental difference between linguists and behavioral scientists is that the former are more inclined to make theoretical assumptions about internal processes than are the latter. Linguists depend on observational data; behavioral scientists depend on experimental evidence. Linguists, psycholinguists, and speech–language pathologists have produced ample observational data on speech–language acquisition; behavioral scientists and behaviorally oriented clinicians have mostly produced clinical treatment data. Linguistic theories are well advanced even if they are constantly changing and thus controversial; the behavioral view of speech–language learning is underdeveloped. However, the fact that linguistic theories change constantly means that those theories may be premature. A dozen or more phonological theories are available, and each theory is a *phonology* unto itself (see Ball & Kent, 1997, for a review). No particular theory is universally accepted, and few, if any, have experimental evidence to support their claims.

New phonological theories are proposed before the full implications of older theories have been tested and evaluated. Most theories have never been tested in clinical applications, partly because their clinical relevance is not clear and partly because any such attempt in an ever shifting theoretical scene is both premature (Yavas, 1998) and risky. Clinicians cannot be blamed if they wait until the dust settles on the theoretical scene.

Summary of the Advanced Unit

• The two major methods of studying speech perception and discrimination in infants—high-amplitude sucking and visually reinforced head turn—are operant conditioning methods; hence, the results show only that infants can be *taught* to discriminate between speech sounds

• Jakobson's (1941/1968) theory proposed that speech sound acquisition follows a universal and innate pattern in which the distinctive features are acquired in a hierarchical manner.

• The theory of natural phonology proposes that natural phonological processes are innate and reflect limitations of the human speech production mechanism.

• Some of the newer phonological theories, especially nonlinear phonological theories, also suggest that phonological acquisition is made possible because children are born with a set of universal phonological principles.

• Cognitive theorists propose that children actively test hypotheses regarding phonological constraints and systems and thus arrive at the adult system.

• The prosodic view suggests that *words,* not phonemes or features, are the initial learning units.

• The linguistic theories of phonological acquisition are varied but share certain common features, including an assumption of the innateness of some basic processes, a rejection of a strong role for environmental variables, assumptions about such cognitive processes as hypothesis testing by infants, a distinction between underlying phonological representations and phonetic realizations, and so forth.

• The behavioral view of speech development is underdeveloped and dated as described in most sources. It generally posits that learning to speak is not essentially different from learning other kinds of skills and that speech and language behaviors are sensitive to environmental reinforcement contingencies.

• Linguists and behavioral scientists differ on such issues as the innateness of phonological processes and the presence of innate templates, the role of the environmental contingencies in speech–language acquisition, the assumption of hypothesis testing by children, the distinction between internal representation and phonetic realization, and the empirical status of phonological processes.

• Because phonological theories are varied, controversial, and ever changing, their clinical application is premature.

Chapter 4

♦ ♦ ♦ ♦ ♦ ♦ ♦ ♦ ♦ ♦ ♦ ♦ ♦ ♦ ♦ ♦ ♦ ♦ ♦

Variables Associated with Articulation and Phonological Development and Performance

Basic Unit

♦ ♦ ♦ ♦ ♦ ♦ ♦ ♦ ♦ ♦ ♦ ♦ ♦ ♦ ♦ ♦ ♦ ♦ ♦ ♦

Variables Related to Articulation and Phonological Development and Performance

The first duty of man is to speak; that is his chief business in this world.

—ROBERT LOUIS STEVENSON

Much of the classic research on the development of articulation, as summarized in Chapter 3, is related to the sequence in which children acquire speech sounds and the chronological ages at which they master speech sounds. More recent research has been concerned with the phonological processes children use and the different ages at which specific processes tend to diminish and disappear. Consequently, we have a wealth of normative information on the acquisition of speech sounds. While collecting normative data, many researchers have wondered what factors promote or retard the acquisition of speech sounds and articulatory performance. A more complete understanding of speech sound acquisition and performance requires a description of variables that may be correlated with their normal or impaired acquisition.

In this Basic Unit, we will summarize the research findings on factors that are associated with acquisition of speech sounds. These factors may be associated with more or less proficient articulation. In the Advanced Unit, we will discuss issues related to concepts and methods used in research and the proposed explanations or theories. We also will critically evaluate the findings and conclusions.

Researched variables associated with the acquisition of speech sounds and articulatory performance may be grouped under (a) anatomic, neurologic, and physiologic factors; (b) motor skills; (c) sensory variables; (d) language skills, (e) such personal characteristics as age and gender; (f) familial prevalence; and (g) tongue thrust.

Anatomic, Neurologic, and Physiologic Factors

Because speech production is a neuromotor event, researchers have investigated oral and neural anatomic factors that may affect the acquisition of speech sounds and articulatory proficiency. It is well known that integrity of the structures and function of the speech production mechanism is essential to normal speech production. Variables that affect speech production also could affect the acquisition of speech sounds in children. For example, problems in neurologic control of the speech mechanism or significant anatomic deviations in structures of speech production could negatively affect the acquisition of speech sounds. Therefore, from the beginning, researchers have been concerned with anatomic, neurologic, and physiologic variables in the acquisition of speech sounds.

Anatomic Structures

The anatomic structures that affect the acquisition and production of speech sounds include the lips, teeth, tongue, hard palate, and soft palate. Intuitively, any abnormality in these structures could negatively affect the acquisition and production of speech sounds. Muscular weakness, deficient neural control of muscles involved in speech production, and growth deficiencies in the oral and facial structures may all cause difficulty in speech sound acquisition.

When abnormalities do exist in the speech mechanism, they vary greatly across children and adults. In some speakers, the abnormality may be minimal; in others, it may be gross. Such variations could produce varied effects on speech sound acquisition. Therefore, it is important to consider the degree of abnormality, not just its presence or absence.

Lips

Lips are important articulators of speech sounds. In producing various speech sounds, the lips come in contact with each other with varying degrees of pressure and force. The bilabial sounds /p/, /b/, and /m/ require such contact. The consonants /w/ and /hw/ and several vowels require lip rounding. If structural abnormalities prevent the approximation of lips or lip rounding, then speech sound acquisition may be delayed or production may be impaired.

Lip size, strength, and mobility normally vary across individuals. There is no evidence to suggest that within normal limits, variations in lip size or function affect the acquisition or production of speech sounds (Fairbanks & Green, 1950). Only gross structural anomalies, such as those found in the cleft of the upper lip, can be expected to produce some effect on speech sound acquisition in children. However, adequately repaired cleft of the lip, especially when done during infancy (which is a common practice), need not be associated with problems in articulatory acquisition. Most difficulties in speech sound acquisition and production are associated with clefts of the hard and soft palate, as described later (Bzoch, 1997).

Even a short and stiff upper lip — a result of ablative surgery for cancer — need not produce significant negative effects on articulation. Speakers with such altered lip structures learn to produce sounds in a compensatory manner to retain normal or near normal speech intelligibility (Bloomer & Hawk, 1973).

Teeth

As described in Chapter 1, the teeth are important articulators. Among the different classes of sounds, teeth are significantly involved in the production of labiodental /f/ and /v/ and linguadental /ð/ and /θ/ phonemes. Teeth also are important in the production of alveolars /s/ and /z/ in that an airstream is directed over the upper incisors.

Teeth may be missing or malpositioned, or the two dental arches may be misaligned. Of these, misalignment of the dental arches, known as **malocclusion,** has received much research attention. Malocclusions are classified as Class I, II, or III. In a **Class I malocclusion,** a few individual teeth are misaligned but the dental arches are generally aligned. In a **Class II malocclusion,** the lower jaw is receded and the upper jaw is protruded. In a **Class III malocclusion,** the lower jaw is protruded and the upper jaw is receded. The normal occlusion, along with Class II and III malocclusions, is shown in Figure 4.1.

 Activity

A child with a receded lower jaw probably has what type of malocclusion?

A child with a protruded upper jaw probably has what type of malocclusion?

Children with missing or misaligned teeth are said to have what type of malocclusion?

The relationship of dental occlusion to articulatory errors generally is not impressive. There is some data showing a preponderance of certain types of dental arch malocclusions in persons with significant articulation problems (Fairbanks & Lintner, 1951). However, much of the available data indicate that mal-

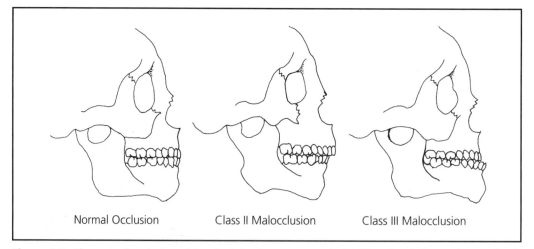

| Normal Occlusion | Class II Malocclusion | Class III Malocclusion |

Figure 4.1. The normal occlusion of the dental arches contrasted with Class II and Class III forms of malocclusions. *Note.* From *Introduction to Communicative Disorders* (2nd ed., Figure 3.12, p. 80), by M. N. Hegde, 1995, Austin, TX: PRO-ED. Copyright 1995 by PRO-ED, Inc. Reprinted with permission.

occlusions may be found in individuals who exhibit normal articulation, as well as in those who exhibit articulation disorders. Malocclusions found in normal speakers suggest that such dental abnormalities are not exclusive causes of articulation disorders.

Based on the evidence, the conclusion is that while they are slightly more common in individuals who have articulation disorders, *dental arch malocclusions themselves do not invariably cause articulation disorders.* Most individuals learn to produce speech sounds correctly in spite of such deviations by using compensatory strategies. To result in articulation errors, malocclusions must be combined with other variables.

Data on missing teeth are similar. A greater proportion of children who misarticulate certain sounds (e.g., /s/, /f/, /ð/ and /θ/) may have missing or abnormally positioned central or lateral incisors (Bankson & Byrne, 1962; Snow, 1961). However, many children with such dental deviations attain normal articulation. Clinical experience suggests that many children who do misarticulate have no significant dental deviations. Therefore, the conclusion is that, although they may be associated with a higher frequency of misarticulations, *missing teeth are neither sufficient nor necessary to cause articulation disorders.*

Tongue

Although the tongue is the most important of the articulators, there is relatively little research on how its size, shape, and mobility affect the acquisition of speech sounds. A variable that was researched to some extent in the past is **ankyloglossia,** which is a short lingual frenum. Ankyloglossia was believed to limit the tongue tip movement necessary to produce certain speech sounds. Although an extremely short frenum may be associated with articulatory errors, there is no evidence to suggest that ankyloglossia is a factor in the majority of children who misarticulate. Within the limits of normal variation, the tongue is an extremely dynamic structure that is capable of rapid and flexible movements necessary to produce speech sounds.

Several investigators have studied the consequences of a glossectomy on speech intelligibility (e.g., Leonard, 1994; Skelly, Spector, Donaldson, Brodeur, & Paletta, 1971). **Glossectomy** is the total or partial surgical removal of a diseased (e.g., cancerous) tongue. Some adults and children who undergo glossectomy may retain surprisingly good articulation, suggesting that a radically altered tongue is nevertheless capable of a range of the fine movements necessary for producing intelligible speech. Adults whose tongue has been partially surgically removed may still attain intelligible speech, though there may be errors of articulation, especially in producing fricatives and plosives (Leonard, 1994). Children with similar surgical excision of the tongue may learn to produce, with systematic treatment, all the speech sounds to a normal or near normal extent. However, in a majority of people who undergo partial or total glossectomy, speech intelligibility may be reduced to varying extents.

Evidence on the normal anatomic variations and surgical alterations of the tongue suggests the conclusion that *the effects of such variations and alterations are surprisingly limited;* while there may be some errors of articulation that negatively affect speech intelligibility, *the speakers learn various compensatory strategies that limit negative effects on speech.* This conclusion underscores the dynamic adaptability of the tongue.

Hard Palate

Limited research in the past suggests that normal variations in the structural dimensions of the hard palate (e.g., its width, length, height) are of no consequence (Fairbanks & Lintner, 1951). However, clefts of the hard palate, if not surgically closed, can be expected to affect speech sound production. Clefts of the hard palate are typically closed within the first 2 years of life with no significant or permanent effects on articulation. Therefore, in the United States, clefts have not been a significant variable in children's misarticulations.

If a cancerous hard palate is surgically removed, totally or partially, speech intelligibility is severely affected. However, patients who undergo this procedure are fitted with a palatal prosthesis to close the opening between the oral and nasal cavities to help improve speech intelligibility.

The evidence on the role of the hard palate in articulation suggests the conclusion that *an absent hard palate, or one with a cleft, may be associated with speech production problems; however, such problems can be corrected with prosthetic devices and surgical procedures.* Normal variations in the size of the hard palate do not seem to promote errors of articulation.

Soft Palate

The soft palate, or the velum, is a part of the velopharyngeal mechanism, which is important in articulation and resonance. The velopharyngeal mechanism couples and uncouples the oral and nasal cavities. Closure of the velopharyngeal port is necessary to prevent unwanted nasal resonance on oral sounds, maintain desirable oral resonance, and build intraoral air pressure to produce certain consonants, known as **pressure consonants.** These include fricatives (e.g., /s/ /f/, /z/), stops (e.g., /b/, /g/, /t/, /k/) and affricates (e.g., /dʒ/ and /tʃ/). **Velopharyngeal inadequacy,** which is difficulty in closing the nasal port for the production of oral sounds, makes it harder to build intraoral air pressure because the air leaks through the nasal cavity.

Velopharyngeal inadequacy results in weak production of pressure consonants. The consonants lack clarity of production and sound imprecise. The speaker tends to compensate for velopharyngeal inadequacy by producing consonants in unusual ways. A common articulatory pattern is to shift the production of consonants to the posterior portion of the oral cavity. Major substitutions that result from compensatory articulation include the following (Bradley, 1997; Bzoch, 1997):

- substitution of such stops as /p/, /b/, /t/, and /d/ with the **glottal stop,** which is produced by a stoppage and sudden release of air at the level of the glottis;

- substitution of linguavelar stops /k/ and /g/ with a **pharyngeal stop,** which is produced by making a pharyngeal contact by the base of the tongue;

- substitution of fricatives and affricates with **pharyngeal fricatives,** which are produced by lingual-pharyngeal contact with an unusual lingual configuration;

- substitution of sibilants with **velar fricatives,** which are produced in the back velar region and sound like a distorted /k/ or /g/; and

- substitution of such stops as /t/, /d/, /k/, and /g/ with **mid-dorsum palatal stops,** which are produced in the same manner the glide /j/ is produced.

In addition to the listed compensatory sound substitutions, velopharyngeal inadequacy results in hypernasality on oral sounds and **nasal emission,** which is an audible air leakage through the nose.

The evidence on the role of the soft palate in articulatory acquisition and production suggests the conclusion that velopharyngeal insufficiency leads to (a) various forms of compensatory articulation resulting in substitutions of sounds produced with an unusual method of production, (b) weak production of pressure consonants, (c) nasal emission, and (d) hypernasality.

✎ Activity

DIRECTIONS: Define the following terms in your own words.

> **Ankyloglossia:** _____
>
> **Glossectomy:** _____
>
> **Pressure consonants:** _____
>
> **Velopharyngeal inadequacy:** _____
>
> **Nasal emission:** _____

Neurologic Factors

Speech production may be negatively affected if neural control of the muscles of speech is impaired. If the peripheral or central nervous system controlling the speech mechanism is damaged, muscles of speech may be weak, uncoordinated, or paralyzed. If such pathologies exist during the years of speech and language acquisition, specific speech sound learning may be impaired. The child may misarticulate multiple sounds. If the neural damage occurs in adults, normally acquired and used speech characteristics may be lost or impaired to varying degrees.

A speech disorder associated with central or peripheral nervous system damage is called **dysarthria.** Weakened, uncoordinated, or paralyzed speech muscles cause a variety of speech problems in both adults and children. In adults, dysarthria is often associated with a variety of neurologic disorders including strokes, tumors, infectious diseases, toxic factors, metabolic disturbances, and brain trauma. In addition to speech sound production problems, dysarthria includes respiratory, voice, resonance, and prosodic problems. Dysarthria is classified into ataxic, flaccid, hyperkinetic, hypokinetic, mixed, spastic, and unilateral upper motor neuron varieties. Dysarthria and its varieties are described in the Advanced Unit of Chapter 6.

Cerebral palsy is a nonprogressive neuromotor disorder in children that in many cases causes communication problems, including articulatory problems. Cerebral palsy is typically described as congenital, although in some cases the brain injury may be sustained any time up to age 16. The speech disorders associated with cerebral palsy also are described as dysarthria. The dysarthric speech of children with cerebral palsy is described in the Advanced Unit of Chapter 6.

Speech disorders also can result from central nervous system damage even when the peripheral neuromuscular mechanism is normal. When the speech motor programming areas, including Broca's area and the supplemental motor area, are damaged, a disorder of speech known as apraxia of speech may result. **Apraxia of speech** is a neurologic communication disorder characterized by a difficulty in positioning the articulators correctly, resulting in such articulatory problems as substitutions, distortions, and omissions of speech sounds. Apraxia of speech with documented neuropathology is demonstrated in adults. However, in children a form of apraxia known as developmental apraxia is described even though no substantial neuropathology is demonstrated. The Advanced Unit of Chapter 6 contains a more detailed description of apraxia.

The study of the normal speech mechanism and its neural control, along with the evidence-based neurogenic communication disorders in children and adults, suggests the conclusion that *the integrity of the neuromuscular mechanism is essential for the normal or typical acquisition and production of speech sounds.* As with any organic deficiency, individuals with an impaired neuromuscular system may develop some compensatory strategies in an effort to produce a better approximation of normal speech.

Motor Skills

That the motor skills of speakers with articulation disorders may be less proficient than those in normal speakers has an intuitive appeal because speech is a neuromotor task. Therefore, researchers have explored the relationship between two kinds of motor skills: general motor skills and orofacial motor skills. Research has generally discredited the notion that compared to those with normal articulation, children with articulation disorders are less proficient in such general motor tasks as finger tapping, ball tossing, and other kinds of gross- or fine-motor skills.

Motor skills executed by orofacial structures have generally yielded evidence that is somewhat inconsistent, although it is suggestive of some deficiency in children who misarticulate. A common clinical procedure in articulation assessment is to ask the client to produce a string of syllables as rapidly as possible. The most popular task is to have the client first repeat /pʌ/, /tʌ/, and /kʌ/ in isolation, and then to repeat /pʌtə/, /tʌkə/, /pʌkə/, and finally repeat /pʌtəkə/. In each case, the clinician typically counts the number of syllables rapidly produced in a given unit of time, usually 10 or 15 seconds. Alternately, the clinician can measure the time it takes for the client to repeat a certain number of syllables. The rapid rate of alternating syllable repetition is known as the **diadochokinetic rate.** The diagnostic use of this procedure is described in the Basic Unit of Chapter 6.

Research on the orofacial motor skills has mostly been concerned with the diadochokinetic rates in children with and without articulation disorders. Children attain the adult diadochokinetic rates variably, between the ages of 9 and 15 years. Generally, children with articulation disorders are likely to have slower rates than the normal diadochokinetic rate. However, children with misarticulations who have normal diadochokinetic rates are frequently seen in speech clinics; therefore, a slower diadochokinetic rate is not a necessary factor in articulation disorders. As we will see in the Advanced Unit, the clinical and theoretical significance of a slower diadochokinetic rate in children with misarticulations is not clear.

The research on motor skills and articulation disorders suggests the conclusion that *deficiencies in motor skills are neither necessary nor sufficient to produce disorders of articulation;* even when such deficiencies are documented, their theoretical and clinical significance is not evident.

Sensory Variables

Investigation into the question of whether sensory functions affect the acquisition and production of articulatory skills has yielded information on one variable that is clearly related and another variable that may be related. The sensory variable that is related to articulatory acquisition and production is hearing. Its clinical implications are known and important to consider in treatment. The sensory variable that may be related to articulation is oral sensation. If oral sensation and articulation are related, treatment implications are questionable or ambiguous.

We will first summarize the research on the relation between articulation and hearing. We will next summarize the available data on oral sensory function and articulation.

Hearing Loss

It is well established that normal hearing is essential to unimpaired acquisition of oral communication, including speech sounds and oral language structures. The child who cannot hear the spoken language of his or her verbal community, or hears it inadequately, does not normally acquire oral language. Two to 3% of school-age children may have a hearing impairment that exceeds 25 decibels (dB) HL (hearing level) (Lundeen, 1991). Therefore, hearing impairment is a significant variable that affects the acquisition of oral communication skills.

Normal hearing is essential for oral speech and language acquisition because of two factors. First, normal hearing makes children aware of the speech and language spoken in their surroundings. It is difficult, if not impossible, to learn what is not heard, seen, or felt. Oral speech and language need to be heard. Second, normal hearing makes it possible to monitor one's own production of speech and language that is being learned. This monitoring is essential to progressively better approximate adult productions. Hearing their own speech, children can self-monitor and further refine their productions. Without the benefit of hearing their own speech, children will be unable to self-monitor.

The terms **hearing impairment** and **hearing loss** mean that there is a hearing problem. Technically, they mean that the auditory thresholds exceed 25 dB HL in the case of adults and 15 dB HL in the case of children. **Hard of hearing,** on the other hand, is a diagnostically more specific term. A person who is hard of hearing has residual hearing that can assist in speech–language acquisition, comprehension, and production. A hard of hearing person is aware of normal conversational speech. However, such a person may need amplification (e.g., a hearing aid). The term *deaf* also is diagnostically specific. Unaware of normal conversation, a **deaf** person is not able to use hearing for speech–language acquisition, comprehension, and production.

Whether hearing impairment affects the acquisition of speech sounds — and if it does, to what extent — depends on several factors. One important factor is the age of onset. The hearing loss may be **congenital,** which means that it is present at the time of birth, or **acquired,** which means that the onset was subsequent to birth. Generally, the earlier the onset, the greater the effect on speech and language acquisition.

Another important factor is the severity of the hearing loss. **Hearing acuity,** which means how well a person hears, is measured in terms of decibels. The **range of normal hearing** varies from 0 dB HL to 15 dB HL in children and from 0 dB HL to 25 dB HL in adults. Even a slight hearing loss, frequently associated with middle ear infections, may cause speech and language delay. Therefore, the upper limit of normal hearing in children is considered 15 dB HL. Typically, the severity of a hearing loss is classified as follows:

- slight impairment: 16 to 25 dB HL
- mild impairment: 26 to 40 dB HL
- moderate impairment: 41 to 70 dB HL
- severe impairment: 71 to 90 dB HL
- profound impairment: 91+ dB HL

Severity of hearing loss often is a function of the type of loss. Sensorineural hearing impairment tends to be more severe than conductive hearing loss. **Sensorineural loss** is associated with pathology in the inner ear or the neural pathways that carry auditory messages to the brain. **Conductive hearing loss** is associated with pathologies in the outer and middle ear; the inner ear and the auditory pathways are normal. Generally, sensorineural hearing loss tends to be more severe than conductive loss. In any case, if the hearing loss is significant for the frequencies of speech (500 to 4,000 Hz), a greater effect on speech and language acquisition is expected.

Still another factor that influences the degree to which hearing impairment negatively affects speech sound acquisition is the age at which clinical services are initiated and the quality of the services the child receives. The earlier the age at which comprehensive, intensive, and regular oral-aural (speech) rehabilitation services are initiated, the lower the negative effects on speech sound acquisition and production.

Children with a significant degree of hearing loss are likely to exhibit a variety of speech problems (Calvert, 1982; Dunn & Newton, 1986; Levitt & Stromberg, 1983). Such children tend to:

- omit final and initial consonants and omit /s/ more consistently;

- produce final consonants too weakly;

- substitute voiced consonants for voiceless consonants, nasal sounds for oral sounds, one vowel for another, and diphthongs for vowels and vowels for diphthongs;

- produce distorted sounds — for example, they may produce stops and fricatives with too little or too much force;

- produce vowels with imprecision, indefiniteness, and often with excessive duration;

- shorten the first or the second vowel in diphthongs;

- produce speech with marked hypernasality, especially in vowels;

- insert unnecessary vowels between consonants (e.g., *selow* for *slow*);

- inappropriately release final consonants (e.g., *mop^h* for *mop*);
- speak at a lower rate (presumably because of longer duration of consonants and vowels);
- pause more frequently;
- show slower articulatory transitions;
- use inappropriate stress on syllables;
- exhibit a harsh and breathy voice;
- speak with a pitch that is too high or too low;
- exhibit inappropriate prosodic features.

Research has shown that people who become deaf after acquiring speech and language tend to omit or distort sounds that are produced with low intensity and high frequency. These include /s/, /ʃ/, /tʃ/, /f/, and /θ/ (Calvert, 1982). In many cases, such people produce consonants in the final position of words with very little force. Consequently, listeners may not hear them.

Some evidence suggests that in nearly one third of children, articulation disorders are associated with **repeated middle ear infections** (Shriberg & Kwiatkowski, 1982a; Shriberg & Smith, 1983). Children with frequent middle ear infections tend to omit the initial consonants or replace them with [h]. They may substitute one nasal sound for another or denasalize nasal sounds. There is some evidence to suggest that most children with middle ear infection may attain normal articulation by age 4, but articulatory errors may persist in nearly a quarter of them (Paden, Matthies, & Novak, 1989).

✎ Activity

DIRECTIONS: Define the following terms in your own words.

Congenital hearing loss: _____

Acquired hearing loss: _____

Sensorineural hearing loss: _____

Conductive hearing loss: _____

Hard of hearing: _____

Deaf: _____

Auditory Discrimination of Speech Sounds

An auditory variable often researched for its relation to speech sound production problems is known as auditory discrimination or perception. Auditory discrimination is tested in various ways. In some studies, children with misarticulations were asked to listen to pairs of words or nonsense syllables and say whether the elements in a pair were the same or different. In those studies, no attempts were made to present sounds that the children themselves misarticulated. Such studies, conducted since the 1930s, have produced contradictory findings. Some suggested that children with articulatory production problems also had difficulty making judgments about sounds they heard. Others failed to replicate those findings, suggesting that despite a problem in speech sound production, children may correctly judge the sounds they hear (see Weiner, 1967, and Winitz, 1984, for reviews of those studies).

Some investigators have wondered whether a more consistent relation between articulatory production and auditory discrimination would emerge if the children were asked to discriminate between the correct and incorrect productions of sounds they themselves misarticulated. In studies using that method, the examiner would provide examples of correct productions and incorrect productions that reflected a child's error. In such a study that involved 131 children with misarticulations, Locke (1980a) reported that 70% of children could discriminate between the correct and incorrect productions of sounds they misarticulated. This means that a majority of children who misarticulated could separate correct and incorrect productions when the examiner presented such productions to them. Similar findings have been reported by other investigators (e.g., Eilers & Oller, 1976).

Thus, the evidence seems to support the conclusion that a majority of children who misarticulate sounds can tell whether someone else produces the same sounds correctly or not. Some children, however, may have difficulty judging the correctness of productions of sounds they misarticulate. As most children can discriminate between correct and incorrect productions, auditory discrimination does not seem to be a strong variable related to production problems in most children. In those who do have both production and discrimination problems, there is no evidence to conclude with certainty that it is the discrimination problem that causes production problems. They may be coexisting problems.

Another, perhaps clinically more useful method of investigating the relation between auditory discrimination and production is to train one or the other and evaluate the status of the untreated skill. That is, one can treat auditory discrimination to evaluate its effects on articulatory production. Alternatively, one can treat articulatory production to evaluate its effects on auditory discrimination. We will return to this issue in our Advanced Unit.

Oral Sensation

There has been some speculation as to whether children with reduced oral kinesthetic sensation may be prone to having difficulty in learning to articulate speech sounds. It is through the kinesthetic sensation that one becomes aware of muscle movement and position. If that sensation is defective, it may be difficult for a child to position and move the oral articulators. Research on this topic is based on that assumption.

Various kinds of stimuli applied to selected oral structures, especially the tongue, may be used to test oral sensation. Small plastic objects of various three-dimensional forms placed on the tongue with no visual information help assess **oral form recognition.** Subjects may be asked to point to the right drawing to identify the shape of the object in the mouth. Also, the tongue may be stimulated at two points to assess what is known as **two-point sensory discrimination.** Finally, the mouth may be **anesthetized** to study the effects of **sensory deprivation** in articulation. Oral form recognition in children with and without articulation problems has been compared to assess the relation between the two variables.

Research has not produced strong or unequivocal evidence to suggest that children with articulation problems have deficient oral form recognition. While some evidence suggests that some children with misarticulation may have poorer oral form discrimination skills (Ringel, House, Burk, Dolinsky, & Scott, 1970), other evidence suggests that those skills are the same in children with and without misarticulations (Arndt, Elbert, & Shelton, 1970).

There also is no strong evidence to suggest that deficient oral form recognition always leads to misarticulations. For example, a neurologically impaired adult with poor oral form recognition skills and poor two-point discrimination may retain good articulation skills (McDonald & Aungst, 1970).

Research on oral form recognition skills is both limited and contradictory. The clinical implication of this line of research is neither clear nor compelling. There is no evidence that children or adults typically depend on an awareness of oral muscle movement and position to articulate speech sounds. Most speakers generally are unaware of specific position and movement of speech muscles as they produce simple or complex speech (Netsell, 1986).

Even if children who misarticulate have difficulty with oral form recognition or two-point discrimination, it does not necessarily follow that articulation training should include oral sensory exercises. When children with misarticulation are trained to have their form recognition scores improve, their articulation may or may not improve. We will return to this issue in the Advanced Unit.

Oral anesthetization is an externally induced variable and may not have much relevance to genetically or neurologically based poor oral sensitivity, which is a possibility that interests researchers or clinicians. Besides, oral anesthetization has been studied mostly in adults, and thus the results do not have a direct bearing on the acquisition of articulation. Generally, the studies of adults have indicated that when the mouth is anesthetized, there is (a) a general increase in misarticulations and a specific increase in misarticulations of fricatives and affricates, (b) difficulty in tongue retroflexion and lip rounding, (c) a more posterior positioning of articulators, (d) a slightly increased duration of consonants, and (e) an increase in intraoral air pressure (Prosek & House, 1975; Gammon, Smith, Daniloff, & Kim, 1971). Although anesthetization is likely to produce these and possibly other effects on articulation, speech remains mostly intelligible.

Language Skills

Language is a larger system that subsumes articulation. Speech sounds are the building blocks of language. Therefore, researchers have wondered whether articulation and phonologic disorders necessarily imply a language disorder as well. Viewed from an opposite angle, when there is a problem in the larger system (i.e., language), there may also be problems in the subsumed system (i.e., the articulation or phonologic system). Researchers have looked at the relation between language and articulation from both angles.

To study the relation between language and articulation or phonological skills, researchers often have analyzed productive language skills of children who have misarticulations. A few studies have tried to assess the relationship between language and articulatory skills by experimental teaching of either language or articulation skills and evaluating the effects of teaching one skill on the other, untreated skill.

The general prevalence data of language and speech disorders throw some light on the potential relation between articulation and language skills. It is known that not all children with language impairment have articulation or phonologic disorders. Similarly, not all children with articulation or phonologic impairment have language disorders. Several studies suggest that up to 80% of children with phonologic disorders may have language problems, and roughly the same number of children with specific language impairment also may have phonologic problems (as summarized in Fey et al., 1994). Children with severe phonologic problems may be more likely to exhibit a concomitant language disorder (Lewis, Ekelman, & Aram, 1989).

There is some evidence to suggest that articulation or phonologic problems of children with specific language impairment may resolve by school age (Whitehurst et al., 1991). A smaller percentage of children with phonologic disorders (10 to 40%) also may have language comprehension problems (Shriberg & Kwiatkowski, 1994). This means that the two problems may coexist in a majority of children showing one or the other problem, but that in a smaller percentage of children, either of the two problems can exist without the other.

Additional observations relative to prevalence of articulation and language disorders also support the view that the two kinds of problems can be independent of each other unless other variables interact with them in such a way as to intertwine them. For example, children who are significantly developmentally delayed and have language impairment may exhibit articulation disorders much more consistently and for a longer duration than children whose articulation disorder is associated with specific language delay. In such cases, language disability and articulation disorders appear to be intertwined, but the two kinds of disorders may be related to the underlying developmental disability rather than to each other.

Research has shown that children with significant articulation and phonologic disorders may use less complex language, shorter utterances, and incomplete sentences. The articulation errors of some children with both articulation and language problems may increase when the children are asked to produce progressively more complex sentence structures (e.g., longer sentences; passive, complex, or compound sentences) or words with a greater number of syllables (longer words). When syntactic complexity is combined with syllabic complexity, a greater increase in errors of articulation may be evident (Panagos, Quine, & Klich, 1979).

Some investigators have tried to assess the relationship between language disorders and articulation disorders by treating one or the other to see if the untreated disorder improves without intervention. The results are somewhat conflicting but generally tend to show that treating language disorders will improve language skills but not phonological skills. Similarly, treating phonologic disorders will improve phonologic skills but not language skills. Each disorder should be treated separately. This complex issue is addressed in the Advanced Unit.

Since the 1930s, researchers have been interested in whether as a form of language skills, **reading skills** are associated with articulatory proficiency. Some of the early studies reported contradictory findings on the relation between reading skills and articulatory proficiency. While some reported that children with articulation disorders have significant reading problems, others reported no such finding.

Earlier research did not take into consideration the potential language problems most children with articulation disorders also tend to exhibit. Reading problems of children with articulation disorders, if documented, may be a part of their impaired language skills. More recent research has suggested this possibility (Lewis & Freebairn-Farr, 1991). Research into the relationship between articulation and reading skills should rule out the presence of language disorders.

In more recent years, decreased **phonological awareness** skills have been implicated with poor reading abilities in young children. This topic is addressed in the Basic Units of Chapters 3 and 7.

Personal Characteristics

Certain personal characteristics of children, especially age, gender, intelligence, and "personality" (of both children and their parents), have been researched for their possible differential association with articulation disorders.

That **age** is a significant factor in articulation learning is a generally accepted notion among speech–language pathologists. Normative data, as reviewed in Chapter 3, indicate that by age 4, most normally developing children will have articulatory skills that resemble those of adults, although improvements may be noted until age 8 or so. Up to that maximum age level, children at lower age levels make more articulatory errors than those in higher levels.

What variables actually contribute to greater mastery of speech sounds in older children (up to the known limits) is not clear, however. Neurophysiological maturation may contribute to articulatory mastery. The influence of environmental feedback and learning also may play a role. It is questionable whether age in itself is a variable that leads to better performance in any skill, including articulatory skill. What happens when neurophysiologic and environmental factors change is probably the true variable associated with increasing age and improved articulatory skill.

Gender is another classic variable associated with articulation and phonologic disorders. Research since the 1920s has shown girls to be slightly superior to boys in speech sound acquisition. In general, girls master sounds sooner than boys, although the difference is typically small (not statistically significant) at most age levels. The more recent research supports the classic findings (Smit, Hand, Freilinger, Bernthal, & Bird, 1990). Survey research since the 1930s also has shown that articulation disorders are more common in boys than in girls.

Intelligence is another personal characteristic that researchers have studied in relation to articulatory proficiency. Various tests of intelligence have been used to correlate I.Q. scores with those on standardized tests of articulation. In some cases, results of speech samples have supplemented articulation test scores. Research, starting with the 1940s, has fairly consistently shown that I.Q. scores that are within the normal limits do not highly correlate with scores on articulation tests. This means that for articulatory acquisition, variations in intelligence *within the normal limits* have only a negligible effect on articulation.

Intelligence that falls *below the normal limit* is a different matter, however. Children whose I.Q. falls below 70 have shown a higher prevalence of articulation disorders. Generally speaking, the lower the I.Q., the higher the prevalence and frequency of articulatory problems. Children who are developmentally disabled (mentally retarded) may learn the sounds in the same sequence as those with normal intelligence, although an increased variability may be evident in the former group. In addition, children with developmental disabilities show a preponderance of consonant deletions and generally inconsistent errors (Shriberg & Widder, 1990).

The **personalities** of children who misarticulate and their parents have been of interest to several researchers. Research into this poorly defined and highly questionable mentalistic construct has not produced anything of clinical or theoretical significance.

The **socioeconomic status** of families has provoked some research on the assumption that it might influence articulation learning in children. In several studies, the occupational status of parents was correlated with articulatory proficiency in their children. Cumulative research evidence suggests that a slightly greater number of children with misarticulation come from families with lower socioeconomic or occupation status.

There is some evidence that any difference in the frequency or prevalence of articulation errors in children at lower socioeconomic levels may disappear by the time the children enter school or soon thereafter (Templin, 1957). In essence, socioeconomic status is only a minor variable in articulation learning and performance.

The influence of **birth order and number of siblings** on articulation learning and performance has interested researchers since the 1950s. It is often stated that the first born and the only child in a family have better articulation skills than subsequently born children. Data to support that claim are weak; in one study, teachers' ratings were used to assess children's articulatory proficiency (Koch, 1956).

There also are contradictory data indicating that number of siblings and articulatory proficiency are unrelated (Wellman, Case, Mengert, & Bradbury, 1931). Unless better designed and current studies demonstrate a more convincing relationship between the two variables, it may be concluded that birth order and number of siblings are not significantly associated with articulation.

In essence, such personal characteristics as age, gender, intelligence within normal limits, socioeconomic status, and personality do not seem to be variables that exert strong influence on articulatory learning and performance. However, below-normal intelligence is significantly associated with articulation disorders.

Familial Prevalence

Familial prevalence of articulation disorders has been researched in more recent years to assess possible genetic bases of articulatory learning and performance. A higher familial prevalence of a speech disorder means that if there is one person with a given disorder, there are likely to be others among blood relatives with the same disorder. To put it differently, the prevalence of a disorder is higher among family members than in the general population. Higher familial incidence of stuttering has been known for many years. Such evidence for articulation disorders has emerged in research conducted since the mid 1980s.

Familial prevalence of articulation disorders may be higher in some families but not in all. For example, Shriberg and Kwiatkowski (1994) have reported that among a group of 62 children with articulation disorders, 39% had one other family member and 17% had more than one family member with articulation disorders. Other research has shown that compared to siblings of children with normal articulation, siblings of children who misarticulate tend to perform more poorly on measures of articulation (Lewis, Ekelman, & Aram, 1989). Furthermore, children of people with a history of articulation disorders perform more poorly on tests of articulation than those whose parents have normal articulation skills (Felsenfeld, McGue, & Broen, 1995).

Tongue Thrust

An issue that generated some controversy in the past because of its hypothesized relation to articulation disorders is tongue thrust, also known as *reverse swallow* or *infantile swallow.* **Tongue thrust** refers to a certain manner of swallowing and tongue placement in the oral cavity during rest, not to the thrusting of the tongue against the frontal teeth, as the term implies. Children younger than 5 years of age normally carry their relatively large tongue more anteriorly than older children and adults; as the oral cavity is enlarged, the tongue is carried more normally (in a relatively posterior position).

Tongue thrust is characterized by (a) a forward gesture of the tongue during swallowing so that the tip of the tongue is in contact with the lower lip; (b) the forward carriage of the tongue in the oral cavity in such a way as to keep the tongue tip against or between the anterior teeth, while the mandible is slightly open; or (c) fronting of the tongue during speech so that the tongue is between or against the anterior teeth, while the mandible is slightly open (Mason & Proffit, 1974). A child may exhibit one or more of these characteristics. The effect on dentition and speech depends on whether one or more characteristics are present.

Tongue thrust may be functional habitual or due to an organic condition. Habitual tongue thrusting is not associated with any structural abnormalities. Organic conditions that cause tongue thrusting are enlarged adenoids or tonsils that partially block the posterior airway passage (American Speech-Language-Hearing Association, 1989; Mason, 1988).

An anterior resting posture of the tongue in the oral cavity may affect the individual placement of teeth. However, when the anterior tongue carriage is combined with tongue thrust swallow, some children may develop a pattern of malocclusion, although more evidence is needed to establish this relationship firmly.

In some children, tongue thrust swallow and a forward tongue resting position may be associated with an articulation disorder, most commonly with a lisp. Distortions of /z/ and /l/ also are common. Interdentalization of /t/, /d/, /n/, and /l/ has been reported as well (American Speech-Language-Hearing Association, 1989).

The American Speech-Language-Hearing Association's 1991 position paper on tongue thrust states that speech–language pathologists who have specialized training in correcting patterns of tongue thrust may offer their services to clients who need them. The reader is referred to that position paper along with the ad hoc committee report on the issue (1989). Treatment for tongue thrust is not provided in many public schools unless there is an accompanying articulation disorder.

Summary of the Basic Unit

- Normal variations in the structure of the lips, teeth, tongue, hard palate, and soft palate *are not significantly associated* with articulatory acquisition or proficiency.

- Significant structural deviations (e.g., a cleft of the palate) *may be associated* with problems in learning speech sounds; velopharyngeal inadequacy results in compensatory articulation, characterized mostly by various forms of sound substitutions.

- Speech sound acquisition and production may be affected if neural control of the speech mechanism is impaired.

- Speech problems associated with central or peripheral nervous system damage are known as **dysarthria.**

- Speech problems due to defective motor planning of speech gestures in the absence of muscular weakness or paralysis is known as **apraxia of speech.**

- General **motor skills** *are not a significant factor* in articulatory and phonologic acquisition.

- Generally, children with articulation disorders have a slower diadochokinetic rate suggesting slower than normal oral-motor skills.

- Deficiencies in motor skills are neither necessary nor sufficient to produce articulatory problems.

- **Hearing impairment** is typically associated with problems in speech sound learning; the extent of the problems depends on the degree of the hearing impairment, the age of onset of the hearing impairment, the quality of aural rehabilitation, the time of initiation, and so forth.

- Severe hearing loss of the **deaf** is associated with various kinds of articulation problems.

- A difficulty in **auditory discrimination** of speech sounds *may be associated* with speech sound production problems in about 30% of children.

- A majority of children with articulation problems do not have difficulty in the auditory discrimination of the sounds they misarticulate.

- **Oral sensation** or **oral-form recognition** *has not been found* to be strongly and consistently associated with articulation problems; oral anesthetization in adults produces articulation problems, although the speech remains intelligible.

- Up to 80% of children with articulation or phonological errors also may exhibit a language disorder.

- Increases in the grammatical complexity of language are associated with increases in articulatory errors.

- Increases in the syllabic complexity of words are associated with increases in articulatory errors.

- When language and articulation disorders coexist, treating only one of them may produce some effect on the other, but it is likely that the effects will not be substantial; more research is needed.

• When language *and* articulation disorders coexist in a child, both should be targeted for treatment.

• Until age 8 or so, higher age levels are associated with better articulation skills.

• Girls are slightly ahead of boys in speech sound acquisition; articulation disorders are slightly more prevalent in boys.

• Intelligence within the normal limits is not a significant factor in articulatory acquisition; below-normal intelligence is associated with disorders of articulation.

• Children with misarticulation do not have a unique personality, nor do their parents.

• A slightly greater number of children with articulation disorders come from families with lower socioeconomic status.

• Birth order and number of siblings are not significantly associated with articulation skills, although some early research suggested otherwise.

• In some families, the prevalence of articulation disorders may be higher than that in the general population; more than half the number of children with articulation disorders report other family members with similar problems.

• Siblings of children who misarticulate and children of parents who have a history of misarticulations may perform poorly on articulation tests.

• **Tongue thrust,** also known as reverse swallow, is characterized by a forward gesture of the tongue during swallowing, a forward carriage of the tongue in the mouth, and fronting of the tongue during speech; the tongue tip may be in contact with the lower lip and the anterior teeth.

• In some children, tongue thrust swallow may be associated with articulation disorders.

Advanced Unit

◆　◆　◆　◆　◆　◆　◆　◆　◆　◆　◆　◆　◆　◆　◆　◆　◆　◆　◆

Research on Variables Associated with Articulation and Phonological Development

As noted, the question of what variables are related to articulatory acquisition in children with and without articulatory problems is of both theoretical and clinical significance. Theoretically, variables related to articulation may be causal factors. However, research on such variables presents numerous challenges to those who wish to draw a cause-effect conclusion. The challenges are both conceptual and methodological. Logical problems in drawing conclusions relative to causes and effects and the methods that are necessary to draw such conclusions require a careful examination.

Research on variables associated with articulatory acquisition and performance has generally been able to identify only a few variables of clinical and theoretical significance. Generally speaking, research on most of the variables is both dated and questionable on methodologic grounds. Some research may be dated because contemporary investigators do not find the variables worth investigating. Research on such variables as oral form recognition; general motor skills; oral anesthetization; structural problems or the dimension of such structures as the hard palate, lips, and teeth; general intelligence; and socioeconomic status has not illuminated the independent variables of articulation. Nor has it provided new insight into the treatment of articulation disorders. The research on variables reviewed in this chapter has not been especially productive partly because of numerous limitations.

In this Advanced Unit, we will examine some of the limitations inherent in research on potential cause-effect relations that investigators have tried to identify. These limitations include: (a) logical and conceptual problems and (b) methodologic problems. We also will address the issue of clinical importance and the implications of such presumed or demonstrated cause-effect relations between various variables and the treatment of articulation disorders.

Logical and Conceptual Problems

The original intent of researchers in this area was to identify potential causes of speech sound acquisition. For instance, they asked such questions as the following: Is intelligence a factor in speech sound acquisition? Are structural deviations in the speech mechanism causes of a failure to normally acquire speech sounds? Is socioeconomic status a significant variable that contributes to better or poorer articulatory performance? Even if the questions were not framed precisely in this manner, the purpose was to find whether each researched variable was a potential cause of better or worse articulatory skill in children. Otherwise, the variables would not interest researchers or clinicians.

For the most part, research has shown that the variables researched are not strongly related to articulation; those that are are related only within a certain range. The major logical and conceptual problems relate to the nature of causation and the appropriate methods of investigating them.

A Factor's Role Within and Outside of Normal Variation

If a factor such as intelligence is a cause of acceptable or unacceptable articulatory skills, it may be so only when it is significantly below normal. Children who are significantly below normal in intelligence do have a higher prevalence of articulation disorders and more severe disorders. And yet articulation disorders are also common in children whose intelligence varies within normal limits. Thus, within normal limits, intelligence does not appear to be related to articulation, but when intelligence is below normal, it certainly is. The same is true of various structural deviations. Dimensional variations of the hard palate within normal limits may not significantly affect articulation, but significant structural anomalies may. Many children with articulation disorders have oral structures that vary within the normal limits. Logically, therefore, it is incorrect to claim that intelligence or oral structures are not related to articulation disorders or to claim that they are. The most accurate claim is that each of those variables is related to articulation when it is on the negative side of the normal range.

Explanation of articulation disorders in children who are within normal limits on variables discussed in this chapter poses a challenge to the theoretician. If certain children with an articulation disorder are normal on the variable investigated, then the cause of that disorder may be a hitherto unsuspected variable. Or the cause of the disorder may lie in the child's faulty learning history. Clinicians generally assume that a communication disorder is treatable. If it is successfully treated, assumption about the role of learning in the maintenance of that disorder is supported to some extent. However, the origin of the disorder may remain a mystery.

Implications of Experimental Manipulation of a Factor in Adults

Another conceptual problem in this area of investigation involves the inference of a relation between two variables when none may exist. Research on the issue of oral sensation illustrates this potential problem. To evaluate the potential effects of oral sensation, some investigators have asked anesthetized adult subjects to produce speech. If the speech is impaired, investigators have inferred that articulation disorders in children may be related to reduced oral sensation.

This inference or implication is unwarranted, however. The results of such a study show only that anesthetization has a negative effect on the articulation of the subjects studied. They have no direct implication for a potential relation between oral sensation and articulation disorders even in children who are demonstrated to have reduced oral sensation. Therefore, it is not possible to conclude that children depend on good oral sensation to acquire sounds or that disorders of articulation are related to poor oral sensation.

Conceptual Problems in Relating Language to Articulation

There are two views on the proposed relation between language and articulation. One view holds that syntactic structure organizes and dominates the phonologic structure; this is known as the *top-down hypothesis* because syntactic structure is a higher level of organization of language. In this view, language disorders are likely to be reflected in articulation and phonologic disorders as well. The other view is that phonologic structure may have an effect on syntactic structure; this is known as the *bottom-up hypothesis* because phonologic structure is a lower level of organization of language (Panagos & Prelock, 1982). In this view, phonologic problems may contribute to language disorders.

On the one hand, research has generally shown that when syntactic complexity increases, articulatory errors also may increase (Panagos, Quine, & Klich, 1979; Schmauch, Panagos, & Klich, 1978). For example, the number of misarticulations may be higher when children with an articulation disorder repeat longer or grammatically more complex sentences than when they repeat shorter or grammatically simpler sentences. In other words, the top-down hypothesis is supported. On the other hand, research also has shown that when syllabic complexity is increased, syntactic errors in children with language disorders also increase. For example, when children repeat sentences containing words with simple syllabic complexity (e.g., *kid,* CVC), they make fewer syntactic errors than when they repeat sentences containing words with more syllabic complexity (e.g., *customer,* CVCCVCV) (Panagos & Prelock, 1982). This is interpreted to mean that phonologic complexity increases syntactic errors in children with language disorders and thus the bottom-up hypothesis also is supported.

The problem with the two apparently opposing hypotheses is that they both seem to be supported. This means, however, that the bottom-up and the top-down hypotheses are nondiscriminatory. That both views are supported means that they each sample only limited data on the relation between language and articulation and that neither hypothesis is valid. The most parsimonious view may be that language and articulation are aspects of a single phenomenon and that complexity in one is likely to compound an existing problem in the other. That any one aspect (e.g., syntactic or phonologic aspect) "controls" all other aspects of language may reflect only a favorite theoretical bias that lacks an empirical basis.

Inferences Based on Treatment of One or the Other Aspect

Children who misarticulate may have additional problems in overall language skills. As summarized in the Basic Unit, such children may exhibit a coexisting language disorder or an auditory discrimination problem. Consequently, some researchers have asked whether treatment of language disorders *or* phonologic disorders in children who have both kinds of disorders will result in improvement in the untreated disorder as well. Other researchers have investigated the parallel question of whether treatment of an auditory speech sound discrimination problem *or* a speech sound production problem will result in improvement in the untreated disorder as well. These questions often are asked in an effort to answer theoretical questions about the relationships between language and articulation and between articulation discrimination and production. The questions, however, have practical implications for the clinician as well. If it is sufficient to treat only one of two problems to effect changes in both, then substantial time and effort are saved.

Treatment of Language Disorders, Articulation Disorders, or Both?

The evidence on the effects of treating language or articulation on the untreated disorder is contradictory. There is some limited evidence that treating language disorders may improve phonologic performance with no direct treatment for articulatory problems (Hoffman, Norris, & Monjure, 1990; Matheny & Panagos, 1978). The evidence supporting the opposite hypothesis that treatment of phonologic disorders may improve language disorders with no direct treatment for language is even more limited. Only the Matheny and Panagos study claims this effect; the Hoffman, Norris, and Monjure study obtained unimpressive effects of phonologic treatment on language skills. In the absence of a strong and replicated effect of phonologic treatment on language disorders, it may be concluded that that effect is minimal at best and clinically not meaningful.

There are data that contradict the just cited evidence that treating language disorders improves the coexisting phonologic disorder. Tyler and Watterson (1991) and Fey and colleagues (1994) have reported that treating language disorders in children with both language and phonologic disorders will improve only language disorders, but not both.

A critical examination of the studies involved suggests that the evidence on the positive effects of language treatment on untreated phonologic disorders is rather weak. Studies that show that language treatment results in articulation improvement also should demonstrate that no unintended articulation practice was a part of the language intervention. Such a demonstration is difficult because language treatment, even if the treatment did not involve specific attention to articulatory performance, may nonetheless involve unintended clinician modeling and client practice of specific speech sounds. In the Matheny and Panagos (1978) study, language treatment involved modeling and imitation of various language structures on repeated trials that may have provided unintended imitation and practice of certain speech sounds.

In the Hoffman, Norris, and Monjure (1990) study, modeling and repeated trial practice were not a factor, as the study used the "whole-language" approach. Unfortunately, the study involved a group design with one subject in each group and no controls for extraneous variables. Consequently, the evidence is both limited and lacking in internal validity. The study did not offer convincing evidence that whole-language treatment positively affected phonologic skills. The lack of strong evidence to show that whole-language treatment is effective even for teaching language skills makes the result even more suspect.

A prudent conclusion is that treating one disorder when both language and articulation disorders coexist in a child may result in clinically significant improvement only in the treated disorder. Therefore, unless stronger evidence is produced and replicated, clinicians should not assume that treating language disorders will change a coexisting articulation disorder with no treatment. Both should be separately targeted.

Treatment of Auditory Discrimination, Sound Production, or Both?

As noted in the Basic Unit, research on the relation between speech sound discrimination and production has produced contradictory findings. Nonetheless, the unambiguous conclusion that discrimination is related to production often is stated (Winitz, 1984), possibly because of strong theoretical biases. Based on such a conclusion, many clinicians believe that it is necessary to treat speech sound discrimination problems to successfully remediate production problems.

Some of the initial studies on training either discrimination or production to assess the effects on the untrained component produced inconsistent results. All possible outcomes have been reported: (a) discrimination training can affect production, (b) production training can affect discrimination, and (c) neither training affects the untrained component (see Williams & McReynolds, 1975, for a brief review of studies). The research design used in those studies did not permit a definitive investigation of the effects of one training on the other. Most were not designed specifically to assess the effects of training one component (discrimination or production) on the untrained component.

The study by Williams and McReynolds (1975) was specifically designed to assess the effect of training one skill on the other skill. The authors provided discrimination training to two subjects and production training to two others. In each case, they probed for changes in the untrained component (production or discrimination). The results showed that discrimination training produced better discrimination but no change in production. Production training, on the other hand, produced changes in both production and discrimination. Those results suggest that it is more efficient to train production because it affects both production and discrimination. The results make sense when one considers that in production training, the child's correct and incorrect responses will be differentially reinforced. A child will not be reinforced for saying *toup* for *soup* but will be reinforced for saying *soup*. It is difficult to imagine that such differential reinforcement will not produce discrimination between correct and incorrect productions. Discrimination training may be inherent to production training, but not vice versa.

Some clinicians provide both production and discrimination training to children who misarticulate. When the results are positive, they then claim that discrimination training is necessary and should be provided concurrently with production training (Rvachew, 1994). This claim is questionable, however, as concurrent training does not separate the effects of the two training procedures. Positive results may be due entirely to production training, discrimination training, or both. In view of the results of the Williams and McReynolds study (1975), it does not seem necessary to train discrimination at all.

The most efficient course of action for the clinician is to train production first and probe for discrimination. In most cases, or even in a certain number of cases, discrimination training may not be needed; production training may have resulted in improved discrimination. If the probes show that discrimination between previously misarticulated sounds and their correct productions is poor even though the sounds are produced correctly, the clinician may consider training discrimination. However, the consequences of poor discrimination when correct production has been achieved have not been addressed. What harm does poor discrimination do? Does a child who cannot tell the difference between *soup* and *toup* not recognize soup? There is little or no evidence that children who do not recognize the difference between speech sounds are actually confused about the relevant objects and events.

Just as the positive results of concurrent training of discrimination and production are not especially revealing, it is not illuminating to show that discrimination training can help improve production training. A clinician can still offer only production training, because production skills are more badly needed than discrimination skills; there is just as good a chance that discrimination, too, will improve without direct training. Only one kind of data can help support discrimination training. Discrimination training may be useful if it is shown that such training will significantly reduce the time and effort required for production training. There are no such data.

Methodologic Problems

A single methodologic limitation makes it difficult if not impossible to draw cause-effect conclusions regarding most variables researched and reviewed in this chapter. This limitation, which stems from the typical method of correlating one variable with another, is addressed in this section. An exception to this limitation is the effects of training one component on the other. If the training of one component and the probing of the untrained component are accomplished within a well-controlled experimental design, the results may have acceptable internal validity.

Research on most variables has not used this experimental strategy. The limitations of the correlation method used in studying the relationship between variables must be kept in perspective when evaluating research on factors related to articulatory acquisition and performance.

Correlation Versus Causation

When two variables (e.g., articulation and intelligence) are simply measured, no variable is experimentally manipulated (except in the case of treatment studies, as noted). Typically, children's articulation is measured along with another variable of interest. In some studies, two groups, one with normal articulation and the other with articulation problems, are formed. Sometimes the group with normal skills is described as the control group and the one with problematic skills is described as the experimental group. However, there is no experimental manipulation in such studies, and the terms *control group* and *experimental group* are misnomers.

Whether only one group (with articulation disorders) or two groups (with and without such disorders) are included, such studies have often looked at some other variable presumably related to articulation. For example, socioeconomic status, intelligence, integrity of the speech mechanism, and so on may be measured in children with articulation disorders (single group) or in children with and without such disorders (two groups). The results of the study are then correlated. If the correlation is positive and statistically significant, it is concluded that the two variables (e.g., articulation and socioeconomic status) are related. A conclusion often implied or even explicitly stated is that the variable investigated is a causal variable. In other words, one might conclude that the variable is one of the causes of misarticulations.

That correlation does not imply causation is common knowledge. A significant positive or negative correlation means that the two factors vary together. A third and unobserved variable may be responsible for the observed covariation. For example, lower socioeconomic status, though correlated with articulatory skills, may have nothing to do with articulation. The parents with lower socioeconomic status also may have less formal education, and that may be causally related to articulation disorders in their children. Please note that this is only an example of an unobserved third variable that *may* be responsible for the observed covariation; it is not suggested here that the educational status of parents is causally related to better or worse articulatory skills in children.

When the correlational method is used in studying the relationship between articulation acquisition and other variables, the most valid conclusion is that certain variables are *associated* with articulatory acquisition and performance. The investigated variables may be causally related, but the data do not support that conclusion.

Summary of the Advanced Unit

• Research on variables that are associated with articulatory acquisition and proficiency is generally intended to find causes of normal and disordered articulation; however, various conceptual and methodologic problems limit the validity of conclusions.

• Much of the research is both dated and of questionable validity; therefore, its theoretical or clinical significance is often clouded.

• Most factors researched do not seem to make a major difference, provided they are within their normal variation; however, those variables may be significant if below normal.

• Experimentally manipulated variables (e.g., oral anesthetization) in adults may affect articulation, but this does not mean that the variable (e.g., oral sensation) is significant in articulatory acquisition and production in children.

• Theoretical concepts that relate language and articulation are generally weak; both the top-down (language structures influence phonologic performance) and the bottom-up (phonologic structures influence language) are supported; therefore, the two hypotheses do not compete and are both based on limited observations.

• The effects of treating a coexisting language disorder on phonologic problems and the effects of treating phonologic problems on the language disorder have been ambiguous and inconclusive; the best clinical practice seems to be to treat both disorders independently. Any study that seeks to evaluate the effects of language treatment on phonologic skills needs to control for unintended practice of speech sounds during language therapy.

• Most children with articulatory production problems do not have auditory discrimination problems; auditory discrimination training helps improve both production and discrimination, whereas discrimination training improves only discrimination. The best clinical practice seems to be to train production first and then train discrimination if necessary; concurrent training of both discrimination and production is inefficient and may be unnecessary in most cases.

• Most studies on the variables associated with articulation acquisition and production have used the correlational method, which suggests only covariation, not causation.

Chapter 5

◆ ◆ ◆ ◆ ◆ ◆ ◆ ◆ ◆ ◆ ◆ ◆ ◆ ◆ ◆ ◆ ◆ ◆

Ethnocultural Variables Affecting Articulation and Phonological Development

Basic Unit

♦ ♦ ♦ ♦ ♦ ♦ ♦ ♦ ♦ ♦ ♦ ♦ ♦ ♦ ♦ ♦ ♦ ♦ ♦ ♦

Ethnocultural Variables of Articulation and Phonological Development

I speak Spanish to God, Italian to women, French to men, and German to my horse.

—CHARLES V (CHARLES THE WISE), 1337–1380

Ethnocultural variations do not always imply language variation. For example, many U.S.-born and -raised children, especially grandchildren, of people who emigrated to the United States may be ethnically heterogeneous but linguistically homogeneous with the native English-speaking population in the United States. On the other hand, a certain number of U.S.-born children of parents who speak a language other than English, and almost all children who emigrated to the United States with their parents whose primary language is other than English, may be both ethnically and linguistically diverse from the majority population. In such cases, linguistic diversity is typically associated with bilingualism.

Ethnocultural variation and the attending linguistic diversity are not limited to recent immigrants. Some U.S.-born, native English-speaking, monolingual persons may be linguistically diverse because of their ethnocultural diversity. African Americans who have lived in the United States for generations are a case in point. Their linguistic diversity is an element in their ethnocultural heritage. To some extent, such diversity may be evident in other ethnocultural groups who have lived in the United States for many generations. For example, although empirical studies are lacking, it is possible that Mexican, Japanese, or East Indian people who have lived in the United States for many generations may retain subtle linguistic differences that are of no social or occupational consequence. To what extent, and after how many generations, the traces of ancestral linguistic heritage fade in a new culture are interesting questions for empirical research.

It is obvious that ethnic background is not a necessary condition for linguistic diversity. Linguistic diversity can thrive within a single ethnic culture. In the genesis of linguistic diversity, relative geographic isolation is a powerful variable. The same language, the same ethnic background, and even broadly the same culture can give rise to linguistic diversity when there is overriding geographic separation. The varied dialects of world languages, spoken by otherwise relatively homogeneous populations, are a case in point. The many dialects of British English and American English are familiar examples of linguistic diversity in the face of broad ethnocultural homogeneity.

Pronounced linguistic diversity poses significant challenges for educators, health care workers, human service professionals, and business people. Obvious and subtle shades of linguistic diversity are interwoven with a host of poorly understood variables related to family, society, and culture. Diversity may be pronounced with bilingual immigrant adults and children whose primary language is other than the dominant language of their adopted country. In the United States, immigrants whose first language is other than English tend to exhibit that pronounced linguistic diversity.

The diversity may be considerable if the children, even though born in the United States, are raised as bilingual speakers by bilingual parents or monolingual, non-English-speaking parents. The extent of diversity may diminish when children born in the United States are raised by English-speaking bilingual parents. The diversity may be minimal or of no consequence if the children are raised as monolingual English speakers by English-speaking monolingual parents.

This chapter is written to help speech–language pathologists who assess language and articulation disorders of children whose primary language is neither English nor general American English, which is often considered to be standard English. To make appropriate assessment and treatment decisions, clinicians need to know about a child's linguistic and cultural background. They need to acquire special expertise in assessing and treating children who speak:

- a language other than English (e.g., Spanish or Hmong);

- English as a second language, acquired some time after the acquisition of their primary language;

- a dialectal variety of American English (e.g., Black English); or

- a different form of English (e.g., Australian English).

In principle, what clinicians need to know is clear. They need to know:

- the language and phonologic characteristics, properties, and rules of the linguistically diverse child's primary language;

- how the primary language affects the learning of the second language; and

- how to determine whether there is a language or phonologic disorder in the child's first language, second language, or both.

However, acquiring such knowledge is not always practical for clinicians. The linguistic diversity of the U.S. population has increased significantly and continues to increase. Clinicians in some states and some regions in certain states face such an enormous linguistic diversity that the demand can be overwhelming. It is not uncommon for speech–language pathologists in certain public schools to face children who speak a dozen or more primary languages that are different from English.

It is sometimes implied that the speech–language pathologists of the majority culture (White Americans) exclusively face this problem. But that is not the case. The problem of providing clinical services to children of diverse backgrounds is faced by all speech–language pathologists. For example, a Hispanic American, an African American, or a Chinese American speech–language pathologist working in an American public school or health care setting faces the same problem. What should a Hispanic speech–language pathologist who speaks Spanish and English do when a child's primary language is other than either of those? What should an African American speech–language pathologist do when a child's primary language is

Hmong? What should any speech–language pathologist do when a child speaks a language other than the one the clinician speaks?

The answer cannot be that all speech–language pathologists should be multilingual. Therefore, there are no easy answers to these questions. Nonetheless, there are many steps speech–language pathologists can take and many professional dispositions they can learn. In this chapter, it is not possible to catalog all the phonological differences between the many languages that are now spoken in the United States; many such differences have not been adequately described. Descriptive research has mostly been concerned with articulatory acquisition and production in (a) African American English (AAE) or Black English, (b) some Native American languages, (c) a variety of Spanish, and (d) certain Asian languages. There is more information on AAE and Spanish and their variations than on any other minority language spoken in the United States.

In this Basic Unit, we summarize the salient information available on children who speak AAE or a language other than English as their primary language. The main purpose is not to exhaustively list the phonologic differences between English and other languages, but to illustrate the point that phonologic differences across languages of interest must be understood. In addition, we summarize basic professional dispositions and guidelines necessary to appropriately assess and treat children with ethnocultural diversity. In the Advanced Unit, we will discuss theoretical issues and clinical research issues.

African American English

Scholars do not agree on what to call the variety of English many African Americans speak. The terms Black English (BE) (Dillard, 1972), Black English Vernacular (BEV), African American Vernacular English (AAVE), and simply African American English (AAE) have all been suggested. African American English is consistent with the name used to describe the ethnic group with which it is predominantly identified; therefore, that term is preferred here (van Keulen, Weddington, & DeBose, 1998).

AAE was once considered a substandard form of White American English or (general) Standard American English (SAE). All scholars, clinical professionals, and such professional organizations as the American Speech-Language-Hearing Association completely reject that view, however. There are significant similarities and differences between the English White Americans speak and the English some African Americans speak. The issue is whether the differences are strong enough to conclude that AAE is a different language. Some scholars have argued that AAE is indeed a language, not just a dialectal variation of English spoken by Whites (van Keulen et al., 1998).

The origin of AAE is not certain. The possible origins of AAE include English spoken by Whites or such independent sources as a creole (Dillard, 1972). Geographically, AAE may have its origins in West Africa, where the Europeans visited for trade. Because there was no common language, a pidgin may have developed that served basic business communication. A **pidgin** is a simplified and limited system of communication that develops out of necessity when two communities with no common language are forced by circumstances to communicate with each other. A pidgin may develop into a **creole,** which is a more complex system of primary communication, with its own phonologic, semantic, syntactic, and pragmatic rules. It is a primary system of communication because it is the only form of communication acquired by children in their typical community. From then on, a pidgin that has become a creole is passed from one generation to the next (Crystal, 1987; Dillard, 1972; Wolfram, 1994). Thus, AAE, which may have started as a pidgin in Africa, may have become a creole among Africans in North America. In time, with greater interaction with SAE, the current forms of AAE may have evolved.

Not all African Americans speak AAE. A few may speak it all the time, some may speak it most of the time, and some speak it occasionally. Some African Americans do not speak AAE at all. A few rural southern Whites use elements of AAE in their speech. Many who speak AAE also speak Standard American English and switch from AAE to SAE or vice versa, depending on the audience, a phenomenon known as *code switching*.

It is now well recognized that AAE has its own phonological, syntactic, semantic, and pragmatic rules. It has a distinct communication style. Many sources provide excellent descriptions of AAE characteristics, rules of usage, and communication style (Dillard, 1972; Hecht, Collier, & Ribeau, 1993; Kamhi, Pollock, & Harris, 1996; Roseberry-McKibbin, 1995; van Keulen et al., 1998; Willis, 1992; Wolfram, 1994). The reader should consult these and other sources for a better understanding of African American culture, family, value system, language structure and use, and communication style.

Assessment of articulation and phonological skills in any child requires, in addition to other procedures, conducting an interview with the family and the child, recording a speech–language sample, and administering standardized or client-specific measures of language and speech. In essence, the clinician should arrange communicative situations to sample speech and language. Therefore, even if the concern is only to assess speech production in a given child, the clinician should know the characteristics and unique properties of the language the child and the family use. An understanding of their communication style and interactional patterns should be appreciated.

In this chapter, for the sake of brevity and special relevance, we will be concerned mostly with phonological aspects of AAE. However, a few critical features of language and communication style will be summarized as well.

Activity

DIRECTIONS: As discussed in the text, describe the primary differences between a **pidgin** and a **creole:**

Africans Americans have a rich linguistic tradition. They can use language effectively, eloquently, and often colorfully. A distinct rhythm and a unique style of communication in individuals may be encouraged in the African American culture. Emotional and gestural expressions may enhance communication to a greater extent than in some other ethnic groups. Public behavior may be more intense and expressive than in other ethnic groups. African Americans may be more inclined to touch or make physical contact during conversation. While eye contact may be a form of verbal expression, rolling the eyes may be considered offensive, and children may not, out of respect for adults, maintain eye contact during conversation.

Children telling stories may include personal judgments and evaluations. A child may prefer to refer to her mother as "Momma" not as "Mother," as the former term is viewed more positively.

Cultural heritage, family relationships, and mutual help and support are highly valued in African American society. Loyalty to family, respect for the elderly, and group efforts for the common good are cultural values. Persons who are not blood relatives may be considered part of the family because of their supportive role and the broader concept of a family. Children may be raised more authoritatively than in other cultural groups, although they are highly valued, well supported, loved, and cared for.

To analyze the phonological characteristics and speech production problems an African American child may have, the clinician needs to take into consideration the language characteristics of AAE. Please see Table 5.1 for a summary of major language characteristics of AAE.

Phonological Characteristics of AAE

Many phonological characteristics are common to AAE and standard English. However, it is important to understand the unique phonological features of AAE so that such features are not misinterpreted as phonological disorders.

Not all speakers of AAE use all its unique phonological features. Wolfram (1986) has shown that the use of certain phonological features may depend on socioeconomic status. Compared to African Americans in lower socioeconomic classes, those in the middle and upper classes use fewer phonological features of AAE. A few features, however, may be used by speakers in all socioeconomic classes, though with varying frequency. For example, omission of the postvocalic r in such words as *sister* (pronounced as *sistə*) may be observed across socioeconomic classes. In contrast, the substitution of /f/ for /θ/ in such words as *bath,* pronounced *baf,* common in middle and lower socioeconomic classes, is uncommon in upper middle and upper socioeconomic classes. Therefore, the lack of /f/ substitution for /θ/ may not suggest that the speaker is not an AAE speaker; it may mean only that he or she is a middle- or upper-class African American.

Table 5.2 lists the major phonological characteristics of AAE. All consonants and vowels found in SAE also are found in AAE. The speech of many AAE speakers may not contain the /ð/, as it is replaced by /d/ in the word-initial position and /v/ or /d/ in the word-medial and -final positions. The /θ/ may be replaced by /t/ or /f/. Most AAE speakers reduce some diphthongs into single vowels, a phonological process known as **ungliding.** Generally, more consonants than vowels differ between AAE and SAE. Consonants in the medial- and final-word positions show greater differences than those in the initial position.

Table 5.1. Major Language Characteristics of African American English

AAE Characteristics	Mainstream American English Statement	AAE Statement
Noun possessives may be omitted.	That's the woman's car. It's John's pencil.	That **the woman** car. It **John** pencil.
Noun plurals may be omitted.	He has 2 boxes of apples. She gives me 5 cents.	He got 2 **box** of **apple.** She give me 5 **cent.**
Third-person singular may be omitted.	She walks to school. The man works in his yard.	She **walk** to school. The man **work** in his yard.
Forms of to be (is, are) may be omitted.	She is a nice lady. They are going to a movie.	**She a** nice lady. **They going** to a movie.
Present tense is may be used regardless of person or number.	They are having fun. You are a smart man.	**They is** having fun. **You is** a smart man.
Person or number may not agree with past and present forms.	You are playing ball. They are having a picnic.	You **is** playing ball. They **is** having a picnic.
Present-tense forms of auxiliary have may be omitted.	I have been here for 2 hours. He has done it again.	**I been here** for 2 hours. **He done** it again.
Past-tense endings may be omitted.	He lived in California. She cracked the nut.	He **live** in California. She **crack** the nut.
Past was may be used regardless of number and person.	They were shopping. You were helping me.	They **was** shopping. You **was** helping me.
Multiple negatives may be used to add emphasis to the negative meaning.	We don't have any more. I don't want any cake. I don't like broccoli.	We **don't** have **no more.** I **don't never** want **no** cake. I **don't never** like broccoli.
None may be substituted for any.	She doesn't want any.	She don't want **none.**
In perfective constructions, been may be used to indicate that an action took place in the past.	I had the mumps when I was 5. I knew her.	I **been had** the mumps when I was 5. I **been known** her.
Done may be combined with a past-tense form to indicate that an action was started and completed.	He fixed the stove. She tried to paint it.	He **done fixed** the stove. She **done tried** to paint it.
The form be may be used as the main verb.	Today she is working. We are singing.	Today **she be** working. **We be** singing.
Distributive be may be used to indicate actions and events over time.	He is often cheerful. She's kind sometimes.	**He be** cheerful. **She be** kind.
A pronoun may be used to restate the subject.	My brother surprised me. My dog has fleas.	My brother, **he** surprised me. My dog, **he** got fleas.
Them may be substituted for those.	Those cars are antiques. Where'd you get those books?	**Them** cars, they be antique. Where you get **them books?**
Future-tense is and are may be replaced by gonna.	She is going to help us. They are going to be there.	She **gonna** help us. They **gonna** be there.
At may be used at the end of where questions.	Where is the house? Where is the store?	Where is the house **at?** Where is the store **at?**
Additional auxiliaries may be used.	I might have done it.	I **might could have** done it.
Does may replace do.	She does funny things. It does make sense.	**She do** funny things. **It do** make sense.

Note. Adapted from *Multicultural Students with Special Needs* (Table 5.1, pp. 52–53), by C. Roseberry-McKibbin, 1995, Oceanside, CA: Academic Communication Associates. Copyright 1995 by Academic Communication Associates. Reprinted with permission.

Table 5.2. The Phonological Characteristics of African American English

	Examples	
AAE Phonologic Feature	Mainstream American English	African American English
/l/ lessening or omission	tool always	too' a'ways
/r/ lessening or omission	door mother protect	doah mudah p'otek
f/ voiceless th substitution in word-final or -medial position	teeth both nothing	teef bof nufin'
t/ voiceless th substitution in word-initial position	think thin	tink tin
d/ voiced th substitution in word-initial and -medial positions	this brother	dis broder
v/ voiced th substitution at word-final position	breathe smooth	breave smoov
Consonant-cluster reduction in initial and final positions	throw desk rest left wasp	thow des' res' lef' was'
Consonant substitutions within clusters	shred strike	sred skrike
Differing syllable stress patterns	guitar police July	**gui** tar **po** lice **Ju** ly
Modification of verbs ending in /k/	liked walked	li-tid wah-tid
Metathetic productions	ask	aks
Devoicing of final voiced consonants	bed rug cab	bet ruk cap
Deletion of final consonants	bad good	ba' goo'
i/e substitution	pen ten	pin tin
b/v substitution	valentine vest	balentine bes'
Diphthong reduction (ungliding)	find oil	fahnd ol
n/g substitution	walking thing	walkin' thin'
Unstressed-syllable deletion	about remember	'bout 'member

Note. Characteristics may vary depending on variables such as geographic region. Adapted from Multicultural Students with Special Needs (Table 5.2, pp. 54–55), by C. Roseberry-McKibbin, 1995, Oceanside, CA: Academic Communication Associates. Copyright 1995 by Academic Communication Associates. Reprinted with permission.

Omission of consonants in word-final position is a notable feature of AAE. However, certain factors influence the omission of consonants (Stockman, 1996; Wolfram, 1991, 1994). For example: The final nasal sound or an oral stop is more likely to be omitted than other consonants. A final consonant in a word is likely to be omitted if the following word begins with a consonant (e.g., the /t/ in *best buy* is more likely to be omitted than the /t/ in *right on*). A consonant that serves a morphemic function is more likely to be omitted if the meaning can still be made clear (e.g., the omission of the plural *s* in such expressions as *two cup*).

Consonant-cluster reduction is a significant feature of AAE. Clustered consonants in the initial position are produced more often than those in the final position. Most consonants in the final position are omitted. There also are a few sound substitutions within initial clusters (see Table 5.2).

Unstressed-syllable deletion is another significant feature of AAE. In such words as *until* and *about,* the initial syllable may be markedly reduced or altogether omitted. Research has shown that the frequency of unstressed-syllable deletion increases with age (Stockman, 1996). This phenomenon also has a pattern. For example, an unstressed syllable is more likely to be deleted if a single vowel forms the syllable shape (e.g., *away*), the preceding word ends in a vowel (e.g., *go away*), or the word is a preposition or conjunction (e.g., *behind, because*). The unstressed syllable is likely to be produced in certain other contexts. For example, the unstressed syllable is produced when the word is a noun, adjective, or verb (e.g., the initial syllable is produced in *begin* but may be deleted in *before*) and when the word has three syllables (e.g., the initial syllable is produced in *depression* but may be deleted in *divorce*) (Stockman, 1996).

In summary, AAE contains most of the same phonemes as SAE. A phoneme inventory is likely to show no or only a few differences between them. The phonemes, however, may be used differently in the two languages. Omissions and substitutions of sounds, often prominent in the word-medial and -final positions, give AAE its most characteristic feature. As we will see in subsequent sections, omission and substitution of phonemes is characteristic of speakers who use English as a second language.

Articulatory Development in Children Speaking AAE

There have been relatively few studies on the acquisition of speech sounds and sound patterns by African American children. Undersampling of African American and other minority children has been a persistent problem in speech and language development studies. For example, most of the classic studies of articulatory development summarized in Chapter 3 have sampled mostly White American children. Therefore, there is a great need for comprehensive studies on articulatory and phonological acquisition in African American children.

It is evident that in studying speech sound development in African American children, the characteristics of AAE should be taken into consideration. For example, such well-known characteristics as final-consonant deletion, cluster reduction, unstressed-syllable deletion, and certain sound substitutions should not be interpreted as evidence of lack of speech development or the presence of an articulation disorder.

In their studies, some investigators have compared African American children's articulatory performance with that of White children of similar age. In such studies, some investigators have evoked and analyzed specific phonological features that characterize AAE. To sample children's articulatory performance, some have evoked various sounds through pictorial stimuli, while others have used standardized tests of articulation. A few other investigators have analyzed selected phonological processes in the conversational speech of African American children. Very few investigators have been concerned with normal or abnormal development of articulatory skills in African American children (Stockman, 1996).

Studies that included African American and White ethnic groups have generally shown that the children in the two groups have similar sound inventories. In each group, errors tend to be higher for younger children than for older children. This trend is consistent with normative data summarized in Chapter 3. This means that, similar to children in other ethnic groups, African American children master speech sounds progressively as they grow older (Stockman, 1996). Though studies are limited, available evidence suggests that African American children develop phonemes roughly in the same sequence as other children. At different ages, the phonetic inventory of African American children may be comparable to that of children of other ethnocultural backgrounds.

Some studies also have shown that African American children make more articulatory errors when the analysis of their speech sample is done from the standpoint of SAE. Most of those "errors" are likely to be characteristics of AAE. Therefore, the conclusion that African American children exhibit a greater number of articulatory errors than comparable White children is not warranted. Children in a lower socioeconomic class may exhibit a slightly higher number of articulatory errors regardless of ethnocultural background. Therefore, it is important that when articulatory performances in different ethnocultural groups are compared, the subjects be from the same socioeconomic class. Other variables that might affect articulatory performance also should be equal across comparative groups.

The speech sounds that African American children tend to misarticulate are, for the most part, the same as those that White children misarticulate. For example, in one study, of the 10 consonants misarticulated, 8 were the same across the two ethnocultural groups (Seymour & Seymour, 1981). The same study also has shown that sound substitutions may be common to children in the two ethnocultural groups. However, African American children tend to exhibit more omissions than White children mostly because such omissions are a feature of AAE. Provided that the special features of AAE are taken into consideration, the normative evaluation of speech sounds for the two groups need not differ in any drastic manner (Seymour & Seymour, 1981).

African American children, similar to children of other ethnocultural backgrounds, show fewer phonological processes as they grow older. However, final-consonant deletion may be an exception to that rule, as such deletions are a feature of AAE. Final-consonant deletion may persist beyond third grade (Haynes & Moran, 1989).

Although much research needs to be done on articulatory development in African American children who speak AAE, limited available data suggest that those children acquire articulatory skills in the same manner as children in other groups. Articulatory acquisition in African American children is susceptible to the same kinds of interference as in other children. For example, such variables as hearing impairment or significant developmental disability may be expected to negatively affect articulatory acquisition in all children. The clinician should interpret all data relative to the articulatory proficiency of African American children in the context of what is known about (a) articulatory acquisition in all children and (b) the characteristics of AAE.

Assessment of Articulatory and Phonological Disorders in African American Children

Assessment of articulatory and phonological disorders in children who speak AAE poses many challenges. Clinicians who wish to assess articulatory proficiency in African American children will find that few or no standardized tests are available. Generally, it is not appropriate to use a standardized test in assessing a child from a minority group when that minority group was not sampled or not sampled adequately in the standardization process.

Some of the available tests of articulation may be highly biased against ethnocultural groups. Some tests may give credit for the child if the item is dialect-sensitive; for example, the second edition of the *Arizona Articulation Proficiency Scale* (Fudala & Reynolds, 1986) allows such credit for African American dialectal variations. However, this test may be more biased against southern African American children than toward the northern (Washington & Craig, 1992). Whether a test gives credit to a child on a dialect-sensitive item or not, the clinician should. For example, an African American child's production of *baf* for *bath* should not signal an articulation disorder. The clinician should examine the test items for dialectal or language-specific variations that may be found in the child who is being assessed.

As warned by Stockman (1996), giving credit to dialect-sensitive items on a standardized test may not solve the problem. When most test items for a given phoneme are dialect-sensitive, giving credit for them may leave few or no items to make a judgment about that phoneme production. Also, single-word articulation tests, regardless of dialect sensitivity, may produce erroneous data. For example, an African American child is less likely to produce certain consonants in isolated words, whereas the same consonants may be produced in continuous speech, especially when the target consonants precede a word that begins with a vowel (Stockman, 1996).

Conversational speech probably is a better measure of phonological skills than are standardized tests. Conversational speech allows the normal speech behavioral patterns to play their role. However, the problem of intelligibility of conversational speech may pose special problems for transcribing the sample.

Some clinicians may depend on parental or community input in determining whether a speech disorder exists in a child who speaks an unfamiliar dialect. Terrel, Arensberg, and Rosa (1992) suggest that parents' speech may be considered a standard against which a child's speech and language skills may be evaluated. Some clinicians believe that if the parents or other caregivers do not think a child has a problem, the clinician should be extremely cautious in diagnosing one (Stockman, 1996).

An appropriate diagnosis of an articulation disorder in children who speak AAE requires data collection from multiple sources, some of which may be unconventional. Careful selection of standardized tests, giving credit to dialect-sensitive items, an extensive conversational speech sampling, a detailed interview of parents or other caregivers, comparing the child's speech to that of the caregivers, and a good understanding of the culture and communication pattern of the child and the family help make an appropriate diagnosis.

Treatment of Articulatory and Phonological Disorders in African American Children

For many African American children, AAE should be the treatment context and treatment goal. Because the speech sound inventory of AAE is, with a few exceptions, the same as that of SAE, all speech sounds of SAE can be potential treatment targets for children who speak AAE. However, specific AAE sound patterns and rules of usage should be considered in selecting treatment target words and in accepting or not accepting productions as correct or incorrect during treatment. For example, an African American child's imitation of the clinician's modeled *bathtub* as *baftub* may be accepted as correct unless the goal is to teach SAE because of parental demand for it. In essence, the acceptable, correct, and clinically reinforced productions will be based on the patterns of articulatory behaviors that characterize AAE.

Unless experimental treatment data or clinical data demonstrate otherwise, clinicians can assume that the basic treatment principles used in treating articulation disorders will be useful in treating African American children as well. Procedural modifications to suit the client may be necessary, as they are with children of all ethnocultural backgrounds. Stimulus materials selected for teaching phonemes should be client-specific, unambiguous, and familiar in the child's environment.

Stockman (1996) suggests that a priority system may be used in selecting treatment targets for African American children. Phonemes whose pattern of usage is the same in SAE and AAE should be the first targets of intervention. The speech intelligibility of an African American child will improve greatly if phonemes that are used in the same manner in both languages are taught first. Stockman suggests that the next set of phonemes to be taught should be those that the child does not use or misuses within the patterns of AAE. Even when the clinical stimulus input is SAE, if the child gives responses that are consistent with AAE usage, the child should be reinforced. The example given earlier of the clinician-modeled *bathtub* and child-imitated *baftub* is a case in point. Specific phonological processes targeted for intervention should be consistent with AAE patterns. For example, in targeting the elimination of final-consonant deletion, only those phonetic contexts in which the final consonant is mandatory in AAE should be taught.

For many AAE speakers, SAE speech sound patterns can be an acceptable goal. If clients face problems because of their use of AAE in social, occupational, or other specific contexts, acquiring the sound patterns of SAE might be a pragmatic decision that the client or the parents may make. In essence, even though there is no speech impairment, a child or an adult who speaks AAE might be socially or occupationally handicapped. In that case, the goal would be to teach an alternative set of speech skills, not to eliminate those associated with AAE. Stockman suggests that clinicians can legitimately offer clinical services when there is a personal, social, or occupational handicap but no speech impairment.

Stockman's (1996) guidelines on clinical intervention are consistent with the general goal of improving the speech intelligibility of the African American child while respecting the integrity of AAE. Learning the phonological patterns of SAE can be a legitimate goal for African Americans who speak AAE, and clinicians should have no problem offering services to achieve that goal.

Some general guidelines for treating children of minority ethnocultural groups are summarized in a later section.

Native American Languages

About 2 million people identified themselves as Native Americans in the 1990 U.S. census (U.S. Bureau of Census, 1992). Many, but not all of them, live on 278 reservations and in 209 Alaskan native villages. Native Americans belong to more than 500 separate tribal groups, each with a distinct culture and language. Each tribe has an autonomous government. Each Native American tribe deals with the U.S. federal government as an independent government. The Native American population is predominantly young: one half of all Native Americans are younger than 21 years of age. Although Native Americans live in all parts of the United States, about 50% of the population lives in the western states. They are most highly concentrated in Arizona, New Mexico, California, Oklahoma, and North Carolina.

Research on the speech and language characteristics of Native Americans is extremely limited. Detailed analysis of phonological characteristics of Native American languages is lacking. This is partly because of the variety of languages and dialects that are spoken by Native Americans in North, Central, and South America. In 1998, the American Indian Web site listed approximately 800 Native American languages. Many sources suggest that there are at least 200 Native American languages in North America (Highwater, 1975).

Many Native Americans, especially the younger people, do not speak their native language. It is estimated that only 50 Native American languages are spoken by more than 1,000 persons (Crystal, 1987); several are spoken by fewer than 10 (Krauss, 1992). For example, Kiowa, a Tanoan language, is spoken by only 18 of a total population of 2,000 persons. Osage, a language of the Siouan family, has only 5 fluent monolingual speakers out of a total population of 2,500 (http://www.sil.org./ethnologue/countries.usa.html). Many younger people are English–Native American bilinguals (whether they are true bilinguals is debatable because their understanding of their native language is usually limited). Only 760,000 Native Americans in North America speak one of the 200 languages. Unfortunately, many Native American languages are extinct, and many more are on the verge of extinction.

The classification of Native American languages in North America is controversial. This may be due to lack of exhaustive study of the many languages Native Americans speak. The estimated number of Native American language families varies from a high of 60 to a low of 3. Highwater's (1975) classification includes 8 language families: Algonquian, Iroquoin, Caddoan, Muskogean, Siouan, Penutian, Athabascan, and Uto-Aztecan. The current American Indian Web site lists 6 families of Native American languages: Eskimo-Aleut, Algonkian-Wakashan, Nadene, Penutian, Hokan-Siouan, and Aztec-Tanoan. Varied spellings are common for some language family names (e.g., Na-Dine, Nadene; Algonquian, Algonkian).

The origin of Native American language families is poorly understood. Native American people's geographic isolation and their habitat, which spread throughout the Western Hemisphere, may have been responsible for the incredible variety of their languages. Experts have found no genetic relationship among the families of Native American languages (Highwater, 1975). For this reason, whether it is appropriate to group these languages under a broad umbrella of Native American languages is not clear.

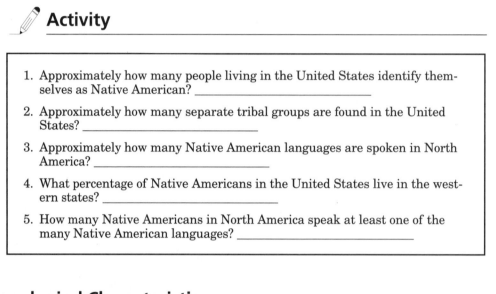

✎ Activity

1. Approximately how many people living in the United States identify themselves as Native American? _____

2. Approximately how many separate tribal groups are found in the United States? _____

3. Approximately how many Native American languages are spoken in North America? _____

4. What percentage of Native Americans in the United States live in the western states? _____

5. How many Native Americans in North America speak at least one of the many Native American languages? _____

Phonological Characteristics of Native American Languages

It is not possible to list the phonological characteristics of Native American languages because of their variety. Most available sources give an overview of Native American phonological characteristics and highlight a few examples from different languages.

Most Native American languages have been undergoing significant changes, some more than others. For example, there is Old Blackfoot and New Blackfoot. In New Blackfoot, the glottal stop of Old Blackfoot is being replaced by a creaky voice, long segments, or both. New Blackfoot has reportedly lost the word-initial /w/ and /h/. In Old Blackfoot, vowels in the word-final position or followed by [x] were devoiced. In the new version, vowels in the word-final position are voiced normally. However, vowels are deleted when they are preceded by glides. Most vowels preceding [x] are voiceless. There are no diphthongs in Old Blackfoot, but they are emerging in New Blackfoot (http://www.teleport.com/~napoleon/blackfoot/phonetics.html).

Blackfoot has no voiced nonsonorant consonants. There are no liquids either. Most stops are released not aspirated, and the length of consonants is contrastive in the language. Blackfoot contains only three vowels: /i/, /o/, and /a/. However, those three vowels have 11 tense and lax allophonic variations. Vowel length is contrastive, but only the tense vowels have length as a feature.

It is not surprising that the phonological properties of Native American languages vary greatly. Because the languages belong to different language families and have little or no genetic linking, many may have independent origins. Some Native American languages have far fewer sounds than English. For example, the Arawakan language has only 17 phonemes (Welker, 1996). Nasalized vowels are a common feature of several Native American languages. To contrast meaning, vowels may be produced with different pitch or tonal quality. In some languages, such as Navajo, vowel length distinguishes meaning. In some languages, vowels may be voiceless. For example, of the three vowels used in the Cheyenne language of the Algonquian family, all may be either voiced or voiceless. Voiceless vowels are whispered (Leman, 1998).

Among the consonants, the glottal stop is one of the few sounds common to most Native American languages. Several Native American languages also have sounds that are produced in the posterior vocal tract. Glottalized consonants, which are produced with a glottal stop and in conjunction with another consonant, also are common to several languages. For example, the word *ts'in* contains a glottal stop and means *bone,* whereas *tsin,* without such a stop, means *tree.* A /k/ that is produced in the uvular region (unlike the English /k/, which is produced at the velum) also is a common feature across several languages. In many Native American languages, /k/ and /q/ are contrastive (Welker, 1996). Consonant clusters are few in Navajo, and no clusters occur in syllable-final position. Navajo also has several sounds that are absent in English (Harris, 1998).

In Native American languages (e.g., in Cheyenne), /p/, /t/, and /k/ are always unaspirated. In some contexts, a /v/ may sound more like the English /w/. For example, in Cheyenne, a /v/ preceding /a/ or /o/ may sound like /w/, although native speakers will recognize it only as /v/.

Articulatory Development in Children Speaking Native American Languages

Reliable and systematic observations of articulatory and phonological development in Native American children are lacking. Because of the paucity of data and the variety of languages spoken, it is difficult to make generalized statements about Native American children's phonological skills, development, and disorders. Minimally, observations have to be extensive and systematic for languages *within each language family.* Presumably, generalized statements would then apply only to languages within a given family.

Native American languages are alive mostly in older people. Many children of Native Americans grow up speaking English and do not acquire their native language. For example, in one screening study of Papago Indian Reservation, the dominant language of 68% of children screened was English. Only 12% of the children spoke Papago as their dominant language at home. The remaining 20% spoke both Papago and English at home (Bayles & Harris, 1982). In Alaska, 17 of the 19 Native American languages are not transmitted to children; in Oklahoma, only 2 of 23 languages are transmitted to children (Crawford, 1996). Each decade in each Native American community, the number of children speaking their Native American language has decreased while those learning English has increased. For example, in the Navajo community, the number of children speaking only English more than doubled from the 80s to the 90s. In other communities, the change has been even more rapid, as the Navajo are known to be the most loyal to their language (Crawford, 1996). Therefore, it is especially difficult to study the development of Native American articulatory skills in children.

A few studies have looked at the English articulatory skills of Native Americans. Bayles and Harris (1982), who administered the *Goldman Fristoe Test of*

Articulation to Papago children, reported that 5% of the 583 children assessed had an articulation disorder. The characteristics of the Papago articulation were taken into consideration in scoring the children's responses. For example, the children were given credit for reduced aspiration and weak production of final consonants.

More systematic studies are needed before a description of the articulatory and phonological acquisition of Native American languages can be offered. Studies need to sample children who speak their native language as their only or their dominant language. As noted, many Native American children acquire English as their dominant language. Some of these children may acquire their native language as a second language. In such cases, acquisition of speech sounds in both English and the native language needs to be analyzed.

Assessment of Articulatory and Phonological Disorders in Native American Children

Assessment of articulatory skills in Native American children poses special challenges. The challenges are greatest when the child's primary language is a Native American language and the clinician lacks expertise in it. Because speech–language pathologists of American Indian background are few, and nonexistent in many parts of the country, it is likely that an assessment of Native American speech sound production will be extremely difficult for most speech–language pathologists. A few areas of the country (e.g., parts of the southwestern United States) tend to have specialists and resources available to assess children of Native American background. In most other parts of the country, people with expertise in Native American phonology are few or nonexistent.

The problem is not immediately solved even when a speech–language pathologist of Native American background is available. That person may or may not speak the particular language of the child to be assessed. Because of the unusual diversity of Native American languages, clinicians in particular regions of the country need to develop resources on the language or languages of Native Americans living in their service area. Currently, various Web sites on the Internet offer a variety of information on Native American languages. Much of the information is not specific to phonological or articulatory aspects of the languages described; however, that may change, and clinicians should monitor those sites to obtain the latest information. Even the sites that do not offer specific information on articulation and phonology do offer plenty of useful information on the Native American culture, language, customs, family, and community life.

It is likely that a local university's linguistic department has a specialist in Native American languages or the particular language spoken in the region. Such a specialist can be a valuable resource, and clinicians who serve Native American children in their clinics should develop a working relationship with such specialists.

It was noted earlier that many Native American children acquire English as their dominant language, and that many of their native languages are either extinct or almost extinct. This sad cultural fact actually makes the job of the speech–language pathologist easier. Most Native American children who need the services of a speech–language pathologist probably need them in English. In such cases, clinicians need to assess the children's articulatory and phonological skills in English. It would still be necessary to understand the cultural background of the child and the Native American communication style (see Table 5.3 for a sum-

Table 5.3. A Summary of Communication Style of Native American People

- Respect is highly valued; one way of signifying respect for another person is to avoid eye contact with that person by looking down.

- Children's communication with adults is respectful and discrete. To show respect, little eye contact is made with adults. Making eye contact is viewed as a way of showing defiance or rudeness.

- Native American mothers, especially those in the Navajo population, may be silent with their infants.

- Most children are taught that one learns more by listening and observing than by speaking.

- Parents often feel that their children's auditory comprehension skills are more advanced than their expressive language skills.

- Speech, language, and hearing difficulties occur five times more frequently among Native Americans than in the general population.

- Children are generally discouraged from speaking the tribal language before they are capable of correct articulation. Opportunities for oral practice in the language may be limited.

- Before they begin using words, some children communicate primarily through pointing and gesturing for a long period of time.

- Among some western Apache Indians, children may be rebuked for "talking like a white man" if they speak English or talk too much in the village.

- Native American etiquette requires a lapse of time between the asking and answering of a question. Some Native Americans believe that an immediate answer to a question implies that the question was not worth thinking about.

- Children often do not answer a question unless they are confident that their answer is correct.

- Children do not express opinions on certain subjects because they first need to earn the right to express such opinions.

- In many groups, it is considered inappropriate for a person to express strong feelings publicly.

- Adults usually express grief around outsiders only during official mourning ceremonies.

Note. Adapted from Multicultural Students with Special Needs (pp. 91–92), by C. Roseberry-McKibbin, 1995, Oceanside, CA: Academic Communication Associates. Copyright 1995 by Academic Communication Associates. Reprinted with permission.

mary of the communication style). Clinicians also should follow the guidelines for working with children who have dual phonological repertoire, described in a later section.

If a Native American child speaks English as a second language, the clinician has to treat that child as bilingual. With the help of resources the clinician has developed on the Native American language and culture, articulation and phonological skills in both the native language and English should be assessed. However, a bilingual child's dominant language may be English or a native language.

The clinician should determine whether there is a phonological disorder in the child's dominant language, in the secondary language, or both. In determining whether there is a disorder in the Native American language, the clinician should know the phonological properties of that language. In determining whether there is a disorder in English, the clinician should credit the child for varied productions of sounds that are consistent with those in the native language. Some of the suggestions offered in the section on Spanish language will be applicable in assessing children who speak both a Native American language and English.

Treatment of Articulatory and Phonological Disorders in Native American Children

Assessment of a Native American child's articulatory and phonological skills will help determine whether the child has a disorder in his or her monolingual Native American language or monolingual English. In the case of a bilingual child, the assessment will help determine whether the child has a disorder in either the dominant language, the secondary language, or both. This kind of differential assessment is essential for planning treatment.

The kind of professional expertise necessary to assess a Native American child also is necessary to offer appropriate treatment. A monolingual English-speaking Native American child's articulation disorders are treated in a way that is similar to treating any other child who speaks only English. However, cultural differences are still important to consider. For example, stimulus materials selected for treatment should be familiar to the child. Target words selected for speech sound training should be useful and prevalent in the child's home and school. The child's and the family members' disposition toward speech disabilities, their cultural values about effective communication, and their educational goals should be the basis of a plan for effective intervention.

If a child needs treatment in a Native American language, only those clinicians who can speak the language can offer it. The clinician who does not speak the relevant language should act as the child's advocate and find appropriate referral sources.

If a Native American child who speaks English as a second language needs articulatory and phonological treatment in that language, the clinician should treat that child as he or she would treat a bilingual child or a child with an African American background. Treatment targets should be consistent with the Native American child's speech and language. For example, if in the child's native language certain consonants are not aspirated, the equivalent aspirated English sounds, if not aspirated, should be acceptable. However, this rule may not hold if the child and the family seek treatment with a goal of acquiring SAE. Then the acceptable productions would be the same as those set for a child whose only language is SAE.

Spanish Language

Children whose primary language is Spanish or who speak Spanish and English, with one of the two being a dominant language, are a significant number among the minority ethnocultural groups. People whose primary language is a form of Spanish belong to different ethnocultural groups. The term *Hispanic* often is used to refer to these groups. According to the U.S. Bureau of the Census (1996), Hispanics are people of Spanish background. Contrary to popular belief, Hispanic is not an ethnic or racial term; it refers only to an individual's Spanish background. Hispanics may be of different races; there are black, brown, and white Hispanic people.

Hispanics, though sharing a Spanish heritage, are not a geographically or culturally homogeneous group; they are varied in the same way Asians are. Hispanics have a wide geographic distribution, spanning both North and South America. Hispanics of Mexican origin constitute the largest group in the United States. Other countries from which Hispanics hail include Puerto Rico, Cuba, Dominican Republic, Spain, Guatemala, El Salvador, Nicaragua, Costa Rica, Honduras, Panama, Colombia, Venezuela, Ecuador, Chile, Bolivia, Paraguay, Uruguay, and Argentina. Such a widespread geographic distribution of Hispanic people comes with varied cultures, customs, language differences, and dispositions toward communication and its disorders.

Hispanics are a growing population in the United States. In 1995, there were 27 million Hispanics in the country. By the year 2000, the number of Hispanics is projected to be 31 million. By the year 2030, the number may exceed 63 million (U.S. Bureau of the Census, 1996).

In the United States, Spanish is the second most common language. Different groups of Hispanics in the United States speak different varieties of Spanish. For example, Mexican Spanish is different from Bolivian Spanish, which is different from Cuban Spanish. In essence, each geographic-cultural group speaks a different variety of Spanish. There are at least six major dialects of American Spanish (Dalbor, 1980). The six varieties are named after their geographic locations: Mexican and Southwestern United States; Central American; Caribbean; Highlandian; Chilean; and Southern Paraguayan, Uruguayan, and Argentinean. In the United States, American Spanish of the Mexican, Puerto Rican, and Caribbean (especially Cuban) varieties is spoken most commonly. More information generally is available on these three varieties of American Spanish.

Hispanic children may be monolingual English speakers, monolingual Spanish speakers, English-Spanish bilingual speakers with good fluency in both, or bilingual speakers with one dominant and one significantly weak language. To assess and treat communication disorders in children of Spanish background, clinicians should have a good understanding of the cultural and linguistic heritage of Hispanics. This chapter summarizes only phonological characteristics, development, assessment, and treatment of children with Spanish background. Therefore, clinicians should consult other sources to gain a broader understanding of Hispanic people and their culture, language, and communication patterns (Kayser, 1995, 1998; Langdon & Cheng, 1992; Perez, 1994; Roseberry-McKibbin, 1995; Yavas & Goldstein, 1998; Zuniga, 1992).

To assess English articulatory skills in children of Hispanic background, clinicians need to know the major language characteristics of Spanish that influence English expressions. It is not possible to provide a detailed description of Spanish language in this chapter. However, a brief summary of some major language differences found in children of Hispanic background is provided in Table 5.4.

Phonological Characteristics of Spanish-Influenced English

Children whose primary language is Spanish but who speak English as their second language may show characteristics of Spanish phonological characteristics. A proper assessment of phonological disorders in such children should take into consideration those variations in English articulation that are presumably due to the characteristics of Spanish, their first language.

Table 5.4. Major Language Differences Found in Children of Hispanic Background

Language Characteristics	Sample English Utterances
Adjective comes after the noun.	The house green. . . .
s is often omitted in plurals and possessives.	The girl book is. . . .
Past-tense -ed is often omitted.	We walk yesterday.
Double negatives are required.	I don't have no more.
Superiority is demonstrated by using mas (more).	This cake is more big.
The adverb often follows the verb.	He drives very fast his motorcycle.

Note. Adapted from Multicultural Students with Special Needs (Table 6.1, p. 67), by C. Roseberry-McKibbin, 1995, Oceanside, CA: Academic Communication Associates. Copyright 1995 by Academic Communication Associates. Reprinted with permission.

The Spanish phonological system is somewhat simpler than that of English (Stockwell & Bowen, 1983). Both languages contain two semivowels. However, English has three times more vowel sounds (15) than Spanish (5). While English contains 24 consonants, Spanish contains only 19. The English consonants /v/, /θ/, /ð/, /z/, and /ʒ/ are absent in Spanish. Some of these consonants may be produced as allophonic variations of consonants that are present in Spanish. For example, a /d/ may be produced as /ð/. Some Spanish consonants, though comparable to English consonants, may be produced differently in the two languages. For example, many Spanish consonants are unaspirated. The Spanish consonants /ɲ/, /λ/, /ɣ/, /χ/, /ř/, and /β/ are absent in English (Perez, 1994).

Some sounds that are grossly similar in English and Spanish are produced differently. For example, /t/ and /d/, which are apical and aspirated in English, are dentalized and unaspirated in Spanish. Compared to English, Spanish has fewer consonants in word-final positions. Only /s/, /n/, /r/, /l/, and /d/ are produced in word-final position. Therefore, omission of final consonants may be more frequently observed in native Spanish speakers who use English.

Spanish and English differ in their use of consonantal blends. Spanish consonantal clusters are fewer and simpler. The /s/ cluster, common in word-initial position in English (e.g., *school*), does not occur in Spanish (e.g., *escuela* for *school*). While medial consonantal clusters are common in both languages, final clusters are rare in Spanish. Both languages contain /l/ and /r/ clusters (Stockwell & Bowen, 1983).

Table 5.5 provides a summary of some of the major characteristics of Spanish-influenced English.

✏ Activity

1. What is the projected number of Hispanics who will live in the United States by the year 2030? _____

2. What are the six major dialects of Spanish spoken in the United States? _____

(continues)

(Continued)

3. How many consonants make up the Spanish language as opposed to English? _____

4. What English consonants are absent in Spanish? _____

5. What are the only consonants in Spanish that can be produced in the final position of words? _____

Table 5.5. Major Articulatory and Phonologic Characteristics of Spanish-Influenced English

Articulation Characteristics	Sample English Patterns
/t, d, n/ may be dentalized (tip of tongue is placed against the back of the upper central incisors).	
Final consonants are often devoiced.	dose/doze
b/v substitution	berry/very
Deaspirated stops (sounds like speaker is omitting the sound because it is said with little air release)	
ch/sh substitution	Chirley/Shirley
d/ voiced th, or z/ voiced th (voiced th does not exist in Spanish)	dis/this, zat/that
t/ voiceless th (voiceless th does not exist in Spanish)	tink/think
Schwa sound inserted before word-initial consonant clusters	eskate/skate espend/spend
Words can end in 10 different sounds: a, e, i, o, u, ɪ, r, n, s, d	sounds at the end of words may be omitted
When words start with /h/, the /h/ is silent.	'old/hold, 'it/hit
/r/ is tapped or trilled (tapped /r/ might sound like the tap in the English word butter).	
There is no /ʤ/ (e.g., judge) sound in Spanish; speaker may substitute y.	Yulie/Julie
Frontal /s/ in Spanish is produced more frontally than in English.	Some speakers may sound like they have a frontal lisp.
The ñ is pronounced like ny (e.g., baño is pronounced bahnyo).	
Spanish has 5 vowels, a, e, i, o, u (ah, ĕ, ee, o, u), and few diphthongs; thus Spanish speakers may produce the following vowel substitutions:	
ee/ɪ substitution	peeg/pig, level/little
ĕ/ă, ah/ă substitutions	pet/pat, Stahn/Stan

Note. Adapted from *Multicultural Students with Special Needs* (Table 6.2, p. 68), by C. Roseberry-McKibbin, 1995, Oceanside, CA: Academic Communication Associates. Copyright 1995 by Academic Communication Associates. Reprinted with permission.

Articulatory Development in Children of Spanish Background

Research on articulatory development in children of Spanish background has used varied methods and subject populations. Some investigators have sampled monolingual Spanish-speaking children, while others have sampled English-Spanish bilingual children with varying degrees of proficiency in each language. A majority of studies have sampled Spanish-speaking children in Mexico and the United States. Other groups on which data have been reported include the Dominican, Puerto Rican, Bolivian, and Venezuelan. Most studies have used the cross-sectional method of simultaneously sampling children from different age groups.

Data on normal phonological acquisition in Spanish-speaking children are accumulating, if slowly. The major studies on articulatory acquisition in children of Spanish background include those by Acevedo (1991), De la Fuente (1985), Goldstein (1988), Goldstein & Iglesias (1996), Gonzalez (1981), Jimenez (1987), Linares (1981), and Mason, Smith, and Hinshaw (1976). However, only a few investigators have analyzed speech sound production in Spanish-speaking or English-Spanish bilingual children with disorders of articulation (Goldstein, 1993; Meza, 1983).

Goldstein (1995) has summarized the results of the studies of normally developing Spanish-speaking or Spanish-English bilingual children as follows. Normally developing infants of Spanish background produce CV syllables containing oral and nasal stops and front vowels. Most Spanish phonemes are mastered by age 4. Dialectal features of the child's community may be evident by age 3. Some phonemes, especially [ð], [χ], [s], [n], [ʧ], [r], and [l], may still be difficult for children at the end of preschool. Consonant clusters also may remain difficult. Such phonological processes as cluster reduction, unstressed-syllable deletion, stridency deletion, and tap or trill /r/ deviations may still be evident at the end of preschool. However, such phonological processes as velar and palatal fronting, prevocalic singleton omission, stopping, and assimilation may no longer be evident in the speech of those children. During the early elementary years, some children may still exhibit errors on the fricatives, affricates, liquids, and consonant clusters (Goldstein, 1995).

Assessment of Articulatory and Phonological Disorders in Children of Spanish Background

Assessment of articulatory and phonological skills of children with Spanish background poses the same challenges clinicians face in providing services to any bilingual client. The standard question is whether to assess the child in Spanish, in English, or both. A disorder in one language is likely to express itself in the other language as well. It is probably unusual to see a child with a significant phonological disorder (not just differences) in one language and normal phonological skills in the other. Therefore, unless the child is a monolingual English speaker of Hispanic (or any other) background, assessment must be completed in both Spanish and English.

Assessing a child's Spanish speech and language skills requires Spanish fluency on the part of the clinician or access to a professionally trained interpreter. This interpreter should speak the same dialectal form of Spanish (e.g., Cuban or

Mexican) and should have training in interpretation and some background in clinical linguistics. The interpreter should provide the stimuli and administer sound evocation procedures in the same manner as the clinician. He or she should have adequate training in response recording and scoring.

Standardized Spanish tests of articulatory and phonological skills may be used. The interpreter the clinician uses should have adequate training in standardized test administration, response recording, and scoring according to the test manual. A few standardized Spanish tests are now available, although they may not be suitable to assess children of all ethnocultural backgrounds who speak Spanish. These tests include the *Austin Spanish Articulation Test* (Carrow, 1974), *Assessment of Phonological Processes–Spanish* (Hodson, 1986b), *Assessment of Phonological Disabilities* (Iglesias, 1978), and *Southwest Spanish Articulation Test* (Toronto, 1977).

Many tests are available if the assessment goal is to sample productions of English phonemes as well. These tests and related procedures are described in Chapter 6. One English test that is also sensitive to certain Spanish patterns of production is the *Fisher-Logemann Test of Articulation Competence* (Fisher & Logemann, 1971). This test samples consonants in the intervocalic positions. Many Spanish consonants are produced in the intervocalic positions. Therefore, the test may help assess articulation differences in English that are influenced by Spanish (Perez, 1994).

Assessment of articulatory and phonological skills should include a comprehensive speech sample. Clinical decisions should not be based solely on the results of standardized tests, as most of them assess phoneme productions in single, isolated words. Dialectal differences and phoneme productions in connected speech are important to assess. Properly structured speech samples, collected with client- and culture-specific stimuli and considerations, also avoid the biases inherent in certain tests.

The assessment data should be analyzed to describe a child's articulatory and phonological skills in Spanish and English. Yavas and Goldstein (1998) recommend that the clinician should describe (a) common and uncommon phonological patterns in the first and the second language, (b) bilingual phonological patterns, (c) interference patterns, and (d) dialectal features. The goal of such a description is to diagnose phonological disorders in bilingual children.

Research on several language families has identified several common and uncommon phonological patterns across languages (see Yavas, 1994, 1998; Yavas & Goldstein, 1998, for a review of studies). For example, such phonological patterns as cluster reduction, final-consonant deletion, final-consonant devoicing, stopping, velar fronting, palatal fronting, liquid simplification, labial assimilation, velar assimilation, nasal assimilation, and weak-syllable deletion are common across many languages, including those belonging to such different families as Germanic (English and Swedish), Romance (Portuguese, Spanish, and Italian), Sino-Tibetan (Cantonese), and Altaic (Turkish). These phonological patterns represent simplified productions of adult models.

Although these are common patterns across languages, a pattern exists in a particular language only if that language has the target pattern. For example, children learning a language that does not have consonant clusters (e.g., Turkish) obviously could not exhibit consonant-cluster reduction. Another notable fact about patterns across languages is that individual sounds may be differently affected within the same process. For example, although liquid simplification or substitution is a common pattern across languages, different sounds may be substituted for the liquids in different languages. In English, /w/ is a typical substitution for /r/. However, /r/ may be replaced by /l/ in Portuguese, /d/ in Spanish, /h/ in Swedish (Yavas & Goldstein, 1998).

Common patterns found in children normally learning different languages also are found in children with articulation and phonological disorders. As in any language, patterns of simplification that persist beyond certain age limits are considered clinically significant. Beyond the common patterns, children who exhibit clinically significant phonological disorders also exhibit some uncommon patterns. Uncommon patterns are those that are found in the speech of children with a diagnosis of articulation disorders but not in the speech of normally developing children (Yavas & Goldstein, 1998). Examples of uncommon phonological patterns given by Yavas and Goldstein include unusual cluster reduction (e.g., *ren* for *train*), initial-consonant deletion (*ep* for *tape*), liquid nasalization (/m/ for /l/ in Portuguese), frication of stops (e.g., *van* for *ban*), nasal gliding (e.g., /j/ for /l/), and delabialization (e.g., /s/ for /b/). Of the several unusual patterns, only two — initial-consonant deletion and backing — have been documented in all languages studied so far. Unusual cluster deletion is also common across languages, except for Turkish. Liquid nasalization was found only in Portuguese and Swedish; frication of stops is evident in English and Spanish; nasal gliding has been documented in Portuguese, Italian, and Swedish; and delabialization is reported only in Swedish (Yavas & Goldstein, 1998). It should be noted, however, that such generalizations may change when other languages are studied.

Identifying bilingual phonological patterns — an important goal of assessment — needs more research. Clinicians cannot make valid clinical judgments based on data gathered separately on English and Spanish phonological acquisition. Clinical judgments should be based on dual phonological acquisition in bilingual children. This is because a monolingual child's phonological acquisition may be different from that of a bilingual child. There is some evidence that bilingual children, normally learning their speech sounds or not, may exhibit patterns that are different from those found in matched monolingual peers in either language (Gildersleeve, Davis, & Stubble, 1996). For example, Spanish-English bilingual children's phonological patterns may be different from those found in children who speak only English or Spanish. Speech of bilingual children, whether normally developing or exhibiting phonological disorders, may be less intelligible and may contain more articulatory errors. Bilingual children are likely to exhibit phonological patterns found in both languages, including those that are unique to each language and those that are common (Gildersleeve et al., 1996).

It is known that the phonological patterns of one language influence the other. Therefore, *describing patterns of interference* from one language to the other is an important goal of the assessment of bilingual children (Yavas & Goldstein, 1998). Weinreich (1953) has described certain patterns of bilingual interference. For instance, a bilingual child may confuse two phonemes in the second language if they are not differentiated in the primary language. A child whose primary language is Spanish may treat the English /d/ and /ð/ as the same, for example, because in Spanish they are not separate phonemes but only allophonic variations. On the contrary, a bilingual child may produce two allophonic variations of the same sound in the second language as two separate sounds because they are separate in the primary language. A child whose primary language is English might produce the Spanish /d/ and /ð/ as separate phonemes because they are separate in English.

Yavas and Goldstein (1998) also suggest that besides segmental interference (interference at the phoneme level), there may be rhythmic interference due to differences in language. Syllable duration errors (syllables that sound too short or too long to a native speaker) and variations in syllable stress patterns (stressing the wrong syllable, failing to stress the right syllable) may be observed because of such differences in the two languages of a bilingual child.

It is common knowledge that learning two languages results in a dialectal variation of the second language. Thus, the *description of the dialectal features* of a bilingual child is yet another important goal of assessment (Yavas & Goldstein, 1998). Because no dialectal variation of any language is a disorder (American Speech-Language-Hearing Association, 1983), a diagnosis of articulatory and phonological disorders is not made on the basis of dialectal variations. As noted previously in the context of African American English, a variation is an error only when it is so in the primary language. If the phonological patterns of the first language were not considered in diagnosing articulatory errors of bilingual children, many with dialectal variations would receive a clinical diagnosis.

In essence, an appropriate assessment of bilingual children's articulatory skills takes into account the features and characteristics of the primary and the secondary languages of the child. Persistence of error patterns beyond expected age ranges is still the main criterion for diagnosis of a disorder. However, distinguishing error patterns from variations due to interference requires a clear knowledge of the structure and use of the two languages a child speaks.

Treatment of Articulatory and Phonological Disorders in Children of Spanish Background

Treatment of articulatory and phonological disorders in bilingual children follows the same general guidelines that were described for African American children. Generally, information on articulatory and phonological patterns in bilingual children is more extensive than that on treatment. No controlled treatment evidence shows that treatment of bilingual children involves unique principles. Until such evidence is produced, it is appropriate to assume that basic treatment principles used in treating monolingual children with articulatory and phonological disorders will hold up in treating bilingual children. The basic treatment principles suggest that all children need various stimulus manipulations, specification of acceptable and unacceptable responses, modeling of correct responses, shaping when necessary, positive feedback or reinforcement for correct production, corrective feedback for incorrect responses, parent training in supporting newly acquired skills in naturalistic settings, and so forth (Hegde, 1998b).

Within the broadly applicable treatment procedures, different procedures may be more or less effective with certain children. Selection of stimuli, for example, should be consistent with the child's home environment and culture. Stimuli unfamiliar to the child may be ineffective or inefficient. Certain kinds of reinforcers may be more or less effective, although we need more controlled data to support that assumption. Now that systematic data are emerging on the different phonological patterns across languages, it is time for clinical researchers to concentrate on treatment research involving bilingual children.

Some general guidelines on treating bilingual children include the following suggestions from Yavas and Goldstein (1998): First, the clinician should treat phonological patterns exhibited with similar error rates in both languages. The deviant patterns may have to be treated in both languages, as they are likely to be exhibited in both. In offering treatment in two languages, the clinician should consider the nature of the two languages in selecting initial treatment targets. For instance, if a language (e.g., Spanish) does not have many final consonants, final-consonant deletion would not be an appropriate initial treatment target.

Second, the clinician should treat phonological patterns that are exhibited in the two languages with unequal frequency. For instance, the final-consonant deletion will affect English and Spanish unequally; the deletion problem will be more serious in English than in Spanish. Nonetheless, the problem will affect intelligibility in both languages. Hence, it is appropriate to treat the patterns in both.

Third, the clinician should treat patterns that are evident in only one language. After treating errors in the two languages that are exhibited with equal and unequal frequency, clinicians should make a quick assessment in the two languages to isolate the deviant patterns in one or the other language. The clinician would then target those patterns for treatment. For example, final-consonant devoicing is likely to be found in both a Spanish-English bilingual child and a monolingual English-speaking child. Therefore, final-consonant devoicing would be a treatment target for those two groups of children. However, that pattern is not commonly found in monolingual Spanish-speaking children, for whom it is not a treatment target (Yavas & Goldstein, 1998).

Asian and Pacific Islander Languages

Currently, Asians are a significant minority population in the United States. Speech–language pathologists working in public schools are likely to encounter many children of Asian background who may be in need of clinical services. Treating language and phonological disorders in children of Asian background poses the greatest challenge to speech–language pathologists because of the incredible variety of languages and dialects that exist in Asia.

People living in Asian countries and the Pacific Islands are ethnoculturally and linguistically so varied that the terms *Asian* and *Pacific Islander* do not do justice to the variety; the terms have only helped create some stereotypes. People living in China, the Indian subcontinent, Southeast Asia, and the Pacific Islands are different from each other. Even within Southeast Asia, the countries are culturally and linguistically varied. For example, Vietnamese, Malaysians, Indonesians, and Thai people have contrasting religions, customs, and languages. Many countries have multiple languages and dialectal variations. China alone has more than 80 languages and countless dialectal variations (Cheng, 1991, 1998). There are more than 20 major languages in India and numerous dialects of each (Shekar & Hegde, 1996). The vast region of Asia is home to many other language families including Sino-Tibetan (e.g., Thai, Yao, Mandarin, and Cantonese); Indo-Aryan, Indo-European or Indic (e.g., Hindi, Bengali, and Marathi); Dravidian (e.g., Kannada, Tamil, Telugu, and Malayalam); Astro-Asiatic (e.g., Khmer, Vietnamese, and Hmong); Tibeto-Burman, (e.g., Tibetan and Burmese); Malayo-Polynesian or Astronesian (e.g., Chamorro, Ilocano, and Tagalog); Papuan (e.g., New Guinean), and Altaic (e.g., Japanese and Korean).

Most Asian-born Americans are bilingual or even multilingual speakers. They speak an English that is influenced by their native language. Therefore, Asian speakers of English will show variations from native English. They also vary from one another in their use of English because of their diverse native languages. Some general characteristics of Asian American English are summarized in Table 5.6.

It is quite possible that some of the characteristics listed in the table do not apply to all Asian speakers. Clinicians should be careful not to entertain linguistic stereotypes about Asian languages or speakers of Asian background.

Table 5.6. Major Characteristics of English Influenced by Asian Languages

Language Characteristics	Sample English Utterances
Omission of plurals	Here are two piece of toast. I got five finger on each hand.
Omission of copula	He going home now. They eating.
Omission of possessive	I have Phuong pencil. I like teacher dress.
Omission of past-tense morpheme	We cook dinner yesterday. Last night she walk home.
Past-tense double marking	He didn't went by himself.
Double negative	They don't have no books.
Subject-verb-object relationship differences/omissions	I messed up it. He like.
Singular present-tense omission or addition	You goes inside. He go to the store.
Misordering of interrogatives	You are going now?
Misuse or omission of prepositions	She is in home. He goes to school 8:00.
Misuse of pronouns	She husband is coming. She said her wife is here.
Omission and/or overgeneralization of articles	Boy is sick. He went the home.
Incorrect use of comparatives	This book is gooder than that book.
Omission of conjunctions	You I going to the beach.
Omission, lack of inflection on auxiliary do	She not take it. He do not have enough.
Omission, lack of inflection on forms of have	She have no money. We been the store.
Omission of articles	I see little cat.

Note. Adapted from Multicultural Students with Special Needs (Table 7.1, p. 81), by C. Roseberry-McKibbin, 1995, Oceanside, CA: Academic Communication Associates. Copyright 1995 by Academic Communication Associates. Reprinted with permission.

Phonological Characteristics of Asian Languages

Because of the wide variety of languages and language families that exist in Asia, it is not possible to describe a single set of phonological patterns of Asian languages. Only certain major phonological characteristics of Asian languages can be highlighted. A list of such characteristics is included in Table 5.7.

Once again, it should be noted that the phonological characteristics listed in the table may not hold true for all speakers of Asian languages. Patterns will vary across speakers because of their different native languages. Because it is not possible to give a detailed description of phonological patterns of hundreds of Asian languages, clinicians who assess Asian children should evaluate their phonological patterns according to those found in the children's first language. Clinicians should develop local resources including information on the phonological characteristics of the Asian languages spoken in their service area and linguistic experts in regional universities who specialize in those languages.

Table 5.7. Major Articulatory and Phonological Characteristics of English Influenced by Asian Languages

Articulation Characteristics	Sample English Utterances	
In many Asian languages, words end in vowels only or in just a few consonants; speakers may delete many final consonants in English.	ste/step	li/lid
	ro/robe	do/dog
Some languages are monosyllabic; speakers may truncate polysyllabic words or emphasize the wrong syllable.	efunt/elephant	
	di versity/diversity	
Possible devoicing of voiced cognates	beece/bees	pick/pig
	luff/love	crip/crib
r/l confusion	lize/rise	clown/crown
/r/ may be omitted entirely	gull/girl	tone/torn
Reduction of vowel length in words	words sound choppy to Americans	
No voiced or voiceless th	dose/those	tin/thin
	zose/those	sin/thin
Epenthesis (addition of uh sound in blends, ends of words)	bulack/black	wooduh/wood
Confusion of ch and sh	sheep/cheap	beesh/beach
/æ/ does not exist in many Asian languages	block/black	shock/shack
b/v substitutions	base/vase	Beberly/Beverly
v/w substitutions	vork/work	vall/wall
p/f substitutions	pall/fall	plower/flower

Note. Adapted from *Multicultural Students with Special Needs* (Table 7.2, p. 82), by C. Roseberry-McKibbin, 1995, Oceanside, CA: Academic Communication Associates. Copyright 1995 by Academic Communication Associates. Reprinted with permission.

Clinicians face different challenges in different parts of the United States. For instance, the Hmong are concentrated in a few states, including California and Minnesota. Chinese and Koreans are concentrated in several metropolitan areas, including San Francisco, New York, and Los Angeles. Asian Indians are concentrated in many metropolitan areas, including the San Francisco Bay area, Los Angeles, Chicago, and New York. Clinicians need to develop resources specific to the Asian languages they are expected to face in their service area. What follows is a description of a few specific phonological characteristics of selected Asian languages, as contrasted with those of English.

Chinese Versus English

Cantonese and Mandarin are the two main dialects of Chinese spoken in the United States. The dialectal variations of Chinese may be mutually unintelligible. Words are written logographically: each word is a graphic symbol, not a combination of alphabets. Across dialects, words are written similarly but pronounced differently. Therefore, even though the spoken forms of a dialect are mutually incomprehensible, the printed forms may be intelligible. Chinese is a tonal language; the same word can have different meaning when spoken with a different vocal pitch. Different meanings may be communicated by the same word by saying it with a high pitch, low pitch, rising pitch, or rising-then-falling pitch.

The Mandarin and Cantonese dialects of Chinese do not contain consonantal blends. Hence, learning English blends can be difficult for a Chinese speaker. Also, unlike English, these two dialects of Chinese have relatively few sounds in word-final position. Cantonese has seven final consonants, and Mandarin has only two. Therefore, Chinese speakers learning English may omit many final English consonants (e.g., *offi* for *office, fi* for *fish*) (Cheng, 1991).

If a sound is similar in Chinese and English, a Chinese speaker may substitute the Chinese sound for the English sound. For example, a Cantonese speaker may substitute /ʃ/ for /s/, as those two sounds are phonetically similar in Chinese. Chinese speakers also may use a Chinese sound as a substitute for a sound that is in English but absent in Chinese. For example, neither Mandarin nor Cantonese contains the English /θ/. Therefore, speakers of these two languages may substitute /s/ for voiceless *th*. Consequently, the speakers may say *sin* for *thin* (Cheng, 1991).

Two other variations found in speakers of Chinese involve stress and intonational patterns. Syllable stress tends to be misplaced in speaking English. An intonational pattern that is more appropriate to Chinese may be heard in the English speech of native Chinese speakers.

South Asian Languages Versus English

South Asia includes the countries of the Indian subcontinent. The region is home to several language families including the Indic languages of the Indo-European (Indo-Aryan) family and the Dravidian languages. Indic languages are spoken mostly in Pakistan, Bangladesh, and northern parts of India. It is a large family of languages and contains such languages as Urdu, Hindi, Punjabi, Marathi, Bengali, Gujarathi, Sindhi, Oriya, and Assamese. Most of them are derived or heavily influenced by Sanskrit, an ancient Indo-European language of India. Although these languages share many features, there are significant differences among them. Of the languages of northern India, Hindi is spoken by the largest number of people. It is the official language of India (Shekar & Hegde, 1995, 1996).

Dravidian languages are spoken mostly in the four states of south India. Kannada, Tamil, Telugu, and Malayalam are the four major languages of the Dravidian family. There has been mutual borrowing among the languages of the Indo-European and Dravidian families.

The sound systems of the Indic and Dravidian languages share many features. For example, Hindi, an Indic language, has five short vowels with long counterparts. Kannada, a Dravidian language, has the same number and variety of vowels. Vowel length is phonemic in both languages. However, Hindi has nasalized vowels, and nasalization of vowels can make a difference in meaning. Kannada, along with other Dravidian languages, does not have nasalized vowels. Syllabic stress is typically not distinctive in most languages of India (Shekar & Hegde, 1995, 1996).

A distinguishing feature of most languages of India is their aspirated stops. Both the Indic and the Dravidian languages have aspirated stops of both the velar (e.g., g^h) and the bilabial (b^h) varieties. Another distinguishing feature is their retroflex consonants. For example, the English /d/, /t/, and /l/ have retroflex variations in most languages of India. Yet another feature of the languages of India is the lack of difference between the English /v/ and /w/ in many contexts. In most languages, /v/ is a bilabial fricative (as against the labiodental fricative in English). When /v/ is followed by a back vowel, it is pronounced as a /w/. These are among the several features of the languages of India that create difficulties for Asian Indians who speak English as their second language (Shekar & Hegde, 1995, 1996).

The languages of India differ in their tonal characteristics. Asian Indians who speak English as their second language may often exhibit a rhythm that is different from the native English rhythm. Because the languages of India are phonetic (each sound is represented in the alphabet of its language), there usually is no confusion between printed words and their pronunciation. Therefore, Asian Indians learning English may find the phonetic realization of printed English confusing or difficult (Shekar & Hegde, 1995). The English of Asian Indians has several other unique characteristics that are described elsewhere (Shekar & Hegde, 1996).

Southeast Asian Languages Versus English

Southeast Asian languages are spoken in such countries as Vietnam, Thailand, Laos, Cambodia, and Burma. Like most other parts of Asia, Southeast Asia is rich in linguistic diversity. Different language families are represented in the region. For example, Vietnamese is a member of the Mon-Khmer branch of the Austro-Asiatic family of languages, as is Khmer, the language of Cambodia. Hmong, another language of the region, is a member of the Sino-Tibetan linguistic family. Thai or Tai, spoken in Thailand, is a member of the Kadai or KamTai language family. All the languages have numerous dialects.

Vietnamese is a monosyllabic tonal language. It has three major dialects, each spoken in a different geographical region. Most educated Vietnamese people speak a formal and an informal variety of their language. Unlike English, Vietnamese does not contain consonantal blends. Syllabic stress is not used to signal difference in meaning. Only a few final consonants are used in the language.

The **Hmong** are originally from southern China, but over the centuries have migrated to Southeast Asia, especially to Laos. Because of their work for the U.S.

Army in the fight with communist Vietnam, the Hmong are now a significant minority in certain parts of this country, predominantly in central California and parts of Minnesota. The Hmong language has two main dialects: White and Green. Although Hmong has 56 initial consonants, it has only one final consonant /ŋ/. Many consonants have aspirated and unaspirated varieties. The sound comparable to English /r/ is a stop, not a liquid. Its aspirated form may sound like /t/, and its unaspirated form may sound like /d/ (Cheng, 1991, 1998). Consonant clusters are produced only in the initial position of words.

Hmong is a tonal language. There are seven tones that help distinguish meaning: high, high falling, mid-rising, mid, low, low breathing, short low, and abrupt end. There are 13 vowels in the White dialect and 14 in the Green dialect, though none is reduced to the schwa. Six basic vowels, two nasalized vowels, and five diphthongs complete the vowel inventory.

English final consonants and final-consonant clusters may pose a particularly serious difficulty for Hmong speakers. They also may pronounce with undue importance English vowels that are unaccented and often reduced to the schwa (Cheng, 1998).

Khmer is the language of Cambodia. However, Cambodians also speak French, Thai, Lao, Chinese, and Vietnamese. One factor that distinguishes Khmer from such other Southeast Asian languages as Laotian and Vietnamese is that it is not a tonal language. As in English, intonational contours vary within and across sentences. Khmer contains mostly disyllabic or monosyllabic words. In disyllabic words, Khmer speakers typically stress the second syllable. The Khmer alphabet is derived from Sanskrit and Pali, the two ancient languages of India. While many classic Khmer words are derived from Sanskrit, most contemporary and technical words are derived from French (Cheng, 1991).

Khmer contains both aspirated and unaspirated consonants. The language contains only 2 fricatives but 50 vowels and diphthongs. Both short and long vowels exist in the language. Khmer has extensive and unusual consonantal clusters. It has 85 initial consonantal clusters but no final clusters. The language contains many initial clusters that do not exist in English, for example: *mty, sd,* and *kn* (Cheng, 1991, 1998).

Some Khmer speakers who speak English as their second language tend to exhibit the following substitutions: /k/ for /g/, /v/ for /w/, /f/ for /b/, /ʧ/ for /s/, and /s/ or /t/ for /θ/. Omission of several final consonants, including /r/, /d/, /g/, /s/, /b/, and /z/ also may be noted in Cambodian English speakers (Cheng, 1991, 1998).

Thai is the official language of Thailand, and many scholars consider it a member of the Tai language family (Comrie, 1990; Hudak, 1990; Strecker, 1990). Thai is heavily influenced by the Sanskrit and Pali languages of ancient India.

Thai has 20 segmental consonants including aspirated consonants (e.g., *k*ʰ, as in the Indic and Dravidian languages of India). All consonants are used in the initial position. Initial-consonant clusters include the following: *pr, pl, phr, tr, thr, kr, kl, kw, khr, khl,* and *khw.* Final-consonant clusters are not used in Thai (Hudak, 1990). The phonemes /r/ and /l/, though distinguished in Thai, may not be distinguished in fast conversational speech. Thus, some Thai people speaking English as a second language may confuse the two English phonemes.

Thai has nine vowels. Each may be short or long. It contains several corresponding diphthongs. The syllabic structures of Thai are associated with distinct tones, as Thai is a tonal language. The tones used in Thai include a low tone, a mid tone, a high tone, a falling tone, and a rising tone (Hudak, 1990). The final syllable in disyllabic and polysyllabic words receives the most prominent stress. Thus, the stress patterns of English as used by a native Thai speaker may be different.

East Asian Languages Versus English

The Philippines, Korea, and Japan are among the East Asian countries from which a significant number of people have migrated to the United States. A brief description of the languages of this region follows.

The people of the Philippines are known as Filipinos. Their language, known as **Filipino,** is extremely varied. At least 75 languages, all belonging to the Malayo-Polynesian group, have been identified. **Tagalog** is the national language of the Philippines. Ilocano and Visayan are among the other major languages spoken in that country of multiple islands.

Tagalog contains 16 consonants, 5 vowels, and 6 diphthongs. It does not contain the following 9 English phonemes: /v/, /z/, /θ/, /ð/, /dʒ/, /f/, /ʃ/, /ʧ/, and /ʒ/. A native Tagalog speaker of English may omit some of those sounds. The Tagalog sounds /p/, /b/, /s/, and /t/ are similar to the English /f/, /v/, /z/, and /ð/. Therefore, a native Tagalog speaker of English may substitute the former set of sounds for the latter.

Korean is the language of Korea. It is a member of the Altaic language family. Koreans in the two countries (North and South Korea) speak the same language. Korean has several mutually intelligible dialects.

The Korean language has 21 consonants and 10 vowels (Kim, 1990). It has no consonant clusters in word-initial or -final position. Therefore, English consonant clusters may be expected to create problems for native Korean speakers. Fricatives and affricates occur only in the word-initial and -final positions. Consequently, a native Korean speaker may have difficulty with English fricatives in word-final position. Korean speakers of English tend to omit word-final fricatives. Korean /r/ and /l/ are allophonic variations of the same phoneme; therefore, in English native Korean speakers may use one for the other (Cheng, 1991, 1998). Also, /l/ does not occur in initial position in Korean speech; it does occur in the initial position in writing, but in speech it is either deleted or pronounced as /n/. In most cases, /h/ in the word-medial (intervocalic) position is deleted (Kim, 1990).

Korean has no labiodental, interdental, or palatal fricatives. Consequently, some native Korean speakers who use English may exhibit the following substitutions: /b/ for /v/, /p/ for /v/, and /s/ for /ʃ/, /t/ for /ʧ/, and /dʒ/ for /ð/.

A distinguishing feature of Korean is the tendency to nasalize a nonnasal stop if it occurs before a nasal sound in a word (Kim, 1990). The stops /k/, /p/, and /t/ are pronounced as /ŋ/, /n/, and /m/, respectively (Kim, 1990). Cheng (1991, 1998) gives the example of native Korean speakers who may say *Banman* for *Batman* in English. Korean vowels do not contrast in length. Therefore, English vowels that do contrast in length may be difficult for native Korean speakers (e.g., /i/ vs. /ɪ/).

Syllable stress is not a characteristic of Korean. Intonational variations, therefore, are minimal. Consequently, when native Korean speakers speak English, the speech may sound flat and monotonous. Expressing meaning through rising intonation, as in asking a question, may be difficult for Korean English speakers.

Japanese, spoken by the entire population of Japan, belongs, somewhat controversially, to the Altaic family of languages. Various scholars have suggested that Japanese is a member of the Indo-European family, the Sino-Tibetan family, or the Dravidian family. Modern written Japanese uses modified Chinese characters. Even though politically shielded from foreign influence or invasion in all its history, Japanese has a surprising number of foreign words, including numerous words from Chinese and several from Korean, Arabic, and Persian (Shibatani, 1990). Japanese is technically not a tonal language, although accentuation in it involves significant pitch differences.

Japanese has five standard vowels: /a/, /i/, /u/, e/, and /o/. Some dialects have up to three additional vowels and others only three. A characteristic of a Japanese vowel that contrasts with that of English is that the Japanese /u/ is unrounded. Another characteristic of Japanese vowels is that high vowels /u/ and /i/ are devoiced (not pronounced) when they are surrounded by voiceless consonants. They are not devoiced in initial position or when they are accented (Shibatani, 1990).

Japanese has 18 consonants. Some double consonants (/kk/ and /pp/) also are present. A significant characteristic of Japanese consonants is the palatalization and affrication of dental consonants. For example, /s/ before /i/ is changed to /ʧ/; /z/ before /i/ or /u/ is changed to /ʤ/; /t/ before /i/ is changed to /ʧ/; and /d/ before /i/ is changed to /ʤ/ (Shibatani, 1990). The /n/ is the only word-final phoneme in Japanese.

Native Japanese speakers using English are likely to substitute /r/ for /l/, /s/ for /θ/, /z/ for /ð/, /j/ for /ð/, and /b/ for /v/. Japanese speakers also may add a vowel to words ending in consonants (e.g., *beddu* for *bed* or *milku* for *milk*) (Cheng, 1991).

Arabic Versus English

Arabic is the language of the Arabs. Arabs are Muslims, but not all Muslims speak Arabic. For example, Muslims in such countries as Pakistan and India do not speak Arabic; they speak an Indo-European language called Urdu. The term *Arab* does not refer to a race, religion, or nationality. Arabs may be of different race (e.g., Negro, Berber, or Semitic), and they live in different countries (M. E. Wilson, 1996).

Arabic is spoken predominantly in countries of the Middle East and North Africa (e.g., Egypt). There are many variations of this language, as it is spoken in such countries as Saudi Arabia, Jordan, Iraq, many smaller Gulf countries in the Arabian peninsula, and such countries as Egypt, Sudan, and Libya in North Africa (W. F. Wilson, 1998).

Arabic is spoken by more than 160 million people worldwide (M. E. Wilson, 1996). It is a member of the Semitic branch of the Afroasiatic family of languages. Hebrew also is a member of this large language family of over 175 languages (Hetzron, 1990). Arabic is a minority language in several countries around the world, including Russia, Iran, and the United States. Variations of the classic Arabic are spoken by Muslims living in many countries in all continents (Kaye, 1990; W. F. Wilson, 1998). Arabic is the official language in 20 countries (M. E. Wilson, 1996).

The standard or classic Arabic has 28 consonants, although some sources indicate 32 consonants (Kaye, 1990; M. E. Wilson, 1996). Arabic has several consonants that are absent in English (e.g., emphatic consonants, voiceless and voiced uvular and pharyngeal fricatives). Five emphatic consonants are /t̲/, /d̲/, /ð̲/, /s̲/, and /q̲/. The first four have nonemphatic cognates, transcribed without the line under them. Emphatic consonants in Arabic are produced with the root of the tongue retracted toward the back wall of the pharynx. The classic Arabic contains three basic vowels (/a/, /i/, and /u/) and their long versions, for a total of six. Modern variations of Arabic have borrowed or evolved such other vowels as /e/ and /o/. Various dialects of Arabic spoken in different countries have somewhat different consonant and vowel systems.

A few other unique characteristics of the Arab phonological system are noteworthy. In many Arab dialects, /q/ may be voiced. The /p/ is absent in the classic Arabic; however, in modern Arabic speech, /b/ that appears before a voiceless consonant may be devoiced to yield a /p/. In most linguistic contexts, many Arab speakers may simply substitute /p/ for /b/. Another sound absent in classic Arabic is /v/.

Stress is an ill-defined phenomenon in most Arabic dialects. Each of the four syllables in a word, for example, may receive stress in different dialects of Arabic. Generally, stress is prominent (a) on the first syllable of a CV syllable, (b) on a long syllable in a word containing only one long syllable, and (c) on the long syllable toward the end of a word that contains multiple long syllables. Because of these differences, English stress patterns may pose special problems for native Arabic speakers who use English.

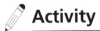

Activity

DIRECTIONS: List some phonological differences between the selected "Asian" language and English.

1. Chinese versus English: _____

2. South Asian languages versus English: _____

3. Vietnamese versus English: _____

4. Hmong versus English: _____

5. Khmer versus English: _____

6. Thai versus English: _____

7. Tagalog versus English: _____

8. Korean versus English: _____

9. Japanese versus English: _____

10. Arabic versus English: _____

Articulatory Development in Children Speaking Asian Languages

It is likely that articulatory development of Asian children in their home countries has been studied to various extents. Unfortunately, much of that information is not readily available. More important, however, is that detailed studies of the articulatory development of children speaking American English and a particular Asian language are not available. This is the kind of information most urgently needed for speech–language pathologists who need to assess and treat Asian American children with articulation and phonological disorders.

A study of phonological acquisition in children speaking Cantonese was reported by So and Dodd (1994). The authors also reported data on children with phonological disorders. Generally, Cantonese children in the study acquired their phonemes at a faster rate than English-speaking children do. Anterior Cantonese phonemes were acquired sooner than posterior phonemes. Oral and nasal stops and glides were acquired before fricatives and affricates. These are consistent with data on acquisition of English phonemes. Cantonese children exhibited phonological processes similar to those found in English-speaking children.

So and Dodd (1994) reported that by age 4-0, Cantonese children exhibited phonological processes relatively infrequently. They generally exhibited phonological processes similar to those exhibited by children acquiring English phonemes. Children with phonological delays or disorders tended to exhibit such phonological processes as cluster reduction, affrication, final-consonant deletion, final-glide deletion, fronting, backing, and assimilation.

A recently published report has described the acquisition of Jordanian Arabic phonemes in children living in Jordan (Amayreh & Dyson, 1998). It should be noted that this was not a report on English-Arabic bilingual children living in the United States. The data showed that, for the most part, the pattern of acquisition of Arabic phonemes was similar to that found for English. At earlier age levels, medial consonants were produced more accurately than final consonants. Stops (e.g., /b/, /t/, /d/, and /k/), fricatives and affricates (/f/, /h/), and sonorants (/m/, /n/, /l/, and /w/) were acquired (75% correct in all positions) the earliest (between the ages of 2-0 and 3-10). Other stops (e.g., /t/, /d/, /q/, /ʔ/) were acquired late (after age 6-4). Acquisition of most other phonemes fell into an intermediate stage (between the ages of 4-0 and 6-4). Arabic children acquired /b/, /t/, /d/, /k/, /f/, and /l/ earlier than the ages generally reported for acquiring the same phonemes in English. On the other hand, five phonemes (/θ/, /ð/, /h/, /r/, and /j/) were acquired later in Arabic than in English (Amayreh & Dyson, 1998).

Assessment of Articulatory and Phonological Disorders in Children of Asian Background

The sheer variety of Asian languages makes it extremely difficult for any clinician, including those of Asian background, to make an appropriate assessment of a bilingual Asian American child's articulatory and phonological skills. In the absence of data on phonological acquisition in many Asian American bilingual children, clinicians can assume that the patterns of development in such children are not radically different from those found in English phonological acquisition. They can make tentative clinical decisions based on their knowledge of phonological acquisition in general. Parental expectations and educational and social demands made on the child will be helpful in making clinical decisions.

An important factor to take into consideration is the potential interference from the first language in the production of English phonemes. Therefore, a general understanding of the phonemes of the particular Asian language of the child and of how they might affect the production of English phonemes is most helpful in assessing a child with a potential articulation or phonological disorder. With the help of an interpreter and available information on the child's first-language phonological system, the clinician needs to determine what phonological patterns observed in English are consistent with those of the child's first language and what patterns are inconsistent and hence deviant. The overall approach and philosophy of assessing a child with an Asian American background would be the same as those advocated for Spanish-speaking or African American children.

Treatment of Articulatory and Phonological Disorders in Children of Asian Background

There is little or no research showing whether certain phonological treatment procedures are effective with children of Asian background. In the absence of such data, clinicians can appropriately use treatment procedures whose effectiveness has been experimentally evaluated. In planning treatment, the clinician should consider the child's language and communication style and the influence of the first language on English.

The general guidelines offered for treating Spanish-English bilingual children are relevant in planning the treatment of articulatory and phonological disorders in children of Asian background. As suggested by Yavas and Goldstein (1998), deviant processes evident in both languages, errors that are unevenly distributed in the two languages, and errors that are unique to each language may all be targets of intervention.

Guidelines on Working with Children Who Have Dual Phonological Repertoire

Children who are bidialectal or bilingual are said to have dual phonological repertoire. *Bidialectal* children speak two dialects of the same language. For example, African American children who speak both African American English and General American English are bidialectal and have a dual phonological repertoire. Children who speak two languages (e.g., Spanish and English or an Asian language and English) are *bilingual*. All children in these two categories have dual phonological repertoire.

In the previous sections of this chapter, assessment and treatment guidelines specific to each ethnocultural group were summarized. In this section, some general guidelines on working with children who have dual phonological repertoire because of their varied ethnocultural and linguistic backgrounds will be summarized.

In assessing and treating children of dual phonological repertoire, the clinician should:

- understand the characteristics of the child's first language, including its phonological, morphologic, syntactic, and pragmatic features and how they contrast with those of English;

- appreciate the communication style of the child and his or her family;

- assess the family resources to obtain and continue treatment services for the child;

- procure help from government or other agencies that support clinical services for the child;

- appraise the family members' dispositions toward and beliefs regarding speech disorders and their causes, as well as the chances of improvement;

- obtain available information on phonological development in the child's first language;

- study the patterns of interference from the child's first language or the varied English dialect (as in the case of an African American child);

- obtain the services of a competent interpreter who speaks the child's native language in completing assessment and treatment planning;

- if necessary, train the interpreter in conversational speech sampling, helping with clinical interviews, and test administration;

- choose standardized tests that have been normed on children from the particular ethnic or linguistic group the child client belongs to;

- avoid tests that are known to be culture-biased or that you suspect to be biased against the child's ethnocultural background;

- let conversational speech samples, preferably involving the parents, other family members, or caregivers, be the primary data for analysis of the child's phonological skills;

- analyze phonological deviations or disorders in light of the first language or first dialect of the child;

- make sure that multiple family members understand treatment recommendations and that they agree with the planned treatment for the child;

- determine the presence of a disorder in both languages or dialects;

- select treatment targets in both languages;

- treat the disorder in the primary language as well as in the second language or dialect;

- assume tentatively that basic treatment principles (e.g., modeling, shaping, positive reinforcement for correct productions, corrective feedback for incorrect productions) may hold true for children of varied ethnocultural backgrounds;

- expect to modify treatment procedures to suit the individual child (e.g., in a given case, although the principle of positive reinforcement may hold, a particular type of reinforcer, such as verbal praise, may be less effective than another type of reinforcer, such as a token);

- carefully collect treatment data to sustain or modify the assumptions made in assessing and treating children;

- target the Standard American English dialect only if the family, the child, or both request it;

- note that according to the position of the American Speech-Language-Hearing Association, no dialectal variation of a language is a deviation or a disorder;

- follow the guidelines given in several professional sources on working with clients of varied ethnocultural background (Battle, 1998; Bernthal & Bankson, 1998; Cheng, 1991, 1995, 1998; Kayser, 1995; Kamhi et al., 1996; Langdon & Cheng, 1992; Roseberry-McKibbin, 1995; Yavas, 1994, 1998; Yavas & Goldstein, 1998).

- develop resources on the language and culture of minority children in the service area; keep a list of linguistic experts at local or regional universities, bilingual speech–language pathologists in the area, and consultants who might be of help;

- identify various Web sites on the Internet that provide information on different languages and cultures;

- watch for new publications in professional journals on language and phonological acquisition in minority children;

- if practical, refer the child to a bilingual speech–language pathologist who speaks the child's language;

- be the child's advocate.

Summary of the Basic Unit

- Each language is spoken in a varied manner. Each variation of a language is a dialect, and no dialect of a language is a basis for diagnosing a language or phonological disorder.

- To assess and treat articulation and phonological disorders in children who are bilingual or bidialectal, the clinician needs to know the characteristics of the primary language.

- A dialectal variety of English that has received much attention is African American English or Black English. AAE is not a substandard variety of Standard American English; it has its own phonological, syntactic, semantic, and pragmatic rules. The origin of AAE may have been a **pidgin,** a simple form of communication that develops between two verbal communities with no common language. A pidgin develops into a more complex **creole** when it is passed on to the next generation as the primary means of communication.

- Native Americans speak a variety of languages, many of them extinct, and most on the verge of extinction. Native American languages belong to different language families. Because of this, their phonological systems vary tremendously. Therefore, clinicians need to develop resources for given languages spoken in their service area.

- After English, Spanish is the second most important language in the United States. People of Spanish background are classified as Hispanic, which does not refer to the race of an individual. Hispanics in the United States have origins in different countries, but most are from Mexico. Children who speak a variety of

Spanish as their primary language and then learn to speak English are likely to show a variety of phonological characteristics from their primary language.

• Asian American children are linguistically and ethnoculturally a diverse group. Children in that group speak many primary languages from different language families, including the Indo-European and Dravidian (languages of India), Sino-Tibetan (languages of China, Thailand), Astro-Asiatic (languages of Vietnam, the Hmong), Tibeto-Burman (languages of Tibet, Burma), and Altaic (languages of Japan, Korea). Clinicians should develop resources on the Asian language or languages spoken in their service area.

Advanced Unit

◆ ◆ ◆ ◆ ◆ ◆ ◆ ◆ ◆ ◆ ◆ ◆ ◆ ◆ ◆ ◆ ◆ ◆ ◆ ◆

Theoretical and Clinical Issues in Bilingual Phonology

In the Basic Unit, we summarized information relative to several minority languages spoken in the United States, along with limited available information on the articulatory and phonological performance of children learning English as a second dialect or a second language. The Basic Unit summarized mostly descriptive information on various languages and their phonological patterns.

In this unit, we will take a look at some theoretical and clinical issues that are relevant to a more complete understanding of the assessment and treatment of articulatory and phonological disorders in children of varied ethnocultural backgrounds.

Theoretical Issues in Bilingual Phonology

Why children learning a second language or speaking a dialectal variation of a language may exhibit what might appear to be errors of articulation has been a topic of much theoretical speculation. Several hypotheses have been advanced to explain phonological deviations or variations found in children learning a second language. These hypotheses may apply very well to children learning a second dialect (e.g., an African American child learning the Standard American English dialect). Phonologists hope that an empirically supported explanation will help us understand the unique patterns of articulations found in the second language or second dialect production and help devise appropriate phonological treatment strategies for bilingual and bidialectal children.

Theoretical explanations in bilingual phonology are based on systematic observation of variations in articulation documented in children acquiring different pairs of languages. One of each pair is a primary language of the child and the other is a second language. The number of cross-cultural phonological studies and professional writings on multicultural and multilingual issues has increased during the past several years (Battle, 1998; Cheng, 1995; Kayser, 1995; Langdon & Cheng, 1992; Roseberry-McKibbin, 1995; Seymour & Nober, 1998; Yavas, 1994, 1998). Studies of ethnocultural children acquiring a different dialect of the same language (e.g., African American children learning standard English) also have increased in recent years (Kamhi et al., 1996; van Keulen et al., 1998).

Many of the theoretical attempts have been concerned with bilingual children. Among the several attempts at explaining phonological deviations or variations found in children acquiring a second language, we will briefly summarize the hypotheses of (a) differentiated or undifferentiated dual phonological patterns;

(b) phonological approximation to the first language (L1), typically described as L1 interference; (c) the critical age for phonological acquisition; (d) hierarchies of phonological difficulty; and (e) universal patterns of phonological productions.

Differentiated or Undifferentiated Dual Phonological Patterns

A child or an adult who speaks two languages may have acquired them simultaneously or successively. **Simultaneous bilingualism** means that the child learned two languages at about the same time. This is most likely to happen when the two parents have different first languages and the child learns the mother's and the father's languages from the beginning. **Successive bilingualism** means that the child first learned one language and then the other. A child who learns Spanish at home and begins to learn English in school illustrates successive bilingualism.

There has been some debate as to whether children who learn two languages simultaneously have separate phonological systems or undifferentiated phonological patterns. Some phonologists have suggested that simultaneously bilingual children develop separate phonological systems from the beginning, whereas others have suggested that the two systems are undifferentiated (see Yavas, 1998, for a review of research and theories). As Yavas suggests, it is likely that in the very beginning, the child, even though learning to speak two languages, has only a single, undifferentiated phonological system. Around age 2, the two systems may become differentiated. Children who learn a different language after the acquisition of their first language probably always maintain a dual phonological pattern. In those children, the effect of the first language on the second is clearly evident.

Successively or simultaneously bilingual children or adults are rarely equally competent in their two languages. Sooner or later, one language assumes dominance in most bilingual people. Even those who have a nativelike phonological competence at the phonemic level in two languages may exhibit some difference at the phonetic (speech sound production) level (Yavas, 1988).

✎ Activity

DIRECTIONS: As discussed in the text, describe the differences between **simultaneous bilingualism** and **successive bilingualism:**

_____

_____

_____

_____

_____

_____

Phonological Approximation to First Language

That a speaker using a second language shows phonological approximations of his or her first language is well recognized. This phenomenon typically is described as *interference* from the first language (Weinreich, 1953; Yavas, 1998). From an empirical standpoint, phonetic productions from an established language generalize to the second language. In other words, productions of the second language approximate those in the first. Among a variety of interferences, underdifferentiation and overdifferentiation of phonemes (Weinreich, 1953), substitution of phonemes, and omission of phonemes are commonly observed.

Underdifferentiation of phonemes in this case is a failure to distinguish two phonemes in the second language if the two phonemes are not distinguished in the first. Our earlier discussion has pointed out several such instances in speakers who speak English as a second language. For example, in Spanish, /d/ and /ð/ are allophonic variations, not separate phonemes; while /d/ is produced in word-initial position after [n], /ð/ is produced in intervocalic positions. However, in English they are separate phonemes. Therefore, native Spanish speakers may not distinguish /d/ and /ð/ when they speak English. Another example is the lack of vowel length contrast in Korean. Consequently, Korean speakers may fail to differentiate English /i/ and /ɪ/ in their speech.

Overdifferentiation of phonemes is making an unnecessary distinction between allophonic variations of two phonemes as separate phonemes. A native English speaker who treats the Spanish /d/ and /ð/ as separate phonemes illustrates such an overdifferentiation.

Substitution of phonemes also is a phenomenon of generalization from the primary language to the secondary language. If certain phonemes are similar across two languages, a bilingual speaker may substitute the sound from the first language for the similar sound in the second language. For example, Chinese speakers tend to substitute /ʃ/ for /s/ because the two sounds are similar in the Chinese language. Because many Spanish consonants are unaspirated, native Spanish speakers who use English may not aspirate aspirated English consonants.

Omission of phonemes, a well-documented phenomenon in some bilingual speakers, illustrates an unusual kind of generalization: a phoneme absent in the primary language is simply omitted in the secondary language, in which that phoneme does exist. Both single phonemes and phonemic blends are susceptible to this kind of generalization. For instance, native Spanish and Chinese speakers tend to omit final English consonants that do not exist in their native language. Similarly, in consonant clusters, the one most likely to be omitted is the consonant that does not exist in the primary language.

Yavas (1998) has provided an excellent summary of various interference patterns found in language learners across a wide variety of languages. According to his summary:

• Native Turkish speakers may devoice final English consonants and delete consonants from initial clusters.

• Native Portuguese and Swedish speakers may exhibit weak-syllable deletion in English.

• Native Italian, Spanish, and Portuguese speakers may delete final English consonants, as their primary language uses more open syllables. For the same reason, speakers of those languages are less likely to exhibit consonant harmony assimilations, a process that is more commonly seen in speakers whose primary language uses more closed syllables (e.g., English). Speakers of those languages also are likely to exhibit prevocalic devoicing and reduced aspiration of aspirated sounds (true for other Romance languages as well).

• Native speakers of syllable-timed languages may exhibit deviant stress patterns in English. This problem is evident in speakers of such languages as Spanish, Italian, and Turkish.

• Native speakers of Spanish may exhibit fricative stopping (e.g., substitution of /b/ for /v/, as Spanish does not have /v/. Spanish speakers also tend to replace the voiceless palato-alveolar fricative /ʃ/ with the affricate /ʧ/.

• Native speakers of Spanish, Portuguese, and Cantonese may confuse the high front vowels /i/ and /ɪ/ (e.g., as in *peach–pitch* and *leave–live*).

It should be noted, however, that interference from the first language does not explain all variations found in second-language production. Phonologists believe that some variations may be due to certain universal patterns of phonological acquisition, described in a later section.

Critical Age for Phonological Acquisition

Research on bilingualism has demonstrated that individuals differ in their bilingual phonological patterns. While some individuals have a near-native phonological pattern in their second language, others exhibit the distinct influence of their first language on their second-language phonological pattern. Some individuals, who have a nativelike command of the grammatical, syntactic, and pragmatic aspects of their second language, may nevertheless exhibit a distinct and varied phonological pattern. Studies have shown that those who write in a second language as competently or even more competently than most native speakers of that language may retain the influence of their first language in their phonological productions (see Patkowski, 1994, for a review of studies).

Based on such observations, some have suggested that the phonological pattern of a second language is more difficult to master than other patterns of that language. In explaining this difficulty, researchers have suggested that there is a critical age for phonological acquisition. Beyond that critical age, it is much more difficult to acquire the phonological aspect than other aspects of a second language. The critical (also called sensitive or optimal) age is thought to be between 18 months and the onset of puberty (somewhere around 12 to 15 years). Some experts have suggested that the upper limit of the critical age period may be as low as age 6. However, most data seem to suggest that at least some people learn their second language with nativelike phonological patterns if the learning begins before age 12 or so (see Yavas, 1998, and Patkowski, 1994, for details and critical review of studies).

By and large, studies have supported the hypothesis that the younger the age at which a second language is acquired, the greater the possibility of nativelike phonological skills. Older people who begin to learn a second language may find it increasingly difficult, if not impossible, to master the phonological patterns of that language. Although this conclusion is relatively uncontroversial, why it is so has been controversial. Some experts believe that there is a biological basis for language acquisition and that there are biological limitations to phonological acquisition in particular. Others believe that there are too many variables that interact, including many environmental variables, to make a strong case for biological restraints on phonological acquisition.

An environmental factor that has not received much attention is the manner of exposure to the second language. Naturalistic exposure to the second language, regardless of the age at which the exposure begins, may encourage more native-like phonological skills than formal instruction. Formal instruction by native speakers of a language may encourage more nativelike phonological skills than similar instruction by nonnative speakers. Age and the manner of second-language acquisition may interact to produce certain effects on the phonological skills. For instance, the most nativelike phonological skills may be acquired if a young child is naturally exposed to a second language and also receives instruction from native speakers of that language. The contribution of several such factors to the acquisition of phonological skills in a second language need to be evaluated.

 Activity

DIRECTIONS: Describe how **age** can affect the phonological acquisition of a second language.

Hierarchies of Phonological Difficulty

Some theorists have tried to explain the difficulties in acquiring second-language phonological patterns on the basis of contrasting phonological features in the first and second languages and thus creating a hierarchy of difficulty. Hierarchies of difficulty are based on the presence or absence of a phoneme in the two languages and on whether their allophonic use is obligatory in given contexts. For example, a child trying to master a sound in the second language that is absent in the primary language will face the greatest amount of difficulty. A child will face much less difficulty if the sound is the same in the two languages and is used in the same obligatory contexts in both (Stockwell & Bowen, 1983).

Critics have found problems with the hierarchies of phonological difficulty (Yavas, 1998). For example, cross-linguistic research has shown that not all the sounds that are absent in the primary language create equal difficulty for the learner of a second language. Some absent sounds are still easier to learn than others. Generally, sounds that are extremely rare in human languages are more difficult than those that are fairly common across languages but absent in a given language. Phonologists use the term *natural* or *unmarked* versus *not natural* or *marked* features to describe these observations. A sound or phonological feature that is frequently found in most languages is called **unmarked;** unmarked sounds or features also are considered **natural.** A sound or a feature that is found infrequently in languages is called **marked;** marked sounds or features also are considered not natural. For example, voiceless stops are unmarked, more natural, and more common in different languages; voiced obstruents are marked, less natural, and less common in languages.

Additional research has shown that sounds that are similar in a first and a second language are more difficult than those that are very different. Sounds of the second language that are the same in the first language are learned with ease. However, similar sounds across the two languages tend to be substituted or distorted. On the other hand, sounds that exist only in the second language may actually be produced in a manner that better approximates the native production of those sounds.

Universal Patterns of Phonological Acquisition

Cross-linguistic studies have generally shown that children acquire the phonemes of their first language in a fairly similar manner (Yavas, 1994, 1998; Kayser, 1995). Children acquiring different languages exhibit similar phonological processes. Yavas (1998) has stated that "in all languages, children reduce consonant clusters, delete and/or devoice final consonants, stop fricatives, front velars and palatals, glide liquids, delete unstressed syllables, and reveal assimilatory changes" (p. 217). However, while both first- and second-language learners exhibit simplifying phonological processes during the period of acquisition, the specific processes they use may be different. For example, the first-language learners tend to exhibit consonant deletion in the case of consonant clusters (e.g., *play* becomes *pey*). However, the second-language learners tend to exhibit epenthesis instead of deletion (e.g., *play* becomes [pəle]).

Phonologists who emphasize the importance of universal patterns of acquisition in understanding phonological acquisition in a first as well as a second language point out that markedness of sounds causes some of the variability found in acquisition patterns. Accordingly, it is not just interference from the first language that affects the pattern of production in the second. Sounds in the second language that are marked (uncommon in languages and hence less natural) may pose greater difficulty than those that are unmarked (common in languages and hence more natural). Therefore, the relative markedness of phonemes creates certain universal patterns of acquisition.

A factor that is less well understood, and one that is of great clinical significance, is individual differences in phonological acquisition. Variations in patterns of development often are as pronounced among children within the same language community as among children between communities. This variability in phonological acquisition within the same language community is not easily explained on the basis of interference or markedness-naturalness. Therefore, clinicians need to pay attention to the individual child's pattern of acquisition or production and make an analysis that is child specific.

✎ Activity

DIRECTIONS: List some phonological processes that have been documented as occurring across languages in normal development.

- _____
- _____
- _____
- _____
- _____
- _____
- _____

Clinical Issues in Bilingual Phonology

Bilingual phonology has been mostly descriptive, comparative, and theoretical. Investigators have mostly been concerned with describing phonological commonalities and differences across languages, comparing such commonalities and differences, and offering hypotheses to explain the documented characteristics across languages. In bilingual phonological research, clinicians find background information necessary to understand a bilingual child's phonological patterns and to make decisions that are consistent with that child's primary language characteristics.

However, clinicians need to go beyond descriptive information on the dual language characteristics a bilingual child might exhibit. The central clinical issues include appropriate assessment techniques and treatment procedures for bilingual children. These issues can be addressed and resolved only by clinical research, not by descriptive, comparative, or theoretical linguistic research.

Assessment Issues and Research Needs

Clinical writing on the assessment of bilingual children has been mostly concerned with assessment techniques. A major issue is whether tests that are standardized on monolingual, English-speaking children are appropriate in assessing children who are bilingual. Clinicians agree that they are not. To remedy the situation, clinicians typically call for development of standardized tests that target particular bilingual children (e.g., bilingual Spanish-English children).

Of the many minority languages in the United States, Spanish has received significant attention because Spanish speakers outnumber other minority language speakers. Various assessment tools are being developed to evaluate bilingual Spanish-English children's language and phonological skills. Continued research is expected to increase the number of available assessment tools. However, the same cannot be said of other minority languages. The variety of Asian languages and the difficulty in sampling an adequate number of children who speak particular Asian languages make it extremely difficult to standardize articulation and phonological tests for those children. Similar problems exist for other minority languages of the United States.

In the absence of standardized measures, and as a supplement to those measures even when they exist, clinicians need to use client-specific procedures. Conversational speech samples are an excellent client-specific measure, especially when the concern is not so much to compare a child's productions with those of his or her peer group as to evaluate his or her current performance. In such cases, absence of norms may not be as handicapping as one might suppose. However, we need more research on naturalistic language sampling, analysis, and clinical decision making based on a child's communication needs and the educational, social, and personal demands the child faces.

Treatment Issues and Research Needs

The most urgent need in bilingual, multicultural phonology is controlled treatment research. While recommendations and guidelines on treating bilingual children abound, controlled research on treatment procedures is lacking.

As suggested in the previous section on guidelines on working with bilingual children, clinicians can assume that the basic treatment principles used in remediating disorders of articulation hold in treating bilingual children as well. Of course, this assumption should be promptly abandoned if controlled treatment research (not just expert opinions or theories) suggests otherwise. Treatment research has generally shown that procedures, not principles, need to be modified to suit individual clients (Hegde, 1998b). For instance, while one child may react positively to verbal praise for correct productions, another may not. However, the child who does not react positively to verbal praise may react well when a token is presented for each correct response. Thus, though the effect of a particular reinforcer may vary across children, the principle of positive reinforcement does not.

There is no evidence to suggest that children of different cultural backgrounds are not susceptible to response-contingent consequences (e.g., positive reinforcers, corrective feedback), though children of different cultural backgrounds may be susceptible to different kinds of consequences, as the example in the previous paragraph suggests. Clinicians tend to assume that bilingual children necessarily require unique treatment procedures, but unless contradicted by experimental data, clinicians can use standard treatment procedures and modify them as found necessary.

The most important consideration in the treatment of bilingual children is the selection of target behaviors. As suggested previously, phonemes that are in error in both languages and those that are in error in the primary language should be the treatment targets. Phonemes that are used differently in the secondary language due to the influence of the primary language should be treated as a matter of *elective* dialectal modification.

Summary of the Advanced Unit

- Children may become bilingual in two ways.

- Some are **simultaneously bilingual,** which means that the two languages were acquired at about the same time.

- Others are **successively bilingual,** which means that one language was acquired before the other.

- Phonological variations found in children who speak two or more languages have been explained on the basis of several factors.

- The hypothesis of **differentiated phonological patterns** states that bilingual children have clearly separate phonological patterns from the beginning.

- The hypothesis of **undifferentiated phonological patterns** states that such children have a single pattern to begin with and only later have a differentiated system. Data seem to suggest that differentiation begins around age 2.

- The hypothesis of **approximation to first language** (interference from the first language) states that children speaking a second language show phonological variations because they try to approximate their second-language phonetic productions to those of their first language. In other words, first-language phonological patterns interfere with the second-language patterns.

- The hypothesis of **critical age for phonological acquisition** states that to acquire nativelike phonological patterns, a child should start speaking the language in question before a certain critical age. The upper limit of this age is thought to be between 12 and 15 years, after which it is difficult if not impossible to acquire the native phonological pattern of a language.

- The hypothesis of **hierarchies of phonological difficulty** states that contrasting features of the first and second languages create varied amounts of difficulty for the child learning two languages.

- The hypothesis of **universal patterns of phonological acquisition** states that children across languages acquire phonological systems in a fairly uniform manner and exhibit such phonological processes as consonant-cluster reductions, deletion of final consonants, devoicing of final consonants, stopping fricatives, fronting velars and palatals, gliding liquids, and so forth.

- There is a great need for developing appropriate client- and primary language–specific assessment tools for evaluating bilingual children.

- In treating bilingual children, clinicians can assume that treatment *principles* do not change, although treatment *procedures* may need to be modified to suit the individual child. Target phonological behaviors should be based on the characteristics of the child's first and second languages.

Chapter 6

◆ ◆ ◆ ◆ ◆ ◆ ◆ ◆ ◆ ◆ ◆ ◆ ◆ ◆ ◆ ◆ ◆

Assessment of Articulation and Phonological Disorders

Basic Unit: General Assessment Procedures with Articulation and Phonological Disorders

Advanced Unit: Description and Assessment of Various Organic and Neurogenic Speech Disorders. 329

Basic Unit

♦ ♦ ♦ ♦ ♦ ♦ ♦ ♦ ♦ ♦ ♦ ♦ ♦ ♦ ♦ ♦ ♦ ♦ ♦

General Assessment Procedures with Articulation and Phonological Disorders

Eloquence is the power to translate a truth into language perfectly intelligible to the person to whom you speak.
—RALPH WALDO EMERSON

A comprehensive and well-structured assessment is extremely important for the eventual diagnosis of any communication disorder. An **assessment** can be described as the process that is followed and the procedures that are used to establish the presence or absence of a disorder. The specific characteristics of the disorder and any possible causative factors are also examined. The clinician's judgment about the absence or presence of a disorder and a description of the nature of an existing disorder lead to a clinical **diagnosis.** It is important to note that not all assessments will lead to diagnosis of a disorder. Some will confirm that a client's skills are clinically appropriate or developing as expected.

To ensure an accurate diagnosis, it is imperative that the clinician carefully consider all of the components typically included in an assessment and alter or modify them so that a particular client's skills are properly observed. Roseberry-McKibbin and Hegde (2000) indicate that the clinician's primary responsibility during an assessment is to determine whether the child referred for an articulation or phonological disorder indeed has a clinical problem and to describe the characteristics of a problem.

Performing the assessment is only the first step in the diagnostic process. On the way to making a diagnosis of normal or disordered articulation or phonological skills, a clinician typically moves through the following steps:

1. *Conducting an assessment.* A case history is obtained, an interview is conducted, formal tests are administered, clinical observations are made, and various clinically relevant data are collected.

2. *Scoring the tests that were administered and consolidating the various data.*

3. *Analyzing the tests and all other relevant data.*

4. *Synthesizing and interpreting the results of the tests and other assessment information.*

5. *Making a clinical decision regarding the presence or absence of an articulation or phonological disorder.* It is at this point that a **diagnosis** is actually made.

6. *Making specific recommendations after a diagnosis has been reached.* Of course, the recommendations will vary according to each client's needs.

The assessment and diagnostic process is an exciting event. The clinician has the opportunity to put forth all of the specialized skills he or she has acquired.

However, the prudent clinician is careful not to diagnose a client when clinical data are merely being collected. At that point in the assessment process, the clinician often begins to suspect that a problem does or does not exist; however, it is not until all of the necessary information has been collected, analyzed, and interpreted that an appropriate diagnosis can be made. Following this scientific principle of reserving opinions until the data "speak" guards the clinician from misdiagnosing a client and making inappropriate clinical recommendations.

Haynes and Pindzola (1998) indicate that there are at least seven important prerequisites to performing an adequate articulation and phonological assessment:

- knowledge of the anatomy and physiology of the speech mechanism;
- knowledge of phonetics;
- knowledge of phonological development;
- knowledge of factors related to articulation disorders;
- knowledge of dialectical variations;
- knowledge of coarticulation; and
- knowledge of the linguistic-articulatory connection.

We have reviewed all of these variables in previous chapters. Also many introduction courses in speech–language pathology are designed to help students meet these prerequisites.

In this Basic Unit we will review the many components of an articulation and phonological assessment. Because of the vast number of elements that are typically included in an articulation and phonological assessment, this Basic Unit is much lengthier than the previous chapters. However, we felt that a thorough examination was important and necessary. Students at this level are often close to making the transition from purely academic courses to clinical practicum. Thus, there is a strong desire for practical information that will help in present or future interactions with clients.

In essence, the primary goal of this Basic Unit is to provide the reader with useful information that can facilitate the clinical process. In the Advanced Unit of this chapter, we will expand on the fundamental assessment principles. We will address assessment issues related to specific clinical populations such as **apraxia of speech, dysarthria,** and **cleft palate.** All the components of assessment discussed in this Basic Unit apply to those special populations; however, there are some specific techniques that are worth examining as well.

General Principles of Assessment

Although a clinician's specific training and own clinical philosophy often dictate what is included in an assessment, there are various principles that are generally followed. Among these are:

- reviewing the client's background;
- planning the diagnostic session;
- selecting appropriate tests;
- preparing the test room;
- conducting an opening interview and explaining the test procedures;
- administering the selected tests;
- assessing related areas;
- conducting a closing interview and discussing the findings;
- making recommendations; and
- writing a diagnostic report.

These components are generally applied to the assessment of all communicative disorders. However, we will tailor them for our purposes to address the assessment of articulation and phonological disorders.

Review the Client's Background

Before a comprehensive assessment can be performed, the examiner must review the client's history for all pertinent background information. A thorough case history can be gathered by (a) reviewing reports written by other professionals, (b) collecting a written case history, and (c) conducting oral interviews with the client and significant others. We will discuss this process in great detail.

Plan the Assessment Session

After a careful analysis of the client's history, the clinician generally has sufficient information to plan the assessment. Appropriate testing instruments and clinical procedures are identified. The clinician also plans the testing sequence to promote an efficient and expeditious assessment. A review of the client's background helps in arranging any special procedures that may need to be used with particular clients. For example, a client with a known history of **tongue thrust** may require a swallowing evaluation with various food textures. Knowing the client's history helps the clinician plan the assessment session(s) by gathering the appropriate materials. A carefully planned assessment can help save both time and money.

Select the Appropriate Test(s) and Activities

The same testing instruments are not appropriate for all clients. The clinician must select tests and activities that help identify an individual client's problems. For example, it is probably unnecessary to administer a lengthy test that targets the use of several phonological processes in a child who reportedly distorts only /s/ and /r/. It would also be inappropriate to administer a reading passage to a young child who has not yet started reading.

Prepare the Testing Area

The setting in which a speech–language pathologist works or the university environment in which services are provided often dictates the clinical testing area. In the typical university clinic, the testing rooms are approximately 7 feet by 9 feet and are often equipped with a one-way **observation mirror.**

At times the one-way mirror can significantly interfere with the testing process; a child facing it may become distracted. If there is any chance that the mirror may become a distraction, it is important to modify the seating arrangement so that the client's back faces the mirror.

It is also important that the clinician keep the testing area free of clutter. We have often witnessed young children become distracted by the clinician's paperwork, objects, and other excessive stimuli. The clinician should place the various testing instruments in a relatively hidden area and retrieve them only as necessary. The clinician also needs to ensure that there is adequate lighting in the testing room. This is especially important when conducting an orofacial examination, since the oral cavity is extremely dark and difficult to see under less than optimal lighting.

Conduct an Opening Interview and Explain the Test Procedures

One of the very first steps of the assessment process is the **opening interview,** also called the **information-getting interview.** At this point the clinician collects important background information from the client or the client's parents. The clinician also seeks clarification of any information provided in the written case history and asks more in-depth questions if necessary. Any information believed to be relevant to the diagnostic process should be obtained during the information-getting interview. It is important that the clinician not rush this part of the assessment. The information collected during the interview is often instrumental in reaching a diagnosis. The process involved in conducting an opening interview will be reviewed in detail in an upcoming section of this Basic Unit.

After the clinician believes that all the necessary background information has been obtained, the next step is to provide a brief explanation of the overall assessment process. The clinician may state something like the following: "Thanks for all of your information. I believe that we have gone over all of the important issues. Before we get started with the actual testing, I just briefly want to explain what we'll be doing. I will spend some time talking with Jenny so that I can listen to her speech. I will also administer a test in which I will show her some pictures, and all she has to do is name the pictures for me. I will also be doing a hearing screening, and I will be looking in her mouth to make sure everything is fine with her oral structures. As I get to know Jenny a little bit better, I may decide to administer other tests, but I'm not quite sure at this point. Every child is unique, and because of this, we always try to tailor our testing so that each child's needs are met. Always feel free to ask me any questions as we go along. After the entire testing is done, I will spend some time with you to explain the results and my recommendations."

Administer the Selected Tests

After the information-getting interview is completed, the clinician administers the selected tests. If **standardized tests** are used, the clinician should adhere closely to the recommended administration procedures to maintain the tests' internal **validity** and **reliability.** If the clinician chooses to alter some of the administration procedures, this should be noted when the results are documented. The clinician may also choose to perform some nonstandardized procedures such as speech and language sampling. Those testing activities will be described in detail in upcoming sections of this Basic Unit.

Assess Related Areas

Other areas typically screened or assessed during an articulation-phonological assessment are the client's hearing, orofacial structures, diadochokinetic syllable rates, level of stimulability, speech rate, and speech intelligibility. The clinician employs specialized procedures to assess all of these related areas. These will be discussed with greater detail in upcoming sections.

Discuss the Findings and Make Recommendations

After all of the testing has been completed and the clinician has analyzed and synthesized the various data collected during the assessment, the next step is to convey this information to the client or the client's parents. The results of the testing and the clinician's recommendations should be discussed in a simple and understandable manner.

The clinician should always *avoid the use of technical jargon* since this may confuse the client or the client's parents, as in the following statement: "Mrs. Williams, the results of the tests show that your daughter has a phonological disorder. She demonstrated significant use of final-consonant deletion, liquid gliding, and velar fronting. A child her age would be expected to have suppressed the use of those processes."

Instead, the clinician should use everyday language that communicates the essence of the diagnosis. The above statement could be reworded as follows: "Mrs. Williams, from the testing I did with your daughter, I was able to confirm that she indeed has a lot of difficulty producing many sounds. Since you brought your daughter in for testing, I'm sure that this doesn't surprise you. The specific disorder that your daughter demonstrated is often called a phonological disorder. What this means is that she seems to have some patterns in the kinds of sound errors that she makes. For example, I noticed that she tends to leave off most of the end sounds in words. She also tends to substitute front sounds for sounds that should be made in the back part of the mouth. Another pattern in her speech is that she uses the *w* sound for the *r* and *l* sounds. These types of sound error patterns are common in young children, but we would not expect a child Jenny's age to show these errors." The statement is longer and may sound much more cumbersome to the trained clinician, but the average layperson needs this type of explanation.

Of course, the clinician should also be careful not to talk down to the client or the client's parents. If the client's parents have a degree in linguistics, for example, it is unnecessary to provide simplified definitions of speech and language terms, since linguists often have that knowledge. During the opening interview, the clinician will get a feel for the client's or the parents' education level and general communication skills and thus alter his or her own communication style accordingly.

Write the Diagnostic Report

After the assessment has been completed and a diagnosis has been made, the clinician must report the findings. This information may be reported verbally to the client's parents, primary care physician, classroom teacher, and so forth to expedite the process. However, for legal and ethical reasons, such reports must be followed up with a detailed written report. We will discuss the details of report writing at the end of this Basic Unit.

Assessment Objectives

In the diagnosis of an articulation and phonological disorder, the clinician must keep in mind several objectives that will aid in determining the presence or absence of a disorder and the nature of the disorder. Roseberry-McKibbin and Hegde (2000) indicate that a clinician's objectives in the assessment of articulation and phonological skills may include the following:

- conducting a speech screening;
- collecting a case history;
- conducting an orofacial examination;
- conducting a hearing screening;
- assessing the child's performance in single-word tests and conversational speech;
- assessing the presence of phonological processes or phonological rules that may help establish patterns of misarticulations;
- evaluating the child's performance in light of developmental norms; and
- evaluating the child's stimulability of the speech sounds that were misarticulated.

We will address all of these objectives and several others as we progress. Our primary goal is that the clinician learn to conduct a comprehensive assessment that will lead to a valid and reliable diagnosis of articulation and phonological disorders.

Conducting a Speech Screening

Overview of Screening Procedures

A **screening** is a pass or failure procedure that can be conducted with a large number of individuals in a relatively short period of time. Nicolosi, Harryman, and Kresheck (1996) define a screening as "any gross measure utilized to separate those who may require specific help in a specific area, such as language, hearing, articulation, fluency, and voice, from those who obviously do not need help" (p. 242). Articulation screenings help identify children who potentially have an articulation or phonological disorder and may require further assessment.

If a client fails a screening, he or she may be referred for a complete appraisal of his or her articulation and phonological skills. Screenings are most widely used in preschool programs, public schools, some colleges and universities, and hospitals. They do not take more than a few minutes to complete.

In the elementary school setting, screenings are typically conducted with children in kindergarten or first grade. Some clinicians also screen children in third grade. As evidenced by the classic information on the development of articulation and phonological skills, mastery of all English sounds would be expected by approximately 8 years, which is the chronological age of most third graders.

Screenings in colleges and universities are commonly performed with students preparing for specific occupations in which adequate communication skills are essential, such as teaching, broadcast journalism, audiology, and speech–language pathology. Screenings in the hospital or other medical setting are generally done with a team of other professionals such as physical therapists, occupational therapists, and nurses. Newly admitted patients may be screened for overall communicative competence by a speech–language pathologist and referred for a complete assessment if appropriate.

Speech–language pathologists may also choose to screen the articulation and phonological status of referred clients to determine if a complete appraisal is warranted. This may save the clinician valuable time since some referrals by other professionals may be well intended but not necessarily appropriate.

Screenings are intended to be a quick and easy measure of speech sound productions. They can usually be completed in 10 to 15 minutes. They can be performed with published testing instruments or nonstandardized measures designed by the examiner or a group of examiners (e.g., speech–language pathologists working for the same public school district or hospital).

Standardized Screening Instruments

Standardized screening instruments are commercially available tests that often include normative data and provide a pass or failure score. Some tests are designed solely as screening instruments, while others are part of a full articulation-phonological or language assessment. Currently, there are various published screening instruments from which the speech–language pathologist can choose. Among these are the following, listed alphabetically.

Denver Articulation Screening Test (DAST)

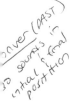

The *Denver Articulation Screening Test* (Drumwright, 1971) is designed to screen the production of 30 sounds in initial- and final-word positions through imitative production. The test also examines the client's intelligibility on a 4-point scale, with 1 being "easy to understand" and 4 being "can't understand." It is tailored for screening sound production skills in Anglo, African-American, and Mexican-American children.

Predictive Screening Test of Articulation (PSTA)

The *Predictive Screening Test of Articulation* (Van Riper & Erickson, 1969) was developed to identify children whose speech is likely to improve without treatment by the end of second grade. It is intended for use with first graders. The PSTA also serves as a screening instrument to identify children who need additional testing. According to Stockman and McDonald (1980), the PSTA's predictive value may be greater for children who misarticulate specific sounds such as sibilants and liquids since these occur more frequently in the test.

Quick Screen of Phonology (QSP)

The *Quick Screen of Phonology* (Bankson & Bernthal, 1990b) was designed to screen 23 consonants and 3 consonant clusters using a picture-naming format. Each stimulus word assesses sounds in initial- and final-word positions. The stimulus items were selected because of their correlation with the norms of the *Bankson-Bernthal Test of Phonology* (Bankson & Bernthal, 1990a). The QSP provides percentile ranks and standard scores for children 3-0 to 7-11 years.

Templin-Darley Screening Test

The *Templin-Darley Screening Test* was designed to screen 22 consonants, 26 consonant clusters, 1 vowel, and 1 consonant-vowel combination. The test stimuli are 50 items from the *Templin-Darley Tests of Articulation* (Templin & Darley, 1969). This screening test provides norms and cutoff scores for children 3 through 8 years of age.

Test of Minimal Articulation Competence (T-MAC)

The *Test of Minimal Articulation Competence* (Secord, 1981c) is a complete assessment instrument that includes a 3- to 5-minute screening test. The Complete Screening portion is designed to screen school-age children for the production of /t/, /k/, /s/, /θ/, /ʃ/, /v/, /tʃ/, /dʒ/, /l/, /r/. Selected picture cards are used to evoke production of the words containing these sounds in pre-, inter-, and postvocalic positions. The Complete Screening also tests production of /ɪɚ/, /ɛɚ/, /ɑɚ/, and /ɔɚ/. The results of the screening are recorded on the T-MAC Record Form, which has the phonetic symbols and words of all the phonemes screened shaded in blue for easy scoring. They can also be scored on the Screening Test Record Form.

The T-MAC offers an additional screening measure designed for preschool children called the *Rapid Screening Test*. This screening assesses all of the English consonants by presentation of picture cards containing the sounds in the intervocalic position of words. The responses may be recorded on the T-MAC Record Form or the Screening Test Record Form. Secord indicates that older children and adults may be screened through selected reading portions of the test.

Fluharty Preschool Speech and Language Screening Test

As can be judged by the title of this test, the *Fluharty Preschool Speech and Language Screening Test* (Fluharty, 1978) is both a speech and a language screening. The speech portion screens 19 sounds using real objects. The test was designed for children 2 through 6 years of age. It provides cutoff scores to indicate the need for further testing.

Nonstandardized Screenings

Speech–language pathologists who prefer to employ unpublished or nonstandardized screening instruments may design their own measures. Informal screenings may be tailored to a specific population and, thus, may be more suitable than standardized screenings at times. Screenings may be designed for a particular group's age or ethnocultural background.

During informal articulation and phonological screenings, the clinician engages the child in brief conversation or may design specific questions that help evoke spontaneous verbal productions. The clinician notes and records any articulation or phonological errors.

Older preschool and kindergarten children may be asked the following during the screening process:

- Tell me your name.

- What is your mommy's (daddy's) name? (Tell me about your mommy and daddy.)

- Tell me about your favorite TV show. (Who is your favorite person in that show?)

- Tell me about your best friend.

- What is your favorite cartoon?

- Tell me about the last movie you saw.

- Tell me what you had for breakfast this morning (or lunch this afternoon).

- Tell me about your favorite vacation trip.

- Tell me about some presents that you have gotten.

- Say your ABCs.

- Count to 20.

- Say the days of the week and months of the year.

If this type of requests or questions fail to evoke the desired verbal productions from a young child, the examiner may use toys or pictures of objects that have the target sounds in their name. If all else fails, the clinician may ask the child to repeat words that contain the target sounds. It is important to remember that an adequate rapport must be established with young children to evoke representative verbal productions. Thus, a screening with a young child may take longer to complete than the average 10 or 15 minutes.

Older school-age children and adults may be asked similar questions. However, the questions should be designed to conform to the interests of a particular age. Assuming that the child or adult has age-appropriate reading skills, he or she may also be asked to read several sentences containing frequently misarticulated sounds such as /r/, /s/, /l/, and /θ/. The adolescent or adult client may also be asked to read a passage with a representative sample of all the English speech sounds, such as the popular "Grandfather Passage" or "Rainbow Passage." Refer to Appendix D for passages that may be used during a screening procedure with older children and adults.

The examiner or group of examiners determines the criterion for passing or failing the designed screening measure. Typically, the client's performance is compared to established developmental norms and the phonological system of his or her linguistic community. Frequently, the need for a more thorough assessment is obvious to the examiner. However, there are occasions when the client's performance on a screening is not clear-cut. In cases when the clinician is in doubt, it is clinically wise to refer the child for a more thorough assessment. This will help ensure that an articulation or phonological disorder does not go unidentified. This is especially important with young children since they are in a developmental stage at which even a few months can make a significant difference in their phonological skills.

Gathering a Case History

As indicated earlier, before a comprehensive assessment can be performed, the examiner must review the client's history for all pertinent background information. A thorough case history can be gathered by (a) collecting a written case history (b) reviewing reports written by other professionals, and (c) conducting oral interviews with the client and the client's parents. The information obtained from a case history can help the clinician better understand the client's problem. Important factors that may contribute to the articulation or phonological disorder (e.g., history of recurrent ear infections) may come to light through this process.

Written Case History Forms

In clinical settings that allow for this, it is important to obtain a written case history. A written case history helps facilitate the assessment process. It provides the examiner with important background information about the client before the initial assessment meeting. This helps the clinician select appropriate testing tools and procedures for a specific client to meet his or her special or unusual needs.

Written case history forms are designed by specific organizations and are most often used in university clinics, outpatient clinics, and private practices. They are completed by the client or the client's caregiver and reviewed by the clinician prior to the initial assessment meeting. Written case history forms address many important diagnostic variables such as the course of the disorder, potential etiological factors for the disorder, and the client's or family's perception of the problem. They provide the clinician with relevant information that helps in planning an expeditious assessment.

Because a standard written case history form used by all speech–language pathologists does not currently exist, clinicians generally develop or adapt forms that address information believed relevant for a given population (Shipley & McAfee, 1998). Although forms vary for child and adult clients, the content of a written case history form commonly includes the following general categories:

- identifying information
- statement of the problem
- speech and language developmental history
- prenatal and birth history
- general developmental history
- medical history
- educational history
- social history
- other related information

According to Shipley and McAfee (1998), the value of a case history form as a preassessment tool may be limited because of various factors such as the following:

- The respondent may provide inaccurate or incomplete information. This may in part be due to a lack of understanding of the terminology on the form.

- The respondent may not have sufficient time to complete the form. It may take a considerable amount of time to collect certain pieces of requested information, such as dates of illnesses or developmental history.

• The respondent may not know or only vaguely recall certain information.

• The respondent may not have complete recollection of the information requested since significant time may have elapsed between the onset of the problem and the speech–language assessment.

• The respondent's ability to recall certain events may be affected by extenuating life events or other circumstances. For example, the parent of an only child will probably remember developmental milestones more clearly than the parent who has several children. The parent of a child with multiple medical, communicative, and academic problems will likely be less focused on specific speech and language development than the parent of a child who has only a communication disorder.

• The respondent's own cultural differences may interfere with accurate provision of necessary information. The respondent may not understand cultural innuendos reflected in the case history's queries (information adapted from pp. 4–5).

In addition to the problems outlined by Shipley and McAfee (1998), there may be other limitations associated with written case history forms. When sending a case history to a client or client's parents, it is assumed that a level of literacy appropriate for completion of the form is present. However, there are occasions when a form is not completed because the respondent is not able to read or write. In addition, clients may feel that their privacy is being invaded by questions that are deemed very personal or private, such as type of occupation, level of education, medical history, and so forth. This is especially problematic in cultures that place a high value on personal or family privacy.

Despite these limitations, the written case history form serves as an important clinical tool that provides valuable information about the client, the potential articulation-phonological problem, the client's or family's reaction to the problem, and the possible etiological factors. A written case history should be obtained if a clinician's employment setting permits it.

Written and Verbal Information from Other Professionals

Clients assessed by the speech–language pathologist may have an educational, medical, or psychosocial history that would reveal important diagnostic information. The client may also have a history of previous assessments by other specialists such as a dentist, psychologist, otolaryngologist, neurologist, audiologist, or speech–language pathologist. Requesting all relevant medical or educational records is an important process in the collection of a thorough case history. This information is often helpful in more thoroughly understanding the disorder before reaching a diagnosis.

The importance of the information provided by other professionals for the diagnosis of an articulation or phonological disorder is not always known until the information is received. Some information may be key to the diagnosis, while other information may be minimally useful. However, the judgment that information from a specific professional may or may not be relevant to the client's diagnosis should be reserved until all of that information has been reviewed (Shipley & McAfee, 1998).

When requesting verbal or written information about a particular client from other professionals, it is important to realize that there are legal and ethical issues that must always be considered. First and foremost, other professionals or agencies should never be contacted for information without the client's or caregiver's consent. Although the consent may be verbal or written, it is most advisable (for legal reasons) to obtain written permission from the client or caregiver. Some agencies and professionals refuse to provide requested information without written consent from the appropriate person.

Opening Interview

To supplement or clarify the information provided in the written case history and the information obtained from other professionals, it is important to conduct a verbal interview. The verbal interview, known as an information-getting interview, opening interview, or intake interview, generally takes place as the initial part of the assessment. It is conducted with the client (if assessing an adult) or a parent (if assessing a young child).

On occasions when assessing an adult client, the interview must be directed to his or her significant other. This may occur when the client cannot verbally supply the necessary information because of severe communication deficits. Out of respect for the client, it is extremely important that in such a case the questions be addressed to both people, even if only the caregiver can respond. Rather than ask such a question as "When did your husband have his stroke?" the clinician should maintain eye contact with both the client and the caregiver and use such questions as "When did you have your stroke?" The caregiver already knows that his or her loved one cannot respond and will likely provide the information spontaneously without further probing from the clinician. For detailed information on interviewing techniques, the reader may consult Emerick and Haynes (1986), Haynes, Pindzola, and Emerick (1992), Shipley (1992), Tomblin, Morris, and Spriestersbach (1994), and Peterson and Marquardt (1994).

General Structure of an Interview

According to Shipley and McAfee (1998) and Shipley (1992), the information-getting interview consists of three phases: the opening, the body, and the closing. In the *opening phase* of the interview, the clinician greets the client, describes the purpose of the meeting, and indicates approximately how much time the assessment will take.

A discussion of the client's history and current status is conducted in the *body of the interview*. At that point, the focus shifts to a discussion of the client's (a) communicative development and current status; (b) medical, developmental, and social history; and (c) educational and vocational history. Information gathered in the written case history is clarified and confirmed.

During the *closing phase* of the information-getting interview, the major points from the body of the interview are summarized and reiterated. The clinician also expresses his or her appreciation for the interviewee's help and indicates what procedures will follow.

Throughout the interview, the clinician asks a combination of *open-ended* and *closed-ended* questions. Open-ended questions allow the interviewee to provide a general and elaborate answer. Many times the respondents' answers to open-ended questions will trigger other questions and will help identify primary concerns that may require further clarification. An example of an open-ended question is "How would you describe your daughter's speech?" Closed-ended questions generally evoke short and direct replies, such as, "Yes" in response to the clinician's query, "Is your daughter's speech difficult to understand?" A question that might prompt a more detailed response is, "Can you describe how understandable your daughter's speech is?"

Interview with Parents and Caregivers

When assessing a child with a suspected articulation or phonological problem, it is extremely important to conduct a well-structured interview with the client's parent(s). The clinician asks questions relevant to a particular case and remains cognizant of why certain questions are asked. Considering the three phases of an information-getting interview, the interview with a parent may proceed as follows.

Opening Phase of the Opening Interview

"Hello, my name is Linda Stevens. I'm the speech–language pathologist who will be testing Jenny's speech today. Another common name for a speech–language pathologist is speech therapist. You may be more familiar with the second term. I would like to begin by asking you some questions about Jenny's speech and other important information about her development. Some of the questions I will be asking may sound familiar from the questionnaire you already filled out. The information that you share with me today will help me get a clearer picture of Jenny's communication skills. Parents are always the best source of information since they spend so much time with their children. If I ask a question that is not very clear, please don't hesitate to let me know and I will try to make it clearer. When you and I are through discussing Jenny's speech, I will spend some time alone with her to do some testing. The entire testing should take about three sessions (assuming the sessions are 30–40 minutes in length). When I'm finished with the testing, I will get together with you again and discuss my findings and recommendations. Do you have any questions before I begin to ask you questions?"

Body of the Opening Interview

"Now I'm going to ask you several questions about Jenny's speech and her overall development. Please remember that all of the questions I'm asking are going to help me determine whether a problem exists, and if it does, whether treatment is appropriate. O.K. let's begin." The questions that follow were selected because they are typical for a client with a suspected articulation or phonological problem. This list is not meant to be all-inclusive and may be altered as necessary. The questions are listed primarily for first-time student clinicians who may need more guidance in conducting an information-getting interview.

Early Speech and Language Milestones

• Was your child a quiet or a vocal infant?

• Did your child coo, babble, or attempt to imitate your sounds? When did these speech behaviors begin?

- When did your child say his first words? Can you recall what the words were?

- When did your child begin to name people and objects?

- When did your child begin to put words together (e.g., *Mommy go*)?

- Were your child's first words and phrases easy or difficult to understand?

Current Communication Status

- Currently, does your child prefer to use speech or gestures to communicate?

- Has your child's speech shown any progress during the last 6 months?

- Is your child aware that his or her speech is different from that of others? If so, how does he or she demonstrate this awareness?

- What have you or other professionals done to help your child speak better?

- At what age was it suspected that your child had a speech problem? Who was the first person to suspect the problem?

- On a range from mild to profound, how severe would you judge your child's problem?

- On a scale of 0 to 100 percent, how understandable would you judge your child's speech?

- On a scale of 0 to 100 percent, how understandable do you think your child's speech is to other family members? How understandable is it to people who are not frequently around him or her?

- Has negative attention been called to your child's speech by any family members or by others? If so, in what way?

History of Professional Intervention

- Has your child's speech ever been evaluated? If so, when and by whom? What were the results? Do you have a copy of the report(s)?

- Has your child ever received speech treatment? If so, when, for how long, for what reason, and with what degree of success? Who was the clinician?

- Has your child ever received any other types of treatments (e.g., audiological evaluation, orthodontic care, or otolaryngological evaluation)? If so, when and for what reason? Who was the professional who provided the care? Do you have a copy of the report(s)?

History of Pregnancy and Delivery

- Did you (the mother) have any illnesses, accidents, or complications while pregnant with your child?

- Did you take any medications while pregnant with your child?

- What was the length of your pregnancy with your child?

- What was the duration of the delivery?

• What was your child's weight at birth?

• Did your child suffer any complications or unusual conditions at birth or shortly after birth?

Current Medical Status and Medical History

• What diseases or serious injuries has your child had? Were there any complications?

• Has your child ever been hospitalized? If so, why?

• What is the present condition of your child's health?

• Does your child have any physical problems? If so, what are they?

• What is the name of your family physician or your child's pediatrician?

• Is your child currently receiving any medication, or is he or she under any medical treatment? If so, what kind and for what reason?

• Has your child ever suffered a severe head injury, trauma, or high fever? If so, please explain.

Academic/School History

• Did your child ever attend a day-care center or nursery school? Did the teachers report any problems or make any recommendations?

• Did your child attend kindergarten? Did the teachers report any problems or make any recommendations?

• At what age did your child begin school?

• What kind of grades or test scores does your child typically achieve?

• Has your child ever been retained a grade in school? If so, which grade? Why?

• Is your child frequently absent from school? If so, why?

• What are or were your child's poorest subjects in school? Best subjects?

• How does your child feel about school and his friends and teachers?

• Has your child ever attended any special classes or received special instruction? If so, why, when, for how long, and where?

Social and Family History

• How does your child interact with other children? Adults?

• Are there any disciplinary problems with your child?

• How does your child get along with others at home?

• Do you have other children? What are their names and ages?

• What interests, hobbies, or other activities does your child have?

• What are your and your spouse's occupations?

- What are your and your spouse's educational levels?

- Is there any other information that might help me better understand your child's problem?

Closing Phase of Opening Interview

"Thank you for all of the helpful information. Now I'm going to spend some time alone with Jenny and test her speech. When I'm completely finished with all of the testing, I'll discuss my findings and recommendations with you."

Interview with Adolescent and Adult Clients

When assessing an older school-age or adult client who has the linguistic and cognitive abilities to participate in the interviewing process, it is important to conduct the information-getting interview with that client. Caregivers of adolescent clients would be interviewed for any information that the client could not supply. An interview with an adolescent or adult client may be conducted as follows.

Opening Phase of the Opening Interview

"Hello, my name is Linda Stevens. I'm the speech–language pathologist who will be testing your speech today. Another common name for a speech–language pathologist is speech therapist. You may be more familiar with the second term. I would like to begin by asking you some questions about your speech and other important related information. Some of the questions I will be asking may sound familiar from the questionnaire you already filled out. The information that you share with me today will help me get a clear picture of your communication or speech skills and your specific needs. If I ask a question that is not very clear, please don't hesitate to let me know and I will try to make it clearer. When we are finished with this part, we will begin the actual testing. The entire testing should take about three sessions (assuming the sessions are 30–40 minutes in length). When I'm done with the testing, I will discuss my findings and recommendations with you. Do you have any questions before I begin to ask you questions?"

Body of the Opening Interview

"Now I'm going to ask you several questions about your speech. Please remember that all of the questions I'm asking are going to help me to determine whether a problem exists, and if it does, whether treatment is appropriate. O.K. let's begin."

The questions that follow were selected because they are typical for an adult client with a suspected articulation problem. This list is not meant to be all-inclusive and may be altered as necessary. Again, it is provided primarily for first-time student clinicians who may need more guidance in conducting an information-getting interview.

- Please describe your concerns about your speech.

- When did the problem begin?

- How did it begin? Gradually? Suddenly?

- To what do you attribute your speech problem?

- Is English your first language? Is it your only language?

- Are there any specific sounds that you know are difficult for you to pronounce?

- How well do your family members understand you?

- How well would you think a stranger would understand your speech?

- Do people ever ask you to repeat yourself? How often?

- Has the problem changed since you first noticed it? Gotten better? Gotten worse?

- Is the problem consistent or does it vary? Are there certain circumstances that create fluctuations or variations?

- How do you react or respond to the problem? Does it bother you? What do you do to make it better?

- Does your speech affect your interactions with others at home, school, work, and so forth?

- Do you believe that your speech has gotten in the way of certain activities?

- Where else have you been seen for the problem? What was suggested? Did it help?

- What other specialists (physicians, teachers, hearing aid dispensers, etc.) have you seen?

- Why did you decide to come in for an evaluation? What do you hope will result?

- Is there anything we have not discussed that you think will help me understand your problem better?

Closing Phase of the Opening Interview

"Thank you so much for all of your information. It will help me in making appropriate recommendations. Now we can go ahead and begin the actual testing. When we are finished with the testing, I will share the results and talk about my recommendations. Do you have any questions?"

Performing an Orofacial Examination

Examination of the orofacial structures is an extremely important component of the assessment process in clients with articulation or phonological disorders. As reviewed in Chapter 4, research has shown that some articulation disorders may be directly related to abnormal structure and function of the orofacial complex. For example, clients with a severe open bite may also present a frontal lisp, and clients with a repaired cleft palate may have **hypernasal** speech. Therefore, when assessing children with an articulation and phonological problem, it is clinically wise to perform a thorough examination of the speech structures. The clinician should determine if the static and dynamic articulators are adequate for speech production. The orofacial examination helps the clinician determine if an articulation or phonological disorder is **functional** or **organic** in nature. An organic disorder is one for which some underlying structural, sensory, or neurological cause can be identified. The articulation problems associated with cleft palate would be an example of an **organic articulation disorder. Functional disorders,** also known as **idiopathic disorders,** are those articulation or phonological disorders for which a cause could not be determined.

Tools and Procedures

Because of the extreme darkness of the oral cavity, the clinician needs a source of illumination such as a small flashlight or penlight. The clinician should always use a glove or finger cot for health and safety reasons for both the client and the examiner. Applicator sticks and tongue blades can be used to flatten the tongue or to probe certain oral structures. It is essential to use individually wrapped applicator sticks and tongue depressors for sanitary purposes. Cotton gauze pads can be used to hold on to the client's tongue if necessary. Additional tools used during an orofacial examination are a small mirror and a stopwatch for **diadochokinetic testing** (to be discussed a bit later in this section).

The clinician should try to make the orofacial examination as pleasant as possible for a client. Some companies such as Super Duper Publications and Speech Dynamics design and market orofacial examination tools with this in mind (e.g., flavored tongue depressors and powder-free examination gloves). Many children are much more compliant if testing of their orofacial structures is done in the context of a game. For example, the clinician and the client can pretend to play "doctor." Children often like to take on the role of the doctor, and they will be much more inclined to let the clinician examine their mouths after they have had an opportunity to examine the clinician's mouth.

Specific Assessments

Structure and Function of the Facial Muscles

Through cursory inspection, the clinician can assess the client's facial expression, size and shape of the head, and overall symmetry of the head and facial structures. Examination of the face is important since it can reveal information about muscle weakness, paresis, and other possible neurological problems of the facial musculature. Also, some genetic disorders have associated facial characteristics that can be identified upon visual inspection.

An assessment of the facial structures can start prior to the actual orofacial examination. The clinician can easily observe the client's face during the opening interview. More direct assessment of the face can be done while at rest and by having the client perform certain movements.

General Symmetry of the Face at Rest:

- Is there drooping at the corner of the mouth?
- Is an eyelid partially or completely closed?

- Is the mandible, or jaw, drooping on one side?

- Are there any abnormal movements (e.g., facial grimaces, spasms, twitching, and so forth)?

- Are there any signs of mouth breathing or drooling?

Symmetry of Face While Making Specific Movements:

- Ask the client to smile. Does the corner of the mouth deviate to one side?

- Ask the client to open the mouth wide. Does the jaw deviate to one side?

- Ask the client to raise both eyebrows. Do the eyebrows rise evenly?

- Ask the client to close the eyes tightly. Do both eyes close evenly?

Structure and Function of the Lips

The lips are important movable articulators for the production of some speech sounds. They are responsible for (a) impounding air for the plosives /b/ and /p/; (b) restricting airflow for the fricatives /f/ and /v/; and (c) shaping the oral cavity for the bilabial consonants and various vowels. Through an adequate labial seal, the intraoral pressure necessary for the production of stops, fricatives, and affricates (**pressure consonants**) can be accomplished.

An assessment of the lips can also start before the actual orofacial examination. The clinician can observe the integrity of the lips while interacting with the client during the opening interview. The lips may be directly examined at rest and by having the client perform certain movements.

Structural Integrity of the Lips:

- Is there drooping at the corner of the mouth?

- Is there an adequate amount of tissue in the lips?

- Do the lips remain closed or apart while at rest?

- Are there any signs of mouth breathing or drooling?

- Does the lip tissue appear healthy?

- Is there any evidence of a repaired cleft lip or other scar tissue?

Functional Integrity of the Lips:

- Ask the client to smile. Does the corner of the mouth deviate to one side?

- Ask the client to pucker. Does the amount of lip puckering favor one side?

- Ask the client to alternate between a pucker and a smile. Does the speech and **range of motion** appear adequate?

- Ask the client to lower and retract the lower lip to approximate the upper lip. Does the range of motion appear adequate?

• Ask the client to puff the cheeks and hold air. Can the client maintain the air in the mouth to at least the count of 5? Is any nasal emission perceived or evident when a mirror is placed under the **nares**?

• Ask the client to say "ooo-eee-ooo-eee" in alternate fashion. Does the range of motion and strength of the lips seem appropriate?

• Ask the client to repeat "pa-pa-pa-pa." Does the range of motion, strength, and lip seal seem appropriate?

Structure and Function of the Tongue

For obvious reasons, the tongue is one of the most important movable articulators. Through its various movements, it helps shape specific consonant sounds by obstructing or channeling the traveling airstream. Subtle movements of the tongue also help create the many vowels of the English language. In addition, the anterior to posterior carriage of the tongue aids in modifying the resonance quality of speech.

Both the structure and the function of the tongue should be evaluated during the orofacial examination. The tongue may be directly examined at rest and by having the client perform specific movements. Ask the patient to open his or her mouth wide. While the mouth is open, shine a penlight or other light source into the oral cavity and assess the size, shape, and condition of the tongue.

Structural Integrity of the Tongue:

• Does the coloration of the tongue appear normal?

• Does the size of the tongue appear appropriate in relation to the client's oral cavity?

• Are there any signs of **atrophy**?

• Are there any abnormal movements such as spasms, **fasciculations,** writhing, twitches, and so forth?

Functional Integrity of the Tongue:

• Ask the client to protrude the tongue as far as possible. Can the client perform that activity without effort? Does the speed and range of motion associated with this movement appear appropriate? Does the tongue deviate to one side upon protrusion?

• Ask the client to maintain the tongue in protruded position to at least the count of 5? Can the client do this without having to rest the tongue on the lower lip? Does the tongue rest or hang over the lower lip?

• Ask the client to protrude his or her tongue and keep it in that position while you apply some pressure on the tip and sides with a tongue blade. As you apply pressure on the tip of the tongue, the left side, and then the right side, instruct the client to resist or "fight" the pressure. Does the strength of the tongue appear appropriate for this activity?

- While the tongue is in a protruded position, ask the client to move the tongue tip up and down, to the right, and then to the left. Ask the client to move the tongue from side to side as quickly as possible. Is the range of motion and excursion appropriate? Are there any signs of **groping,** uncoordinated movements, or weakness?

- Ask the client to retract the tongue. Does the speed and range of motion associated with that movement appear adequate?

- Ask the client to open the mouth and lift the tongue so that the lingual **frenulum** can be observed. Is there any sign of **ankyloglossia** (tongue-tie)?

- Ask the client to repeat "la-la-la-la." Does the range of motion, strength, and excursion of the tongue seem appropriate?

- Ask the client to repeat "ka-ka-ka-ka." Does the range of motion, strength, and excursion of the tongue seem appropriate?

- Ask the client to repeat "ka-la-ka-la." Can the client move the tongue from a posterior to anterior position without difficulty to produce the alternating syllables?

Structure of the Hard Palate

The hard palate, along with the soft palate, divides the nasal and oral cavities. It serves as a point of constriction for various sounds, including /r/, /j/, /ʃ/, /ʒ/, /tʃ/, and /dʒ/. The clinician can ask the patient to open his or her mouth wide. Since the hard palate is static, the clinician's goal is to assess its structural integrity. While the mouth is open, a penlight or other light source can be directed into the oral cavity. The size, shape, contour, and condition of the hard palate should be observed.

Structural Integrity of the Hard Palate:

- Does coloration of the hard palate appear normal along its midline?

- Does the height and width of the hard palate vault appear normal? It is important to keep in mind that the shape of the hard palate varies from one person to another. Consider the width and height in respect to sound production. Does there appear to be enough space for appropriate contact of the tongue against the hard palate?

- Are there any signs of repaired or unrepaired clefts, **fistulas,** or **fissures**?

- Are there any signs of surgical removal of any portion of the hard palate?

- Are there any **prostheses** (e.g., dentures, obturators, or palatal lifts) present?

Soft Palate Structure and Function

Because the soft palate is a dynamic articulator, it should be examined according to its structure and function. The velum is the point of articulation for the back sounds /k/, /g/, and /ŋ/. Through its dynamic function, it contributes to velopharyngeal closure for adequate oral resonance and to velopharyngeal opening for nasal resonance. Through its valving action, the velum is extremely important for the buildup of intraoral pressure for stops, fricatives, and affricates. Weakness, paralysis, or structural problems related to clefts, fistulas, or surgery may lead to **velopharyngeal incompetence** or **velopharyngeal insufficiency.**

It is important that the clinician assess the velum while the client's head is level and centered since that is its typical position during normal talking (Hall, 1994). Inspection of the velum while the head is tilted back or to one side may distort the relationship of the various structures in the mouth. The client's mouth should be level with the clinician's eyes. The client should be instructed to open his or her mouth about three-quarters of the maximum opening and to flatten rather than protrude the tongue while the clinician shines a penlight or other light source into the oral cavity. This will help in observing the natural movements of the velum and other related structures.

Structural Integrity of the Soft Palate:

• Does coloration of the soft palate appear normal along its midline? The normal coloration is white and pink.

• Is the **uvula,** the posterior-most portion of the velum, normal or bifid? A **bifid uvula** may indicate a possible submucosal cleft, especially if a bluish midline tint is also observed.

• Are there any signs of repaired or unrepaired clefts, fistulas, or fissures?

• Are there any signs of surgical removal of any portion of the soft palate?

• Are there any prostheses (e.g., dentures, obturators, or palatal lifts) present?

• Does the velum appear symmetrical? Asymmetry may indicate muscle weakness or paralysis.

• Does the length of the velum appear sufficient for adequate posterior movement in **velopharyngeal closure**? This is often an estimate on the part of the clinician since ultimately it is the patient's connected speech productions that help determine if velopharyngeal closure is indeed appropriate.

Functional Integrity of the Soft Palate:

• Does the client's speech sound normal, **hypernasal,** or **hyponasal** during conversational speech? Are the pressure consonants produced correctly? Are there any unusual substitutions such as **pharyngeal fricatives** and glottal stops for pressure consonants?

• Ask the client to produce isolated sounds, syllables, or words loaded with nonnasal consonants. Place a small mirror under the client's nostrils as the client produces the nonnasal consonants. Clouding or fogging of the mirror may indicate **hypernasality** or **nasal emission.** It is important to instruct the patient not to exhale as the sounds or words are produced, to rule out normal exhalation as the cause for the mirror fogging.

• Ask the client to produce a prolonged /a/. Does the velum move up and back to meet the pharyngeal wall? A sterile depressor may be used to hold down the tongue if the oropharynx is not visible.

• Ask the client to make repeated productions of /a/. Does the velum move up and back to meet the pharyngeal wall?

Teeth and Other Related Structures

As reviewed in the Basic Unit of Chapter 1, the teeth are important static structures that serve as a point of articulation for the tongue in the production of four English sounds: /f/, /v/, /θ/, and /ð/. The teeth also play an important role in the production of /s/, /z/, /ʃ/, and /ʒ/ in that the airstream necessary for those sounds is directed over the upper incisors. In the Basic Unit of Chapter 4, we also reviewed the potential speech problems that may result from missing or malpositioned teeth or **malocclusion** of the upper and lower dental arches.

Although, as stated in Chapter 4, the relationship of dental occlusion and missing teeth to articulatory errors generally is not impressive, the clinician should routinely examine a client's teeth to rule out abnormal dentition or malocclusion as a potential causative factor.

Integrity of the Teeth and Dental Arches:

• Ask the client to open the mouth. Are there any teeth missing? Are the teeth jumbled, tilted, or malpositioned? Are there full or partial dentures in place? The following terms may apply to the relative position or integrity of individual teeth in the upper or lower dental arches (Hall, 1994):

  • *labioversion*—a tooth that tilts outward toward the lip
  • *buccoversion*—a tooth that tilts outward toward the cheek
  • *linguaversion*—a tooth that tilts inward toward the tongue
  • *edentulous space(s)*—a missing tooth or missing teeth
  • *supernumerary or extraneous teeth*—too many teeth

• Ask the client to bite down gently and separate the lips so that the teeth can be observed. The clinician may have to use a tongue blade to lift and pull the lips to observe the client's occlusal relationship.

• What is the molar occlusal relationship? From a lateral view, the first molars should be in contact with each other. The relationship of the upper and lower dental arches is assessed in reference to the first molars. Refer to Figure 4.1 for normal and abnormal occlusal relationships of the teeth and upper and lower jaws.

  • *Normal occlusion.* The lower first molar is approximately half a tooth ahead of the upper first molar. Very few individuals have a normal occlusion (Hall, 1994).
  • *Neutrocclusion* (Angle's Class I malocclusion). The upper and lower dental arches are in normal occlusion; however, individual teeth are misaligned, rotated, or jumbled.
  • *Distocclusion* (Angle's Class II malocclusion). The lower dental arch (mandible) is too far back in relation to the upper dental arch (maxilla). This typically can be observed when the mouth is closed; the person has a receding chin.
  • *Mesiocclusion* (Angle's Class III malocclusion). The lower dental arch (mandible) is too far forward in relation to the upper dental arch (maxilla). This can also be observed when the mouth is closed. In this case, the person has a protruding chin.

• What is the occlusal relationship of the teeth? The relationship of the upper and lower front teeth is observed (incisors, cuspids, and bicuspids). This should be done from a frontal view.

- *Open bite*—a lack of contact between the upper and lower front teeth. The upper front teeth fail to make contact with the lower front teeth despite normal occlusion of the first molars. A central space is created.

- *Overjet*—excessive horizontal distance between the surfaces of the incisors. A normal distance of 1–3 mm of the upper central incisors in relation to the lower central incisors can be expected.

- *Closebite*—excessive vertical overlapping of the upper front teeth over the lower front teeth. The upper teeth cover more than the usual half to one-third of the lower teeth. Occlusion of the molars is normal.

- *Crossbite*—lateral overlapping of the upper and lower dental arches. The lower jaw is either to the right or to the left of a normal, central position in relation to the upper jaw.

- Judge the general condition of the teeth (e.g., hygiene, cavities, breaks, and so forth).

Diadochokinetic Syllable Rates

Diadochokinetic syllable rates, also known as **alternating motion rates (AMRs)** and **sequential motion rates (SMRs),** refer to the speed and regularity with which a person produces repetitive articulatory movements (Hegde, 1996a). Such measurements help assess the functional and structural integrity of the lips, jaw, and tongue through rapid repetitions of syllables. Alternating motion rates are measured through successive repetition of the same syllable (e.g., /pʌ-pʌ-pʌ/, /tʌ-tʌ-tʌ/, /kʌ-kʌ-kʌ/). Sequential motion rates assess rapid movement from one articulatory posture to another by the repetition of different syllables (e.g., /pʌtəkə-pʌtəkə-pʌtəkə/).

During diadochokinetic testing, the client's speech mechanism is overworked, since in natural speech people rarely use their most rapid rate of speech (Hall, 1994). (This statement obviously would exclude people who work as public or private auctioneers since their job depends on the use of a very rapid, yet regular rate of speech.) Shipley and McAfee (1998) describe two methods that are often used to measure a client's diadochokinetic syllable rates:

- The client is asked to rapidly repeat a selected syllable. The clinician then counts the *number of syllable repetitions* the client produces within a predetermined number of seconds (typically 5 seconds).

- The client is asked to rapidly repeat a selected syllable. The clinician then counts the *number of seconds* it takes the client to repeat a predetermined number of syllables (typically 20 repetitions).

Fletcher (1972, 1978) offers some norms for the production of syllable rates by children. His study included a total of 384 children from 6 to 13 years of age. Each of the age groups included 24 boys and 24 girls. The children were asked to repeat /pʌ/, /tʌ/, /kʌ/, and /pʌtəkə/ as rapidly and accurately as possible while the number of seconds required for 20 repetitions was recorded. We emphasize that Fletcher's data should be viewed with caution since the number of children included in the sample was rather small, statistically speaking. The following results were obtained:

Age	Average Number of Seconds								
	20 reps					**15 reps**			**10 reps**
	pʌ	tʌ	kʌ	fʌ	lʌ	pʌtə	pʌkə	tʌtə	pʌtəkə
6	4.8	4.9	5.5	5.5	5.2	7.3	7.9	7.8	10.3
7	4.8	4.9	5.3	5.4	5.3	7.6	8.0	8.0	10.0
8	4.2	4.4	4.8	4.9	4.6	6.2	7.1	7.2	8.3
9	4.0	4.1	4.6	4.6	4.5	5.9	6.6	6.6	7.7
10	3.7	3.8	4.3	4.2	4.2	5.5	6.4	6.4	7.1
11	3.6	3.6	4.0	4.0	3.8	4.8	5.8	5.8	6.5
12	3.4	3.5	3.9	3.7	3.7	4.7	5.7	5.5	6.4
13	3.3	3.3	3.7	3.6	3.5	4.2	5.1	5.1	5.7

As Fletcher's data show, children's diadochokinetic syllable rates seem to increase with age. Such increase is likely related to a child's gradual neurological and physiological development as he or she grows older. Other sources have indicated that approximately 5 to 7 repetitions per second for AMRs and 2.6 to 7.5 repetitions per second for SMRs can be expected in normal adults (Hegde, 1996a).

Diadochokinetic rates are most clinically significant in the assessment of motor speech disorders, including **apraxia of speech, dysarthria, developmental apraxia of speech,** and other articulation disorders due to poor oral motor movements. Adults with apraxia of speech and children with developmental apraxia of speech may display significant breakdown in appropriate sequencing of syllables. Adults or children with dysarthria may show irregular, slow, labored, or accelerated syllable rates secondary to muscle weakness, paralysis, or incoordination. These disorders will be discussed further in the Advanced Unit of this chapter.

The following procedures can be used to measure a client's diadochokinetic rates, including alternating and sequential motion rates:

- *Instruct the patient:* "Please take a deep breath and say [pʌ-pʌ-pʌ] as long and as evenly as you can." Model the response for the client to imitate: "Try doing it like me. . . ." (AMRs)

- *Instruct the patient:* "Please take a deep breath and say [tʌ-tʌ-tʌ] as long and as evenly as you can." Model the response for the client to imitate: "Try doing it like me. . . ." (AMRs)

- *Instruct the patient:* "Please take a deep breath and say [kʌ-kʌ-kʌ] as long and as evenly as you can." Model the response for the client to imitate: "Try doing it like me. . . ." (AMRs)

- *Instruct the patient:* "Please take a deep breath and say [pʌtəkə-pʌtəkə-pʌtəkə] as long and as evenly as you can." Model the response for the client to imitate: "Try doing it like me. . . ." (SMRs)

For all of these, the client is allowed to continue for about 3 to 5 seconds or until a predetermined number of repetitions are recorded. The clinician then compares the response rates to normative data.

Appropriate Referrals

If anything of medical significance is observed during the orofacial examination it is important to refer the client to an appropriate professional. For example, the clinician may refer the client to an orthodontist if an occlusal or bite problem is judged to affect articulation. A referral to a pediatrician may be warranted if tonsilitis, or inflammation of the tonsils is suspected. If hyponasality or hypernasality is observed, a referral to an otolaryngologist is generally appropriate. The types of referrals that may arise from an orofacial examination are too many to review specifically. The implications of the results of the orofacial examination and diadochokinetic testing will be addressed in the analysis of assessment information portion of this Basic Unit.

Conducting a Hearing Screening

Although conducting a full **audiological evaluation** is within the scope of practice of only an audiologist, the speech–language pathologist may screen a client's hearing. The primary purpose of an **audiological screening** is to determine the client's auditory function and to identify a potential peripheral hearing loss that might be related to the client's communicative problem. As addressed in the Basic Unit of Chapter 4, hearing loss is a known etiological factor of articulation and phonological disorders.

Therefore, it is extremely important to gather some information about the client's hearing status during the assessment. We prefer to do a hearing screening before administering a group of tests that generally require adequate audition on the part of the client. This information helps us anticipate any modifications that will need to be made, such as altering the volume of our own voice to a level that facilitates the client's understanding of the tasks presented. Audiological screenings are commonly performed through pure-tone audiometry.

Pure-Tone Audiometry

When a pure-tone audiometer is used, the client's hearing is most often screened by presenting pure-tone stimuli at 500, 1,000, 2,000, and 4,000 Hz (**Hertz**) at a preset intensity level, usually 20 or 25 dB (**decibels**). Although the typical intensity level is 20 or 25 dB, it may be altered to compensate for the level of ambient noise in the testing environment. The frequencies tested are considered the most important for speech reception, and the intensity level is usually sufficient to compensate for excessive environmental noise. A more conservative criterion may be used with children by screening their hearing for 500, 1,000, 2,000, 4,000, and 8,000 Hz at 15 dB. This more stringent criterion may reduce the risk of missing a child with a mild hearing loss (Shipley & McAfee, 1998, p. 408).

Public Schools–Related Issues

Although it is within the scope of practice of the speech–language pathologist to screen the client's auditory function, hearing screenings in the public schools are commonly performed by the school nurse. Different states and school districts may have varying policies about what professional can and should perform audiological screenings. If the speech–language pathologist is not allowed to conduct screenings, it is important to develop a good working relationship with the school nurse so that all relevant information is exchanged when needed.

Appropriate Referrals

A client who fails the audiological screening or for whom a hearing loss is suspected should be referred to an audiologist for a complete audiological evaluation. It is important to inform parents that their child's failure of a hearing screening is not necessarily indicative of a hearing loss. The clinician should stress that a complete audiological evaluation is recommended to rule out the possibility of a hearing loss, which may have important diagnostic and treatment implications. For insurance coverage purposes in most states, an audiologist will likely need a physician referral before he or she can conduct a reimbursable assessment. A clinician should alert a client's parents that unless they plan to pay privately for the procedure, they should contact their child's physician for a referral. See Appendix E for a sample referral letter to an audiologist.

Administering Standardized Articulation and Phonological Tests

The assessment of articulation disorders typically involves the use of standardized testing measures commonly known as fixed-position or single-word articulation tests. Traditional articulation tests provide information about the client's productions in relation to the types of errors and the word positions in which the errors occur. More specifically, they describe the client's sound system according to substitutions, omissions, distortions, and additions in the initial, medial, and final positions of words. Single-word articulation tests generally sample consonants and consonant clusters. Although less common, some also test vowels and diphthongs.

There are many similarities shared by standardized articulation tests. However, there are also some important differences from one test to another. Therefore, a clinician unfamiliar with a particular test should devote some time to reviewing the administrative procedures. Most commercially available tests provide norm-based guidelines that can be used to diagnose the presence of an articulation disorder and its severity.

More recently, several formal tests have been developed to assess children's use of phonological processes. These tests are intended to meet the diagnostic needs of children who present with multiple misarticulations and are highly unintelligible. They differ from traditional articulation tests in that they focus on the patterned misarticulations across words rather than individual phonemes in specific word positions. The assumption behind these tests is that some children may not have problems with the motor aspect of sound production but may demonstrate difficulties with the underlying sound system or phonological rules. Therefore, the use of assessment batteries that test for the presence of phonological processes may provide a clearer understanding of the child's phonological system. This may, in turn, help in the development of a more efficacious treatment program for the client.

Evoking Procedures

Most articulation and phonological tests are designed to be relatively quick measures. The client is typically shown a card and instructed to name the pictured object. Commercially available instruments frequently provide the examiner with additional prompts to evoke the target response if the client is unable to name the picture upon visual confrontation. If the child is unable to name the picture with the use of alternative prompts, most standardized tests allow the examiner to model the production for the client to imitate. The use of modeling should be recorded for later analysis.

Controversy exists about whether asking the child to repeat the examiner's production changes the testing results. Some researchers have documented that responses obtained by having the child name the picture will be more representative of his or her typical responses than will utterances obtained through imitation (Carter & Buck, 1958; Kresheck & Socolofsky, 1972; Siegel, Winitz, & Conkey, 1963; Smith & Ainsworth, 1967; Snow & Milisen, 1954). However, other research has failed to report a significant difference between picture naming and imitation productions (Paynter & Bumpas, 1977; Templin, 1947). To counteract the possible effects of imitation, some suggest the use of delayed imitation (Hegde, 1996a; Newman & Creaghead, 1989). With **delayed imitation,** the clinician casually names the picture and then moves on to the next stimulus word. After a few minutes the picture is presented again in hopes that the client can now name it without the need for **immediate imitation cues.** Despite varying thoughts on the use of imitation, the examiner using a standardized testing instrument must follow formal testing procedures. If the test allows for imitation, then the examiner should feel comfortable using that prompting technique. However, if the use of imitation invalidates the test results, the examiner should avoid the use of imitation and record the client's responses according to the test manual instructions. The clinician should be careful to document any divergence from the standardized procedures.

Response Recording

As the child produces the target responses, the clinician must record the productions on the recording form or protocol provided by the particular test. The recording method used may vary across examiners. According to Bankson and Bernthal (1998), "The recording systems used by clinicians may vary according to the purpose of testing, the transcription skills of the examiner, and personal preferences" (p. 238). Three methods of recording responses are as follows: (a) the correct/incorrect system, (b) the type-of-error method, and (c) the whole-word phonetic transcription method. These are listed from the method that yields the least amount of information to the method that provides a maximum amount of information.

Correct/Incorrect Method

The most simplistic method of response recording is the correct/incorrect or $(+/-)$ system. Using this system, a response is judged as either correct or incorrect based on the examiner's perception of the accuracy of the sound production. This type of recording method does not yield much clinically relevant information; it simply identifies the sounds that are articulated correctly or misarticulated by the client.

It does not identify the types of errors and does not allow for a pattern analysis of the client's production. This method is most appropriate for screenings rather than lengthy assessments.

Types of Errors

In the second method of response recording, errors are identified as omissions, distortions, substitutions, or additions in the initial, medial, and final positions of words. This method is one of the most commonly used by clinicians. A correct production of the target sound is typically indicated by using a plus mark or by leaving the item blank. Newman and Creaghead (1989) suggest that if the response is correct, that should be noted by leaving the item blank to prevent possible misinterpretation of marks during later analysis.

Sound **distortions** may be noted by recording a capital *D* on the recording form, indicating that the sound was distorted. However, when used alone, this symbol does not address the severity of the distortion. To indicate the severity of the distortion, a rating system may be used. Milisen (1954) used a rating of 3 when the distorted production was interpreted to be so severe that it would attract the attention of most listeners. The severe distortion would also make it difficult to recognize the sound. A rating of 2 was used to note a mild distortion of a sound (distorted to a degree that it would attract the attention of many laypeople but would not be difficult to recognize). Milisen gave a rating of 1 to the normal production of sounds. Another rating system that may be used to denote the level of distortion is as follows: D_1 (mild distortion), D_2 (moderate distortion), and D_3 (severe distortion) (Pendergast, Dickey, Selmar, & Soder, 1969). The clinician can also use **narrow phonetic transcription** to record the type of distortion in addition to the level of distortion.

Sound **substitutions** are identified by phonetically transcribing the sound that was substituted for the target phoneme. For example, if the target sound is /k/ in the word *cup* and the child says [tʌp], then a /t/ is recorded. On forms that provide a space for response recording, it is necessary to transcribe only the sound substituted for the target phoneme. When a recording form is not used, a sound substitution is typically written as follows: $^t/_k$, $^p/_f$, or $^d/_g$, for example. The top symbol denotes the sound that was actually produced, while the bottom symbol indicates the target sound. In other words, $^t/_k$ indicates that a /t/ was produced in place of a /k/. It is not uncommon for the symbols to be inadvertently reversed. Care must be taken to avoid that.

Omissions are recorded with a minus sign (−) or a zero (0) in the appropriate space. A minus sign is preferred because it is easy to confuse a zero (0) with the /o/ or /θ/ phonetic symbol. Although less common, some children add sounds to the target words. For example, a child may say "gerin" for *green* or "stopa" for *stop*. **Additions** are best recorded by transcribing the client's entire production.

Most standardized articulation tests document the child's productions according to the type-of-error recording system. This method, although more specific than the correct/incorrect system, also has some limitations. These will be addressed under our discussion of whole-word phonetic transcription.

Whole-Word Phonetic Transcription

In whole-word phonetic transcription, the examiner phonetically records the client's entire production. The focus of transcription is not the production of a particular sound in a specific position, but the production of the whole word. All sounds in the word are considered. This method of transcription has many advantages, since some children may produce a target sound correctly but misarticulate another sound within the word. This error would not be depicted if the correct/incorrect or type-of-error systems were used.

To illustrate this point, let us consider that the word *cup* was used to evoke the production of /k/ in the initial position. If the child said "ku" for *cup,* the production would be marked *correct* if using either the correct/incorrect or the type-of-error recording system because the child produced the target sound /k/ correctly. However, if the entire word were considered, an error production would be identified. Even though the target sound was produced correctly, the nontarget /p/ was omitted in the final position. This error would be recognized only if the whole-word phonetic transcription recording system was used. This method of transcription is most appropriate for the identification of phonological processes or other patterned misarticulations. From this information, the child's errors can also be identified as substitutions, distortions, omissions, and additions across word positions.

Description of Commonly Administered Articulation Tests

The following sections will serve as a review of the most popular formal articulation tests that are commercially available. Again, these tests share many features, but some of the administration procedures do vary. Therefore, it is recommended that the examiner carefully review the standardized administration procedures prior to their administration.

Photo Articulation Test (PAT)

The *Photo Articulation Test–Revised* (Pendergast, Dickey, Selmar, & Soder, 1969) is made up of 72 colored photographs. Each of eight sheets contains 9 pictures. The last 3 pictures are designed to assess connected speech. Together the eight sheets of pictures test all consonants in initial, medial, and final positions, all vowels, and all diphthongs. The clinician explains to the client, "I am going to show you some pictures, and I want you to tell me what they are as I point to them." The test takes approximately 15–20 minutes to administer.

The client's responses are recorded as follows: if the sound is produced correctly, no mark is recorded; if a sound is omitted, a minus sign is recorded; if another sound is substituted, the phonetic symbol representing the substitution is recorded; and if the sound is distorted, the severity of the distortion is indicated as D_1 (mild), D_2 (moderate), or D_3 (severe), and the distortion is described under the "Comments" section.

The PAT also includes a deck of 72 individual photographs that can be used in three different ways. The test deck can be used when testing individuals with visual problems, or with subjects who would have difficulty with the presentation of more than one picture at a time. The individual cards can be used for **contextual testing.** For example, if the client erred on the /l/ sound in the initial position during articulation testing, the picture of "lamp" can be placed following the picture of "nails" to assess the influence of /n/ on the production of /l/. Furthermore, the test cards can be used in actual therapy to evoke sounds.

The PAT is designed to test the articulation proficiency of children 3 to 8 years old. Normative data are provided for that age population. The test was developed with 684 Caucasian children, and the reliability and validity scores were reported to be high. Although the test is designed for young children, it can be administered to adult clients. The use of actual photographs rather than line drawings makes it appealing for testing adult clients. One weakness of the PAT is that some of the photographs are dated and not apt to evoke the target response. For example, a picture of roller skates is used to evoke the /sk/ blend. Children today are more familiar with roller blades than roller skates.

A third edition of this popular test was released in 1997. The *Photo Articulation Test–3* (PAT–3) (Lippke, Dickey, Selmar, & Soder, 1997) is an updated version of the original test. The photographs are new and modernized. This edition was standardized on a larger number of children than the original version. Administration procedures are similar; however, the scoring method is less detailed. More interpretive information is provided in the third edition (i.e., age equivalents, percentiles, and standard scores). See Figure 6.1 for a copy of the PAT–3 recording form.

Fisher-Logemann Test of Articulation Competence

The *Fisher-Logemann Test of Articulation Competence* (Fisher & Logemann, 1971) was designed to provide a distinctive feature analysis of the client's phonologic system. The client's consonant productions are analyzed according to place of articulation, manner of articulation, and voicing. Vowel productions are assessed according to tongue height, place of articulation, degree of tension, and lip rounding. The test uses 109 colored picture stimuli displayed on 35 cards to evoke the target productions. Together they test 25 consonants, 23 consonant blends, 12 vowels, and 4 diphthongs.

The client is instructed to look at the pictures and name what is seen. The authors include some phrases for prompting if pictures are not readily identified. The following system is used to record the client's responses: if the client produces the target sound correctly, no entry is made; if the sound is omitted, a minus sign is marked; if another sound is substituted, the phonetic symbol reflecting the substitution is recorded; and if the sound is distorted, an allophonic transcription is made. For example, if /s/ is dentalized, it would be recorded as [s̪].

The Fisher-Logemann is somewhat unique in that it does not use the typical initial-, medial-, and final-position system to analyze sound productions. Rather, it analyzes the phoneme according to syllabic function in prevocalic, intervocalic, and postvocalic positions.

The authors do not provide validity and reliability measures in the manual. They simply state that all test therapists expressed favorable views on the general linguistic basis of the test, the organization of the record forms, and the instructions in the manual. The age range tested is from 3 years to adult. The test takes approximately 20 minutes to administer.

Goldman-Fristoe Test of Articulation (GFTA)

The *Goldman-Fristoe Test of Articulation* (Goldman & Fristoe, 1986) assesses a client's articulation of consonant sounds in initial, medial, and final positions and consonant blends. The test also evaluates connected speech on a limited basis by

			Consonants					Vowels/Dipthongs				
			Sound Production			Errors				Sound Production	Errors	
Age	Sound	Words	I	M	F	Tongue	Lips					Comments
3.5	p	pie[1], apples[2], cup[3]						aɪ	pie[1]			
	m	monkey[4], hammer[5], comb[6]						o	comb[6]			
	w	witch[7], flowers[8]						ɪ	witch[7]			
	h	hanger[9]										
	b	book[10], baby[11], bathtub[12]						ʊ	book[10]			
	d	dog[13], ladder[14], bed[15]						ɔ	dog[13]			
	n	nails[16], bananas[17], can[18]						ə	bananas[17]			
	j	yes, thank you										
4	k	cat[19], crackers[20], cake[21]						ɚ-ə	crackers[20]			
	g	gum[22], wagon[23], egg[24]						ʌ	gum[22]			
	t	table[25], potatoes[26], hat[27]						æ	hat[27]			
	f	fork[28], elephant[29], knife[30]										
5	ŋ	hanger[31], swing[32]										
	dʒ	jars[33], angels[34], orange[35]										
6	ʃ	shoe[36], station[37], fish[38]						u	shoe[36]			
	l	lamp[39], balloons[40], bell[41]						ɛ	bell[41]			
	ʒ	measure, beige										
	v	vacuum[42], TV[43], glove[44]						ju	vacuum[42]			
	tʃ	chair[45], matches[46], sandwich[47]										
7	s	saw[48], pencil[49], house[50]						aʊ	house[50]			
	s bl	spoon[51], skates[52], stars[53]										
	z	zipper[54], scissors[55], keys[56]										
	l bl	blocks[57], clock[58], flag[59]						ɑ	blocks[57]			
	ð	(this/that[60]), feathers[60], bathe										
	r bl	brush[61], crayons[62], train[63]						e	train[63]			
8	θ	thumb[64], toothbrush[65], teeth[66]						i	teeth[66]			
	r	radio[67], carrots[68], car[69]										
		[Story] [70–72] ___ voice quality ___ fluency						ɔɪ	boy[70]			
		___ language use ___ intelligibility of connected speech						ɝ-ɚ	bird[70]			
		Totals										Raw Score Total

key: (+) *no error;* (–) *omission, sound substitution, distortion;* (i) *imitated sounds*

Figure 6.1. The *Photo Articulation Test–3* Sample Recording Form. *Note.* From *Photo Articulation Test* (3rd ed.), by B. A. Lippke et al., 1997, Austin, TX: PRO-ED. Copyright 1997 by PRO-ED, Inc. Reprinted with permission.

having the client paraphrase two picture stories. Vowels and diphthongs are not tested. Forty-four single-item and large colored pictures on an easel serve as the test stimuli.

The target productions are evoked by instructing the client, "You are going to see some pictures here. I want you to tell me what you see as I turn the cards." The client's responses are recorded in the following manner: if the sound is produced correctly, the cell is left blank; if the sound is omitted, a minus sign is marked; if the sound is distorted, the number 2 is used to indicate a mild distortion or 3 to indicate a severe distortion; if another sound is substituted, the phonetic symbol depicting the substitution is used; and if a sound is added, the addition is indicated by writing the additional sound plus the correct sound. Approximately 20 minutes are required for complete administration of the test.

The GFTA also includes a stimulability assessment of each misarticulated phoneme in syllables, words, and sentences. This feature, along with testing connected speech, adds to the uniqueness of the test.

Templin-Darley Tests of Articulation

Unlike other articulation tests, the *Templin-Darley Tests of Articulation* (Templin & Darley, 1969) are actually a group of tests including the "Diagnostic Test (Picture and Sentence Forms)," "Screening Test," and "Iowa Pressure Test." The "Iowa Pressure Test" is specifically designed to test the adequacy of the velopharyngeal mechanism by testing the pressure consonants in clients with a significant history of cleft palate, dysarthria, or other disorder that may be accompanied with inadequate velopharyngeal closure.

The "Diagnostic Test" is designed to obtain a representative sample of the client's articulatory proficiency. It includes 57 semicolored cards containing several drawings on a single card. The picture stimuli elicit 141 speech sounds including consonant sounds, consonant blends, vowels, and diphthongs. Carrier phrases are provided on the back of each card to prompt the production of the target word. The *Templin-Darley* permits examiner modeling if the carrier phrases provided fail to evoke the target production or if the child is unfamiliar with the picture stimuli.

The authors suggest the following procedures for recording the client's productions: if the sound is produced correctly, a checkmark (✓) is used; if another sound is substituted, the phonetic symbol depicting the sound that is substituted is recorded; if the sound is omitted, a minus sign is marked; if the sound is distorted, an (x) is marked; and if nasal emission is perceived, it is indicated by (NE). Scoring and interpretation are performed by counting the number of correct productions and comparing them to established norms.

The test also calls for a rating of the client's intelligibility of contextual speech by the examiner according to: (a) readily intelligible, (b) intelligible if the listener knows the topic, (c) intelligible now and then, and (d) completely unintelligible. Errors noted in contextual speech but not identified on the articulation test are recorded in the corresponding section of the protocol sheet.

Test of Minimal Articulation Competence (T-MAC)

Secord developed the *Test of Minimal Articulation Competence* (T-MAC) in 1981. This test uses a picture confrontation format for the identification of articulation errors on: 24 consonant phonemes according to prevocalic, intervocalic, and postvocalic syllabic functions; frequently occurring /s/, /r/, and /l/ blends; 12 vowels; and 8 diphthongs consisting of 4 phonemic diphthongs and 4 **centering diphthong** variations of /ɚ/ (Secord, 1981c, p. 1). The test has a total of 107 illustrations that lead to a measure of 44 phonemes.

The T-MAC is a comprehensive evaluation that has many different components including the following:

- a picture test stimuli with a built-in easel;
- a reading version of the picture test for older children and adults;
- a sentence test to assess connected speech;
- a picture and reading screening test (described earlier); and
- a rapid screening test (described earlier).

The picture test stimuli are most appropriate for young children who cannot read, while the reading version can be administered to older children and adults. The reading version helps assess the client's production of the target sound in connected speech. The various versions of the test can be recorded and scored on the same record form.

The record form contains all of the test words corresponding to the picture stimuli. The tests words plus suggested phrases to prompt the target production are printed on the examiner's cards. Most of the pictures can be easily identified, while a few may require special prompting on the part of the examiner. For example, our own experience in administering this test has shown that children often have difficulty identifying the picture for the target words *dishes* and *toothache,* among a few others. Prompts such as "After you finish dinner, you wash the . . ." help facilitate production of the target production.

The client's articulation errors are recorded on the Test Record Form in the appropriate scoring boxes. The author suggests the traditional system for recording articulation errors according to types of errors. The following is specifically suggested:

- *Substitution.* Record the phoneme substituted for the target sound.
- *Distortion.* Record an X_1 for a mild to moderate distortion and an X_2 for a severe distortion. The X represents the target sound.
- *Omission.* Record a $(-)$.
- *Addition.* Record a $(+)$ and the added phoneme.

In addition to the test stimuli, the T-MAC provides the examiner with a list of words that can be used to assess speech sound **stimulability.** Secord (1981c) defines stimulability as the client's ability to correctly produce the previously misarticulated sounds upon maximum auditory and visual stimulation (p. 9). The T-MAC has an intricate scoring system that guides the clinician in diagnosing the severity of the disorder.

Commonly Administered Phonological Processes Tests

The following sections serve as a review of some of the most popular commercial tests that help evaluate the use of phonological processes by young children. Like the articulation tests, these tests share many features. However, because some of the administration procedures vary, it is recommended that they be carefully reviewed prior to their use.

Assessment of Phonological Processes–Revised (APP–R)

Hodson developed the *Assessment of Phonological Processes* (APP) in 1980 and revised the original version in 1986. *The Assessment of Phonological Processes–*

Revised (Hodson, 1986a) is unique among phonological tests in that it was not designed to identify phonological disabilities. Rather, its purpose is to identify priorities in the treatment of unintelligible children.

The APP–R uses objects, pictures, and body parts to elicit 50 target responses by having the client name the various materials as they are presented. Unfortunately, the objects are not supplied in the assessment measure. However, they are common household objects that can be easily collected by the examiner. Picture cards are included for things that are not collectible such as for the word *smoke.* The test is structured to score over 40 phonological processes. The client's transcribed production of the 50 stimulus words is scored for the presence of various processes listed in a matrix format. For ease in scoring, any sound changes that cannot occur on a particular target word are darkened on the boxed matrix across the word as a hint to the examiner that such errors should not be considered. For example, for the target word *page,* the "Omission of Consonant Sequences" box on the matrix is blacked out since this word does not contain consonant sequences (clusters) and thus such an error could not occur. The APP–R divides the phonological processes into six general categories: omissions, class deficiencies, phonemic substitutions, assimilations, voicing alterations, and place shifts. A box for Other Error Patterns/Preferences is also provided.

Analysis of the APP–R derives a Frequency of Occurrence Score, Percentage of Occurrence Score, Severity Rating, and Composite Deviancy Score. According to the information in the test manual, the APP–R can usually be administered in 20 minutes; however, an additional 30 minutes may be needed to analyze the information.

The *Assessment of Phonological Processes–Spanish* (AAP–S) (Hodson, 1986b) is available for Spanish-speaking children. The Computer Analysis of Phonological Processes: Version 1.0 (Hodson, 1985) is a computer version of *The Assessment of Phonological Processes–Revised.* The computerized format can help clinicians who have access to a computer speed up the analysis portion of the assessment.

Bankson-Bernthal Test of Phonology (BBTOP)

In 1990 Bankson and Bernthal developed the *Bankson-Bernthal Test of Phonology* (1990b). The test was designed to describe consonant productions and the use of phonological processes in preschool and early school-aged children. A picture-naming format is used to elicit 80 stimulus words designed to analyze the following phonological processes: assimilation, fronting, final-consonant deletion, weak-syllable deletion, gliding, cluster simplification, depalatalization, deaffrication, and vocalization. The stimulus words also provide opportunities for occurrence of all the consonants in the initial and final position of words with the exception of /ʒ/ and /ŋ/.

The client's word productions are recorded as follows: if the word is produced correctly, the number 1 is placed in the Word Correct Box; if the word is produced incorrectly, a zero (0) is placed in the Word Correct Box and the client's actual production is transcribed in the appropriate space; and if the word must be modeled for elicitation, the Modeled Box is checked and the appropriate score and transcription are recorded.

After the test is administered in its entirety, it is analyzed in various ways. The number of correct productions is determined, and the total is entered in the space provided in the recording sheet. The Consonant Inventory analyzes individual consonants according to word-initial and word-final position. The Phonological Processes Inventory helps the examiner determine the phonological processes used by the client. The protocol conveniently lists examples of incorrect productions commonly associated with individual processes in phonetic transcription. The examiner then compares his or her transcription with those provided in the Phonological Processes Inventory, circles any transcription that matches the client's production, counts the number of occurrences of each process, and records it at the bottom of the page in the space provided. If a process other than those provided occurs, it is transcribed and scored accordingly.

The BBTOP provides normative data for children between 3 and 6 years of age. Between 120 and 190 children were used as normative samples for each age group (3, 4, 5, and 6). Although the test is standardized for children between the ages of 3 and 6, it can also be administered to older school-age children with severe phonological or articulation problems.

The Khan-Lewis Phonological Analysis (KLPA)

The *Khan-Lewis Phonological Analysis* was developed by Khan and Lewis in 1986. It uses the 44 words from the *Goldman-Fristoe Test of Articulation* Sounds in Words subtest as testing stimuli. The KLPA was designed to identify the phonological processes that account for various types of errors by preschool children. These include 12 developmental, as well as 3 nondevelomental processes: deletion of final consonants, initial voicing, syllable reduction, palatal fronting, deaffrication, velar fronting, consonant harmony, stridency deletion, stopping of fricatives and affricates, cluster simplification, final devoicing, liquid simplification, deletion of initial consonants, glottal replacement, and backing of velars.

The picture stimuli of the *Goldman-Fristoe Test of Articulation* serve to evoke the sample for analysis. Rather than recording the client's productions according to omissions, substitutions, distortions, and additions, the clinician transcribes them in their entirety. The transcribed words are placed on the KLPA score form, where sound changes are scored on a multipaged protocol. The protocol lists common sound changes associated with phonological processes for the examiner's convenience. It provides the following measures: Developmental Phonological Processes Rating, Speech Simplification Rating, Percentile Rank, Age Equivalents, and a Composite Score. In combination with the GFTA, the *Khan-Lewis Phonological Analysis* makes possible a phonetic and phonological analysis of the client's articulatory system.

The KLPA was designed to assess the speech of children ages 2 through 5. However, the authors indicate that this analysis may also be used to identify specific phonological processes for remediation in children 6 years and older. The test was normed on 927 children between the ages of 2-0 and 5-11 at 41 sites in various cities. A total of 852 children were selected from the original 927 to develop the test's normative data. According to the authors, the sample represented the United States population with regard to sex, race or ethnic group, and geographic region.

Assessment Link Between Phonology and Articulation (ALPHA)

In 1986, Lowe developed the *Assessment Link Between Phonology and Articulation*. It gives the examiner the option of scoring the client's production using a traditional (omission, distortion, substitution) or a phonological processes format, or both. The test elicits 50 target words by using delayed sentence imitation along with black-and-white line drawings.

The client's productions are transcribed onto the test protocol using whole-word phonetic transcription. This method of transcription allows for a traditional analysis as well as a phonological analysis of the client's production. The transcribed productions are then scored for sound changes in word-initial and word-final positions. The words are also analyzed for the occurrence of phonological processes. Fifteen phonological processes are arranged in a scoring matrix located across from the transcriptions. Boxes are provided that can be checked for the occurrence of a process for each target word. Boxes for processes that are not likely, or impossible, to occur for a target word are shaded. The phonological processes examined by the ALPHA are: consonant deletion, syllable deletion, stridency deletion, stopping, fronting, backing, alveolarization, labialization, affrication, deaffrication, voicing changes, gliding, vowelization, cluster reduction, and cluster substitution.

The ALPHA was designed for administration to children 3 years of age and older. It is a normed test that was standardized with a total of 1,310 subjects, ages ranging from 3 years, 0 months, to 8 years, 11 months. The manual indicates that the population on which the test was normed was obtained from midwestern rural, suburban, and inner cities. The normed subjects came from residential areas that included professionals and physical laborers.

Phonological Process Analysis (PPA)

Weiner (1979) describes the *Phonological Process Analysis* as a speech sampling procedure especially useful in assessing the speech of highly unintelligible children. The test uses delayed imitation and sentence recall along with action picture presentation to elicit the target words both as single words and in the context of sentences. For example, in testing deletion of final consonants, the client is presented with an action picture and told, "Here is a hat. Uncle Fred is standing on his ____. What is Uncle Fred doing?"

The PPA analyzes various phonological processes and categorizes them according to syllable structure, harmony, and feature contrast processes:

Syllable Structure Processes

- deletion of final consonants
- cluster reduction
- weak-syllable deletion
- glottal replacement

Harmony Processes

- labial assimilation
- alveolar assimilation
- velar assimilation
- prevocalic voicing and final-consonant devoicing
- manner harmony
- syllable harmony

Feature Contrast Processes

- stopping
- affrication
- fronting
- gliding of fricatives

- gliding of liquids
- vocalization
- denasalization
- neutralization

The proportion of occurrence of the tested processes is determined along with the frequency of occurrence of nontest processes (times processes occurred when not specifically being tested). Also, the PPA has a Phonetic Inventory, which identifies which sounds were produced and which were not.

Natural Process Analysis (NPA)

The *Natural Process Analysis* was developed in 1980 by Shriberg and Kwiatkowski. This test is designed to analyze eight phonological processes: final-consonant deletion, velar fronting, stopping, palatal fronting, liquid simplification, regressive and progressive assimilation, cluster reduction, and unstressed-syllable deletion. These processes were selected for analysis because they were judged to be natural processes (meaning that they occur in the phonological system of normally developing children); occur frequently in preschool and school-aged children with delayed speech; and can be scored reliably by clinicians.

Continuous speech samples collected by the examiner serve as the information for analysis. The authors suggest several activities for collecting a representative speech sample, including: having the client describe activities on sequence story cards; asking the client to tell a story using pictures in books; prompting the client to talk about personal interests and experiences; having the client comment while playing with familiar and unfamiliar toys; asking the client to comment on the arrangement of some objects and figures; and having the client comment on a familiar story being viewed through a toy movie viewer. Care must be taken by the clinician to ensure that all speech sounds have an opportunity to occur during these speech-evoking activities.

The connected speech sample is tape-recorded live for later analysis. Between 80 and 100 different words from the sample are transcribed onto the NPA transcription sheet. The words are analyzed both phonetically and phonologically. Using a phonetic analysis, the client's inventory of sounds is assessed and compared to normative data. Also, the sounds that are produced correctly at least once, sounds that are produced somewhere, and sounds that are never produced are identified using the phonetic analysis.

The words are also coded for phonological processes using NPA Coding Sheets. The phonological processes being used, the stage of development the processes are in, and what phonetic contexts (if any) influence the occurrence of the process are determined. Five of the processes are marked to indicate their level of occurrence as follows: always occurs when the opportunity is there, sometimes occurs, or never occurs. The NPA is not normed, but the authors provide a detailed appendix on the acquisition of phonology for a comparative analysis.

Advantages and Disadvantages of Standardized Tests

Several advantages associated with formal tests make their use extremely attractive. Among one of the biggest advantages is the relatively short amount of time it takes for their complete administration. Assuming that the examiner is working with a cooperative client, a standard test can usually be completed in 15 to 25 minutes. For clinicians with a high client caseload, such as school practitioners, time is valuable, and test procedures that are too lengthy are simply not practical.

A second advantage of formal tests is that they provide a representative sample of most, if not all, English consonants and several phonological processes, depending on the nature of the test. Articulation tests are structured so that all English consonants are tested in the initial, medial, and final positions of single words. Phonological process exams are organized so that the majority of natural phonological processes are sampled. Most clinicians do not have time to collect the many stimulus items that would be needed to obtain a representative sample of sound productions and phonological processes if informal measures were used.

A third advantage of formal or standardized tests is that the examiner has knowledge of the intended production or the target form. With highly unintelligible children this is extremely important since the occurrence of specific error types or underlying phonological processes can be identified only when the target production is known. This allows for a comparison of the child's actual production and the target word form. In conversational speech there is a high probability that unintelligible productions cannot be analyzed for the presence of specific error types or phonological processes because the target production cannot be reliably identified.

Despite the many advantages of formal tests, there are also several limitations that need to be considered. Paradoxically, many of the factors that make these tests attractive also contribute to their weaknesses. Probably the biggest disadvantage of most standardized or formal tests is that they assess sound production in single words. However, most children and adults do not talk in isolated word units. Thus, this activity may not be representative of the client's productions in connected speech. Research has repeatedly shown that some children produce more errors in connected speech than in single words (Dubois & Bernthal, 1978; Faircloth & Faircloth, 1970; Healy & Madison, 1987; Johnson, Winney, & Pederson, 1980; Morrison & Shriberg, 1992).

Healy and Madison (1987), in particular, found (a) that connected speech samples revealed a significantly higher number of errors than single-word samples did; (b) that connected speech samples revealed a higher number of omissions, substitutions, and distortion errors than single-word samples did; and (c) that 35% of all errors in connected speech were produced differently at the single-word level (p. 134). Andrews and Fey (1986) reported a similar problem for the occurrence of phonological processes in single-word versus connected speech samples. They noted a higher incidence of phonological processes in connected speech for most of their subjects.

In our own clinical practice we have witnessed young children who do fairly well on standard articulation or phonological exams but show a significant phonological breakdown during conversational speech. This has particular implications for the diagnosis of a disorder, in that potential articulation and phonological disorders may go undiagnosed if formal tests are used exclusively.

Shipley and McAfee (1998) summarize other drawbacks of formal tests that should be considered:

• *These tests usually elicit phonemes in only one phonetic context within a preselected word.* Even if the client produces the sound correctly, there may be other contexts and words in which the client cannot produce the target sound correctly. Or, an error may be elicited that is not reflective of a general pattern in other contexts.

• *Some articulation tests examine only consonants* — yet accurately produced vowels are also important for well-developed speech.

• *These tests provide only an inventory of the sounds sampled.* They do not yield predictive information, such as whether a sound error might be outgrown.

• *The reliability of findings may be questionable with disorders that result in variable sound production.* For example, a key feature of apraxia is inconsistently produced sounds. Many patients with apraxia produce a sound or word correctly one time and incorrectly the next. With a variable disorder, the clinician who samples a given word once or only a few times may draw conclusions that are misleading (pp. 134–135).

Collecting a Connected Speech Sample

As stated earlier, because people do not talk in isolated speech units, the client's production of sounds during single-word tests may not be representative of his or her articulation and phonological proficiency during connected speech. Therefore, it is extremely important to supplement the information obtained from standardized articulation or phonological tests with a thorough sample of connected speech. This will help the clinician obtain a more valid picture of the client's phonological system (Dubois & Bernthal, 1978; Faircloth & Faircloth, 1970; Johnson, Winney, & Pederson, 1980; Newman & Creaghead, 1989; Morrison & Shriberg, 1992; Stoel-Gammon & Dunn, 1985).

The collection of extended speech samples provides the clinician with important data from which a thorough analysis can be performed. If an adequate and representative speech sample is collected, the clinician can perform the following types of analyses:

- a traditional analysis of sound productions to determine the occurrence of sound omissions, substitutions, distortions, and additions;

- a pattern analysis to determine the use of phonological processes or patterned misarticulations;

- a phonetic inventory analysis to determine the sounds that are part of the child's phonetic repertoire;

- a syllable structure analysis to determine the word shapes used by the child;

- a speech intelligibility analysis to determine the child's level of intelligibility during known and unknown contexts;

- a consistency analysis to determine the consistency or inconsistency with which sounds are produced in error.

These types of analyses will be discussed in detail in the analysis of assessment information section of this Basic Unit.

Obtaining Extended Speech Samples: Strategies To Use with Children

Gathering a connected speech sample that is representative of a child's typical productions is not an easy feat. The clinician is merely a stranger to the child, and more often than not the client may be hesitant to talk. Resistance is not always manifested by crying and storming out of the testing room; some children demonstrate their refusal by simply not talking to the examiner. In our experience, the latter can be even more frustrating for the clinician, especially for the inexperienced clinician. What do you do when a child refuses to talk?

When collecting a sample, try to imagine yourself as a 3-year-old who at such a young age has more than likely experienced significant failure with communication. Your mother or father has promised to take you to a "fun place" but instead carts you to an unfamiliar room where a perfect stranger welcomes you with a smile. In this room there are tongue depressors, flashlights, and swab sticks, as well as various toys. The place looks suspicious; you get the feeling that someone wants something from you. Then this unfamiliar person starts to ask you weird questions like "How was your trip here?" "Would you like to play with my toys?" "Can you tell me about your friends?" Oh, no. Suddenly you realize that he or she wants you to talk. You do the only thing that seems logical, the only thing that you have control over. You shut down and remain quiet.

The sampling process can be very intimidating for a young child. However, there are some things that clinicians can do to facilitate a child's interaction. Many times clinicians make simple mistakes without even realizing it. The following are some suggestions that can help structure the testing process so that a child is more willing to engage in conversation with the clinician (Lowe, 1994; Shriberg & Kent, 1995):

• Before the appointment for the conversational speech sample, interview the parents to determine the child's interests (e.g., favorite toys, TV shows, friends, foods, etc.).

• Once the child's interests have been determined, prepare the clinic room with toys and games that the child is familiar with and enjoys.

• Avoid playing 20 Questions as soon as the child enters the testing room. Instead, manipulate the environment so that the atmosphere is relaxed and unintimidating. Participate in parallel play with the child without any verbal interaction. Establish an opportunity for the child to initiate a conversation. For example, you may place one of the child's favorite toys so that it is visible but out of reach.

• As the child warms up to the activity, you may use toys and objects to evoke connected speech productions, or you may use objects that help evoke the production of specific speech sounds. Use a variety of materials and introduce different topics that will evoke a representative sample of word shapes, phonological processes, and phonemes. Because all English phonemes do not occur with the same level of frequency, it is extremely important to arrange situations that will evoke less frequently occurring sounds.

• If you are audiotaping, be casual about the presence of the tape recorder. Most children will accommodate to a tape recorder. Children who notice it may ask,

"What's that?" We have found that most children will be satisfied by a brief explanation such as "Oh, I'm recording your voice." Some children also enjoy hearing themselves on tape. At times, hearing their recorded speech motivates them to interact more.

• Remember to capitalize on the presence of the child's parents or siblings. If possible, record the child's speech with significant others. The child may be more willing to talk with a family member. Also, this allows you to compare the child's productions across different social situations.

The clinician will usually use toys, objects, books, and pictures to evoke connected speech productions from the child. Again, because some sounds occur with less frequency during spontaneous speech, specific objects that represent those sounds may be used to evoke their production. For example, a toy fish may be used to evoke *sh* in the final position of words.

Some experts recommend collecting at least 80–100 words for a representative sample (Ingram, 1981; Shriberg & Kwiatkowski, 1980), while others recommend a minimum of 200 words (Weiss, Gordon, & Lillywhite, 1987). Depending on the client's language abilities and willingness to talk, between 50 and 150 utterances usually are sufficient to obtain the recommended number of words (Stoel-Gammon & Dunn, 1985). This can usually be accomplished in 20 to 30 minutes, depending on the client's level of interaction. Ultimately, the clinician must decide the number of words and utterances needed for a representative sample of a particular client's articulation and phonological skills in connected speech.

Recording the Sample

It is extremely important to audiotape the connected speech sample for later analysis to increase the accuracy of the examiner's transcription. It is very difficult, if not impossible, to reliably transcribe continuous speech at the time of the assessment. It is especially difficult with highly unintelligible children who have multiple misarticulations. Care must also be taken to ensure a high-quality sample that can be accurately transcribed. This is critical when gathering a sample for the analysis of a client's articulation and phonological skills.

One of the most frustrating situations for a clinician is to gather what appeared to be a great sample only to find out that it is essentially useless because the quality of the tape does not permit a reliable analysis. Shriberg and Kent (1995) provide an excellent outline of several procedures that can be followed to maximize the quality of audiotape recordings. Their recommendations include the following:

• Use a high-quality audiotape recorder with an impedance-matched external microphone. It is strongly recommended that built-in microphones not be used because they do not provide the fidelity needed for phonetic transcription.

• Before collecting the sample, learn the basic features of the recorder.
   • Where does the power cord plug into the recorder?
   • Where does the remote microphone plug into the recorder?
   • How do you set the recording speed?

- What knobs or buttons control loudness of recording and/or playback?
- Does the recording mode require simultaneous depression of two buttons?
- How does the pause control work?
- How does the remote off/on switch on the microphone work?

- Use the manual volume control, not the automatic volume control. Automatic volume controls will distort beginnings and endings of speech and include unwanted background noise.

- Prior to taping, record the speaker's name and the complete date on the tape. It is also useful to record this information at the end of the tape when you have finished recording. Be sure to write this information clearly on the tape container and on the label.

- Place the microphone 6 to 8 inches from the speaker's lips. To avoid popping noises, angle the microphone to point at the speaker's nose rather than the mouth. Adjust the volume control so that the speaker's vowels cause the needle on the VU (volume unit) meter to peak just below the distortion area. The consonants should be sufficiently audible to discriminate subphonemic features, such as unaspirated and frictionalized stops. Be sure that your utterances can be heard easily upon playback, with the speaker's voice somewhat louder than yours (adapted from p. 374, Appendix E).

Allen (1984) also recommends that noise sources be avoided as much as possible because they frequently affect the quality of the recording. Noisemaker toys can be very attractive to the child, but they can wreak havoc during later analysis of the information. Soft toys and books and cloth-covered tabletops should be used instead. These will help mute excessive noise.

Another situation that can create problems for reliable data analysis is the erroneous faith that many clinicians have in their ability to remember what a child said during the sample. Clinicians often trust that they will remember the context of the child's utterances as the sample is being collected. However, it is not uncommon to listen to an audiotape at a later time only to find that an analysis cannot be made because the target productions are not known and cannot be deciphered. A simple way to avoid this situation is to **gloss** or restate the child's attempt into the tape. This will serve as a cue during transcription of the sample. When glossing the child's productions, the clinician should do so in a natural, conversational style. For example, if a child says, "Ant a," while pointing to a toy car, the clinician can gloss the production by saying, "Joey, did you say you wanted the toy car?" It is not necessary to gloss every word, only those that the clinician determines may be difficult to understand at a later date.

It is also important to realize that as useful as audiotaping is for analysis of a conversational speech sample, it does have some limitations. One such limitation is that audiotaping by definition records only auditory input. However, speech production is not solely an acoustic process. The listener may perceive some sounds as acoustically correct that were produced with motoric alterations. Those articulatory alterations would not be identified on the tape recording. Making special notations of such articulatory behaviors might counteract this problem. For example, lingual dentalization, lip rounding, unreleased stops, minor sound distortions, and other facial gestures accompanying speech production can be noted by the clinician.

Transcribing the Sample

After a conversational speech sample has been collected, the clinician must decide the phonetic detail with which it will be analyzed. Some children's productions may require a more thorough analysis than others, depending on their error patterns.

When recording sound substitutions, it is often sufficient to use **broad phonetic transcription.** For example, if a child says, "My gagi buy me a koy [my daddy buy me a toy]," the clinician can record the substitutions as g/d (initial and medial positions) and k/t (initial position). However, some children may use sounds that are not part of the English language, or they may distort certain sounds. Some misarticulations may be due to adaptation or assimilation errors. In such cases, it is more appropriate to use **narrow phonetic transcription** with diacritic markers or non-English sound symbols. Examples of narrow phonetic transcription include the following:

- [d̪ɑg/dɑg] (dentalized alveolar stop)
- [z̥u/zu] (devoiced alveolar fricative)
- [βɛri/bɛri] (bilabial fricative for bilabial stop substitution)
- [dɑɣi/dɑgi] (velar fricative for velar stop substitution)

The first two are examples of narrow phonetic transcription through the use of the diacritic marker [̪] indicating dentalization of [d], and [̥] indicating devoicing of [z]. The latter two represent substitutions of non-English sounds for English sounds—[ɣ/g and β/b]. Please refer to Table 2.2 for several diacritic markers and special symbols that can be used for narrow phonetic transcription.

Advantages and Disadvantages of Connected Speech Samples

Conversational speech samples are extremely important for a complete appraisal of a child's articulation and phonological skills. A sample can be used to perform various types of analyses including a phonological analysis and a phonetic inventory analysis. There are many advantages to collecting a continuous sample. However, there are also some disadvantages that should be highlighted.

Among the many advantages of connected speech samples is that they are more representative of the child's true phonological skills since they prompt children to communicate as they would in daily interactions. Most children do not communicate in single words (unless they are at the one-word stage in their linguistic development) as tested by many single-word tests. Connected speech samples that are adequately scripted also allow for multiple occurrences of various speech sounds, phonological processes, and syllable shapes, unlike most single-word tests. Furthermore, the child's phonetic inventory, consistency of errors, level of intelligibility and stimulability can be determined from a connected speech sample. Other variables affecting overall intelligibility, such as rate of speech, loudness, and utterance length, may come to light during this activity.

Some of the disadvantages associated with connected speech samples prevent their widespread use in various settings and by all clinicians. One of the biggest disadvantages is the time required to collect, transcribe, and analyze a connected speech sample. Many clinicians with a high caseload simply do not have the time to perform such a thorough analysis. Also, some children may be resistant to talk during the testing process despite the clinician's well-structured efforts, though allowing time to gain rapport with the client or using the client's family in the sampling process can help counteract this problem. Furthermore, a connected speech sample gathered from a child who is highly unintelligible is difficult to analyze because the adult model is not always known. Glossing the child's utterances and structuring the setting so that the target words are known may alleviate this problem to some extent.

Conducting Stimulability Testing

After a client's articulation and phonological skills have been thoroughly examined, clinicians may choose to test the level of stimulability for some or all of the incorrect sounds. **Stimulability** refers to the client's ability to make a correct or improved production of a misarticulated sound when given a model or additional stimulation by the examiner. Some standardized articulation tests such as the *Goldman-Fristoe Test of Articulation* and the *Test of Minimal Articulation Competence* offer a section for stimulability testing, while others do not. If using a formal test that does not include a stimulability section, the clinician can easily devise an informal assessment measure. See Appendix F for a list of words and sentences that can be used for stimulability testing of all English consonants.

If there are so many sounds produced in error that time does not permit stimulability testing with all of them, a clinician can limit testing to those sounds that are potential therapy targets. Stimulability testing can be done of sounds in isolation, or in syllables, words, or sentences. The client's performance during stimulability testing often dictates the most complex linguistic level that will be examined. The following steps can be used during this procedure:

1. The clinician instructs the client, "Joey, I want you to watch my mouth and listen to me closely. I want you to say exactly what I say. . . ."

2. The examiner then draws the client's attention to his or her mouth while providing an exaggerated model of the target sound.

3. After providing a model of the target sound in isolation, words, or sentences, the clinician instructs, "Joey, can you make the sound just like I made it? Please try it for me."

4. The examiner delivers some verbal praise or other type of reinforcer for the client's cooperative behavior and attempt at producing the sound. Verbal praise or other reinforcer is provided whether the sound was produced correctly or not. For example, "Joey, thank you for trying so hard. You did a very good job."

Although currently there is no standard for what type of stimulation should be provided during stimulability testing, most examiners minimally assess the client's improved production after the clinician's model. However, other types of stimulation can be used (e.g., visual cues, auditory cues, **kinesthetic** cues). The information obtained from stimulability testing is clinically significant in that it helps the clinician identify the kinds of cues and prompts that can be used in therapy to facilitate correct production of a sound. The following lists the various types of stimulation that can be used during stimulability testing. They are arranged from least to maximal level of stimulation.

• Model Only: "Joey, listen closely as I say the word c̲ow. Now you say c̲ow."

• Model + Visual Cue: While in front of a mirror, the clinician says, "Joey, look how the back of my tongue touches the roof of my mouth way in the back when I say the word c̲ow. You try putting your tongue back there when you say c̲ow. Joey, say c̲ow."

• Model + Tactile Placement Cue: The clinician assists the client's placement of the back of the tongue against the velum with a tongue depressor or other instrument and provides an auditory model. "Joey, when I say the word c̲ow, my tongue is way in the back when I make the *k* sound. Let me help you make that sound. . . ."

• Model + Any Combination of Cues: The clinician provides an auditory model plus a combination of visual, tactile, and phonetic placement cues.

The prognostic and therapeutic implications of stimulability testing will be discussed further in the analysis of assessment information portion of this Basic Unit.

Performing Contextual Testing

Another type of assessment that can be done with clients suspected of having an articulation or phonological disorder is contextual testing. **Contextual testing** is a special procedure that can help identify a facilitative phonetic context for correct production of a particular phoneme. A **facilitative phonetic context** is a surrounding sound or group of sounds that has a positive influence on the production of a misarticulated phoneme. As reviewed in the Basic Unit of Chapter 2, in connected speech, sounds have an articulatory influence on each other, and through contextual testing it is the clinician's goal to find a phonetic context that helps evoke correct production of the selected phoneme.

The concept of contextual testing is not new. Spriestersbach and Curtis (1951) found that many children who misarticulated /s/ and /r/ produced them correctly in a specific phonetic context (e.g., /s/ in the context of /sp/and /r/ in the context of /tr/). Van Riper and Irwin (1958) also suggested that certain phonetic environments facilitate the correct production of a phoneme. They indicated that there are **key words** in which a phoneme can be produced more effectively. They emphasized that if a key word is discovered, the clinician can make use of such a facilitative context to stabilize the client's production of a target sound once therapy is initiated.

Since then other researchers have substantiated the notion that sounds influence each other during connected speech (Curtis & Hardy, 1959; Gallagher & Shriner, 1975a, 1975b; Hoffman, Schuckers, & Ratusnik, 1977; Zehel, Shelton, Arndt, Wright, & Elbert, 1972). However, the idea that phonemes can be affected by sounds that precede or follow them within a word or an utterance is primarily attributed to Eugene McDonald. This is probably due to McDonald's development of his now classic test, the *Deep Test of Articulation* (McDonald, 1964).

Commercially Available Resources

Deep Test of Articulation

The *Deep Test of Articulation* (McDonald, 1964) examines the articulation of sounds in many different phonetic contexts. McDonald termed this type of assessment "deep testing" because each consonant is tested in approximately 40–60 different phonetic contexts in a syllable-arresting (terminates the syllable) or syllable-releasing (initiates the syllable) position. This test is often referred to as *McDonald's Deep Test* (MDT). It is not an articulation test per se because it does not examine phoneme production according to error types in initial-, medial-, and final-word positions. Rather, it is intended as a supplement to formal articulation tests or connected speech samples to more deeply examine error sounds previously identified.

Each of the stimulus items on the MDT has two **abutted** words. One of the words contains the target phoneme in either an arresting or a releasing position. The abutted words are said together as a single bisyllable unit (e.g., "hat-s̲un," "be̲d-thumb," and "co̲m̲b-moon"). The purpose of the MDT is to deep test each target sound to discover the phonetic contexts in which it can be produced correctly. The test includes a sentence and a screening form in addition to the picture form. The picture form is appropriate for young children and clients with reading skills below third grade. The sentence form may be administered to older children and adults who read at least at the third-grade level. The examiner must be very familiar with the test to secure its appropriate administration. Poor familiarity with the administration procedures typically leads to its faulty administration.

Clinical Probes of Articulation Consistency

Secord (1981a) developed another commercially available instrument for contextual testing. The *Clinical Probes of Articulation Consistency* (C-PAC) assess the production of phonemes in a variety of phonetic contexts including pre- and postvocalic positions. Through a variety of C-PAC probes, sounds are also assessed in initial, medial, and final clusters. The production of sounds in sentences and conversation (storytelling) is also examined. Individual probes are provided for each consonant and the vocalic /ɜ˞/. Approximately 100 responses are evoked for each sound when all of the different phonetic contexts are tested. The probes can be used to measure consistency of production and to identify phonetic contexts that can be used as starting points in therapy (Newman & Creaghead, 1989).

Informal Contextual Testing Procedures

In addition to commercially available resources, other procedures may be used for contextual testing. The clinician may carefully review a connected speech sample for contexts in which a target sound is produced correctly. This parallels Van Riper and Irwin's (1958) concept of **key words** described earlier. On occasion, facilitating contexts not apparent in single-word tests or abutted word pairs can be found in conversational speech (Bankson & Bernthal, 1998).

Speech Discrimination Testing

The relation of auditory or speech discrimination skills to articulation and phonological disorders was reviewed in the Basic Unit of Chapter 4. Studies have been conducted to determine if children could discriminate between the correct and incorrect productions of sounds they themselves misarticulated. Word pairs reflecting the child's error and the correct production have been used to determine if indeed the child can "perceive" or "discriminate" the difference between the target production and his or her error production. As reviewed in Chapter 4, a study by Locke (1980a) revealed that a high percentage of children could discriminate between the correct and incorrect productions of sounds they misarticulated when the examiner presented such productions. Eilers and Oller (1976) reported similar findings. Clinical experience with children who have articulation and phonological disorders supports the notion that they can often identify errors intentionally made by the clinician as errors that they make. We have frequently encountered children who attempt to correct the clinician when they are confronted with their own errors. For example, the first author can recall the following conversation with a young client:

CLIENT: "I have a pet **wabbit.**"

CLINICIAN: "Oh really, you have a pet **wabbit.**"

CLIENT: "No, I have a pet **waabbit.**" (The child was a bit louder and emphasized the target sound although still in error. She also seemed somewhat indignant that I would make such an error.)

CLINICIAN: "That sounds interesting, but I don't know what a **wabbit** is."

CLIENT: "You know . . . a **waabbit.** It hops." (At this point, the child provided me with a definition of rabbit, just in case I did not know what the word meant.)

CLINICIAN: "Oh, you mean a pet **rabbit.** I get it."

CLIENT: "Yeah, a pet **wabbit.**" (The client seemed relieved that I finally figured out what she was saying.)

In this example, the child clearly had the auditory discrimination abilities to identify correct and incorrect productions of the sound even though she could not articulate it correctly. This client's problem lay with the motor aspect of the sound.

On other occasions we have witnessed clients who clearly could not distinguish the difference between the error sound and the target sound. We have found this to be most pronounced in children and adults for whom English is a second language. As reviewed in Chapter 3, the ability to discriminate sound contrasts (e.g., /fa/ and /va/) that are nonnative decreases after the first year of life and continues to deteriorate into adulthood. Clients who have difficulty with auditory discrimination of their own error productions and target sounds often make such comments as "I can't tell the difference between what you said first and what you said second." Some children may say, "I can't tell when it's right or when it's wrong." In such instances, the clients' poor auditory discrimination between their own sound errors and the target sounds clearly has an impact on their production. This is contrasted from the above example in which the problem seemed to lie primarily with the motor aspect of the sound.

Although research studies have not substantiated poor auditory discrimination skills as a strong factor in articulation or phonological disorders, testing for it could be done if the clinician suspects that it may be a problem in a particular client. We recommend that such testing be done after the sound production errors have been clearly identified. The clinician can use minimal contrasting pairs to determine if the child can distinguish between his or her own error productions and the target productions. For example, if the client frequently substituted /i/ for /ɪ/, the clinician could design contrasting word pairs that would assess the discrimination between those two sounds (e.g., *bit–beet, mitt–meat, ship–sheep*).

If poor speech discrimination skills of specific sound contrasts are identified, we strongly recommend *against* the inclination to exclusively focus therapy on auditory discrimination training. As discussed in the Advanced Unit of Chapter 4, studies have documented that speech discrimination training alone does not lead to better production, while production training leads to changes in both production and discrimination (Williams & McReynolds, 1975; Shelton, Johnson, & Arndt, 1977). The reader is referred to Winitz (1989) for a thorough examination of auditory considerations in treatment.

Analyzing and Interpreting the Assessment Information

After the assessment has been completed, the clinician has a wealth of information that must be analyzed. For student clinicians, especially first-time clinicians, this is one of the most overwhelming aspects of the assessment and diagnostic process. We have often heard our own student clinicians make such comments as "What needs to be done with all of this information?" and "Where do I begin?"

Students often fail to realize that the diagnosis of an articulation or phonological disorder goes beyond the administration of tests and the collection of a speech sample, among other things. Data collection is only the first step in making a diagnosis and generating specific treatment recommendations. It is only through data analysis and interpretation that the clinician is able to answer such questions as:

- Does an articulation or phonological disorder exist?
- If a problem does exist, what is the nature of the problem?
- What is the severity of the disorder?
- What are the possible compounding or potentially related factors?
- Is treatment appropriate?
- What is the prognosis for improvement?

Analysis of Speech Sound Production

The sound segment information obtained during the assessment can be scored and analyzed in two ways: through an independent analysis or through a relational analysis (Stoel-Gammon & Dunn, 1985). In an **independent analysis,** the child's speech productions are described without reference to the adult model. Rather, the clinician examines the data according to the sounds that are part of the child's phonetic inventory according to their position of occurrence and their articulatory features. The clinician can also determine the syllable structures and word shapes that are within the child's repertoire and the operating **phonotactic** constraints.

In an independent analysis, the child's productions are not described in terms of errors. The clinician simply determines what the child can do. Although this type of analysis can be used with all clients, it is clinically most useful with very young children since their productions do not always parallel adult word forms. It can also be used with children who are so unintelligible that the adult target cannot be easily identified.

The second type of analysis is termed **relational analysis** because the clinician compares or relates the child's production to the adult target form within a specific linguistic community. By comparing the child's production with the standard or adult word form, the clinician can identify: (a) the types of errors according to substitutions, omissions, distortions, and additions in specific word positions; (b) any absent phonological rules or distinctive features; and (c) the operating phonological processes.

A *combination* of an independent and a relational analysis leads to a thorough examination of the assessment data. However, the extent to which the information is examined is highly dependent on the particular child's phonological skills. Through a relational analysis, the clinician can compare the child's production with the standard adult model and, thus, perform a traditional sound-by-sound analysis, a manner-place-voicing analysis (MPV), a distinctive feature analysis, and a phonological process analysis.

Traditional Analysis

Elbert and Gierut (1986) employed the term *traditional analysis* to describe one of the earliest methods of analyzing articulation and phonological information. This method of analysis considers two variables:

- the position in which the sounds are misarticulated (initial, medial, or final); and

- the type of errors made (omissions, distortions, additions, or substitutions).

This method is most appropriate for children with a few articulation errors and relatively good speech intelligibility. The nature of the problem tends to be phonetic (articulatory) rather than phonological.

On occasion, error patterns can be identified in the child's productions even with this most simplistic way of analyzing the data. For example, the clinician could identify that a child's articulation errors are primarily omissions in the initial position of words. Another child may demonstrate lateral distortions of all sibilants. Yet another child may display substitution errors that affect all or nearly all alveolar sounds. Most single-word articulation tests analyze the assessment information according to error types in initial-, medial-, and final-word positions (e.g., *Photo Articulation Test–3, Test of Minimal Articulation Competence, Goldman-Fristoe Test of Articulation*).

Although the term *traditional* is employed in reference to this method of analysis, clinicians today continue to examine the client's productions in this fashion. This may be the only information needed to clearly identify the extent of the articulation problems for some children. We often incorporate this method into our own clinical practicum. It is a relatively quick procedure that often yields practical information with children demonstrating only a few errors. A traditional analysis can also be used with children who have multiple misarticulations; however, it may not produce all the information needed for a clear understanding of the extent and nature of the articulation or phonological disorder. Refer to Appendix G for a form that can be used for a traditional analysis of single-word or connected speech productions.

Pattern Analysis

Through a **pattern analysis,** the clinician tries to identify any patterned or systematic modifications in a child's speech production errors. If regularities are observed, the clinician often categorizes them into descriptive rules or processes (e.g., final-consonant deletion, velar fronting, and so forth). A pattern analysis is most appropriate with children who have multiple misarticulations.

Place-Voicing-Manner Analysis. One of the most basic types of pattern analysis is the place-voicing-manner (PVM) method. This type of analysis considers a child's misarticulations in relation to the phonetic features of place, voicing, and manner. One of the single-word articulation tests previously described, the *Fisher-Logemann Test of Articulation Competence,* incorporates this type of analysis.

A place-voicing-manner analysis can help the clinician derive patterns in the sound production errors of some clients. Through this type of analysis the clinician may discover that a child frequently substitutes alveolar sounds for palatal and velar sounds, which is a problem with *place of articulation.* This error pattern would be stated as "The client frequently substitutes alveolar consonants for palatals and velars." A pattern that affects the *manner of production* may be observed in a client who substitutes fricatives for stops, or glides for liquids. Multiple substitutions of voiceless for voiced consonants would be described as an error pattern affecting the *voicing feature* of sounds. A PVM analysis may be performed from the information obtained in a single-word test or the connected speech sample. It is not a complicated type of analysis, and it can be done relatively quickly (Elbert & Gierut, 1986).

Clinicians often use the PVM analysis method in clinical practice. After identifying particular substitution patterns, the clinician may choose to teach one or many **exemplars** of the affected sound class. For example, if velars are frequently substituted by alveolars, the clinician may choose to teach one of the velar sounds within the class and then probe for generalized productions to the untaught sounds. Or, the clinician may choose to teach all velars /k/, /g/, /ŋ/ simultaneously. This topic will be discussed further in the Basic Unit of Chapter 7. Appendix H provides a worksheet that can be used to perform this type of pattern analysis.

Distinctive Feature Analysis. In the early 1970s the description of sounds according to their distinctive features became extremely popular. Recall that "distinctive features" refer to unique characteristics that distinguish one sound from all other sounds. Examples of these are the voice, nasal, posterior, anterior, and sonorant features. This theoretical notion quickly made its way to the assessment and treatment of articulation and phonological disorders.

Using this classification system, children's multiple misarticulations are grouped according to the presence or absence of particular features. For example, analyses of the assessment data may reveal that a child's phonological system lacks the posterior, strident, or sonorant feature, resulting in incorrect productions of sounds that require that feature. At other times, the clinician may note that a group of sounds that share a feature (e.g., sonorants, stridents, nasals) are consistently produced incorrectly or substituted for another class of sounds. If this approach is followed, the goal of therapy then becomes to teach the absent phonological features or the operating rules. Because of the complexity of this method of analysis and its questionable clinical relevance, it is not frequently used in the assessment or treatment of articulation and phonological disorders.

Phonological Process Analysis. One of the most current classification systems in the assessment of phonological disorders is the **phonological process analysis** approach. In this type of pattern analysis, the child's sound errors are classified according to operating phonological processes. As reviewed in Chapter 2, phonological processes are descriptive terms used to identify patterned misarticulations in children's speech. Such terms have been used to describe sound production errors in children with both normal and disordered phonological skills. This type of analysis is often used with highly unintelligible children who have multiple misarticulations.

In the Basic Unit of Chapter 2 we identified the phonological processes most frequently addressed in the phonology literature according to (a) syllable structure processes, (b) substitution processes, and (c) assimilation processes. Syllable structure processes include final-consonant deletion, syllable deletion, cluster reduction, and epenthesis. Examples of substitution processes are stopping, velar fronting, liquid gliding, and depalatalization. Assimilation processes are varied and include labial assimilation, nasal assimilation, prevocalic voicing, and postvocalic devoicing.

Patterns of misarticulations that differ from the more commonly observed phonological processes have been identified in children with normal and disordered phonological skills. These patterns occur infrequently in children with normal phonological skills, and thus they are termed *unusual* or *idiosyncratic phonological processes* (Grunwell, 1997a, 1997b; Leonard, 1985; Stoel-Gammon & Dunn, 1985). Examples of idiosyncratic processes include the replacement of late-developing sounds for early sounds, the use of nasal sounds for /s/ and /z/, click substitutions, and the substitution of stops for glides (Grunwell, 1997a, 1997b; Bankson & Bernthal, 1998; Stoel-Gammon & Dunn, 1985). The reader is referred to Chapter 2 and Appendix C for a description of various phonological processes.

Phonological processes can be assessed according to their frequency of occurrence and their percentage of occurrence. In **frequency of occurrence,** the clinician simply identifies the number of times a particular process occurs in the child's speech sample. **Percentage of occurrence** would be more specific; in that type of analysis the clinician determines the number of times the child uses a particular phonological process in relation to the total number of opportunities to use that process. For example, a frequency of occurrence may reveal that a child used velar fronting on 5 occasions. However, the significance of that information would be enhanced if the percentage of occurrence were also known, if it were known, for example, that the child used that process in 5 out of 8 total opportunities (63% percentage of occurrence) rather than, say, 5 of 30 total opportunities (17% percentage of occurrence). To calculate a percentage of occurrence the clinician needs to determine the total number of opportunities for the use of a specific phonological process, in addition to the total number of actual occurrences. The following formula may be used:

Total Number of Occurrences of a Process ÷ Total Number of <u>Opportunities</u> for the Process = Percentage of Occurrence

Most formal phonological processes instruments provide the clinician with the total number of opportunities for the use of each process tested. The clinician then identifies the actual occurrences by administering the test and recording the client's responses. This predetermined information helps the clinician identify the total percentage of occurrence for each process tested. Calculating a percentage of occurrence is a much more difficult task for a conversational speech sample; the clinician must take the time to ascertain not only the number of times the process occurred but also the total number of opportunities for the occurrence of each process under analysis. Determining the number of opportunities for the use of various processes in a conversational sample can be extremely time consuming. Most clinicians do not have the luxury of such time. Thus, a percentage of occurrence is most often determined from a formal instrument rather than a connected speech sample.

An important clinical issue related to the use of phonological processes is the question of when a child's sound production errors constitute a pattern. Although the literature is inundated with definitions for a variety of phonological processes, the same is not true for criteria that can clearly identify the presence of a process. McReynolds and Elbert (1981a) made the valid point that one occurrence of an omission or substitution error under the definition of a particular process does not signify the presence of a process. They also advanced one of the few sets of criteria available to clinicians today for the identification of phonological processes.

McReynolds and Elbert suggest that to qualify as a process, an error must have an opportunity to occur in at least four instances and must occur in at least 20% of those opportunities. For example, if the child's speech sample contained 10 words with velar consonants, the process of velar fronting would be identified only if the child demonstrated at least 2 instances of an alveolar-for-velar substitution. One of the problems with McReynolds and Elbert's criterion is that it is rather inclusive. For example, if a child substituted [w] for /r/ in 2 of 8 total /r/ production opportunities, then the phonological process of liquid gliding would be identified since the 20% criterion was met. It is questionable whether two instances of a sound substitution could constitute a phonological process.

A more stringent criterion is offered by Hodson and Paden (1991), who suggest that a phonological process must have at least a 40% occurrence before it is selected as a treatment target. Processes that occur in less than 40% of opportunities would be monitored but not addressed in therapy. It should be noted that Hodson and Paden's criterion is intended for the identification of phonological processes that are in need of remediation rather than for the classification of specific phonological processes. Lowe (1996) has suggested that the minimal requirements for qualifying a sound change as a phonological process are that (a) the process must affect more than one sound from a given sound class, and (b) the sound change must occur at least 40% of the time.

Because of the lack of clear criteria for the identification of phonological processes, clinicians often rely on their own professional judgment. The development of quantitative criteria is an important area for further research. It would also be useful to develop a standard definition for individual phonological processes so that if a specific quantitative criterion is used, it can be compared from one source to another.

Another consideration in the identification of phonological processes is that children rarely use a single phonological pattern on a specific word. Rather, they often produce word forms that reflect the co-occurrence of multiple processes. For example, a child who produces [wat] for the word *lock* demonstrates the use of liquid gliding and velar fronting on a word. Also, a single production error can be identified as an instance of various processes. For example, the production of [tut] for *shoot* could potentially be identified as stopping, depalatalization, and alveolar assimilation. The clinician would obviously have to look beyond the production of a single word to identify the phonological processes that are part of the child's phonological system. The worksheet in Appendix I can be used for the identification of phonological processes.

Analysis of Related Information

Orofacial Examination and Diadochokinetic Testing

We previously described the procedures in conducting an orofacial examination and those involved in diadochokinetic testing. This information is important and helps the clinician rule out any organic, structural, or neurological variables as the underlying cause of an articulation or phonological disorder. Although most often the cause of an articulation or phonological disorder is unknown, it should be standard practice to examine the structure and function of the speech mechanism to avoid missing any potential structural, functional, or neurological problems. Interpretation of the information obtained during an assessment can lead to a more thorough diagnosis. Various observations and their clinical implications are described below.

Face at Rest and During Specific Movements

Observations

- Drooping at the corner of the mouth on one side at rest.
- Partially or completely closed eyelid at rest.
- Drooping of the mandible on one side at rest.
- Abnormal facial movements (e.g., facial grimaces, spasms, twitching, and so forth).
- Deviation of the corner of the mouth to one side when smiling.
- Deviation of the jaw to one side when opening mouth.
- Uneven rising of the eyebrows when asked to raise both eyebrows.
- One eye stays open or closes only partially when asked to close eyes tight.

Implications

All of these may be signs of neurological damage or facial weakness.

Lips at Rest

Observations

- Drooping at the corner of the mouth on one side.
- Evidence of a repaired cleft lip or other scar tissue.
- Lips apart while at rest.
- Mouth breathing or drooling.

Implications

Drooping of the corner of the mouth may be a sign of neurological damage. A repaired cleft lip or other scar tissue is indicative of structural damage; however, it may or may not affect articulation. Lips that remain apart during rest may indicate a restricted nasal passageway or **myofunctional imbalance.** Drooling may result from neurological damage or anterior posturing of the tongue at rest.

Lips During Specific Movements

Observations

- Deviation of the corner of the mouth to one side during smiling.
- Deviation of the lips to one side during puckering.
- Inadequate range of motion while alternating between a pucker and a smile.
- Inadequate labial seal or escape of air when impounding air.
- Inadequate range of motion, strength, and lip seal during repetition of "pa-pa-pa."

Implications

All of these may be signs of neurological damage or labial weakness.

Tongue at Rest and During Specific Movements

Observations

- Abnormal coloration of the tongue.
- Inappropriate size of the tongue in relation to the oral cavity.
- Signs of **atrophy.**
- Abnormal movements such as spasms, **fasciculations,** writhing, twitches, and so forth.
- Slow, imprecise, uncoordinated, or groping movements of the tongue during protrusion, retraction, lateralization, or diadochokinetic tasks.
- A short or restricted lingual frenum that would indicate **ankyloglossia** or tongue-tie.

Implications

A grayish color of the tongue may indicate muscular weakness or paralysis, while a bluish tint may result from excessive vascularity or bleeding (Shipley & McAfee, 1998). A tongue that is too small (**microglossia**) or one that is too big (**macroglossia**) in relation to the client's oral cavity may lead to sound distortions. Signs of atrophy and any abnormal movements such as twitching or fasciculations may indicate neurological damage. Slow, imprecise, uncoordinated, or groping movement of the tongue may also indicate neurological damage or lingual weakness. A short lingual frenum or ankyloglossia may or may not affect the production of alveolars and palatals.

Hard Palate

Observations

- Abnormal coloration of the hard palate along its midline.
- An abnormally high and narrow hard palate.
- Signs of repaired or unrepaired clefts, fistulas, or fissures.
- Signs of surgical removal of any portion of the hard palate.
- Presence of prostheses (e.g., dentures, obturators, or palatal lifts).
- Prominent rugae on the alveolar ridge.

Implications

A whitish, bluish tint along the midline of the hard palate may indicate a submucosal cleft, while an abnormally dark or translucent color is a symptom of a palatal fistula. Repaired clefts or fistulas may be associated with sound distortions or substitutions. Surgical removal of the hard palate may affect articulation, while prosthetic devices can help counteract some of these problems. Prominent rugae on the alveolar ridge are associated with tongue thrust (Shipley & McAfee, 1998).

Soft Palate at Rest and During Specific Movements

Observations

- Abnormal coloration of the soft palate along its midline.

- Presence of a bifid uvula.

- Signs of repaired or unrepaired clefts, fistulas, or fissures.

- Signs of surgical removal of any portion of the soft palate.

- Presence of prostheses (e.g., dentures, obturators, or palatal lifts).

- Asymmetry of the velum at rest.

- Hypernasal or hyponasal quality during conversational speech.

- Clouding or fogging of a mirror placed under the nares during the production of nonnasal sounds.

- Inadequate movement of the velum during prolongation or repetition of /a/.

- Deviation of the uvula to one side at rest or during sound production.

Implications

The normal coloration of the soft palate is pinkish. A whitish, bluish tint along its borders may indicate a submucosal cleft. A bifid uvula, especially when accompanied by a bluish tint of the soft and hard palates, is also a symptom of a submucosal cleft. Repaired cleft palates and surgical removal of part of the soft palate may affect sound articulation and resonance. A prosthesis may be in place to help alleviate some of the problems associated with velopharyngeal insufficiency or inadequacy. Asymmetry of the velum and deviation of the uvula to one side may indicate muscular weakness or paralysis. Hypernasality or nasal emission may result from neurological impairment or structural anomalies.

Teeth and Other Related Structures

Observations

- Missing, jumbled, tilted, or malpositioned teeth.
- Malocclusion of the molars.
- Malocclusion of the incisors.

Implications

Missing teeth, malocclusions, and bite problems may or may not affect articulation. See Chapter 4 for a description of normal and disordered occlusion and its implications on speech production.

Medical History Analysis

From the written case history, information-getting interview, and review of reports written by other professionals, the clinician usually gains a good understanding of a client's current health status and medical history. Occasionally, clients bring a history of medical diagnoses and interventions that can affect the diagnosis of articulation or phonological disorder. For example, a client with a history of a repaired cleft lip and palate may manifest articulation errors that can be explained by the one-time presence of such structural anomalies. Clients with a history of cerebrovascular accident (stroke) may have incurred neurological damage that could account for the presence of dysarthria or apraxia of speech. Furthermore, children with a history of recurrent otitis media and fluctuating hearing loss may display sound distortions, substitutions, and omissions typically associated with hearing loss. Not all children have an articulation or phonological disorder that can be accounted for by the presence of some structural, functional, or neurological damage; however, when the underlying cause of the disorder can be clearly identified or suspected, the clinician should make reference to such in the diagnostic report.

Phonological Knowledge Analysis

Elbert and Gierut (1986) advanced the notion of **phonological knowledge.** This refers to the child's presumed knowledge or understanding of the phonological rules of the adult system. Assessment of the child's knowledge is accomplished through careful analysis of his or her productions. In essence, the authors propose that the greater the consistency of correct productions in varied contexts, the higher the level of phonological knowledge. Likewise, the lower the consistency of correct productions, the lower the level of phonological knowledge. Elbert and Gierut have identified the types of phonological knowledge along a continuum progressing from Type 1 to Type 6.

• **Type 1:** The child produces the sound correctly in all word positions and for all morphemes. The sound is never produced in error.

• **Type 2:** The child produces the sound correctly in all word positions and for all morphemes. However, an occasional error may occur due to an *optional* phonological rule.

• **Type 3:** The child produces the sound correctly in all positions. However, certain words or morphemes that were acquired in error are retained (**fossilized forms** or **frozen forms**).

• **Type 4:** The child produces the target sound correctly for all morphemes in a particular word position. However, errors continue in other word positions.

• **Type 5:** The child produces the sound correctly only in some word positions and some morphemes. The sound would be produced in error in all morphemes in other word positions (Types 3 and 4 combined).

• **Type 6:** The child never produces the sound correctly in relation to the adult form.

Elbert and Gierut (1986, pp. 64–65) recommend the following procedures for assessing a child's productive phonological knowledge:

1. Obtain a representative sample of the child's spontaneous speech. The sample should include both connected speech and elicited single words. The speech samples should also:

• sample all target English;
• sample sounds in each word position;
• sample sounds in a number of different words;
• sample each item more than once;
• provide an opportunity for the child to produce potential minimal pairs; and
• provide an opportunity for the child to produce potential morphophonemic alternations.

2. Establish a child's phonological knowledge by considering:

• the breadth of the distribution of sounds, including the phonetic and phonemic inventories, and the distribution of sounds across word positions and across target morphemes;
• the application of phonological rules—phonotactic constraints, allophonic rules, or neutralization rules; and
• the nature of the child's lexical representations—either adultlike or nonadultlike.

3. Determine the types of knowledge observed for a given sound, sound class, or overall sound system.

4. Rank a child's phonological knowledge on a continuum, ranging from most to least knowledge of the target sound system.

5. Select target sounds for treatment based upon a child's phonological knowledge.

6. Select an order of treatment, proceeding either from most to least phonological knowledge or least to most phonological knowledge.

7. Predict a child's generalization learning patterns depending on his or her phonological knowledge and the order of intervention.

The treatment implications of a child's phonological knowledge will be addressed in Chapters 7 and 8.

Developmental Analysis

In a developmental analysis, the information obtained from standardized tests or a connected speech sample is compared to well-established developmental norms. Such comparison allows the clinician, in part, to determine whether the child's articulation errors are common to most children of his or her chronological age or are beyond the average age of mastery. The typical acquisition of articulation and phonological skills is a relatively lengthy process, and children cannot be expected to master production of all sounds or suppress all phonological processes at the same time. Some children suspected of having an articulation or phonological disorder by parents, teachers, or significant others may simply be producing age-appropriate errors. In such a case, the child's articulation or phonological skills would be considered normal rather than disordered.

Speech–language pathologists working in the public school system rely heavily on normative data to make eligibility decisions. Children who appear to be following the normal course of development would not be considered adequate candidates for speech pathology services. This can help the clinician maintain a manageable caseload in a work setting that is known for serving an extremely high number of clients.

In the Basic Unit of Chapter 3 we discussed at great length the normal development of individual phonemes, distinctive features, phonological processes, and speech intelligibility. Students may refer to this information when making a developmental analysis. The methodological issues of several large-scale studies discussed in Chapter 3 and the inherent problem of using group data for the evaluation of an individual's performance should always be taken into account. The clinician should always remember that developmental data are only one of several variables considered in the diagnosis of articulation and phonological disorders.

Stimulability Analysis

As previously discussed, stimulability testing can be done after a complete articulation assessment has been performed. Sounds that were misarticulated are evoked by having the child imitate the clinician's production or by providing additional stimulation such as auditory, tactile, or visual prompts. The information obtained from stimulability testing is important for several reasons. It can serve as a valuable prognostic indicator of the client's progress in therapy. Also, through stimulability testing, the clinician can identify the types of stimulation and the linguistic level that are most appropriate in the treatment of specific sounds. For example, if the client was found to be stimulable at the syllable level for a particular sound, the clinician could choose to start therapy at the word level of production. Also, if modeling was not sufficient to evoke correct production of the sound, the clinician could try to establish the sound through the use of other types of prompts (e.g., phonetic placement cues). Furthermore, the results of stimulability testing are among the many variables clinicians consider in the selection of target sounds for training. This information will be further reviewed in the Basic Unit of Chapter 7.

Intelligibility Analysis

The conversational speech sample collected during the assessment can be analyzed in regard to the client's speech intelligibility. How understandable the client is during connected speech production is an important variable that should be considered. Misarticulations often affect speech intelligibility, and thus the primary goal of therapy in most cases is to make the client more understandable.

Clinicians can make a professional judgment of speech intelligibility during natural conversational interactions with the client. This type of analysis is subjective, but experienced clinicians rely on years of practice in making such judgments. The following statement reflects this type of analysis: "This examiner judged the client's speech intelligibility to be 50–60% intelligible during known and unknown contexts." Other clinical rating systems can be used to identify the degree of intelligibility. Bleile (1995) describes two rating scales of intelligibility as follows:

3-Point Clinical Judgment Scale of Intelligibility

- 1   Readily intelligible
- 2   Intelligible if topic is known
- 3   Unintelligible even with careful listening

5-Point Clinical Judgment Scale of Intelligibility

- 1   Completely intelligible
- 2   Mostly intelligible
- 3   Somewhat intelligible
- 4   Mostly unintelligible
- 5   Completely unintelligible

A more objective analysis should also be performed to supplement the clinician's initial impression of intelligibility. This can be done for both known and unknown conversational contexts. The following steps can be taken in making an objective analysis of the client's speech intelligibility:

1. *Collect a connected speech sample.* The sample that was collected to assess the client's production of sounds can be used. However, it is important that the clinician select a portion of the sample that was not specifically used for sound production analysis, since the purpose at this point is to assess speech intelligibility.
2. *Transcribe the sample.* Do not make a concerted effort to understand the child as you did during sound production transcription. Rather, listen to the utterance once and transcribe accordingly. This would more closely resemble listening in the natural environment, since the average listener would not have the luxury of

recording the child's productions and listening to the sample several times. Write out each word for each utterance. The words may be written orthographically.

3. *Use a symbol that helps depict an unintelligible word.* A slash (/) may be used. We frequently use a squiggle mark, such as (〰).

4. *Calculate intelligibility for words.* Divide the total number of intelligible words by the total number of words. For example: 105 **intelligible words** ÷ 250 **total (intelligible + unintelligible) words** = 42% intelligibility for words.

5. *Calculate intelligibility for utterances.* Divide the total number of intelligible **utterances** by the total number of utterances (an utterance is considered intelligible only if the entire utterance can be understood). For example: 62 **intelligible utterances** ÷ 200 **total (intelligible + unintelligible) utterances** = 31% intelligibility for utterances.

Weiss, Gordon, and Lillywhite (1987) suggest the following method for calculating a client's speech intelligibility:

1. Randomly select 200 consecutive words from the client's tape-recorded contextual speech sample and compare them with established developmental norms for intelligibility (refer to information on speech intelligibility in Chapter 3).

2. Play back the recorded sample, listen to the sample, and count the number of unintelligible words.

3. Subtract the number of unintelligible words from 200 and divide the remaining number by two.

4. The answer is the intelligibility percentage score for the client.

Severity Analysis

Assuming that a child indeed has an articulation or phonological disorder, the clinician should judge the severity of the disorder as part of a clinical diagnosis. Severity refers to the degree of impairment in a particular client, which may range from slight to profound. Some standardized tests such as the *Test of Minimal Articulation Competence* (Secord, 1981c) provide clinicians with the necessary information to derive a severity score; however, others do not. In cases when formal testing instruments are not used or do not include a severity analysis portion, clinicians often rely on their own professional judgment for determining the severity of the disorder.

Clinicians consider several variables that may impact the severity of the disorder, including the child's speech intelligibility, the number of error sounds or active phonological processes, the consistency of the errors, and the child's age. In general, it can be expected that the higher the number of error sounds or active phonological processes and the higher the consistency of the errors, the lower the client's speech intelligibility. And the lower the client's speech intelligibility, the more severe the disorder. Although currently there is no standard application of terms, clinicians often use the terms *slight, mild, mild-moderate, moderate, moderate-severe, severe, and profound* to indicate the degree of impairment.

In an attempt to provide a more objective measure of severity, Shriberg and Kwiatkowski (1982c) developed a metric system that considers the **percentage of consonants correct** (PCC) as an index of degree of impairment. They outlined the following procedures for determining the PCC for a particular client (information adapted from p. 267):

1. Collect a Speech Sample

   • Tape-record a continous speech sample of at least 50–100 words.

   • Determine the meaning of the utterances to ensure accurate transcription. The child's utterances may be glossed to aid later analysis.

   • Identify and exclude any dialectical differences, casual speech pronunciations, or allophonic variations.

2. Consider Exclusion Criteria

   • Consider only intended consonants in words. All vowels, including /ɚ/ and /ɝ/, should be excluded. Exclude the addition of a consonant before a vowel since the intended production is the vowel (e.g., [hon] for *on* is not scored).

   • The second or successive repetition of a consonant should not be included. Only the first production should be scored (e.g., in "ba-balloon," score only the first /b/).

   • Words that are partially or completely unintelligible should be excluded. Words whose gloss is highly questionable should also be excluded. Score only intelligible words or words that can be reliably identified.

   • Target consonants that occur in the third or successive repetitions of adjacent words should be excluded unless articulation of the word changes. For example, the consonants in only the first two words of the series [kæt], [kæt], [kæt] are counted, while the consonants in all three words are counted in the series [kæt], [kæk], [kæt].

3. Determine Incorrect Consonant Productions

   • The following consonant sound changes are scored as incorrect:

   (a) deletions of the target consonant

   (b) substitutions of another sound for a target consonant, which includes replacement by a glottal stop or a cognate

   (c) partial voicing of initial target consonants

   (d) distortions of a target sound, no matter how subtle

   (e) addition of a sound to a correct or incorrect target consonant (e.g., [karks] for *cars*).

   • Initial /h/ deletion (e.g., [i] for *he*) and final n/ŋ substitutions (e.g., [rin] for *ring*) are counted as errors only when they occur in stressed syllables. They are counted as correct when they are produced in unstressed syllables (e.g., [fidɚ] for *feed her* and [rʌnin] for *running*).

   • Score dialectical differences and casual speech productions based on the consonant the child intended (e.g., [aks] for *ask* is correct in African-American English, but [ats] for *ask* is incorrect).

   • Allophonic variations should be scored as correct (e.g., [waɾɚ] for *water*).

4. Calculate the Percentage of Consonants Correct

   • The PCC is calculated by using the following formula:

   Number of Correct Consonants ÷ Number of Correct *Plus* Incorrect Consonants × 100 = PCC

- Example:

$$50 \text{ consonants produced correctly} \div 200 \text{ total consonants}$$
$$\text{attempted} \times 100 = 25\% \text{ (PCC score)}$$

5. Determine the Severity Level

The following scale is used to determine the severity of the disorder:

- 85–100% mild
- 65–85%   mild-moderate
- 50–65%   moderate-severe
- < 50%   severe

According to Lowe (1994), the PCC may be used not only as a severity rating, but also as a means of monitoring progress. The PCC is an objective way of determining the severity of a disorder. It may also provide clinicians with a quantitative criterion by which the efficacy of a treatment can be evaluated.

Contextual Testing Analysis

Contextual testing is performed to determine if certain phonetic contexts facilitate the correct production of a target phoneme. Through formal and informal contextual testing, facilitative phonetic contexts for a phoneme may be identified. It should be emphasized that this type of testing does not help determine the need for treatment. Rather, it helps establish a possible starting point in therapy. The clinician can use published instruments such as the *Deep Test of Articulation* (McDonald, 1964) and *Clinical Probes of Articulation Consistency* (Secord, 1981a) or collect a speech sample to identify any facilitating contexts. The clinician then analyzes the information and determines if any sounds that precede or follow the target sound help evoke a correct or improved production. At times, patterns of production may be identified that are clinically significant. For example, the clinician may determine that /s/ and /z/ are produced correctly when they precede or follow any alveolar sound. The clinician can promote early success in therapy by taking advantage of such a facilitative context. Stimulus pictures can be paired so that /s/ and /z/ are preceded by alveolar sounds (e.g., *hat–sun, dad–zoo, moon–soap*). Also, through careful analysis of the speech sample, the clinician may identify *key words* for correct production of the target sound. Such key words can be used to promote early success in therapy.

Phonetic Inventory Analysis

A **phonetic inventory analysis** helps the clinician identify the consonants and vowels the client can make without consideration for the contrasting effects of the sound in adult words. The point of interest with this type of analysis is not whether the sound was used in the appropriate linguistic or phonetic context, but whether the client demonstrated the motor ability to make the sound. Figure 6.2 illustrates a typical phonetic inventory analysis form for consonants in the initial, medial, and final position of words. A chart for vowels is also provided. *The Khan-Lewis Phonological Analysis* (Khan & Lewis, 1986) is a standardized assessment instrument that includes a phonetic inventory analysis component.

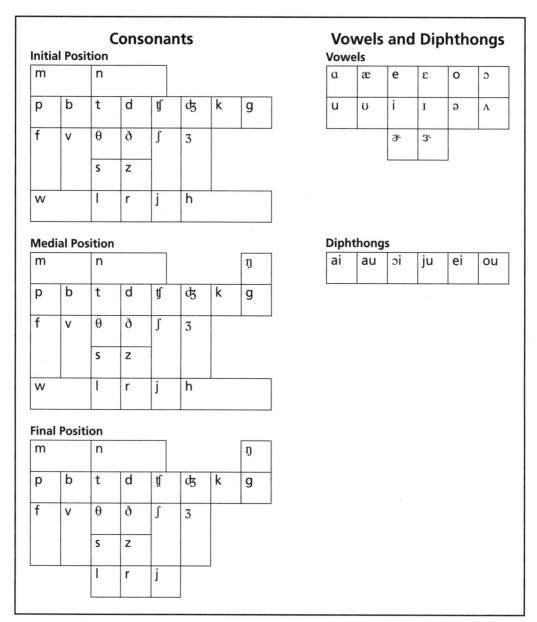

Figure 6.2. Phonetic inventory analysis model chart.

The client's phonetic inventory can be determined from the information obtained on single-word articulation tests, phonological process assessments, or a connected speech sample. Lowe (1994) advanced the following rules for performing a phonetic inventory analysis when using a phonetic inventory model chart (see Figure 6.2):

• Sounds that occur at least three times are circled and considered part of the child's productive inventory.

• Sounds that occur one or two times are considered marginal and can be marked using parentheses or underlining. According to Lowe, "These sounds are not given full status, as the clinician may have transcribed incorrectly or the production may have been a fluke" (p. 143).

The client's phonetic inventory can provide relevant clinical information. The clinician may discover that the client's productive phonetic inventory is limited to only a few sounds, which can help explain the high number of misarticulations or phonological processes in the child's speech. A child with a limited phonetic inventory would likely have multiple sound omissions or substitutions. The clinician may also discover a difference in the child's productive phonetic inventory from one word position to another. For example, the child may produce all stops in the initial position, but those sounds may not be part of the child's phonetic inventory in the final position. Thus, the clinician may choose to train the child in the production of stops in the final position of words to increase his or her use of various syllable shapes. Furthermore, through the use of a phonetic inventory analysis form it may become apparent to the clinician that the client's production of sounds is restricted to certain sound classes or types of sounds (e.g., stops and glides). Through the use of such a form the clinician often gets a visual representation of the client's productive inventory of sounds.

Making a Diagnosis

Once the various types of analysis have been completed, the clinician typically has enough data to make a diagnosis. It is at this point that the clinician decides whether an articulation or phonological disorder exists. If a disorder is present, the clinician also describes the severity and nature of the disorder. In general, the assessment may lead to one of two **diagnoses:** (a) normal articulation and phonological skills, or (b) disordered articulation and phonological skills.

The clinician may decide that a child's sound productions are normal in the following situations:

• *The errors identified are related to second-language interference, bilingualism, or the use of a particular dialect.* Recall from Chapter 5 that articulation and phonological differences are not considered disorders, unless the client demonstrates errors that would not be expected when the dialectical or linguistic variations are taken into account. Dialectical or phonological differences may or may not affect a child's speech intelligibility, social interactions, and academic performance.

• *The errors fall within the normal developmental range of mastery for a particular age group.* In the normal acquisition process, children demonstrate articulation and phonological errors that cannot be considered disordered. Research has consistently established that the development of articulation and phonological skills is a gradual process. A 2-year-old child, for example, would be expected to have many more errors than the average 6-year-old. If those two children demonstrated the same errors, the younger child could potentially be diagnosed as having normal articulation skills, whereas the older child's productions would likely be considered delayed or disordered. This depends on the errors, of course.

• *The errors are so slight or subtle that, for all intents and purposes, they would not call undue attention to the speaker or be perceived as disordered by the average layperson.* Some individuals may demonstrate slight or very mild sound distortions that may be evident to the trained ear of the speech–language pathologist but not to the average listener. Such errors would probably not affect the individual's social, academic, or vocational life. Some sound classes are particularly vulnerable to distortion: sibilants (lisping), liquids (vowelization), and nasals (hyponasality).

It should be emphasized that in all three cases, the client's or family's perception of the problem becomes extremely important. If the client or the client's family believes that the articulation errors are or may become "handicapping" in the future, the clinician may need to reconsider the diagnosis and the treatment recommendations. Adults in certain vocations, such as public speaking, television and radio broadcasting, teaching, and acting, may want or be required to enunciate precisely.

Also, children and adults whose articulation errors are the result of bilingualism or dialectical differences may seek out speech therapy because their social, vocational, or academic life is affected by their nonstandard English productions. Speech therapy services may be warranted in such a case. However, clinicians in the public school setting need to adhere to state and federal guidelines that may prohibit the provision of speech–language pathology services solely on the basis of dialectical differences or second-language acquisition of English. Children whose errors fall within the normal range of development may or may not be "handicapped" by the presence of certain errors.

If the clinician decides that indeed the client has an articulation or phonological disorder, a description of the disorder is appropriate. For example, the types of errors most commonly observed might be identified, or the clinician can make reference to the active phonological processes. In addition, the clinician may choose to offer a more specific diagnosis in regard to the type of the disorder. Although such a distinction was not always made, clinicians today are more inclined to label a child's sound production errors as either an *articulation disorder* or a *phonological disorder.*

As reviewed in the Basic Unit of Chapter 2, in clinical practice, the term **articulation disorder** is most often applied in the following situations:

• the child has a few errors for which a pattern or derivable rule could not be identified;

• the sound errors could be attributed to some underlying structural, functional, or neurological problem; or

• the child has difficulty producing only one or two specific sounds (e.g., frontal lisp of /s/ and /z/ or distortion of /r/).

The term **phonological disorder** is most often used to describe sound production errors for which some underlying rule or principle could be identified. The child with a phonological disorder may present with multiple misarticulations, various phonological processes, poor intelligibility, limited syllable shapes, and a restricted phonetic inventory. A phonological disorder may be identified from a manner-place-voicing analysis, distinctive feature analysis, or phonological process analysis. In essence, the child appears to have problems with the acquisition of certain phonological rules or the suppression of phonological processes.

Other specific diagnostic terms such as *apraxia of speech, dysarthria, tongue thrust,* and *developmental apraxia of speech* may be used with clients who demonstrate a sufficient number of characteristics associated with those speech disorders.

An estimate of the severity of the disorder is also very important. For parents, other professionals, and third-party payers this is often one of the most important elements of the diagnosis. However, because there is no standard way of measuring severity, speech–language pathologists frequently rely on their clinical intuition to make a diagnosis. As discussed earlier, many variables can affect the severity of the articulation or phonological disorder. These include the client's speech intelligibility, the total number of misarticulated sounds or active phonological processes, the client's age, the frequency of occurrence of the incorrect sounds, and the presence of any structural or neurological problems. We believe that speech intelligibility has the highest connection to the severity of the disorder. In general, the lower the client's intelligibility, the more severe the articulation or phonological disorder. As mentioned previously, the terms *mild, mild-moderate, moderate, moderate-severe, severe,* and *profound* are frequently used to designate the severity of the problem. Again, because there is no standard way of measuring severity, such judgments are subjective. Clinicians, however, do not apply such labels at random. Rather, they analyze the assessment information, consider all the variables, and make a clinical judgment.

If any structural or neurological factors are believed to contribute to the articulation or phonological disorder, the clinician should make note of those in the diagnostic report. For example, the child's disorder may result from structural problems associated with cleft palate and malocclusions, neurological problems associated with apraxia of speech, dysarthria, or cerebral palsy, or sensory problems associated with hearing loss.

Assuming that a disorder is identified, diagnostic statements may be written as in the following examples. A diagnostic statement is generally one of the last portions of the written report. The style and format in which it is written varies from one clinician to the other.

• Dee Dee demonstrated a severe articulation disorder as well as severe delay in receptive and expressive language. Dee Dee's articulation errors primarily consisted of labial and lingual sound distortions. The restriction of tongue and lip movement noted in the orofacial examination may be contributing to misarticulation of these sounds.

• Sammy has a mild articulation disorder associated with tongue thrust behavior. Sammy's specific sound errors included interdentalization of /s/, /z/, /ʃ/, and /ʧ/. His speech intelligibility was not affected by his misarticulations.

• Suzie has a mild articulation disorder characterized by a lateral lisp of /s/ and /z/. Her speech intelligibility was minimally affected by her articulation errors. No structure or function problems of the speech mechanism were noted during the orofacial examination that could help explain her articulation errors.

• Frank exhibited a mild-moderate phonological disorder characterized by final-consonant deletion, syllable deletion, and velar fronting. Frank's phonological disorder may be related to his history of middle ear infections and moderate conductive hearing loss.

• Christina has a mild articulation disorder characterized by distortions of the /r/ and /l/ phonemes in all word positions. Christina's voice was also judged to have weak oral resonance due to minimal mandibular and labial movements during speech.

• Bobby exhibited a moderate articulation disorder characteristic of developmental apraxia of speech (DAS). Error patterns leading to the diagnosis of DAS included the following: sound transposition errors, sound perseveration errors, increased articulation errors with increased word length, and substitution errors primarily affecting fricatives and affricates.

• Edith demonstrated a moderate-severe articulation delay characterized by several omission, substitution, and distortion errors.

• John exhibited moderate flaccid dysarthria characterized by distortion of the stops, fricatives, and affricates. Other characteristics of flaccid dysarthria noted in John's speech included hypernasality, a hoarse-breathy vocal quality, and general weakness of the speech musculature.

• Geraldine has a severe phonological disorder characterized by stopping of fricatives and affricates, vowelization of postvocalic /l/ and /r/, and partial reduction of /s/, /l/, and /r/ clusters. Geraldine's overall speech intelligibility was clinically judged to be 50% when the conversational context was known. This level of intelligibility is severely delayed for a child Geraldine's age.

• Mark demonstrated age-appropriate articulation skills. Although several errors were noted on the *Goldman-Fristoe Test of Articulation* and a spontaneous speech sample, they were within normal developmental limits for a child of Mark's chronological age.

Determining the Prognosis for Improvement

A prognosis is a statement that estimates the extent of progress that can be expected in therapy. The initial prognosis is based upon the *available* information at the time of the assessment. Various **prognostic variables** can aid the clinician in making a professional judgment about the client's anticipated progress. Prognostic variables are factors that can positively or negatively influence the client's improvement of his or her articulation and phonological skills. The initial prognosis may change over the course of time.

A well-written prognostic statement has at least three major components: (1) a goal statement, (2) a judgment of success, and (3) the prognostic variables that lead to the prognosis. The *goal statement* makes reference to what skill(s) the child is expected to achieve. This part should be clearly written. For example, the statement "The prognosis is good" is not acceptable since it does not indicate what the child is expected to learn or achieve. A better statement would be "The prognosis for correct production of /s/ is excellent."

The above example hinted at the next component of a prognostic statement: the *judgment of success*. This is a clinical judgment that makes reference to how well the client is expected to do in therapy. The terms *poor, fair, good,* and *excellent* are often used in clinical practice. This prediction is based on the various variables that come to light during the assessment. Prior clinical experience often helps clinicians make such a determination. However, even the most experienced and wisest of clinicians has been proven wrong on occasions. A client who was initially judged to have a poor prognosis might do extremely well in therapy, whereas another client believed to have an excellent prognosis may demonstrate very limited progress.

When making a prognosis or a decision about the expected outcome, the clinician may consider several variables. These variables help the clinician decide whether the client has an excellent, good, fair, or poor prognosis for the attainment of a specific goal. It is emphasized, though, that because of the uniqueness of each clinical case, there is not a certain set of variables associated with each judgment of success. Ultimately, the clinician must use his or her professional judgment to arrive at a decision. Client-centered *prognostic variables* include the following:

Variable	Underlying Assumption
Severity	The more severe the disorder, the poorer the prognosis. The less severe the disorder, the better the prognosis.
Chronological age	The younger the client at the time of treatment, the better the prognosis. It may be easier to remediate articulation or phonological errors in a young child than an adolescent or adult.
Motivation	The less motivated the person, the poorer the prognosis for improvement. The client who is highly motivated is more apt to have an "attitude" of learning. Such a patient will likely follow through with assignments, therapy suggestions, and so forth. This variable is most significant with older elementary school children, adolescents, and adults. Young children may be much more motivated by external factors manipulated by the clinician.
Stimulability	The more stimulable the client for an improved or correct production of the target sounds, the better the prognosis. A client with low stimulability may not do as well in therapy. However, this logical conclusion has not been strongly supported. Some children with poor stimulability do very well in therapy and vice versa.
Inconsistency	Inconsistency in sound production errors is often considered a positive prognostic variable. If the errors can be produced correctly at least some of the time, they may be more amenable to correction once therapy is initiated.
Associated behaviors	Any behavior that may interfere with the client's progress in therapy is thought to have a negative impact on prognosis. A child with a limited attention span or poor cooperation, for example, may not learn as quickly as a child who is willing and ready to learn.

Treatment history	A child with a history of limited progress or poor maintenance of previously learned behaviors may be thought to have a poorer prognosis than a child absent of such history. Not all children come with a history of speech–language pathology services. Thus, this variable may not apply to all clients.
Family support	The stronger the support extended by the client's family, the better the prognosis for improvement. Research has continually documented that if the client's family takes an active role in therapy, the likelihood is higher that the client will maintain the skills learned in the clinical environment.

Clinicians have the ethical responsibility to provide the client or the client's family with a prognosis for improvement. However, the clinician should be careful not to guarantee the results of treatment. Principle of Ethics I, Rule of Ethics F, found in the Code of Ethics of the American Speech-Language-Hearing Association strictly prohibits clinicians from guaranteeing the results of any treatment procedures. However, a "reasonable statement" of prognosis can be made (American Speech-Language-Hearing Association, 1994).

Written prognostic statements are part of a thorough diagnostic report. The following are provided as examples of prognostic statements. However, it should be emphasized that the style in which such reports are written often varies from one clinician to the other. These examples are provided primarily to illustrate inclusion of the goal statement, judgment of success, and prognostic variables.

• *Example Statement for Excellent Prognosis:*
Jamie's prognosis for improved production of /s/ and /z/ with therapy was judged excellent based on the following variables: the mild nature of her articulation disorder, her stimulability for correct production of the target sounds, her cooperative behavior and good attention span during the assessment, the absence of any structural problems, and the high level of support from her parents.

• *Example Statement for Good Prognosis:*
Based on John's age (4 years, 2 months), his cooperative behavior, and his stimulability for correct production of some of the target sounds, his prognosis for improved phonological skills and increased speech intelligibility was judged to be good with therapy this semester.

• *Example Statement for Fair Prognosis:*
Jerry was very cooperative during the assessment and has good family support. However, her prognosis for improved articulation skills and increased speech intelligibility with therapy was judged fair at this time because of her age (13 years), the severity of her disorder, and the extent of her hearing loss. Her prognosis will be reevaluated according to her performance once treatment is initiated.

• *Example Statement for Poor Prognosis:*
Ron's prognosis for improved articulation skills was judged poor based on the severe nature of his disorder, his uncooperative behavior during the testing process, his short attention span, and a reported history of limited progress. However,

in that this clinician has not personally worked with Ron before, his prognosis will be reevaluated throughout the course of treatment.

Making Treatment Recommendations

Regardless of the results of the assessment and the clinical diagnosis, the clinician is obliged to make specific recommendations. The clinician must decide whether speech–language pathology treatment is appropriate for a particular client. Not all children or adults tested for an articulation or phonological disorder require clinical intervention. In essence, there are four possible scenarios that can help the clinician decide whether speech–language pathology treatment should be recommended or provided:

- *The child has* _normal articulation or phonological_ *skills and thus* _treatment is not recommended_.
The child's errors may be within normal developmental limits, they may be related to linguistic or dialectical differences, or they may be so subtle that the child's social, vocational, or academic life is not significantly affected. In such cases, treatment should not be recommended. However, some clients with dialectical differences or subtle articulation errors may feel handicapped by what they consider a "disorder." In such cases, the clinician may need to reconsider his or her recommendations.

- *The child's articulation skills appear to be following the* _normal course of development_, *and therefore* _treatment is not recommended_. *However, a reassessment after a specified period of time may be warranted.*
Some children may be following the normal course of development, and thus treatment is not recommended during the initial evaluation. However, the clinician may recommend that the child's articulation and phonological skills be reevaluated to ensure that indeed the errors were developmental rather than disordered. This type of recommendation is most common with young children who are still in the developmental process and who the clinician suspects may simply need time to fully acquire an adult phonological system. This recommendation would be inappropriate with older children, since most children can be expected to have adultlike articulation and phonological skills by 8 or 9 years of age. The clinician may recommend that the child's articulation and phonological skills be reevaluated 3, 6, 9, or 12 months after the initial evaluation. New diagnostic decisions and treatment recommendations may be made at that time.

- *The child has an* _articulation or phonological disorder_, *but* _treatment is not recommended_.
Although the above statement may seem contradictory, there are occasions when a client indeed has an articulation or phonological disorder but the clinician may decide against recommending treatment. An example would be a young child with an unrepaired cleft palate whose articulation errors result from his or her structural anomalies. Although a disorder is present, speech–language pathology services may be contraindicated until the child's cleft is surgically repaired. A clinician may also choose not to recommend treatment if a client has a clinical history of poor motivation, limited improvement, or a poor prognosis for improvement. The case scenarios leading to this recommendation are too vast to summarize, but the clinician should be prepared for this clinical situation.

- *The child has an <u>articulation or phonological disorder</u> and <u>treatment is recommended</u>.*

If the clinician decides that the client indeed has an articulation disorder and treatment is appropriate, other more specific recommendations should also be made. For example, the clinician should decide how often the client will receive clinical services and how long the sessions will last. Often, the clinician has very little control over this decision, since his or her place of employment may have set policies. For example, in an outpatient clinic clients are often provided services three times a week and sessions generally last 45 minutes. In university clinics services are arranged twice a week, and the clinic director often decides on the length of sessions.

The clinician also needs to determine which sounds or phonological skills will be targeted in therapy. The target behavior selection process is outlined in great detail in the Basic Unit of Chapter 7. If appropriate, other recommendations may be made, such as referral to an otolaryngologist, orthodontist, medical doctor, audiologist, or speech–language pathologist who has a particular specialty.

Conducting an Information-Giving Interview

After the assessment has been completed, it is important to conduct a **closing interview,** which is also known as an **information-giving interview,** with the client and the client's caregivers. During the interview, the findings of the assessment process are discussed and the clinician makes specific recommendations. The information-giving interview is typically conducted in person, but there are occasions when it must be done over the telephone. It is important to review the information in a clear and concise fashion that is understandable to the client and/or the caregiver. The use of technical jargon should be avoided, and illustrations may be used to facilitate understanding of a complicated issue. Like the opening interview, the information-giving interview typically consists of three phases: an *opening,* the *body,* and a *closing* (Shipley, 1992).

In the opening phase of the interview, the clinician introduces the purpose of the meeting, indicates how much time the session will take, reports whether adequate information was obtained during the assessment, and describes the client's behavior during the assessment (if reporting to caregivers).

The major findings and conclusions from the assessment are reported in the body of the interview. Specific recommendations are made. The clinician must remember to use understandable language, being careful to avoid technical jargon. If technical terms must be used, it is important that the clinician define those terms in simple language. The clinician should emphasize the major points so that the listener is able to understand and retain the information presented. Again, visual illustrations should be used if needed to simplify complicated information.

During the closing phase the clinician summarizes the major findings, conclusions, and recommendations discussed during the body of the interview. It is important that the clinician ask if the listener has any further questions, thank the listener for his or her help and interest, and describe the next steps that will need to be taken according to the recommendations that have been made. A closing interview may proceed as follows when the three phases are considered.

- *Opening Phase of the Information-Giving Interview:*
"First of all, I'd like you to know that I really enjoyed working with Stephanie

today. She is a delightful little girl, and she worked very hard for me. I feel that I was able to get all of the information I needed. Now, I'd like to spend the next 20 to 30 minutes with you to discuss my findings and my recommendations."

- *Body of the Information-Giving Interview:*

"Mrs. Williams, from the testing I did with Stephanie, I was able to confirm that she indeed has significant difficulty producing many sounds. Since you brought your daughter in for testing, I'm sure that this doesn't surprise you. The specific disorder that your daughter demonstrated is often called an articulation disorder. What this means is that she substitutes some sounds for other sounds, leaves certain sounds out of her words, or distorts sounds. Stephanie had the most difficulty making the *f, v, s, z, sh, ch, th, r,* and *l* sounds. Because she is not able to make all of the appropriate sounds, she is a bit difficult to understand. I felt that I understood about 50% of what she says, which is in agreement with how much you are able to understand.

"I don't believe that Stephanie would outgrow these errors on her own, and if she does, it may take a long time. I'm concerned that her social interactions and academic performance may be affected by her sound errors. Therefore, I'm recommending that she receive speech–language pathology services. The goal of therapy would be to teach her specific sounds so that she becomes easier to understand. I recommend that she receive therapy three times a week for about 30 to 40 minutes per session. Although I cannot guarantee how well she will do or how long it will take for her to become more understandable, I believe that her prognosis is good because she is so young, she seems very motivated, and she doesn't have any language or behavioral problems that could get in the way of her learning. Also, you seem very interested to help her at home. I cannot overly emphasize the importance of parent involvement in therapy. In general, children whose parents take an active role in the therapy process tend to do better than children whose parents are not involved. I will guide your involvement in therapy."

- *Closing Phase:*

"Again, from my testing, I found that Stephanie has an articulation disorder. She is not able to make many sounds that she would be expected to make at her age. A good sign though is that she was able to make all of the sounds with probing. For example, when I showed her how to do so, she made the /s/ sound in words like *sun* perfectly. I again emphasize that I cannot tell you how long it will take for Stephanie to learn to make all her sounds. We need to take it one step at a time. But I will keep you informed about her progress frequently and will also involve you in therapy when appropriate. Do you have any questions about what I have discussed? I really appreciate all of the information you shared with me and all of your help. I will call you on Monday to arrange a schedule for Stephanie's therapy. Is there a time and day that would work best for you?"

Writing a Diagnostic Report

Once the assessment has been completed and a diagnosis has been made, the clinician writes a diagnostic report summarizing all of the relevant information. The diagnostic report provides written documentation of the clinical findings and the treatment recommendations. Because the clinical report becomes an official, and sometimes legal, document, it is important that the clinician devote quality time for its preparation. Also, other professionals often gain some perspective of the clinician's knowledge and competence from the diagnostic report. Reports containing several grammatical errors, a poor style, and confusing wording may leave a negative impression on the reader.

The exact format, style, length, and degree of detail of clinical reports frequently vary from setting to setting. For example, diagnostic reports written in the university setting are much lengthier and more detailed than those written in any other clinical setting. Our own experience in various clinical settings has given us firsthand knowledge of the vast differences in the way diagnostic reports are written. Across settings, diagnostic reports may vary from formatted check-off lists, to one-paragraph reports, to six-page reports. The clinician should be flexible and adhere to the regulations of his or her university program or work setting.

It should be emphasized, however, that although the length, format, and style of reports do vary from one setting to another, general principles of good writing should be followed. The reader is referred to Hegde (1998a) for a thorough review of scientific and professional writing in speech–language pathology. Also, diagnostic reports share common features. Regardless of the degree of detail, most reports include the following general categories: identifying information, background information, histories, assessment information, diagnostic statement, and treatment recommendations. The reader is referred to Appendix J for sample diagnostic reports.

Summary of the Basic Unit

- An **assessment** is the process that is followed and the procedures that are used to establish the presence or absence of a disorder and to describe any associated factors. The clinician's judgment about whether a disorder does or does not exist and a description of its nature leads to a clinical **diagnosis.**

- An assessment is only the first step in the diagnostic process. It is the initial step, in which clinical data are collected. These data are then analyzed and interpreted.

- There are various prerequisites to performing an adequate articulation and phonological assessment, including knowledge of the anatomy and physiology of the speech mechanism, knowledge of phonetics, and knowledge of dialectical variations.

- Some general procedures in the assessment of articulation and phonological disorders include reviewing the client's background, planning the assessment session, selecting appropriate testing instruments, making recommendations, and writing a diagnostic report.

- An **articulation or phonological screening** is a pass or fail procedure that helps the clinician determine whether a more thorough assessment is warranted. Screenings are intended to be quick and can usually be completed in 10 to 15 minutes. Screenings for articulation or phonological disorders can be performed with children in preschool, kindergarten, or third grade. They may also be conducted with students preparing for specific voice-dependent professions or with referred clients. Screening can be a formal or informal procedure.

- A **case history** is important to determine any information related to a potential articulation or phonological disorder. A thorough case history can be obtained by collecting a written case history, reviewing information written by other professionals, and conducting oral interviews with the client or the client's parents. The **information-getting** or **opening interview** consists of three phases: **opening phase, body,** and **closing phase.**

• An **orofacial examination** helps the clinician determine if there are any underlying structural, sensory, or neurological problems that could account for the articulation or phonological disorder. The orofacial examination helps the clinician distinguish functional articulation disorders from organic articulation disorders. Diadochokinetic testing is typically a part of the thorough orofacial examination.

• An **audiological screening** is usually a part of the assessment of articulation and phonological disorders. It helps determine the client's auditory function and identify any potential peripheral hearing loss. The hearing screening is conducted at 500, 1,000, 2,000, 4,000 Hz at 25 dB HL.

• The child's speech productions can be assessed by **standardized articulation tests** and **phonological processes tests.** The clinician can record errors using three methods: correct/incorrect, type of error, and whole-word transcription. The first provides minimal clinical information; the second is commonly used when a child has a few sound production errors; and the last is most often used to determine rules or patterns in production.

• Children's articulation and phonological skills are also assessed in **conversational speech.** The clinician collects a representative speech sample. In general, children display more errors in conversational speech than in single-word productions.

• **Stimulability testing** helps the clinician determine whether the client can make a correct or improved production of the error sounds when given a model or additional stimulation (e.g., tactile, visual, auditory, and kinesthetic cues).

• The clinician can perform **contextual testing** to determine if any facilitative phonetic contexts can be identified that evoke correct production of an error sound. The clinician can use informal procedures or formal testing instruments such as the *Deep Test of Articulation* or *Clinical Probes of Articulation Consistency*.

• The clinician conducts **auditory discrimination testing** with children who are suspected of having auditory or speech discrimination problems that may be affecting the articulation of specific sounds.

• After all relevant assessment information has been collected, the clinician analyzes the various data. The clinician can perform an independent analysis or relational analysis. In an **independent analysis** the child's speech productions are described without reference to the adult model. In a **relational analysis** the clinician compares the child's productions to the adult model and determines error types or patterns of production.

• The clinician can perform a **traditional analysis** according to the types of errors in initial-, medial-, and final-word positions. This method of analysis is appropriate with children who exhibit a few articulation errors. A **pattern analysis** may be performed with children who have multiple misarticulations. A place-voicing-manner, distinctive feature, or phonological processes analysis may be performed.

• The clinician analyzes all relevant information such as that obtained during oro-facial examination, stimulability testing, and contextual testing.

• The clinician determines the client's **speech intelligibility** and makes a clinical judgment of **severity.**

• After analyzing and interpreting all of the relevant data, the clinician makes a clinical **diagnosis,** determines the **prognosis** for improvement, and makes specific **treatment recommendations.**

• The clinician then conducts an **information-giving** or **closing interview** with the client or the client's parents and follows up with a written **diagnostic report.**

Advanced Unit

♦　♦　♦　♦　♦　♦　♦　♦　♦　♦　♦　♦　♦　♦　♦　♦　♦　♦

Description and Assessment of Various Organic and Neurogenic Speech Disorders

I n the Basic Unit of this chapter we addressed the various components of a thorough assessment. Various principles of assessment were reviewed that can be successfully applied to various speech disorders. In this Advanced Unit, we will briefly consider the assessment of various speech problems associated with specific disorders or special populations: apraxia of speech, developmental apraxia of speech, dysarthria, cerebral palsy, cleft palate, and hearing impairment. In general, these disorders are associated with structural, sensory, or neurological variables that can help explain their presence.

Our intent is not to offer an exhaustive presentation of the special procedures that can be used in the assessment of these disorders. That would be impossible to do in a single chapter. Rather, we would like to introduce the reader to various organic or neurogenic speech disorders that will in all likelihood be further addressed in other courses in speech–language pathology. For example, the assessment and treatment of speech disorders associated with cleft palate are typically addressed in a graduate seminar focusing on the study of craniofacial anomalies; the assessment and treatment of apraxia and dysarthria may be addressed in a graduate seminar on motor speech disorders.

The format of this unit varies somewhat from that of previous chapters. We provide a definition for each disorder, outline some information related to its etiology, describe the assessment objectives, and discuss some assessment techniques or procedures that can be used with each disorder. Because our goal is to keep what could become very complicated information understandable and easy to read, we have chosen to use a sort of outline format with frequent bullets. The reader is referred to the Advanced Unit of Chapter 1 for a review of the anatomy and neuroanatomy of speech production.

Apraxia of Speech in Adults

Definition of Apraxia of Speech

Apraxia of speech is a motor programming disorder resulting from neurological damage. It is characterized by a difficulty in the execution of volitional movements in the absence of muscular weakness, paralysis, or incoordination. The person with apraxia has adequate muscle strength, but brain damage creates problems in the programming of skilled, smooth, and deliberate motor movements. The lack of muscle weakness, paralysis, or incoordination differentiates apraxia of speech from **dysarthria.** Dysarthria results from disturbances of muscle control due to weakness, paralysis, or incoordination that interfere with one or more of the speech parameters (i.e., respiration, phonation, resonance, articulation, and prosody).

Three types of apraxia that affect the motor movements important for speech and communication have been described in the literature: oral apraxia, limb apraxia, and verbal apraxia (Shipley & McAfee, 1998; Love & Webb, 1996). In **oral apraxia,** the client has problems executing volitional nonspeech movements of the oral muscles. For example, the client may be able to stick out his or her tongue automatically (nonvolitional) to lick an ice cream cone, but when asked to pretend to lick an ice cream cone (volitional), the motor programming problems become evident.

Limb apraxia is characterized by volitional movement difficulties of the arms and legs. The client, for instance, may have trouble waving good-bye or picking up a spoon on command despite having the necessary muscular strength. **Apraxia of speech,** also known as **verbal apraxia,** is an impaired ability to program and execute volitional movements for the production of phonemes and words. Verbal apraxia may occur singly or in combination with oral and limb apraxia. If a client exhibits characteristics of oral apraxia, there is typically a concomitant verbal apraxia. However, a client with verbal apraxia may or may not have an accompanying oral apraxia. Shipley and McAfee (1998) indicate that apraxia of speech is the most common type of apraxia, while limb apraxia is the least common. Thus, our discussion of etiology and assessment information will be limited to apraxia of speech.

Etiology and Nature of Apraxia of Speech

Apraxia of speech is most often caused by neurological damage in the dominant cerebral hemisphere for speech and language, which is the left hemisphere for most people. Although there is controversy about the exact site of lesion leading to apraxia of speech, the most probable site of damage is the third frontal convolution of the left hemisphere. This area is known as **Broca's area,** which is also associated with language expression. Thus, apraxia of speech is often accompanied by **aphasia,** an acquired language disorder. Recently, damage to the **insular lobe** (island of Reil) and the parietal lobe has also been implicated in apraxia of speech (Love & Webb, 1996; Bhatnagar & Andy, 1995). Although the exact site of lesion is not known, it is generally accepted that a lesion leading to apraxia of speech is not discrete.

The most common etiology of the neurological damage leading to apraxia of speech (about 58% of cases) is a single left hemisphere stroke (Hegde, 1996a). Other etiologies include:

- degenerative diseases such as **multiple sclerosis, primary progressive aphasia,** and **Creutzfeldt-Jakob disease;**
- traumatic injury to the left hemisphere during a motor vehicle accident;
- surgical trauma to the left hemisphere during tumor removal, **aneurysm** repair, or **hemorrhage** evacuation;

- tumors present in the left hemisphere; and

- seizure disorder.

In about 4% of cases the etiology is undetermined (Hegde, 1996a).

The specific characteristics associated with apraxia of speech vary from client to client. However, there are some **salient** features that help the clinician differentially diagnose apraxia from other **neuromotor speech disorders.** Not all clients exhibit all of the possible symptoms, and the severity of the disorder may range from mild to profound in relation to its effect on verbal communication. Speech production errors associated with apraxia of speech primarily affect articulation and prosody. Hegde (1996a) summarizes these characteristics as follows (adapted from information on pp. 57–60):

General Characteristics

- The client displays good awareness of the speech problems. The client is often surprised and frustrated by his or her errors.

- Volitional sequencing of movements required for speech are notably affected.

- **Automatic speech** (e.g., counting, reciting the alphabet, social greetings, singing a familiar tune, and so forth) is much less affected than spontaneous or **volitional speech.**

- The client displays highly variable speech errors. Different kinds of errors occur on repeated attempts. The same word may be produced correctly on one occasion but incorrectly on subsequent trials.

- Some clients display the use of a reduced rate of speech, which usually develops as a self-discovered compensatory strategy for improved speech production.

Articulation Errors

- Substitutions, distortions, and omissions of speech sounds are observed. Substitutions are the most common type of articulation errors, although all types of errors can occur. Some errors perceived as substitutions may actually be severe sound distortions.

- The greatest number of substitutions involves place of articulation errors. Manner of production, voicing, and oral/nasal distinctions are less frequently observed, usually in that order.

- There are fewer errors on bilabial and lingua-alveolar consonants than on other sound classes according to place of articulation.

- There are more errors on fricatives and affricates than on other sound classes according to manner of production.

- There are more errors on consonant clusters than on singleton consonants.

- Vowel errors are less frequent than consonant errors, although they occur in some clients.

- **Anticipatory substitutions** (when a phoneme that occurs later in the word affects one that occurs earlier) may be observed. Examples include "tat" for *cat,* "pospital" for *hospital,* and "nen" for *men.*

- **Regressive substitutions** (when a phoneme that occurs earlier in the word affects one that occurs later) may be observed. Examples include "tatle" for *table,* "dred" for *dress,* and "parp" for *park.*

- **Metathetic errors** or the switched position of phonemes in words can occur. Examples include "tephelone" for *telephone,* "amulinum" for *aluminum,* and "Fran Sancisco" for *San Francisco.*

- The number and frequency of errors increase as the linguistic complexity of the productions increases.

- Delayed initiation of speech can be observed.

- There is usually trial-and-error **groping,** searching, and struggling behavior associated with speech attempts. This becomes most evident during spontaneous or volitional speech.

- The initial position of sounds may be more difficult than other word positions.

- There is a higher frequency of errors on infrequently occurring sounds.

- Nonsense syllables are more difficult for the client to produce than meaningful words.

- The client typically displays attempts at **self-correction,** although they are frequently unsuccessful. This may contribute to groping behaviors and **false starts.**

- Impaired imitation of modeled words occurs in some cases; in most cases, imitative performance may be comparable to, or better than, spontaneous production.

Prosodic Problems

- A reduced rate of speech is generally observed.

- The client has difficulty in increasing or changing the rate of speech when instructed.

- Silent pauses between words may be observed.

- There is an increased duration in the production of consonants and vowels.

- The client may exhibit even stress on syllables.

- The combination of prosodic problems may limit variations in intonation. The client's speech may have a **monotone** quality

- There is an even loudness of speech or a restricted range of intensity.

- There is a restricted range of pitch.

- Overall dysprosody may be observed.

- Silent pauses occur, especially when speech is to be initiated.

- Repetitions due to **false starts** and attempts to correct articulatory errors are observed.

- The client's speech problem may be perceived as a foreign accent because of the differences in prosody.

Assessment Objectives for Apraxia of Speech

There are multiple objectives in the assessment of apraxia of speech. These include the following:

1. To assess the client's articulatory proficiency in volitional or purposeful speech.

2. To assess the client's prosodic skills.

3. To assess other communication skills including the client's auditory comprehension, verbal expression, and reading and writing skills. Assessment of these skills will help the clinician develop a client-specific plan of treatment.

4. To distinguish apraxia of speech from other motor speech disorders including dysarthria and neurogenic fluency disorders.

5. To distinguish apraxia of speech from neurogenic language disorders including aphasia and **dementia.**

6. To identify potential treatment targets and possible compensatory communication strategies.

7. To make a clinical judgment of prognosis.

8. To describe the client's strengths and intact skills. This will help the clinician develop a plan of treatment that capitalizes on what the client can do.

9. To suggest potential **neuropathology.** This may be extremely beneficial in determining medical treatment of the underlying etiology if the cause of the neurological damage leading to apraxia of speech is not already known.

Assessing Clients with Apraxia of Speech

In the assessment of apraxia of speech, the clinician can follow some of the general procedures outlined in the Basic Unit of this chapter. However, there are some other procedures and activities appropriate for diagnosing apraxia of speech in clients who are suspected of having this speech disorder. For example, because clients with apraxia of speech display particular difficulty on diadochokinetic testing, the clinician can devote ample time to that procedure and note any specific characteristics of apraxia that become evident (e.g., metathetic sound errors, anticipatory errors, grouping of the articulators, and false starts). The clinician can also pay special attention to the client's production errors on automatic speech tasks and imitative tasks, bearing in mind that clients with apraxia of speech typically show greater difficulty on imitative speech tasks.

The clinician can start by collecting a spontaneous speech sample to assess the client's articulatory performance in connected speech productions. The sample should be tape-recorded for later analysis since it may be difficult to identify all of the symptoms while collecting the sample. The clinician should pay special attention to any struggling, groping, or searching behaviors that may suggest motor programming problems. Repetitions, other forms of dysfluencies, delayed reaction time, attempts at self-correction, facial grimacing, and articulatory errors should also be noted.

Next, the clinician can ask the client to perform a variety of tasks progressing from simple to complex, as in the following lists. The activities are purposely arranged to overwork the client's speech system so that the characteristics of apraxia, if present, become apparent. (The tasks in the first list may need to be modified so that they are ethnoculturally sensitive. For example, recent immigrants may not know "Happy Birthday" or the "Pledge of Allegiance").

Assess Production of Automatic Speech Tasks

- *Instruct the client:* "Please count to 20."

- *Instruct the client:* "Please name the days of the week starting with Sunday."

- *Instruct the client:* "Please name the months of the year starting with January."

- *Instruct the client:* "Please sing 'Happy Birthday to You.'"

- *Instruct the client:* "Please say the 'Pledge of Allegiance.'"

Assess Imitative Production of a Single Speech Sound

- *Instruct the client:* "Please say /a/ as long and as evenly as you can." Model the response for the client to imitate, "Do it like me . . ."

- *Instruct the client:* "Please say /i/ as long and as evenly as you can." Model the response for the client to imitate, "Do it like me . . ."

Assess Diadochokinetic Alternating and Sequential Motion Rates (AMRs and SMRs)

- *Instruct the client:* "Please say [pʌ-pʌ-pʌ] as long and as evenly as you can." Model the response for the client to imitate, "Try doing it like me . . ." (AMRs)

- *Instruct the client:* "Please say [tʌ-tʌ-tʌ] as long and as evenly as you can." Model the response for the client to imitate, "Try doing it like me . . ." (AMRs)

- *Instruct the client:* "Please say [kʌ-kʌ-kʌ] as long and as evenly as you can." Model the response for the client to imitate, "Try it like me . . ." (AMRs)

- *Instruct the client:* "Please say [pʌ-tə-kə] as long and as evenly as you can." Model the response for the client to imitate, "Try it like me . . ." (SMRs)

Assess Imitative Production of Single Words

- Select words that represent all of the English consonants in at least one position.

- *Instruct the client:* "Please repeat these words after me":

hot	love	pop	back	hope	cat	lamp	night	dog	store	men	fire
good	jail	red	soft	take	vest	wet	your	zebra	ant	door	eel

Assess Imitative Production of Multisyllable Words
(Wertz, LaPointe, & Rosenbek, 1991)

- *Instruct the client:* "Please repeat these words after me":

several	television	refrigeration	*Encyclopedia Britannica*
tornado	catastrophe	responsibility	Boston, Massachusetts

artillery	gingerbread	unequivocally	Minneapolis, Minnesota
linoleum	probability	parliamentarian	San Francisco, California
snowman	thermometer	statistical analysis	regulatory commission

Assess Imitative Production of Words of Increasing Length
(Shipley & McAfee, 1998)

- *Instruct the client:* "Please repeat these words after me":
  - love–loving–lovingly
  - please–pleasing–pleasingly
  - jab–jabber–jabbering
  - zip–zipper–zippering
  - soft–soften–softening
  - hope–hopeful–hopefully
  - strength–strengthen–strengthening

Assess Repeated, Imitative Production of Words
(score each production) (Wertz, LaPointe, & Rosenbek, 1991)

- *Instruct the client:* "Repeat the word I say five times. I'll say it first, and then you repeat it five times":
  - artillery
  - impossibility
  - disenfranchised
  - catastrophically
  - disenchanted

Assess Imitative Production of Sentences
(Wertz, LaPointe, & Rosenbek, 1991)

- *Instruct the client:* "I'm going to say some sentences. I want you to repeat them after me. If you need me to say the sentence over, please ask me to do so before you get started":
  - The valuable watch was missing.
  - In the summer they sell vegetables.
  - The shipwreck washed up on the shore.
  - Please put the groceries in the refrigerator.
  - Please tell the gardener to fertilize the plants.
  - I do not understand the reasons for repeating it.

Standardized tests available for the diagnosis of apraxia include the *Apraxia Battery for Adults* (Dabul, 1986), the *Comprehensive Apraxia Test* (DiSimoni, 1989), and the *Test of Oral and Limb Apraxia* (Helm-Estabrooks, 1992). The diagnosis of apraxia of speech is made when some neuropathology is identified and the client displays speech programming difficulties with inconsistent errors, groping and struggling behavior during speech production, notable difficulties in spontaneous and volitional speech versus automatic speech, and prosodic problems. The severity of the disorder may range from mild to profound.

Developmental Apraxia of Speech

Definition of Developmental Apraxia of Speech

The childhood equivalent of apraxia of speech is known as **developmental apraxia of speech** (DAS). This childhood developmental speech disorder is also termed **developmental verbal apraxia** (DVA). Although this diagnostic label has quickly made its way into the repertoires of many clinicians, it is not without controversy.

The label *developmental apraxia of speech* is a borrowed term from the adult-acquired neuromotor speech disorder we described earlier. Many researchers find it difficult to accept DAS as a neuromotor speech disorder because to date no neurological lesions have been documented that could help explain the speech production problems in children diagnosed with developmental apraxia of speech. In adults, apraxia of speech is a known manifestation of lesions to Broca's area and the sensorimotor cortex in the left hemisphere, and thus is widely accepted as a neurological disorder.

The use of the term developmental apraxia of speech with young children emerged primarily as a descriptive diagnosis. Some researchers and clinicians noted that a specified group of children with articulation disorders demonstrated similar symptoms to those of adults with apraxia of speech. Several similarities and differences have been advanced between the childhood and adult disorders (e.g., Rosenbek & Wertz, 1972). However, Hall, Jordan, and Robin (1993) indicate that in their clinical experience, "the most important similarity that exists between the groups, and between the individuals within the groups, is the lack of volitional control of the oral mechanism for speech production" (p. 3).

We are not against the use of the term developmental apraxia of speech or developmental verbal apraxia so long as they are employed as *descriptive* diagnostic labels. The appropriate use of the term can indeed be beneficial in meeting the assessment and treatment needs of this special group of children. However, we fervently disagree with the use of the label as an indicator of etiology or associated neuropathology. Simply because a group of children presents with similar speech characteristics to those found in adults with a known neurological disorder does not imply that the cause of their disorder is also neurogenic based. Clinicians need to be careful not to make such ungrounded speculations and inadvertently communicate that as the cause of the disorder to significant others, parents, and other professionals involved in the child's life. Perhaps as neuroimaging technology becomes even more sophisticated and as even subtle changes in the human brain can be detected, our understanding of the disorder will change. However, considering our current knowledge, the label DAS should be used with caution.

Etiology and Nature of Developmental Apraxia of Speech

Developmental apraxia of speech is essentially a childhood articulation disorder of unknown etiology. Although it is defined as a disorder of motor control, the underlying neurological cause for the associated symptoms has not been advanced to date (Velleman & Strand, 1994). Many of the potential causes are admittedly theoretical (Hall, Jordan, & Robin, 1993). Developmental apraxia of speech may be found in children with several associated disabilities, including mental retardation, cerebral palsy, global developmental delay, attention deficit disorder, and sensorineural hearing loss (Hegde, 1996a).

The speech characteristics associated with developmental apraxia of speech are at times inconsistent and contradictory from one source to another. Also, some of the characteristics on which the diagnosis is made are not unique to DAS since they can be used to diagnose children with functional articulation and phonological disorders (Hall et al., 1993). In our review of the existing literature on this topic, Hall et al. (1993) appeared to offer one of the most extensive reviews of the speech characteristics most often associated with DAS. The information that follows is a summarized presentation of their thorough examination (adapted from pp. 9–48).

Speech Characteristics

• Moderate to severe speech intelligibility problems.

• Connected speech productions that are more unintelligible than would be expected based on the child's performance in single-word tests.

• Variable speech intelligibility depending on the length and complexity of the utterances.

• Range of severity of the disorder on a continuum of mild to severe. An estimate of severity may depend on several variables, including the child's intelligibility, level of stimulability, change over time, degree of developmental lag, and ability to control the environment through the use of speech.

• Inconsistent or variable sound errors when the same word is produced on repeated trials. Inconsistency is an important diagnostic variable.

• Unusual articulation errors, which are defined as errors that are not usually found in children with functional articulation disorders or normal articulation. These include:

> • addition errors (e.g., /gərin/ for *green,* /klæt/ for *cat,* and /kwink/ for *queen*);
>
> • prolongation errors (e.g., /be:by/ for *baby* and /s:ʌn/ for *sun*);
>
> • production of sounds that are nonphonemic in English (e.g., glottal plosives and bilabial fricatives); and
>
> • repetition of sounds and syllables.

• Usual or typical errors of articulation, which are defined as errors that may also occur in children with functional articulation disorders or in the normal acquisition process. These include:

> • predominance of omission and substitution errors, although distortion and addition errors also occur and distortion errors may predominate in some older children;
>
> • errors more common on fricatives, affricates, and consonant clusters;
>
> • possibility of developmental errors on fricatives and affricates continuing longer than in children with functional articulation problems or normal articulation;
>
> • voicing and devoicing errors; and

- vowel omissions and misarticulations, which are characterized primarily by distorted vowels and diphthong reduction.

• Resonance problems, which may be characterized by hyponasality, hypernasality, or nasal emission. These problems are likely due to poor motor control of the velopharyngeal mechanism.

• Prosodic problems manifested by **aprosody** (flat prosody) in some children, **dysprosody** (presence of variation in frequency and duration, but inappropriate use of them) in some children, and the inappropriate use of stress patterns.

• Increased frequency of dysfluencies, although information on specific types and their frequencies is not available. Dysfluencies may be related to associated linguistic problems or the presence of groping and searching behavior.

Sound and Syllable Sequencing Problems

• Difficulty producing sounds in correct sequence.

• Difficulty sequencing the sounds in syllables or words, even if the individual phonemes are within the child's phonetic inventory.

• Increased difficulty in producing multisyllabic words.

• Difficulty in sequencing phonemes on diadochokinetic speech tasks.

• An increase in the number of sequencing errors as the complexity or length of the utterance within a speech task increases.

• **Metathetic** or sound reversal errors (e.g., /mæks/ for *mask* and /ʃɪf/ for *fish*).

Groping Behaviors and Silent Posturing

• Silent posturing errors, which are defined as static articulatory postures without sound production. For example, although the child may position the lips for articulation of /b/, no sound is associated with the production.

• Groping errors, which are an active and ongoing series of movements of the articulators in an attempt to find the appropriate placement or position for the production of a sound or sounds.

• Silent posturing and groping may not be present in all children diagnosed with DAS. They may be more commonly observed in older school-age children.

• Groping and searching behavior may become evident during diadochokinetic testing.

Associated Problems

• Generally slow progress in therapy.

• **"Soft" neurological signs** often presumed from the child's fine- and gross-motor incoordination.

• Presence of oral apraxia or difficulty with volitional nonspeech tasks.

• Slowed **diadochokinetic syllable rates.**

• Decreased oral awareness (**oral astereognosis**).

- Expressive language problems, with relatively better receptive language skills.
- Associated learning disability in some children.
- Family history of speech and language problems in some children.

Assessment Objectives for Developmental Apraxia of Speech

As with adult apraxia of speech, there are multiple objectives in the assessment of developmental apraxia of speech. These include the following:

1. To assess the child's articulation skills and speech intelligibility across varied tasks and situations.
2. To assess other communication skills, including the child's auditory comprehension, verbal expression, and reading and writing skills. Assessment of these skills will help the clinician develop a client-specific plan of treatment.
3. To assess other aspects of communication including resonance, prosody, and fluency.
4. To assess the child's oral motor skills during speech and nonspeech tasks.
5. To describe the nature of the child's speech production problems and make an estimate of severity.
6. To distinguish developmental apraxia of speech from other speech disorders such as a functional articulation disorder or a phonological disorder.
7. To identify potential treatment targets and possible compensatory communication strategies.
8. To make a clinical judgment of prognosis.
9. To describe the client's strengths and intact skills. This will help the clinician develop a plan of treatment that capitalizes on what the client can do.

Assessment Techniques for the Diagnosis of Developmental Apraxia of Speech

In the assessment of apraxia of speech, the clinician can follow some of the general procedures outlined in the Basic Unit of this chapter. Some procedures and activities are more appropriate for diagnosing developmental apraxia of speech in children who are suspected of having this speech disorder. Many of these are similar to those described under "Apraxia of Speech in Adults." Haynes (1985, p. 261) recommends that the clinician minimally assess the following parameters:

- expressive and receptive language skills;
- articulatory proficiency, including simple and complex isolated phonemes, polysyllabic words, and connected speech utterances;
- oral diadochokinetic syllable rates;
- volitional nonspeech movements of the oral muscles, both in isolation and in sequence; and
- orosensory perception and oral awareness.

After collecting a thorough case history and screening the child's hearing, the clinician can start the actual assessment by collecting a spontaneous speech sample to assess the child's articulatory performance in connected speech productions. The sample should be tape-recorded for later analysis since it may be difficult to identify all of the symptoms at the time of the assessment. Because the child with DAS often presents nonphonemic or atypical errors, Hall et al. (1993) recommend that clinicians "hone their listening and transcribing skills to accurately record the productions they are assessing" (p. 16). As with apraxia of speech in adults, the clinician should pay special attention to any struggling, groping, and searching behavior that may be suggestive of motor programming problems. Sound prolongations, other forms of dysfluencies, delayed reaction time, silent postures, attempts at self-correction, and articulatory errors should also be noted.

The clinician can then ask the client to perform a variety of activities such as those in the following lists. Such activities have been designed to help the clinician differentially diagnose developmental apraxia of speech from other types of articulation or phonological disorders in children by evaluating specific skills.

Assess Nonimitative Speech Production Skills

• Obtain nonimitative productions of a set of single words that sample all phonemes. The clinician may use object- or picture-naming tasks or a standardized articulation test (e.g., *Goldman-Fristoe Test of Articulation* or *Test of Minimal Articulation Competence*) to evoke nonimitative productions. Stimulus materials should be readily identifiable and appropriate for the child's age to decrease the need for modeling by the clinician.

> ▶ **Examples:**
>
> pen baby dog fire gum horse cat light mop nose table soap

• Phonetically transcribe the utterances and speech sound errors. Make **whole-word transcriptions** to identify any patterns in production errors or coarticulatory errors (e.g., anticipatory errors, regressive errors, metathetic errors).

• Observe and record any signs of speech motor programming problems (e.g., groping, dysfluencies, false starts, struggling behavior).

• Observe and record speech production problems as the length of the word increases.

• Use stimulus materials described under "Apraxia of Speech in Adults" and modify the materials to suit the child or use parallel stimulus items selected from the child's vocabulary.

Assess Imitative Speech Production Skills

• Model individual sounds and syllables and ask the child to imitate them.

• Initially, hide your oral movements; if the child cannot imitate, show the normal movements.

• Model a series of shorter or longer words and ask the child to imitate them.

▶ **Examples:**

bat	expensive
hat	attacking
coat	cafeteria
bed	playground
look	computer
fast	principal

• Model a series of shorter or longer sentences and ask the child to imitate them.

▶ **Examples:**

The cat is big.	The cat in the box is black and white.
My mom is nice.	My mother gave me a present for my birthday.
Who wants cake?	I asked everyone, "Who wants chocolate cake?"
I like candy.	My favorite candy is milk chocolate.
I have a toy.	Yesterday, I bought a toy car at the toy store.

Assess the Consistency and Variability of Errors

• Sample speech productions in varied phonetic contexts. The clinician may arrange informal tasks or may administer formal instruments such as the *Deep Test of Articulation* (McDonald, 1964) or *Clinical Probes of Articulation Consistency* (Secord, 1981a).

• Sample speech production in imitative and spontaneous modes. The clinician may identify the words the child produces spontaneously and then ask the client to imitate the same words. Any differences in production are noted.

• Sample production of the same phoneme (in the same word) in multiple trials. Any articulatory differences in the production of the sound from one trial to the other are recorded.

Assess Diadochokinetic Syllable Rates, Including Alternating and Sequential Motion Rates (AMRs and SMRs)

• *Instruct the child:* "Please say [pʌ-pʌ-pʌ] as long and as evenly as you can." Model the response for the client to imitate, "Try doing it like me . . ." (AMRs)

• *Instruct the child:* "Please say [tʌ-tʌ-tʌ] as long and as evenly as you can." Model the response for the client to imitate, "Try doing it like me . . ." (AMRs)

• *Instruct the child:* "Please say [kʌ-kʌ-kʌ] as long and as evenly as you can." Model the response for the client to imitate, "Try it like me . . ." (AMRs)

• *Instruct the child:* "Please say [pʌ-tə-kə] as long and as evenly as you can." Model the response for the client to imitate, "Try it like me . . ." (SMRs). The word *buttercup* may be substituted for [pʌ-tə-kə] with children who have difficulty following through with repetition of [pʌ-tə-kə].

• Record any groping or struggling behaviors observed during this task. Then compare the scores obtained for a particular child with established developmental data for the production of diadochokinetic syllable rates in children (Fletcher, 1972, 1978).

Assess Intelligibility of Speech

• Assess intelligibility from the conversational speech sample; use the procedures described in the Basic Unit of this chapter.

• Assess intelligibility at different levels (syllables, words, phrases, and sentences).

Assess Resonance Problems

• Assess hypernasality, hyponasality, and nasal emission by clinical judgment.

• Use a mirror to judge nasal emission in the production of nonnasal sounds.

• Visually inspect the velopharyngeal mechanism as part of the orofacial examination.

• When necessary or feasible, use mechanical instruments to diagnose resonance problems.

Assess Prosodic Problems

• Clinically evaluate the appropriateness of pitch and loudness variation.

• Clinically evaluate the stress patterns.

Assess Fluency and Dysfluencies

• Count the frequency of each dysfluency type exhibited in the speech sample.

• Count the frequency of each dysfluency type exhibited in an oral reading sample.

A well-recognized formal instrument for the assessment of developmental apraxia of speech is the *Screening Test for Developmental Apraxia of Speech* (Blakeley, 1980). The diagnosis of developmental apraxia of speech is primarily based on the child's problems in sequenced speech movements not attributable to other factors (e.g., paralysis or cerebral palsy), significant problems of speech intelligibility, articulatory groping and other characteristics of disordered speech motor control, and prosodic problems (Hegde, 1996a).

Dysarthria

Definition of Dysarthria

Dysarthria is a neuromotor speech disorder affecting one, various, or all parameters of speech production: respiration, phonation, resonance, articulation, and prosody. Dworkin (1984) identified dysarthria as "disorders of phonation, articulation, resonation, and prosody which occur singly or in combination as a result of weakness, paresis, incoordination, and/or abnormalities in the tone of the muscles of the speech mechanism . . . and are due to impairment of the central nervous system, peripheral nervous system, or both . . ." (p. 264). You will notice that Dworkin uses the word **disorders** versus **disorder** in his definition of dysarthria. This is because dysarthria is actually a **group** of motor speech disorders resulting from neurological damage. Each dysarthria is slightly (or sometimes dramatically) different from the other. The special symptoms or problems associated with each dysarthria depend on the site of the lesion within the nervous system.

Etiology and Nature of Dysarthria

It should be emphasized that dysarthria is one of the diagnostic labels used to identify a speech disorder of neurological origin. Dysarthria is not the cause of the disorder but rather the speech disorder itself. The etiology of dysarthria is the actual central or peripheral nervous system damage sustained by an individual. Again, the exact nature of the disorder depends on where along the nervous system the damage was incurred.

The varied etiologies that have been associated with dysarthria include degenerative, vascular, traumatic, infectious, neoplastic, congenital, and toxic factors. Among the many degenerative neurological diseases are multiple sclerosis, Parkinson's disease, myasthenia gravis, amyotrophic lateral sclerosis (ALS), Wilson's disease, progressive supranuclear palsy, dystonia, Huntington's disease, and Friedreich's ataxia. Nonprogressive, or acute onset, disorders include stroke, infections such as Guillain-Barré, traumatic brain injury, surgical trauma, encephalitis, and toxic effects from alcohol, drugs, and other environmental factors. Congenital conditions such as cerebral palsy and Moebius syndrome are also associated with dysarthria.

The exact site of lesion within the nervous system and the variation in the etiological factors result in different types of dysarthria. The four most common sites of lesion leading to dysarthria are (a) the lower motor neuron system, (b) the upper motor neuron sytem (unilateral or bilateral), (c) the cerebellar system, and (d) the extrapyramidal system (basal ganglia) (Hegde, 1996a). Neurological damage along these systems may lead to weakness, flaccidity, spasticity, incoordination, rigidity, reduced range of movement, and the presence of involuntary movements. Each system is commonly associated with specific pathophysiological symptoms. For example, damage to the extrapyramidal system almost invariably leads to the presence of involuntary movements, and muscular weakness and flaccidity are most often associated with damage to the lower motor neuron system.

The major speech deficits associated with the dysarthrias can be subdivided according to respiratory problems, phonatory disorders, resonance disorders, articulation disorders, prosodic disorders, and other associated symptoms (adapted from Hegde, 1996a, pp. 181–183).

Respiratory Problems

- The client may exhibit forced inspirations or expirations that interrupt speech.

- Audible or breathy inspiration may be apparent during quiet breathing and speech production.

- The client may exhibit a grunt at the end of an expiration.

Phonatory Disorders

- The client's pitch may be too high or too low.
- The client may exhibit abrupt variations in pitch, which often result in pitch breaks.
- The client may lack variations in pitch, which results in monopitch and lack of inflection.
- The client may have a shaky or tremulous voice.
- **Diplophonia,** which is the simultaneous production of both a lower and a higher pitch, may be apparent while the client is asked to sustain a vowel or during spontaneous speech productions.
- The client's voice may be too soft or too loud, depending on the type of dysarthria. The client may also exhibit sudden and excessive variations in loudness.
- The client may demonstrate a lack of variation in loudness, which results in **monoloudness.**
- The client may exhibit loudness decay (progressive decrease in loudness), which results in speech that is too soft toward the end of utterances.
- The client may have a harsh, rough, gravely voice.
- The client may have a hoarse and "wet" voice, which is sometimes termed "liquid-sounding" hoarseness.
- The client may exhibit a continuously breathy voice.
- The client may have strained-strangled, effortful phonation.
- The client may display a sudden and uncontrolled cessation of voice.

Resonance Disorders

- The client's speech may be perceived as hypernasal.
- The client's speech may be perceived as hyponasal.
- Nasal emission may be perceived or confirmed with special testing.

Articulation Disorders

- The client's production of consonants is imprecise or distorted.
- The client may exhibit prolonged productions of phonemes.
- The client may repeat the production of phonemes.
- The client exhibits irregular breakdowns in articulation.
- The client may exhibit vowel distortions.
- The client's production of pressure of consonants may be weakened.

Prosodic Disorders

- The client's speech rate may be slower than the normal.
- The client may exhibit an overall fast rate of speech.
- A progressive increase in rate in certain segments of speech may be observed.

- The client may have a variable rate of speech.
- The client's phrase length may be shorter than expected, which may be related to respiratory difficulties.
- The client may exhibit reduced stress on stressed syllables or excessive stress on unstressed syllables, depending on the type of dysarthria.
- The client may demonstrate an equal stress on stressed and unstressed syllables.
- There may be a prolongation of intervals between words or syllables and inappropriate pauses (silent intervals) in speech.
- The client may exhibit short rushes of speech.

Other Characteristics

- Slow diadochokinetic rate or alternating motion rates (AMRs).
- Fast diadochokinetic rate or AMRs.
- Irregular diadochokinetic rate or AMRs.
- **Palilalia** (compulsive repetition of one's own utterances) with increasing rapid rate and decreasing loudness.

Global Characteristics of Verbal Communication

- Decreased intelligibility of speech due to the problems of respiration, articulation, resonation, and phonation.
- "Bizarreness" of speech because of its unusualness or peculiarity.

Not all dysarthrias show the same characteristics. Thus, at least seven types of dysarthrias have been identified by various researchers: flaccid, spastic, ataxic, hypokinetic, hyperkinetic, unilateral upper motor neuron, and mixed (Darley, Aronson, & Brown, 1969a, 1969b, 1975; Duffy, 1995; Rosenbek & LaPointe, 1985; Yorkston, Beukelman, & Bell, 1988). Each possesses some primary characteristics that differentiate it from the others. Variations in etiologic factors and speech characteristics allow for this typological classification. Darley, Aronson, and Brown (1969a, 1969b, 1975) are considered pioneers in the classification of dysarthria because of their extensive research in this area. Their standard classification system divides dysarthria into six types: (1) flaccid, (2) spastic, (3) ataxic, (4) hypokinetic, (5) hyperkinetic, and (6) mixed. More recently, Duffy (1995) identified a seventh type, unilateral upper motor neuron dysarthria.

Flaccid Dysarthria

The specific cause of **flaccid dysarthria** is **lower motor neuron damage** to the cranial or spinal nerves that supply the speech muscles. This is also known as **bulbar palsy.** Damage to the **motor nuclei** (cranial or spinal nerve nuclei), the cranial nerve, the muscle itself, or the **myoneural junction** (synaptic junction between the nerve and the muscle) all can lead to lower motor neuron damage. In essence, the final common pathway for muscle contraction is damaged. Possible etiologies include any disease that affects a part of the **motor unit** (i.e., motor nuclei, cranial nerve, myoneural junction, or muscle), such as:

- cerebrovascular accident — brain stem stroke;

- infection — polio, herpes zoster, secondary infections in AIDS clients;

- tumors;

- demyelinating disease — Guillain-Barré syndrome, myotonic muscular dystrophy;

- congenital conditions — Moebius syndrome, cerebral palsy;

- disease — myasthenia gravis, botulism;

- palsies — Bell's palsy, progressive bulbar palsy;

- trauma — traumatic brain injury during motor vehicle accident; surgical trauma during brain, laryngeal, facial, or chest/cardiac surgery; injury to the laryngeal branches of the vagus nerve.

The primary speech characteristics of flaccid dysarthria include hypernasality, nasal emission, imprecise articulation (plosive and fricatives are especially affected because of poor intraoral pressure), breathiness, harsh voice, audible inhalation or inspiratory stridor, monopitch, monoloudness, and the production of short phrases. Although these can all characterize flaccid dysarthria as a whole, there are some differing speech characteristics according to the exact nerve or motor nuclei damaged (adapted from Hedge, 1996a, pp. 197–198):

- **Trigeminal (V) Nerve.** Bilateral damage causes significant problems with articulation involving bilabial, linguadental, and alveolar sounds; vowels may also be distorted.

- **Facial (VII) Nerve.** Unilateral and bilateral damage can cause problems with articulation primarily involving bilabial and labiodental sounds; pressure consonants may be weak or imprecise.

- **Glossopharyngeal (IX) Nerve.** Isolated damage is uncommon but most usually associated with damage to the Vagus (X) nerve. Thus, its effects on speech are not clearly delineated.

- **Vagus (X) Nerve.** Bilateral damage to the Vagus nerve may lead to breathiness, diplophonia, reduced pitch, pitch breaks, reduced loudness, short phrases, and mild to moderate hypernasality. Unilateral damage of the Vagus nerve is not common. If there is unilateral damage, the effects on phonation and resonation will be mild.

- **Hypoglossal (XII) Nerve.** Damage typically leads to problems with articulation.

- **Spinal Nerves.** Damage to the spinal nerves innervating the respiratory muscles (e.g., intercostals, diaphragm, etc.) may have an effect on respiration, leading to poor volume, imprecise consonants, short phrases, and impaired prosodic control.

- **Multiple Cranial Nerves.** A combination of the many effects discussed may result, depending on what nerves are involved.

Some associated neurologic characteristics of lower motor neuron damage are hyporeflexia (reduced reflexes), muscle atrophy (shrunken muscles over time), fasciculations (small spontaneous muscle contractions especially on the tongue muscles), hypotonicity (decreased muscle tone or flaccidity), muscle weakness, and possible swallowing disorder. The presence of these often helps a neurologist diagnose the presence of lower motor neuron damage.

Spastic Dysarthria

The cause of **spastic dysarthria** is **bilateral upper motor neuron damage.** This is also known as **pseudobulbar palsy.** The etiologies associated with bilateral upper motor neuron damage are cerebrovascular accident, tumor, infection, congenital conditions such as cerebral palsy, traumatic brain injury, and surgical trauma. The speech characteristics associated with spastic dysarthria are very different from those of flaccid dysarthria. In flaccid dysarthria the speech symptoms are a result of poor muscle contraction or decreased tone, whereas spastic dysarthria is typically associated with too much muscle contraction and tone. Some of the primary characteristics include hypernasality, imprecise articulation (consonants and vowels), a harsh voice (strained-strangled vocal quality), effortful grunting at the end of vocalizations, an excessively low pitch, pitch breaks, monoloudness, reduced stress, excess and equal stress (inappropriate stress on monosyllabic words and the unstressed syllable in polysyllabic words), a slow rate of speech, and the presence of short phrases.

As with lower motor neuron damage, there are some associated neurologic characteristics that may help a neurologist or other specialist diagnose the presence of upper motor neuron damage. These include *hyperreflexia* (increased reflexes), *hypertonicity* (increased muscle tone or *spasticity*), muscle weakness, limited range of movement, slowness of movement, hyperactive gag reflex, impaired movement patterns, loss of fine or skilled movement, and possible swallowing disorder.

Ataxic Dysarthria

Ataxic dysarthria results from neuropathological **damage to the cerebellum or the cerebellar control circuits.** The cerebellum and its control circuits are extremely important for regulated and coordinated muscular movements. The cerebellum ensures that muscular movements, including those necessary for speech, have the appropriate force, speed, strength, and range. There are various etiologies for the neurological damage leading to ataxic dysarthria, including cerebrovascular accident (cerebellar stroke), degenerative diseases (Friedreich's ataxia, olivopontocerebellar atrophy), tumor in the cerebellum or associated structures, toxic conditions (alcohol abuse, drug toxicity), inflammatory conditions (meningitis, encephalitis), traumatic brain injury, and surgical trauma.

The primary characteristics of ataxic dysarthria are imprecise articulation, irregular articulatory breakdowns, distorted vowels, prolonged phonemes, prolonged intervals between words or syllables, excess and equal stress, harsh voice (similar to a coarse voice tremor), monopitch, monoloudness, loudness control problems, variable nasality (occasional hypernasality and nasal emission), a slow rate of speech, and a general "drunken" speech quality.

Some of the associated neurologic characteristics that aid in the diagnosis of cerebellar damage are the presence of an abnormal *stance* (standing pattern) and *gait* (walking pattern), the instability of the trunk and head, the presence of *intention tremors,* a rotated or tilted head posture, hypotonia (reduced muscular tone), and ocular movement abnormalities (**nystagmus**). In addition, the client typically presents with various movement disorders: over- or undershooting of targets; discoordinated movements; and jerky, inaccurate, slow, imprecise, and halting movements.

Hypokinetic Dysarthria

Hypokinetic dysarthria is a neuromotor speech disorder associated with **basal ganglia (extrapyramidal system) damage.** Various diseases and neurological disorders leading to the neurological damage resulting in hypokinetic dysarthria have been identified. These include Parkinson's disease, progressive supranuclear palsy, Alzheimer's disease, Pick's disease, vascular disorders resulting in multiple or bilateral strokes, repeated head trauma, inflammation, tumor, antipsychotic or neuroleptic drug toxicity, and hydrocephalus. Of these, Parkinson's disease is the most common etiology of hypokinetic dysarthria. However, only about 50% of clients with Parkinson's disease have hypokinetic dysarthria. In Parkinson's disease degenerative changes occur in the substantia nigra, leading to a deficiency in dopamine, a **neurotransmitter,** in the caudate nucleus and the putamen portions of the basal ganglia.

The primary speech characteristics of hypokinetic dysarthria are imprecise articulation, repetition of phonemes, repetition of syllables (palilalia) in about 15% of cases, mild hypernasality in about 10–25% of cases, reduced vital respiratory capacity, irregular breathing, faster rate of respiration, hoarse voice, continuously breathy voice, tremulous voice, low pitch, monopitch, monoloudness, reduced stress, inappropriate silent intervals, short rushes of speech, variable and increased rate in segments, and short phrases. Clients do not always present with all of these speech characteristics, and the exact symptoms may vary from one client to the next.

Since Parkinson's disease is the most frequent etiology of hypokinetic dysarthria, we will describe some neurologic characteristics frequently associated with Parkinson's disease. These include:

- rest tremor;

- *pill-rolling* movements between the thumb and forefinger;

- rigidity;

- *bradykinesia* — reduced speed of movement;

- *hypokinesia* — decreased amplitude of movement;

- **masked facies** — lack of facial expression, infrequent blinking, lack of smiling, reduced hand and facial movements during speech;

- **micrographia** — small handwriting, in which letters get smaller as writing progresses;

- abnormal posture — stooped and leaned slightly forward; involuntary flexion of the head, trunk, and arms; problems changing positions;

- **festinating gait**—short, slow, shuffling steps; tendency to begin slow and then take short, shuffling steps; and

- swallowing disorders.

Hyperkinetic Dysarthria

Hyperkinetic dysarthria is an inclusive diagnostic label for a variety of speech disorders resulting from **damage to the basal ganglia (extrapyramidal system).** The exact site of lesion within the basal ganglia is not known. Damage to this neuromotor system may result in a variety of involuntary movement disorders including tremor, chorea, athetosis, dystonia, myoclonus, and tics. These are all considered **hyperkinetic** (too much) movement disorders. The symptoms associated with hyperkinetic dysarthria frequently parallel the client's specific movement disorder. Although the exact site of lesion is not always known, some pathological changes associated with chorea include loss of neurons from the globus pallidum, caudate nucleus, and cerebral cortex. Lesions of the putamen have been associated with athetosis.

A known cause of hyperkinetic dysarthria is Huntington's chorea, an autosomal-dominant, inherited disease with an age of onset typically in the 50s. It is progressive and fatal. A similar disorder to Huntington's chorea is Sydenham's disease, a noninherited childhood disease. However, the symptoms in that case may clear up within 6 months. Other possible causes of basal ganglia damage leading to hyperkinetic dysarthria are vascular disease (subcortical strokes), trauma, tumors, metabolic disorders, antipsychotic and neuroleptic drug toxicity, encephalitis, and Tourette's syndrome.

The speech characteristics associated with hyperkinetic dysarthria are variable depending on the specific type of hyperkinetic movement disorder (i.e., chorea versus athetosis versus dystonia). Among these are imprecise articulation, distorted vowels, inconsistent articulatory errors, voice tremor, intermittent strained voice, voice arrests, harsh voice, intermittent hypernasality, slow rate, excess loudness variations, prolonged inter-word intervals, inappropriate silent intervals, equal stress, audible inspiration, forced and sudden inspiration and expiration, and involuntary vocal noises (e.g., coughing, barking, snorting, and cussing). Involuntary vocal noises are most often associated with Tourette's syndrome.

The movement disorders associated with extrapyramidal damage are:

- **orofacial dyskinesia**—abnormal and involuntary movements of the facial musculature;

- **myoclonus**—involuntary jerks of body parts, which may occur singly or be repetitive;

- **tics** of the face and shoulders;

- **tremor**—involuntary trembling and quivering at rest;

- **chorea**—random, rapid, and apparently meaningless movements;

- **ballism**—abrupt and severe contractions of the extremities;

- **athetosis**—writhing involuntary movements;

- **dystonia**—abnormal postures resulting from contractions of antagonistic muscles; and

- **spasmodic torticollis**—intermittent dystonia and spasm of the neck muscles.

Mixed Dysarthria

Mixed dysarthria is a combination of two or more pure dysarthrias. The neuropathology associated with this dysarthria is varied and often multiple, leading to mixed symptomatology. **Flaccid-spastic dysarthria** is the most common, accounting for approximately 42% of all mixed dysarthrias. The disease most often associated with it is amyotrophic lateral sclerosis (ALS), which results from both upper and lower motor neuron damage. **Spastic-ataxic dysarthria** is the second most common mixed dysarthia, occurring in about 23% of cases. The disease most often associated with this type of mixed dysarthria is multiple sclerosis, which results from demyelination of various neural tracts of mainly white matter (upper motor neuron, cerebellar systems).

Another type of mixed dysarthria is **ataxic-spastic-hyperkinetic dysarthria,** which is very rare and most often associated with Wilson's disease. This disease results from a toxic-metabolic disorder due to a deficiency of a copper binding protein. It can lead to cerebellar, upper motor neuron, and extrapyramidal system damage. Dietary and chemical regimens can restore the copper balance and the client may return to normal functioning.

The possible etiologies resulting in mixed dysarthria are varied, including multiple strokes; degenerative diseases such as amyotrophic lateral sclerosis; demyelinating diseases such as multiple sclerosis; vascular diseases; toxic-metabolic diseases such as Wilson's disease; tumor; and infection.

Because of the varied etiology and symptomatology associated with mixed dysarthria, the speech characteristics are variable. We will address these according to the type of mixed dysarthria, as follows:

Flaccid-Spastic (amyotrophic lateral sclerosis)

- imprecise consonants
- distorted vowels
- harsh voice
- strained-strangled voice
- breathy voice
- short phrases
- hypernasality

Spastic-Ataxic (multiple sclerosis)

- defective articulation
- hypernasality (25% of cases)
- impaired loudness control
- harsh voice
- breathy voice (37% of cases)
- inappropriate pitch control

- impaired emphasis—inappropriate judgments of rate or phrasing, pitch and loudness variation for emphasis, and increased stress on usually unstressed words and syllables
- excess and equal stress (14% of cases)

Ataxic-Spastic-Hyperkinetic (Wilson's disease)
- imprecise articulation
- irregular articulatory breakdown
- slow rate
- reduced stress
- monoloudness
- monopitch
- inappropriate silent intervals
- harsh voice
- strained voice
- inappropriately low pitch
- hypernasality

Unilateral Upper Motor Neuron Dysarthria

Duffy (1995) described **unilateral upper motor neuron dysarthria** (UUMD) as a motor speech disorder caused by a **unilateral lesion to the upper motor neurons that supply the cranial and spinal nerves involved in speech.** The name of the dysarthria is descriptive of its etiology.

The most frequent neuropathology associated with UUMD is a cerebrovascular accident in the right or left hemisphere. It frequently coexists with aphasia or apraxia if the lesion is in the left hemisphere. If the damage is in the right hemisphere, it is most often associated with cognitive-linguistic-perceptual problems.

Because most of the speech muscles, with the exception of those in the lower face, are bilaterally innervated, a unilateral upper motor neuron lesion of either hemisphere does not result in the severe effects associated with bilateral upper motor neuron damage. However, the symptoms of UUMD can range from mild to severe depending on the extent and recency of the neurological damage.

The major symptoms of UUMD are unilateral lower facial weakness, unilateral tongue weakness, unilateral palatal weakness, and hemiplegia or hemiparesis. Because of the effects of unilateral upper motor neuron damage on the facial, lingual, and palatal muscles associated with speech, this dysarthria is frequently associated with imprecise production of sounds, irregular articulatory breakdowns, a harsh voice, reduced loudness, and hypernasality.

Assessment Objectives for Dysarthria

The assessment objectives for dysarthria are similar to those discussed under apraxia of speech and developmental apraxia of speech. Specific objectives for diagnosing this speech disorder include the following:

1. To determine whether dysarthria is indeed the diagnosis. If it is, to determine the specific type of dysarthria.

2. To determine the specific respiratory, phonatory, articulatory, and prosodic characteristics of speech.

3. To determine the presence of any accompanying disorders such as aphasia, apraxia, right hemisphere brain syndrome, dementia, and dysphagia.

4. To assess or consider any associated neurological symptomatology that could aid in differential diagnosis of the specific type of dysarthria (e.g., hemiparesis, gait, involuntary movements, and so forth).

5. To judge the severity of the disorder.

6. To assess the family's perception of the problem.

7. To identify potential treatment targets and possible compensatory communication strategies.

8. To make a clinical judgment of prognosis.

9. To describe the client's strengths. This will help the clinician develop a plan of treatment that capitalizes on what the client can do.

10. To suggest potential neuropathology. This may be extremely beneficial for the medical treatment of the underlying etiology if it is not already known at the time of the speech assessment.

Assessing Dysarthria

In the assessment of dysarthria, the clinician can follow some of the general procedures outlined in the Basic Unit of this chapter. The clinician should gather a comprehensive history and conduct a thorough interview. Requesting information about the client's health or medical status is extremely important since most clients with dysarthria come with a history of medical intervention. The client may also have a current neurological diagnosis. It is important to get a clear idea of the course of the disorder (e.g., acute onset, progressive worsening, sudden or steady improvement, and so forth) and any associated behavioral changes. This may help in the differential diagnosis of the dysarthrias.

Assess Connected Speech Production

The actual assessment can start by taking a conversational speech sample, which may be initiated during the interview process. The clinician makes note of the client's speech characteristics and any other obvious behavioral or neurological symptoms. The clinician can also assess connected speech during oral reading. The client may be asked to read the "Grandfather Passage" or "Rainbow Passage" aloud while the sample is audio- or videotaped. These passages are arranged so that all of the English consonants are sampled.

Assess the Speech Production Mechanism

Because dysarthrias are associated with muscular weakness, paresis, or incoordination, it is important to conduct a thorough orofacial examination. The clinician can assess the speech production mechanism during the following nonspeech activities:

• Observe the face at rest, taking note of facial symmetry, tone, signs of tension, droopiness, expressive or masked facies, and the presence of involuntary movements and tremors.

• Observe the movements of the facial structures by asking the client to puff the cheeks, retract and round the lips, bite the lower lip, blow, smack the lips, open and close the mouth, maintain an opened posture of the mouth, and so forth.

• Observe the client's emotional expressions, paying close attention to any involuntary vocal behaviors such as cussing, screaming, crying, laughing, and so forth.

• Take note of the client's jaw at rest, its range of movement and tone, its deviation to one or the other side during movement, and any resistance as you try to close or open it.

• Observe the tongue by asking the client to protrude it and move it from side to side as fast as possible, lick his or her lips, push the cheeks out with it on each side, resist your attempts to push the protruded tongue back, and so forth.

• Observe the velopharyngeal mechanism as the client says "ah," while taking note of the movement of the soft palate (e.g., symmetry, tone, range, speed, and so forth).

• Assess nasal airflow by holding a mirror under the nares as the client prolongs the vowel /i/. Because this vowel does not have nasal resonance, the mirror should remain clear during its production, unless the client is hypernasal. However, the clinician should instruct the client to temporarily stop normal breathing so that this variable is eliminated as a factor of mirror fogging.

• Assess laryngeal functions by asking the client to cough. Take note of a weak cough associated with weak adduction of the vocal cords, inadequate breath support, or both.

Assess Diadochokinetic Alternating and Sequential Motion Rates (AMRs and SMRs)

The clinician measures the speed and regularity with which the client makes repetitive and sequential movements. Alternating motion rates and sequential motion rates help assess the functional and structural integrity of the lips, jaw, and tongue during speech movements. They are of diagnostic value in the assessment of motor speech disorders, including apraxia and dysarthria.

• *Instruct the client:* "Please take a deep breath and say [pʌ-pʌ-pʌ] as long and as evenly as you can." Model the response for the client to imitate, "Try doing it like me . . ." (AMRs)

• *Instruct the client:* "Please take a deep breath and say [tʌ-tʌ-tʌ] as long and as evenly as you can." Model the response for the client to imitate, "Try doing it like me . . ." (AMRs)

• *Instruct the client:* "Please take a deep breath and say [kʌ-kʌ-kʌ] as long and as evenly as you can." Model the response for the client to imitate, "Try doing it like me . . ." (AMRs)

- *Instruct the client:* "Please take a deep breath and say [pʌ-tʌ-kʌ] as long and as evenly as you can." Model the response for the client to imitate, "Try doing it like me . . ." (SMRs)

- For all of these, the client is allowed to continue for about 3 to 5 seconds. The clinician records the sample and then compares the response rates to normative data. The normative data for AMRs—[pʌ-pʌ-pʌ], [tʌ-tʌ-tʌ], and [kʌ-kʌ-kʌ]—range from 5 to 7 repetitions per second in adults. The normative data for SMRs—[pʌ-tə-kə]—range from 3.6 to 7.5 repetitions per second in adults. Slowness or accelerated response rates may suggest neuromotor problems.

Assess Possible Respiratory Problems

- Observe how the client's posture might affect breathing. Take note of difficulties such as a slouched posture, poor trunk control, and so forth.

- Observe the client's breathing patterns while at rest and during speech activities. Take note of rapid, shallow, or effortful breathing, signs of shortness of breath, irregular inhalation and exhalation, and so forth.

- Observe the client's loudness in connected speech. Rosenbek and LaPointe (1985) indicate that loudness characteristics in connected speech are the "best" perceptual cues to a client's adequacy of respiration (p. 113). They make this statement because loudness is controlled primarily by the muscles and structures of respiration. The clinician should always consider the ambient noise and the loudness level appropriate to a specific situation when making a perceptual judgment about a client's loudness control.

- Rosenbek and LaPointe (1985) suggest the following activities to test the strength, tone, and coordination of the diaphragm, chest, and abdominal muscles:
  - Ask the client to sniff.
  - Ask the client to pant.
  - Ask the client to make an abrupt loudness change on a prolonged /a/ (from very soft to very loud) without changing pitch or opening his or her mouth wider.
  - Ask the client to produce a loudness pattern by gradually increasing and then decreasing the loudness of a sustained vowel (e.g., /i/, /a/, /u/).

- The clinician may assess the client's ability to alter loudness by creating sufficient physical distance that would require the client to talk louder to be heard.

Assess Possible Phonatory Problems

- The clinician asks the client to take a deep breath and then say "ah." The client is asked to sustain "ah" as steadily and as long as the air supply lasts.

- The clinician makes a perceptual judgment of the appropriateness of the client's pitch during conversational speech. The client's pitch level is evaluated in relation to his or her age and gender. The clinician can also take note of the following:
  - pitch breaks and abrupt variations in pitch
  - normal or absent variations in pitch; monopitch
  - voice tremors
  - diplophonia

• The clinician judges the appropriateness of vocal loudness, taking note of a voice that is too soft or too loud. The clinician also takes note of loudness that is inappropriately variable.

• The clinician should also take note of loudness decay and normal or abnormal alternations in loudness; monoloudness.

• The clinician judges the quality of the client's voice, taking note of harshness, hoarseness, and breathiness. The clinician also takes note of the severity and consistency of those qualities.

• The clinician judges whether the client's voice production is abnormally strained, strangled, and effortful. The clinician also takes note of sudden cessation of voice.

Assess Possible Resonance Problems

• The clinician makes a perceptual judgment of hypernasality during connected speech productions. The presence of hypernasality cannot always be reliably detected through clinical judgment.

• The clinician makes a perceptual judgment of hypernasality by tape-recording the client's production of:

  • prolonged vowels accompanied by low- and high-pressure oral consonants (e.g., /a/ with *pop* and /u/ with *Lulu*)

  • sentences that are devoid of nasal sounds (e.g., *He must go to the store; Why are girls so sweet? Who ate the cookie?*)

• The clinician instructs the client to produce selected phrases and sentences devoid of nasal sounds while holding and releasing the nose. Reduced hypernasality while holding the nose suggests hypernasality and velopharyngeal incompetence.

Assess Possible Articulation Problems

• The clinician assesses the client's production of English consonants and consonant clusters by administering a standardized test. Either the *Photo Articulation Test* (Pendergast et al., 1969) or *Photo Articulation Test–3* (Lippke et al., 1997) is a good choice for adult clients because the testing stimuli are actual photographs of objects. Standardized administration and analysis procedures are followed.

• The clinician can supplement the results of the standardized testing by collecting a conversational speech and oral reading sample. This is important with dysarthric clients since articulatory precision tends to lessen as the complexity of the task increases. The connected speech samples can be assessed for distortion, omission, and substitution errors. A pattern analysis can be performed to determine the classes of sounds that are misarticulated.

• The clinician evaluates the duration of consonant sounds, taking note of prolongation of phonemes.

• The clinician records any consonant repetitions (some dysarthrias are characterized by phoneme repetition).

- The clinician takes note of irregular articulatory breakdowns in conversational speech.

- The clinician assesses the precision with which vowels are produced. Vowel errors are usually characterized by distortions.

- The clinician judges the adequacy of pressure consonants (i.e., stops, fricatives, and affricates). These are especially difficult for dysarthric clients due to respiratory or resonatory problems.

Assess Possible Prosodic Problems

The client's difficulty with respiration, phonation, resonation, and articulation aspects of speech production invariably will have an effect on his or her prosodic features. The clinician can make a perceptual judgment of prosody by doing the following:

- Measuring the client's rate of speech (ROS). An objective analysis of words per minute or syllables per minute can be made from a conversational speech sample. A clinical judgment can also be made by evaluating the client's rate of speech as normal, slower than normal, or excessively fast. Even though some clients do not present with an excessively fast rate of speech at the time of the assessment, their ROS may be judged to be at a level that compromises articulatory precision or overall speech intelligibility.

- Judging whether the client's ROS is highly variable, taking note of progressive rate increases in some speech segments.

- Measuring the client's phrase length in selected portions of conversational text and judging their adequacy.

- Evaluating the stress patterns in the client's speech, taking note of inappropriate patterns including even stress, lack of stress, and undue stress on normally unstressed syllables.

- Taking note of pauses in speech and judging whether they occur at appropriate or inappropriate junctures or are too long.

- Taking note of any short rushes of speech.

There are a few standardized tests available for the assessment of dysarthria. These include the *Frenchay Dysarthria Assessment* (Enderby, 1983), the *Assessment of Intelligibility of Dysarthric Speakers* (Yorkston, Beukelman, & Traynor, 1984), and the *Dysarthria Examination Battery* (Drummond, 1993). A diagnosis of dysarthria is made when there is clear evidence of peripheral or central nervous system damage, when there is an associated medical-neurological diagnosis, and when the client exhibits speech characteristics that support a diagnosis of dysarthria (Hegde, 1996a). Differential diagnosis according to a dysarthria subtype is based on the specific neuropathology identified by a medical specialist, specific speech characteristics identified during the speech assessment, and any associated motor characteristics.

Cerebral Palsy

Definition of Cerebral Palsy

Cerebral palsy is a nonprogressive neuromotor disorder resulting from brain damage before, during, or shortly after birth. Because of the early onset of this disorder, it is often described as a **congenital** condition. This description is used even if the damage occurs after birth. The brain damage does not get worse as the child gets older; however, a child's capability for functional movement may deteriorate over time (Long, 1994). Cerebral palsy may be classified according to when the brain damage occurs as: **prenatal** (before birth), **perinatal** (during birth), or **postnatal** (after birth). The incidence of cerebral palsy is estimated at about 2 in 1,000 live births (Hegde, 1996a; Flexer, Gillette, & Wray, 1997; Love & Webb, 1996). It should be noted that even though cerebral palsy is a child-onset disorder, it is also found in adults since a person diagnosed with cerebral palsy in childhood will eventually become an adult.

Etiology and Nature of Cerebral Palsy

There is no single etiology for cerebral palsy (Long, 1994), and the actual cause is unknown in about 40% of cases (Hegde, 1996a). *Prenatal factors* associated with cerebral palsy are multiple. They include the following: exposure to radiation, interuterine infections including HIV, exposure to drugs, exposure to metal toxicity, fetal anoxia or deprivation of oxygen, damage caused by blood infiltration in the nervous system, cerebral hemorrhage, chromosomal abnormalities, abrupted placenta or premature detachment of the fetus, and brain growth deficiency. All of these factors may cause injury to the nervous system of the developing fetus.

Complications during the child's delivery have been listed as *perinatal factors*. These include trauma to the child's brain during the delivery, which occurs only in a very small percentage of cases, cerebral hemorrhage during the birthing process, and anoxia. *Postnatal factors* include premature birth, asphyxia, sepsis (blood toxicity or microorganisms in the blood), cerebral hemorrhage, inflammatory diseases of the brain (encephalitis and meningitis), and head trauma.

Because the severity and exact nature of the disorder vary across clients, various systems have been used to classify the types of cerebral palsy. A system focusing on the distribution of limb paralysis uses the following categories:

- **Quadriplegia**—paralysis involving the trunk and all four extremities
- **Diplegia**—paralysis of the corresponding extremities on both sides of the body
- **Paraplegia**—paralysis of the lower trunk and both lower extremities
- **Hemiplegia**—paralysis of one side of the body
- **Monoplegia**—paralysis of a single extremity

This classification system is limited in that it does not highlight the type of paralysis associated with the disorder. A classification system based on the neuromuscular characteristics of cerebral palsy or the damaged neurological system results in the following categories:

- **Spastic.** This type is the most common, occurring in about 50% of children with cerebral palsy. It is related to pyramidal system lesions and is characterized by increased muscle tone, an exaggerated stretch reflex, and slow, effortful, jerky, voluntary movements.

- **Athetoid.** Athetoid cerebral palsy occurs in only about 10% of all cases. It is a result of extrapyramidal lesions and is characterized by the presence of slow, writhing involuntary movements when volitional actions are attempted, fluctuating muscle tone from normal at rest to hypertonic with voluntary movements, and increased involuntary movements with stress or distraction.

- **Ataxic.** Ataxic cerebral palsy also is less common, occurring in 5–10% of diagnosed cases. It is caused by damage to the cerebellum or its control circuits. It is characterized primarily by a disturbed equilibrium resulting in balance problems. The child's reflexes and muscle tone are normal, however.

- **Rigid.** Rigid cerebral palsy occurs in a very small percentage of cases, about 1%. Rigidity is caused by pyramidal damage and lesions to higher cortical centers of motor control. It is characterized by simultaneous contraction of all muscle groups, producing constant muscle tone. Persons with rigid cerebral palsy also present with slow, effortful voluntary movements.

- **Mixed.** Mixed cerebral palsy is a combination of more than one type. The most common combination is that of spastic and athetoid cerebral palsy, resulting from both pyramidal and extrapyramidal lesions. Although the paralysis is mixed, one type usually predominates. This type occurs in about 30% of all cases.

The two classification systems described above focus primarily on the neuromotor symptoms of the disorder. However, cerebral palsy is often associated with many other problems, including speech and language disorders. Communication problems are not present in all children with cerebral palsy. It is generally recognized that the degree of neuromotor involvement will have a direct bearing on the degree of communicative impairment (Hegde, 1996a). Children with mild cerebral palsy may not have any significant communication problems, while those with severe cerebral palsy may be so affected that verbal communication is not functional. Love and Webb (1996) indicate that approximately 75–85% of children with cerebral palsy show obvious speech problems.

The speech disorders associated with cerebral palsy are considered developmental dysarthrias. Their characteristics are similar to those discussed under adult dysarthrias; however, their onset is congenital rather than acute. All aspects of speech may be affected, including respiration, phonation, resonance, articulation, and prosody. However, articulatory problems are most frequently noted.

The person's impaired speech production is directly related to his or her neuromotor disorder. However, speech difficulties may also arise from some related sensory problem such as hearing loss. The child's speech is generally characterized as jerky, effortful, labored, and irregular. Speech intelligibility is reduced as a result of poor articulation along with decreased loudness control, respiratory inefficiency, poor intraoral pressure, and hypernasality. We will review the speech symptoms associated with cerebral palsy according to articulatory, resonatory, phonatory, respiratory, and prosodic problems (adapted from Hegde, 1996a, pp. 120–122):

Articulatory Problems

(Some symptoms may contradict each other, which highlights the different types of neuromotor involvement associated with cerebral palsy.)

- generally, more severe articulation problems with athetosis than with spasticity;
- generally inefficient or imprecise articulation as a result of affected muscle strength, tone, speed, and range of movement;
- slurred speech quality, especially with ataxic cerebral palsy;
- significant difficulty with tongue-tip sounds, especially with spastic or rigid cerebral palsy;
- articulatory conspicuousness, especially in athetoid cerebral palsy as a result of involuntary movements;
- difficulty phonating or prolonging sounds;
- predominance of omissions over substitutions or distortions;
- greater difficulty with sounds in word-final position than in other positions;
- such phonological processes as cluster reduction, stopping, depalatalization, fronting, and gliding; and
- less articulate speech in connected productions than in single words.

Resonatory Problems

- hypernasality due to velopharyngeal dysfunctions;
- nasal emission due to velopharyngeal dysfunctions; and
- poor oral resonance due to difficulties with controlling intraoral breath pressure.

Phonatory Problems

- weak voice;
- poor volume in some cases;
- poor control of loudness, which may result in irregular bursts of loudness;
- loss of voice toward the end of sentences and phrases, which may result in a whisper;
- high pitch in some cases;
- strained vocal quality in some cases due to hyperadduction of the vocal folds; and
- breathiness in some cases due to hypoadduction of the vocal folds.

Respiratory Problems

- persistence of rapid breathing rate beyond the first year of infancy (as compared to the normal slowdown as children mature);

- possibly excessive diaphragmatic activity and reduced activity of the chest and neck muscles;
- flattening or flaring of the rib cage;
- indented (sucked in) sternum; and
- air waste during speech production, resulting in short phrases or weak productions of final segments of sentences.

Prosodic Problems

- monotone;
- monoloudness;
- lack of smooth flow of speech; and
- general dysprosody as a result of respiratory, phonatory, resonatory, or articulatory difficulties.

Associated Problems

- slow and jerky jaw movements;
- impaired or discoordinated tongue movements during speech production; and
- slow diadochokinetic syllable rates.

Other problems associated with cerebral palsy may confound the client's speech difficulties, including hearing loss, mental retardation in about 50% of cases, attentional deficit, language disorders, and general learning disorders. All of these may also have an impact on the diagnosis of articulation and phonological disorders, the prognosis for improvement, the selection of treatment objectives, and the general course of treatment.

Assessment Objectives for Cerebral Palsy

There are multiple objectives in the assessment of the speech disorders associated with cerebral palsy. Because of the known benefits of early intervention, it is not uncommon for the assessment process to begin before the first birthday with children who are suspected of having cerebral palsy. Specific assessment objectives include the following:

1. To work closely with other professionals involved in the assessment and rehabilitation of the child with cerebral palsy. Clinicians should remember that the assessment of a child with cerebral palsy is a team effort involving medical specialists, nurses, psychologists, audiologists, educators, social workers, physical therapists, occupational therapists, and so forth.

2. To assess several developmental nonspeech or prespeech abilities in the young child that provide a foundation for the acquisition of later articulation skills. These include the following:

   - head control with stability of the neck and shoulder girdle, because stability provides for later mobility of the oral structure;

- a coordinated pattern of respiration and phonation, which is related to development of abdominal muscles; and

- babbling practice, which may serve as a foundation for the development of later articulation and phonological skills (Air, Wood, & Neils, 1989, p. 283).

3. To assess the communication deficits typically associated with cerebral palsy. The clinician should assess the child's speech, language, and communication skills.

4. To assess the child's strengths and intact skills. This will help the clinician develop a plan of treatment that capitalizes on what the client can do.

5. To conduct follow-up assessments as needed, since the child with cerebral palsy will need long-term care.

6. To determine the child's potential for the use of alternative or augmentative communication systems if verbal communication is not a feasible option.

Assessing Children with Cerebral Palsy

Observe and Obtain Information on Neuromotor Functions

- Obtain or request reports from the child's physicians or neurologist.

- Take note of the listed neurological symptoms during the assessment.

- Consult with other specialists involved in the assessment process such as physical therapists, nurses, occupational therapists, and so forth.

Observe and Obtain Information on Motor Development

- Use a developmental scale or checklist to assess the child's motor and general behavioral development.

- Obtain systematic information from the parents about the child's motor developmental milestones.

- Consult with other specialists involved in the assessment process, such as physical therapists, nurses, and occupational therapists, who may have some knowledge of the child's motor development.

Obtain Information on Mental Development

- Obtain a copy of the child's psychological report.

- Make clinical judgments based on your assessment of speech and language development.

Assess Speech Disorders and Speech Intelligibility

- Administer an assessment scale that provides information about the areas of prespeech behavior in which the child with cerebral palsy may have difficulty (Air, Wood, & Neils, 1989). The *Prespeech Assessment Scale* (Morris, 1975) is one such measure. This instrument, which is usually administered by a team of professionals, can provide the clinician with information about:

- the influence of abnormal body tone and movements on the speech mechanism;

- the presence of any structural deviations and deformities of the speech mechanism, as well as other parts of the body;

- the child's facial expressions, which may be affected by poor muscle tone;

- the child's general feeding, sucking, chewing, biting, and swallowing behaviors;

- the child's control of the oral mechanism for imitation of nonspeech and speech movements;

- the child's breathing patterns and breathing rates as related to control over phonation;

- the presence of any early articulatory behaviors such as cooing and babbling; and

- the variability, spontaneity, and speed of the child's articulators during the production of early articulatory gestures.

• Take an extended speech and language sample if the child is verbal. Analyze the information according to any articulation errors, speech intelligibility, patterns in production, and so forth.

• Obtain a speech sample that involves the child and the parent or another family member to distinguish any differences in speech production across social situations.

• Administer a formal articulation or phonological assessment such as the *Goldman-Fristoe Test of Articulation* (Goldman & Fristoe, 1986) or the *Bankson-Bernthal Test of Phonology* (Bankson & Bernthal, 1990a). Assess the errors according to standard procedures. Also determine any patterns in the child's misarticulations.

• Make clinical judgments about speech intelligibility for single words and sentences and with or without contextual cues; make a more detailed analysis of articulation skills when intelligibility is reduced.

• Take into consideration any oral structural deviations (e.g., tongue weakness, asymmetries in the tongue and soft palate, abnormalities of the jaw, unusually high palate, malocclusions).

• Take into consideration functional oral-motor problems (e.g., oral apraxia; lateral tongue deviations; sluggish movement of the tongue; uncontrolled movements of the facial muscles; chewing, sucking, or swallowing problems).

• Analyze the speech samples for individual sound errors and for patterns of errors suggesting phonological processes (e.g., final-consonant deletion, cluster reduction, fronting).

Assess Prosodic Problems

• Take note of the stress patterns, intonation, rate of speech, and pauses.

• Make clinical judgments about prosody.

• List any prosodic problems noted.

Assess Voice and Respiratory Problems

• Make clinical judgments about vocal loudness and pitch and their social adequacy and appropriateness for age and gender of the client.

• Judge whether variations in loudness and pitch are smooth and normal or jerky and abnormal.

• Take note of voice quality (harshness, hoarseness, breathiness, strained-strangled).

• Take note of any difficulty in voicing that may be due to vocal folds that are either hyperadducted or hyperabducted.

• Judge the adequacy of breath support for speech.

• Take note of any breathing abnormalities.

Assess Resonance Problems

• Observe the presence of hypernasality, hyponasality, nasal emission, and reduced oral resonance. A mirror may be used to determine the presence of hypernasality and nasal emission as discussed under the assessment of dysarthria.

• Consider the resonance data along with information on the child's velopharyngeal functioning.

Assess Oromotor Dysfunctions

• Complete a detailed orofacial examination.

Assess the Need for Augmentative or Alternative Communication

• Assess the child's oral communication potential.

• If the child's communication potential is low, also assess the child's potential for a variety of alternative and augmentative communication devices that might be used. This may be done with a team of professionals, including an occupational therapist and a physical therapist.

Cerebral palsy is a medical diagnosis consistent with a history of damage to the developing brain. It is associated with various neuromotor symptoms, behavioral patterns, and communication problems associated with brain damage before or soon after birth. The speech–language pathologist's primary responsibility to children with cerebral palsy is to assess their speech, language, and communication problems.

Cleft Lip and Palate

Definition of Cleft

In relation to the speech production mechanism, a **cleft** is a structural malformation affecting the tissues, muscles, and bony processes of the upper lip, alveolar process, hard palate, soft palate, and uvula (Air, Wood, & Neils, 1989). Such a congenital anomaly most often results in an opening in the hard palate, the soft palate, or both. Although less common, clefts of the upper lip also occur.

Cleft lip and cleft palate occur during embryonic development. For a variety of reasons, the growth and fusion of the palatal and lip structures are disrupted. Normal closure of the lips generally occurs in the 5th or 6th week of gestation, while the hard and soft palates tend to fuse at about the 8th or 9th week of gestation (Golding-Kushner, 1997). Because of their separate embryonic points of fusion, cleft lip and palate do not always coexist. It is not uncommon for a child to have a cleft palate and an intact lip or vice versa. Cleft lip with or without palatal involvement is thought to have a different etiology than an isolated palatal cleft.

The incidence of cleft palate is 1 in 600 to 750 live births (Hegde, 1996a; McWilliams, Morris, & Shelton, 1990). However, incidence rates have been reported to vary across different cultural groups, with the highest incidence occurring in North American Indians, followed by Japanese, Chinese, White, and African American children. Interestingly, incidence statistics have shown that clefts of the lip and palate affect males twice as often as females, while isolated cleft palate occurs twice as often in females as in males. In overall cases, nearly half of all children affected demonstrate a cleft of the lip and palate, one quarter show a cleft of the lip only, and another quarter show a cleft of the palate only.

The presence of a cleft palate with or without a cleft lip may be associated with various communication disorders including articulation and phonological problems. Less severe clefts that are medically and surgically managed early in life may not produce significant communication disorders. However, the more severe the malformations and the more delayed the surgical and medical intervention, the greater the severity of communication disorders. Communication disorders may be more common in children with clefts that are part of a genetic syndrome.

Etiology and Nature of Cleft Lip and Palate

The etiology of cleft lip and palate is extremely complex. This structural disorder is often considered to be of multifactorial origin. Clefting has been associated with autosomal-dominant syndromes such as Apert syndrome, Stickler syndrome, van der Woude syndrome, Waardenburg syndrome, and Treacher Collins syndrome. Other syndromes associated with cleft lip and/or palate are Pierre Robin syndrome, Crouzon syndrome, and Shprintzen syndrome. Environmental teratogens such as excessive alcohol consumption, illegal drug use, and prescription drug use (e.g., anticonvulsants and thalidomide) during pregnancy have also been associated with cleft lip and palate.

There are many classification systems used to describe clefts. Each has its limitations, and none is accepted universally (Hegde, 1996a). A cleft of the lip can be categorized as complete or incomplete depending on its extension. An incomplete cleft of the lip will be only a minor notch or may extend almost to the nostril, while a complete cleft includes all of the lip and continues into the floor of the nostril (McWilliams et al., 1990). A cleft lip can be unilateral (on only one side, which is usually the left) or bilateral (on both sides). A cleft of the lip can occur with or without a cleft of the palate (McWilliams et al., 1990), as mentioned.

Cleft palate can involve the hard and soft palates. The anterior two-thirds of the roof of the mouth makes up the hard palate, while the posterior one-third makes up the soft palate. The hard palate has a bony foundation and a muscular overlay. The soft palate is composed only of muscle and mucosa.

There are various communication disorders associated with cleft lip and palate. These may originate from the structural abnormalities associated with clefts. They may also stem from a problem or combination of problems that can accompany this disorder (e.g., middle ear infections, hearing loss, mental retardation, and velopharyngeal incompetence). We will review the speech symptoms associated with cleft lip and palate according to articulation and phonological disorders, laryngeal and phonatory disorders, and resonance disorders. The severity of the speech disorder associated with cleft lip and palate runs along a continuum. Isolated cleft lip rarely results in misarticulations, while bilateral complete clefts of the hard and soft palates lead to the most severe speech problems (Hegde, 1996a).

Articulation and Phonological Disorders

• The child generally has greater difficulty with voiced sounds than with unvoiced sounds.

• The child with cleft palate has particular difficulty with sounds that require a buildup of **intraoral pressure,** which results in weak production of fricatives, affricates, and stops (**pressure consonants**).

• The child may substitute nasal sounds for nonnasal sounds. These may not be true substitutions, however. The added nasal resonance may be due to **velopharyngeal inadequacy,** which is difficulty in closing the nasal port for the production of oral sounds. This would be a resonance disorder rather than an articulation disorder.

• The child may exhibit audible or inaudible nasal emission while producing voiceless sounds.

• The child may demonstrate some distortion of vowels.

• The child may exhibit **compensatory errors.** These are sound substitutions made by the child in an attempt to remedy the inadequate closure of the velopharyngeal mechanism. Many of these substitutions are non-English sounds made with posterior movements of the tongue to stop the air or to produce friction noise. These include the following:

- substitution of glottal stops /ʔ/ for stop consonants;

- substitution of laryngeal stops for stop consonants and laryngeal fricatives for fricatives (This involves posterior movement of the tongue so as to move the epiglottis toward the pharynx to block the air or to create friction noise.);

- substitution of pharyngeal stops (/ʡ/ unvoiced; /ʕ/ voiced) for stop consonants and pharyngeal affricates for palatal affricates (This substitution involves posterior movement of the tongue to make contact with the pharynx to build up pressure that is suddenly released or to constrict the air to create friction.);

- substitution of posterior nasal fricatives for fricatives /Δ/ (This is accomplished through the use of the posterior dorsum of the tongue and the soft palate to create friction noise.);

- substitution of mid-dorsum palatal stops (/ɟ/ voiced; /ɟ/ unvoiced) for /t/, /d/, /k/, and /g/ (The child builds pressure by raising the mid-dorsum of the tongue to the hard palate.);

- substitution of mid-dorsum palatal fricatives for fricatives and mid-dorsum palatal affricates for affricates (This is created by moving the mid-dorsum toward the hard palate to create friction of the built-up pressure.);

- production of nasal fricatives for various sounds (These are also called *nasal snorts, nasal rustles,* or *nasal friction.*);

- substitution of velar fricatives (/χ/, unvoiced; /ɣ/ voiced) for velar stops /k/ and /g/.

• Children with cleft palate may exhibit reduced speech intelligibility to varying extents depending on the number and type of articulation errors.

Laryngeal Pathologies and Phonatory Disorders

(Most phonatory disorders may be due to velopharyngeal inadequacy, which leads to hyperfunction of the voice.)

• In general, there is a higher prevalence of voice or phonatory disorders in children with cleft palate.

• In general, there is a higher frequency of vocal nodules. This may stem from undue strain on the vocal cords as the child attempts to compensate for articulation errors by producing pharyngeal and laryngeal sounds.

• There may be hypertrophy and edema (swelling) of the vocal folds.

• The child's voice may be hoarse.

• The child's voice may be too soft. This may stem from the child's inability to increase vocal intensity because of velopharyngeal inadequacy.

• The child's voice may be monotonous due to limited pitch variation.

• The child's voice may have a strangled vocal quality due to excessive effort and tension in producing voice to avoid hypernasality.

Resonance Disorders

• The child may present with hypernasality on vowels and voiced oral consonants due to inadequate velopharyngeal closure and restricted mouth opening.

• The child may present with hyponasality (reduced nasal resonance on nasal sounds).

• The child may present with denasality (near absence of nasal resonance on nasal sounds).

Associated Problems

• The child may have velopharyngeal incompetence resulting in inadequate closure of the velopharyngeal port.

• The child may have a history of recurrent middle ear infections.

- The child may have a diagnosed hearing loss. Hearing loss occurs in approximately 50% of children with cleft palate. These are typically conductive hearing impairments associated with recurrent middle ear infections or eustachian tube dysfunction. Language problems may be more severe and more persistent in children who have associated hearing loss.

- The child may have a significant language disorder resulting from a cleft that is part of a genetic syndrome.

- The child may present with generally delayed language development. However, significant improvement may occur as the child grows older, and the child may attain normal language by about age 4.

Assessment Objectives for Cleft Lip and Palate

There are multiple objectives in the assessment of the speech disorders associated with cleft lip and palate. Since cleft palate is a congenital structural disorder, the initial assessment is usually performed soon after the child's birth. Many hospitals have a craniofacial clinic where children with congenital disorders are assessed by a team of specialists (e.g., pediatrician, nurse, dentist, orthodontist, speech–language pathologist, physician, counselor, audiologist, and so forth). The surgical repair of cleft lip and palate is done by a team of medical specialists. The speech–language pathologist is an integral member of the multidisciplinary team to identify the communication problems in a particular child. Specific objectives for the assessment of speech problems associated with cleft lip and palate include the following:

1. To work closely with other professionals involved in the assessment and treatment of the child with cleft lip and palate. Clinicians should remember that the assessment of children with cleft lip and palate is a team effort involving many specialists.

2. To determine the communication disorders typically associated with cleft lip and palate. The clinician should assess the client's speech, language, and communication skills, along with the orofacial structures.

3. To make periodic assessments of communication and its potential disorders to generate information that might help plan surgical intervention.

4. To suggest communication treatment targets if speech problems persist after surgical intervention.

5. To assess the child's strengths and intact skills. This will help the clinician develop a plan of treatment that capitalizes on what the child can do.

Assessing Children with Cleft Lip and Palate

In the assessment of communication problems associated with clefts of the lip and palate, the clinician can follow some of the general procedures outlined in the Basic Unit of this chapter. The clinician should collect a comprehensive history and conduct a thorough interview. The client's health background is extremely important since most clients have a history of medical and surgical intervention.

Some children may have a history of recurrent otitis media or eustachian tube dysfunction and concomitant hearing loss. The clinician should get clear information on the child's speech and language development.

Assess Connected Speech Production

The actual assessment can start by taking a conversational speech sample, which may be initiated during the interview process. The clinician makes note of the client's speech characteristics and any other obvious behavioral or structural symptoms. Assuming the client can read, the clinician can also assess connected speech during an oral reading task. The clinician should select a reading passage that is appropriate for the child's age and reading level. The sample may be audio- or videotaped for later analysis.

Assess the Speech Production Mechanism

Because clefts of the lip and palate are associated with structural and physiological problems, it is important to conduct a thorough orofacial examination. The procedures for conducting an orofacial examination discussed in the Basic Unit of this chapter can be used for assessment of the speech production mechanism in children with cleft palate. The clinician should pay special attention to unrepaired clefts of the lips, the hard palate, and the soft palate. If the clefts have been surgically repaired, the clinician can make a judgment about the adequacy of the repair. It is important to remember that movements of the soft palate during sustained production of /a/, a typical activity during the orofacial examination, may not always be a valid indicator of soft palate movement in connected speech or the adequacy of velopharyngeal closure. Perceptual judgments of hypernasality or hyponasality may be more appropriate to judge velopharyngeal closure in connected speech.

Assess Possible Articulation and Phonological Problems

- The clinician can arrange activities that sample the production of sounds of special relevance to evaluate the effects of clefts on speech. The clinician can select words and sentences that contain stops, fricatives, and affricates (pressure consonants). As described earlier, those sounds are particularly difficult for children with cleft lip and palate.

- The clinician can administer the *Iowa Pressure Test,* which is a special subtest in the *Templin-Darley Tests of Articulation* (Templin & Darley, 1969). This subtest is designed to sample the production of sounds that are particularly difficult for children with cleft palate and dysarthria, or any other disorder associated with velopharyngeal insufficiency. Any patterns in the child's misarticulations should be identified. It is important to note the use of **compensatory substitution errors** since these are commonly observed in children with cleft palate.

- The clinician assesses the child's stimulability for improved production of the error sounds. Children with cleft palate may need a combination of auditory, visual, tactile, and kinesthetic cues to facilitate correct production of the sounds misarticulated during testing.

• The clinician should keep in mind that children with cleft palate may have difficulty with the motor production of sounds because of their underlying structural problems; however, they may also exhibit developmental phonological rules or patterns in their productions (e.g., final-consonant deletion, syllable deletion, velar fronting, and so forth).

Assess Possible Phonatory Problems

• After listening to the child's speech, the clinician may determine whether a detailed voice assessment is needed.

• The clinician should judge the client's voice to determine if it is breathy, harsh, hoarse, excessively soft, and so forth.

• The clinician should make note of any vocally abusive behaviors such as excessive coughing, throat clearing, snorting, and use of compensatory articulatory gestures that may place undue strain on the vocal folds.

Assessing Possible Resonance Disorders

• The clinician should assess hypernasality and nasal emission since this is often associated with cleft palate. The clinician makes a clinical judgment based on the client's productions in connected speech.

• The clinician can observe the velopharyngeal mechanism as the client says "ah," while taking note of the movement of the soft palate (e.g., its symmetry, tone, range, speed, and so forth).

• The clinician can assess nasal airflow by holding a mirror under the nares as the client prolongs the vowel /i/. Because this vowel does not have nasal resonance the mirror should remain clear during its production, unless the client is hypernasal. However, the clinician should instruct the client to temporarily stop normal breathing so that this variable is eliminated as a factor of mirror fogging.

Although the initial assessment and subsequent surgical management of cleft lip and palate are under the realm of the medical specialists, the speech–language pathologist is the professional primarily responsible for assessing the child's speech, language, and communicative problems.

Hearing Impairment

Definition of Hearing Impairment

As discussed in Chapter 4, hearing loss is a known variable of impaired articulation and phonological skills. We have chosen to further discuss this topic in this Advanced Unit because of the unique assessment and treatment needs of children with hearing loss and any concomitant speech and language problems. **Hearing impairment** or **hearing loss** refers to reduced **hearing acuity,** which can range from mild to profound. The following categories are frequently used relative to the degree of hearing loss and severity of the disorder:

- slight hearing loss: hearing thresholds in the 16–25 dB HL range
- mild hearing loss: hearing thresholds in the 26–40 dB HL range
- moderate hearing loss: hearing thresholds in the 41–70 dB HL range
- severe hearing loss: hearing thresholds in the 71–90 dB HL range
- profound hearing loss: hearing thresholds that are 91 dB and above

Depending on the severity of the hearing loss, a person may be considered **hard of hearing** or **deaf.** A child whose hearing loss falls between 16 and 90 dB HL is considered hard of hearing, as previously described. A child whose hearing thresholds are 90 dB or higher is considered deaf.

Etiology and Nature of Hearing Impairment

The causes of hearing loss are multiple and varied. Most causes are organic, although some people may experience **psychogenic** hearing loss. The most common types of hearing loss are (a) conductive, (b) sensory-neural, and (c) mixed.

Conductive hearing loss is characterized by the interrupted transmission of sound to the cochlea. The interruption may occur in the outer or middle ear, but the latter is more common. The prevailing cause of middle ear dysfunction in children is *otitis media*. Otitis media is more commonly known as middle ear infection. Recurrent otitis media may lead to temporary or permanent conductive hearing loss. The most common cause of conductive hearing loss in adults is osteosclerosis. This is a disease of the middle ear ossicles in which the footplate of the stapes attaches to the oval window, preventing transmission of sound to the inner ear. Other causes of conductive hearing loss include:

- *otitis externa,* or inflammation of the external auditory canal, which is frequently referred to as "swimmer's ear";
- *collapsed ear canal,* which is most common in elderly females;
- *osteomas,* or benign bony tumors of the external auditory canal;
- *disarticulation* of the auditory ossicular chain;
- *aural atresia,* or a closed external auditory canal; and
- *stenosis,* or narrowing of the external auditory canal.

Sensori-neural hearing loss is an inclusive term depicting the type of loss that results when the hair cells of the cochlea or the fibers of the acoustic nerve (CN VIII) are damaged. More specifically, damage to the hair cells constitutes a *sensory loss,* while damage to the acoustic nerve is best described as a *peripheral neural loss.* This type of loss is permanent, since the hair cells of the cochlea or fibers of the acoustic nerve cannot regenerate once damaged.

Sensory loss is common in the elderly because damage to the hair cells in the cochlea is part of the normal aging process. The term **presbycusis** is used in reference to hearing loss associated with the effects of aging. Other causes of sensory hearing loss include:

- exposure to excessively loud noise.;
- vascular accidents that restrict cochlear blood supply;
- viral and bacterial infections such as meningitis and maternal rubella;
- ototoxicity, or damage from drugs; and
- mechanical injury to the cochlea.

Fetal alcohol syndrome, maternal drug addiction, congenital disorders, and low birth weight have also been implicated in sensory hearing loss. Isolated peripheral neural loss is relatively rare. It may result from a tumor of the VIIIth cranial nerve, which is the most common of the cranial tumors. Demyelinization, or damage to the myelin sheath of the acoustic nerve, may also result in this type of hearing loss.

A combination of conductive hearing loss and sensori-neural hearing loss leads to what is commonly termed **mixed hearing loss.** Mixed hearing loss may result from a combination of the causes described for pure conductive and pure sensori-neural hearing loss.

There are many communication disorders associated with hearing loss. The specific communication disorder depends on a variety of factors. These include (a) the degree of hearing loss, (b) the child's age at the time of the loss, (c) the kind and quality of intervention, (d) the age at which intervention was initiated, (e) the extent of family support, and (f) the presence of other physical, cognitive, and sensory problems. The speech problems associated with hearing loss are described according to information presented by Hegde (1996a, pp. 236–238).

Articulation Problems

- Omission of final consonants and consonant clusters
- Omission of /s/ across word positions
- Omission of initial consonants
- Substitution of voiced consonants for voiceless consonants
- Substitution of nasal consonants for oral consonants
- Vowel substitutions
- Distortion of sounds, especially of stops and fricatives
- Imprecise production of vowels
- Increased duration of vowels
- Addition of sounds, especially an intrusive schwa between consonants in blends (e.g., /bəlu/ for /blu/)
- Breathiness before the production of vowels
- Inappropriate release of final stops (e.g., /stapʰ/ for /stop˹/)

Voice and Resonance Problems

(These are most pronounced in the deaf.)

- High-pitched voice
- Harshness
- Hoarseness
- Nasal emission on voiceless consonants
- Hypernasality on voiced consonants and vowels
- Hyponasality on nasal consonants
- Breathiness
- Lack of normal intonation

Prosodic Disturbances

- Generally limited fluency
- Increased rate of dysfluencies

- Slow rate of speech
- Inappropriate pauses
- Abnormal flow of speech
- Abnormal rhythm of speech
- Abnormal intonation patterns

Associated Problems (language and reading problems)

- Generally limited vocabulary
- Poor comprehension of word meanings
- Lack of understanding of multiple-meaning words
- Difficulty understanding abstract, metaphoric, and proverbial phrases
- Slower acquisition of grammatical morphemes
- Omission of several grammatical morphemes
- Slower acquisition of verb forms
- Shorter sentences
- Fewer varieties of sentence types
- Pragmatic language problems
- Lack of elaborated speech
- Insufficient background information
- Occasional irrelevance of speech
- Poor reading comprehension
- Writing that mirrors the verbal language problems listed

Assessment Objectives

Several objectives should be considered when assessing the communication disorders of deaf and hard of hearing children. The clinician should keep in mind that it is an audiologist or other medical professional who actually diagnoses the type and severity of the hearing loss. The child may be followed by a team of specialists including audiologists, teachers of deaf and hard of hearing children, a regular classroom teacher, a social worker, a psychologist, and so forth. The speech–language pathologist's primary responsibility is to assess the speech and language problems that may result from the hearing loss, as follows:

1. To assess the child's articulation skills and speech intelligibility across varied tasks and situations.

2. To assess other aspects of speech including voice, resonance, and prosody.

3. To assess other communication skills including the child's auditory comprehension, verbal expression, and reading and writing skills. Assessment of those skills will help the clinician develop a client-specific plan of treatment.

4. To describe the nature of the child's speech production problems and make an estimate of severity.

5. To identify potential treatment targets and possible compensatory communication strategies.

6. To make a clinical judgment of prognosis.

7. To describe the client's strengths and intact skills. This will help the clinician develop a plan of treatment that capitalizes on what the client can do.

Assessing Speech Problems Associated with Hearing Impairment

In assessing communication problems associated with hearing loss, the clinician can follow the general procedures outlined in the Basic Unit of this chapter. A comprehensive history should be collected, and a thorough interview should be completed. The client's developmental and medical background is extremely important. It is crucial that the clinician become familiar with the client's type and degree of hearing loss and inquire about the age of onset of the disorder. Clients with congenital or **prelingual** hearing loss may exhibit more severe communication problems than clients whose loss is acquired or **postlingual.** The type and extent of educational, therapeutic, and medical intervention should be determined.

Consider Possible Problems with Auditory Perception or Speech Discrimination

• The clinician should consult with an audiologist to determine what information the child can receive from a speech signal presented without visual cues (Elfenbein, 1994).

• In collaboration with an audiologist, the clinician can administer a formal instrument to assess the client's auditory perceptual skills across a wide range of activities. The *Test of Auditory Comprehension* (TAC) (Trammell et al., 1976) is an example of such an instrument. The TAC contains the following ten subtests:

  • Subtest 1: Discriminates between linguistic and nonlinguistic sounds.

  • Subtest 2: Discriminates between linguistic, human nonlinguistic, and environmental sounds.

  • Subtest 3: Discriminates between stereotypic messages.

  • Subtest 4: Discriminates between single-element core-noun vocabulary words presented in a sentence.

  • Subtest 5: Recalls two critical elements from a sentence.

  • Subtest 6: Recalls four critical elements from a sentence.

  • Subtest 7: Sequences three events from a story.

  • Subtest 8: Recalls five details from a story.

  • Subtest 9: Sequences three events from a story presented with a competing message.

  • Subtest 10: Recalls five details from a story presented with a competing message.

• The client's auditory or speech discrimination skills should always be considered in light of associated language and cognitive problems.

Assess the Speech Production Mechanism

Deaf and hard of hearing people may or may not exhibit problems of the speech production mechanism. If the client's hearing loss is part of another disorder (e.g., cleft palate, cerebral palsy), the clinician may need to perform a comprehensive orofacial examination. If the client's speech problems are a result of the hearing loss only, a less detailed orofacial examination may be sufficient. The procedures for conducting an orofacial examination outlined in the Basic Unit of this chapter can be used with deaf and hard of hearing children to rule out any problems with the speech production mechanism.

Assess Possible Articulation and Phonological Problems

• Administer a standardized articulation or phonological test such as *The Goldman-Fristoe Test of Articulation* (Goldman & Fristoe, 1986) or *The Assessment of Phonological Processes–Revised* (Hudson, 1986a). Follow standardized administration procedures.

• Analyze the information to identify any error patterns or phonological processes.

• Pay special attention to the typical errors exhibited by deaf and hard of hearing people.

• Be prepared to use narrow phonetic transcription to fully capture the extent of the client's errors since many are sound distortions.

Assess Connected Speech Production

The clinician should collect a conversational speech sample to supplement single-word articulation tests. Children who are hard of hearing, like children with normal hearing, may demonstrate better articulation skills in single-word tests than in connected speech. Assuming the client can read, the clinician can also assess connected speech during an oral reading task. The clinician should use passages that are appropriate for the client's age and reading level. The speech sample can be analyzed for articulation and other speech problems. Misarticulations should be determined, along with any evident phonological patterns or processes. The child's speech intelligibility can be determined from the conversational speech sample.

Assess Possible Voice and Resonance Problems

• Clients who are hard of hearing may exhibit voice or resonance problems that may warrant further assessment.

• The child may present with hoarseness, nasal emission, hypernasality, hyponasality, or poor oral resonance.

• The clinician can use procedures discussed under other disorders to confirm any voice or resonance problems.

The child who is hard of hearing is followed up by a team of professionals, including medical specialists, educators, and psychologists. The speech–language pathologist is only one member of the treatment team. Close communication should always be maintained between the speech–language pathologist and other professionals. The clinician should consult closely with the audiologist and educators of deaf and hard of hearing children. The primary responsibility of the SLP is to thoroughly assess the speech, language, and communication problems associated with hearing loss.

Summary of the Advanced Unit

- The speech–language pathologist may be involved in the assessment of clients with speech disorders of an organic or neurogenic origin.

- **Apraxia of speech** is a motor programming disorder resulting from neurological damage. The damage is typically in the third frontal convolution of the frontal lobe in the left hemisphere, although other areas have been implicated.

- The etiology of the neurological damage resulting in apraxia of speech is predominantly cerebrovascular accident, although other etiologies have been identified.

- Apraxia of speech is associated with groping and searching behaviors, articulation problems, and prosodic problems. The client displays significant articulatory breakdown during volitional speech. Automatic speech (i.e., common social greetings, counting, singing, and so forth) is less difficult.

- **Developmental apraxia of speech** is the childhood equivalent of acquired apraxia of speech in adults. It is a descriptive disorder of unknown etiology in most cases. Children with apraxia of speech may exhibit speech characteristics similar to that of adults with apraxia of speech. The behavior most common to the two is the lack of volitional control of the oral mechanism for speech production.

- **Dysarthria** is actually a group of motor speech disorders (dysarthrias) associated with muscle weakness, paralysis, or discoordination. There are various types of dysarthria, including: spastic, flaccid, hyperkinetic, hypokinetic, ataxic, unilateral upper motor neuron, and mixed. Specific speech characteristics accompany each type of dysarthria.

- Several etiologies have been associated with dysarthria, including cerebrovascular accident, infectious diseases, tumor, degenerative diseases, and trauma.

- All aspects of speech production may be affected in dysarthria, including articulation, phonation, resonation, respiration, and prosody.

- **Cerebral palsy** is a nonprogressive neuromotor disorder resulting from brain damage before, during, or shortly after birth. At least five subtypes of cerebral palsy have been identified: spastic, athetoid, ataxic, rigid, and mixed.

- Speech characteristics associated with cerebral palsy are similar to those found in dysarthria. They may vary from one type of cerebral palsy to another.

- A **cleft** is a structural malformation affecting the tissues, muscles, and bony processes of the upper lip, alveolar process, hard palate, soft palate, and uvula. The terms **cleft lip** and **cleft palate** are frequently used.

- The etiology of cleft lip and palate is multifactorial. The damage occurs early in the embryonic stage of development. The incidence of cleft palate is 1 in 600 to 750 live births. Incidence rates have been reported to vary across cultural groups.

- The child with cleft palate may exhibit articulation and phonological problems, resonance problems, and voice problems.

• **Hearing impairment** or **hearing loss** refers to reduced **hearing acuity,** which can range from mild to profound. The terms **hard of hearing** and **deaf** are differentiated by the extent of hearing loss in an individual. The most common types of hearing loss are **conductive, sensori-neural,** and **mixed. Psychogenic** hearing loss has been identified, but it is less common.

• Clients with hearing loss may exhibit problems with articulation, resonance, prosody, and voice.

Chapter 7

♦ ♦ ♦ ♦ ♦ ♦ ♦ ♦ ♦ ♦ ♦ ♦ ♦ ♦ ♦ ♦ ♦

Treatment of Articulation and Phonological Disorders

Advanced Unit: Treatment of Various Organic and Neurogenic Speech Disorders......455

Basic Unit

♦ ♦ ♦ ♦ ♦ ♦ ♦ ♦ ♦ ♦ ♦ ♦ ♦ ♦ ♦ ♦ ♦ ♦ ♦ ♦

Basic Principles and Procedures in the Treatment of Articulation and Phonological Disorders

It is not sufficient to know what one ought to say, but one must also know how to say it.

—ARISTOTLE

Chapter 6 emphasized the importance of a thorough assessment. Clinicians consolidate their specialized skills to secure an accurate diagnosis of the client's articulation and phonological skills. By collecting, analyzing, and interpreting various data, the clinician discovers the communication skills that for whatever reason have not developed normally in a particular child.

Once a diagnosis has been reached, the clinician makes specific recommendations. If clinical services are recommended, an individualized treatment program is developed and the clinician selects treatment procedures appropriate for the remediation of articulation and phonological disorders. Over the past several years, various treatment approaches have emerged that claim to meet the needs of children with articulation and phonological disorders. In Chapter 8 we will explore many of those treatment approaches in great detail. However, the focus of this Basic Unit will be on the general sequence of treatment that can be successfully applied across clients and clinical populations. We believe that the child's intervention needs are best met when the treatment sequence minimally includes the following components:

1. selection of client-specific target behaviors, commonly known as treatment goals and objectives;

2. establishment of pretreatment information through baseline measures;

3. selection and preparation of adequate stimulus materials;

4. identification and use of successful sound-evoking techniques;

5. development and implementation of an individualized treatment program;

6. incorporation of various strategies that help strengthen the client's generalized responses and maintenance of the target behaviors;

7. involvement of the client's family and significant others in the treatment process;

8. completion of a follow-up assessment and the provision of booster treatment as necessary;

9. use of specific treatment activities that help maximize the client's performance.

The goal of this Basic Unit is to provide the reader with a thorough understanding of the many components involved in the treatment of articulation and phonological disorders. We will begin with the target selection process and end with a discussion of several strategies that can be used to ensure maintenance of the learned sounds or phonological skills. In the Advanced Unit, more specific procedures for the treatment of organic and neurogenic speech disorders such as **apraxia of speech, cleft palate,** and **cerebral palsy** will be provided as a general introduction to the remediation of those disorders.

Selecting Potential Target Behaviors

One of the most important components of articulation and phonological therapy is the selection of functional target behaviors. **Target behavior** is a standard term that refers to any skill or action that is taught to a client, patient, or student (Hegde & Davis, 1995). Specific to articulation and phonological disorders, target behaviors are the precise skills taught by the clinician to improve the client's sound production skills, phonological skills, speech intelligibility, and overall communication effectiveness. In most clinical settings, target behaviors are termed *treatment goals* and *objectives*.

Short-Term Objectives and Long-Term Goals

Target sounds and phonological skills for training are selected after the assessment and diagnostic process is completed and the client's specific needs are identified; long-term goals and short-term objectives are outlined. **Short-term objectives** refer to skills that can be trained in a relatively short period of time (e.g., 2 weeks, 1 month, 3 months). They are steps toward achievement of the long-term goal. **Long-term goals** are more broadly defined communicative behaviors that the client needs to learn to improve his or her overall communication competence (e.g., age-appropriate articulation skills, improved phonological skills, improved intelligibility, self-correction skills). It takes a longer period of time to reach a long-term goal.

In clinical practice, long-term goals are the articulation or phonological skills that the client is expected to learn by the end of a specified treatment period (e.g., one semester in most university settings and one year in most public school settings) (Bleile, 1995). Short-term objectives help support the long-term goals. The ultimate long-term goal is always maintenance of the learned articulation and phonological skills in the client's natural environments across varied situations. This will be discussed further toward the end of this Basic Unit.

General Considerations

As previously described, the assessment data provide the clinician with the information needed to identify the sounds that are misarticulated and the phonological processes or rules that are active in the child's system. However, because children with articulation and phonological disorders misarticulate many sounds or use several phonological processes at the same time, the clinician must select and prioritize the order of treatment. Adequate long-term goals and short-term objectives can be established only if the client's individual needs are carefully considered.

Hegde and Davis (1995) identify four guidelines for the selection of potential target behaviors that can be applied across communication disorders. Before proceeding with various suggestions specific to articulation and phonological disorders, we believe it is important to discuss these four variables because of their client-specific basis in the selection of target behaviors. In recent years, our profession has increasingly acknowledged the importance of adapting therapy to meet the functional needs of individuals. We now know that if speech–language therapy services are to have long-lasting effects, clinicians must teach target behaviors that are meaningful in the client's life. Hegde and Davis (1995) make the following recommendations:

1. *Select behaviors that will make an immediate and socially significant difference in the communicative skills of the client.*

- Select target behaviors that will improve the client's social communication, academic achievement, and occupational performance.

- In treating a child with misarticulations, select those sounds that are most frequently used in conversation and misarticulated by the child and whose correct production will improve intelligibility the most.

2. *Select the most useful behaviors that may be produced and reinforced at home and in other natural settings.*

- Such behaviors are likely to be sustained over time.

- Behaviors that fulfill the needs of the client tend to be produced and reinforced in the home and other natural settings.

- Behaviors that help the client meet the demands made on him or her also tend to be produced and maintained in natural settings.

3. *Select behaviors that help expand the communicative skills.*

- Teach words that may easily be expanded into phrases and sentences.

4. *Select behaviors that are linguistically and culturally appropriate for the individual client.*

- Find out what kinds of vocabulary, language structures, and pragmatic communication patterns are valued in the culture and family.

- Talk to the parents, spouses, and other family members before you finalize the target behaviors for clients with diverse cultural backgrounds (adapted from pp. 170–171).

We strongly believe that a clinician who takes a client-specific approach to therapy can better meet the needs of clients and their entire family constellation. We also believe that the clinician who truly embraces this treatment philosophy is more sensitive toward the client's cultural and linguistic differences. If the individual needs of particular clients are to be met, their cultural and linguistic diversity should always be considered.

Considerations for the Selection of Phonological Processes and Individual Sounds

In working with articulation and phonological disorders, many experts have suggested various criteria that may be considered in the selection of individual sounds and phonological rules or processes. We will begin by reviewing the criteria recommended for the selection of phonological processes. We will then highlight the many guidelines that have been set forth for the selection of individual target phonemes. We emphasize that these recommendations are mere guidelines, not fixed rules. It is the individual clinician who ultimately must consider all of the variables and the impact that they will play on the client's communication skills.

Phonological Processes

Through a phonological process analysis, the clinician identifies the processes that are active in the child's phonological system. The **percentage** or **frequency of occurrence** for each process can also be determined. However, at this point the clinician may not have yet decided which processes are the most appropriate for remediation. Therefore, the next step is to prioritize the treatment targets so that the child's communication needs are met.

There are many factors that need to be considered in selecting phonological processes for intervention. Traditionally, one of the most widely used variables has been developmental acquisition data delineating the average ages of phonological process use and suppression.

Although information on normal development is a valid variable, it should not be deemed the sole criterion in the selection of phonological processes. As indicated earlier, each child has unique and individual needs that may not be met if developmental norms are used exclusively. It is important to remember that developmental norms are a statistical representation of the average performance of an entire age group. By definition, norms neutralize individual uniqueness and variations. Lowe (1994) indicates that norms are "useful for determining delays in development or eligibility for a remedial program, but they are probably not the best resource for choosing intervention targets" (p. 176). With this in mind, we will regard developmental norms as one of the many criteria that should be considered.

Edwards and Bernhardt (1973) suggest three very important guiding principles for the selection of phonological processes. Their three suggestions are as follows:

1. Select processes that affect intelligibility the most.
2. Select processes that are less stable.
3. Select processes that are most common in young children.

In 1983, Edwards expanded on some of the original guidelines and provided a very detailed list. Although Edwards and Bernhardt (1973) advocated the application of their three principles in the order provided, Edwards (1983) later acknowledged that it is not possible to delineate an exact sequence in the selection of processes. Instead, she provided several principles that can be used as general guidelines. No specific order was emphasized. The following summarizes Edwards's four principles (information adapted from pp. 39–41):

Compare c.
contrast treatment
of articulation
phonological
disorders
children

- **Principle #1.** Choose processes that result in early success or that would be relatively easy to remediate. The underlying assumption is that an active phonological process may be more amenable to remediation if the child has already shown suppression of the process to some extent.

  - Select processes that are optional — in other words, whose frequency of occurrence is less than 100%.

  - Select processes that occur only in certain **phonetic environments.**

  - Select processes that affect sounds that are within the child's **phonetic inventory.** These are sounds that the child can produce to some extent, though not always in the appropriate linguistic context to create a contrast between words.

  - Select processes that affect sounds for which the child is **stimulable.** These are sounds that the child can make correctly with additional stimulation, typically in the form of modeling.

- **Principle #2.** Choose processes that are "crucial" for the individual child.

  - Select processes that are deviant, unusual, or **idiosyncratic.** For example, velarization, lateralization, frication of stops, and glottal replacement may make good initial targets since they call attention to the child's speech.

  - Select processes that contribute significantly to the child's reduced **intelligibility.** *Stopping,* for example, may have a significant effect on the child's speech intelligibility since it can affect a large set of sounds.

  - Select processes that result in extensive **homonymy.** Homonymy leads to the loss of linguistic contrast between two or more words (e.g., child produces [pɪt] for *his, fish,* and *sit* due to the effects of stopping of fricatives).

  - Select processes that are used consistently by the child.

- **Principle #3.** Choose "early" processes or processes that affect early sounds.

- **Principle #4.** Choose processes that interact. Processes that interact may create complex substitutions based on more than one rule change. Work on processes that affect the greatest number of sound segments.

Edwards's (1983) principles are extensive yet broad enough to allow for individual variability and client uniqueness. They should be used carefully and tailored to meet the needs of individual clients.

Hodson and Paden's (1983, 1991) work in the area of phonology has received much acclaim over the past several years. They are thought to have played a key role in shifting therapy from a traditional motor approach to a more linguistic-based approach in children diagnosed with a phonological process disorder versus an articulation disorder. As part of their selection criteria, Hodson and Paden (1991) first consider processes that have a **percentage of occurrence** of at least 40%. They indicate that "children who are using a phonological process less than 40% of its opportunities seem to be well on the way toward developing that particular pattern on their own. Phonological processes that occur less than 40% of the time therefore are not targeted at the outset. They are reviewed periodically during readministration of the APP-R and may become targets later if they seem to be *frozen* at a particular percentage near 40%" (pp. 69–71). Percentages of occurrence are calculated via administration of the *Assessment of Phonological Processes– Revised* (Hodson, 1986a).

Although on the surface Hodson and Paden's statements seem logical, the reality of their assumptions can be ascertained only through experimental manipulation of **dependent** and **independent variables.** Therefore, until more empirically valid data are available, we cannot recommend that a clinician assume that processes that occur less than 40% of the time will likely suppress over time without special intervention. If other variables indicate that a process occurring less than 40% is an important initial therapy target, the clinician should select such process without hesitation.

Hodson and Paden (1983) further prioritize phonological processes into four levels reflecting intelligibility: Level 0, Level I, Level II, and Level III. Level 0 processes include those that affect intelligibility the most, whereas Level III patterns have a minimal effect on intelligibility. Thus, lower-level patterns would always take priority over higher-level processes. Lower-level processes take priority even if higher-level processes have a higher percentage of occurrence.

According to Hodson and Paden (1983), *Level 0 patterns* are characterized by omission of obstruents and liquids. Although less common, Level 0 may also reflect omission of glides and nasals. *Level I patterns* include omission of syllables, prevocalic singletons (usually obstruents but sometimes sonorants), postvocalic singletons (usually obstruents), and cluster deletion. Major substitution patterns in Level I include fronting of velars and backing. Other patterns included in Level I are prevocalic voicing, prevocalic devoicing, reduplication, vowel deviations, and idiosyncratic (child-specific) rules. Omissions in *Level II patterns* include cluster reduction and stridency deletion (especially in clusters), while major substitutions include stopping, liquid gliding, and vowelization. Last, *Level III patterns* are characterized by nonphonemic alterations such as tongue protrusion (including both frontal lisp and dentalization) and lateralization, major phonemic substitutions such as affrication, deaffrication, palatalization, depalatalization, "th" shifts, and devoicing of final obstruents.

Individual Sounds

Whether a child is diagnosed with an articulation disorder or a phonological process disorder, the clinician must select a set of phonemes that will be taught to improve the child's communication skills. If the child is diagnosed with a phonological process disorder, the sounds affected by the process need to be targeted for direct training. For example, if the child uses the phonological process of stopping, it can be predicted that many fricative sounds will be affected. Therefore, those fricative sounds would have to be taught to decrease the use of stopping. However, because many sounds within a particular class can be affected at the same time, the clinician must determine which of those sounds will be taught first.

How does a clinician determine which sounds should be taught first? For beginning clinicians this is one of the most difficult steps in the therapy process. As part of our clinical supervision, we often ask clinicians to outline a general plan of treatment before they actually write a comprehensive treatment program. We also ask them to meet with us so that we can discuss their plan. In discussing a client diagnosed with an articulation or phonological disorder, one of the tasks that we require from clinicians is that they explain why they chose certain sounds for teaching. Many clinicians will eventually confess that they are not sure why.

When student clinicians provide a rationale without prompting on our part, most frequently it is based on developmental norms. Answers such as "These are sounds that the child should have," and "Most kids are making these sounds by this age" are common. With coaxing, clinicians can supply answers based on other variables, such as, "I think these sounds will make him more intelligible" and "These are the sounds that were stimulable during the assessment."

In defense of student clinicians, the selection of target sounds is not an easy process. Many experts have provided guidelines that can be used as selection criteria. We will highlight many of these in the following sections. It is our goal that a discussion of these suggestions will facilitate the clinician's selection of target sounds for training.

In addition to guidelines for the selection of phonological processes, Edwards (1983) offers the following criteria for the selection of target phonemes for training:

- Choose target sounds that are in the child's phonetic repertoire.
- Choose sounds for which the child is stimulable.
- Choose sounds that should improve intelligibility.
- Choose frequently occurring sounds.
- Choose sounds that are acquired early.
- Choose high-value sounds — that is, sounds that will have an impact for the child; for example, sounds that might cause the child embarrassment if used incorrectly.
- Choose sounds that should be relatively easy to produce in the position of concern.

Weiss, Gordon, and Lillywhite (1987) discuss several factors that influence the selection of sounds for training. You will notice that some of these are similar to the criteria advocated by Edwards (1983). Weiss et al. recommend that a clinician select the error phoneme:

- that is the earliest to develop;
- that is the most stimulable;
- that is produced correctly in a **key word;**
- that occurs most frequently in speech;
- that is most consistent;
- that is visible;
- for which the client has been most criticized or penalized;
- that the client most desires to correct;
- whose production is least affected by physical deviations;
- that is the same for a group of clients.

Elbert and Gierut (1986) also provide various suggestions for the selection of target sounds. Their selection criteria are rather unusual, however, in that they base them on a set of predictions. They describe a prediction as a twofold process that acts interdependently. The clinician first predicts specific sound changes that will occur in a child's phonology, and then uses that information to select target sounds for treatment.

Elbert and Gierut (1986) developed their predictions from their extensive review of the available research on sound generalization. They emphasize that these predictions "provide a synthesis of the various kinds of sound changes that clinicians can expect to occur in a child's phonology" (p. 105). The important clinical significance of this is that the clinician who understands the sound corrections that can be expected to occur due to the process of generalization will select sounds that "will induce the greatest changes in the child's system" (p. 104). This may reduce the number of sounds that the clinician needs to teach directly, which, in turn, maximizes the training process. The set of predictions offered by Elbert and Gierut, as derived from their extensive review of the literature, are outlined below (1986, adapted from pp. 105–107). They recommend using these singly or in combination when selecting target behaviors for training.

1. PREDICTION: *Teaching one member of a cognate sound pair will result in the use of the other sound in the pair.*
- Example: A child does not produce [s] or [z] correctly.
- Treatment: Teach [z] production.
- Prediction: Production of [s] will also improve.

2. PREDICTION: *Teaching one allophone will result in the production of other related allophones.*
- Example: A child does not accurately produce [r], [ɝ], or [ɚ].
- Treatment: Teach [ɝ] production.
- Prediction: Production of [r] and [ɚ] will also improve.

3. PREDICTION: *Teaching a distinctive feature in the context of one sound will result in the use of that feature in other untreated sounds.*
- Example: A child does not accurately produce [f, v, s, z, ʃ].
- Treatment: Teach [+strident] feature by contrasting [s] and [θ].
- Prediction: Untreated sounds with the [+strident] feature [f, v, z, ʃ] will also improve.

4. PREDICTION: *Teaching sounds in the final position of morphemes will result in more accurate production of the sounds in inflected intervocalic contexts.*
- Example: A child does not produce [s] accurately.
- Treatment: Teach [s] word-finally in the context of words like *kiss, miss, hiss.*
- Prediction: Production of [s] will improve intervocalically in words like *kissing, missing,* and *hissing.*

5. PREDICTION: *Teaching stops in word-final position will lead to more accurate production in word-initial position.*
- Example: A child does not produce [k] or [g] in any word position.
- Treatment: Teach production of [k] and [g] in word-final position.
- Prediction: Production of [k] and [g] in word-initial position will also improve.

6. PREDICTION: *Teaching fricatives in word-initial position will result in more accurate production of fricatives in word-final position.*
- Example: A child does not produce [f] or [v] in any word position.
- Treatment: Teach production of [f] and [v] in word-initial position.
- Prediction: Production of [f] and [v] in word-final position will also improve.

7. PREDICTION: *Teaching fricatives will result in more accurate production of stops.*

- Example: A child does not accurately produce the fricatives [f, v, s] or the stops [d, k, g].
- Treatment: Teach production of [f, v, s].
- Prediction: Production of the stops [d, k, g] will also improve.

8. PREDICTION: *Teaching voiced obstruents (stops, fricatives, affricates) will result in accurate production of voiceless obstruents.*

- Example: A child does not accurately produce [ʧ] or [ʤ].
- Treatment: Teach production of [ʤ].
- Prediction: Production of [ʧ] will also improve.

9. PREDICTION: *Teaching sounds that are stimulable results in more accurate production than teaching sounds that are not stimulable.*

- Example: A child does not produce [θ] or [ð] but is stimulable on production of [θ].
- Treatment: Teach production of [θ].
- Prediction: Production of [ð] may improve, but production of [θ] will still be better.

10. PREDICTION: *Sounds that are phonologically "known" will be produced more accurately than sounds that are phonologically "unknown."*

- Example: A child has knowledge of stops in all positions but uses an optional rule of word-final deletion. The child does not use affricates in any position.
- Treatment: Teach production of affricates, which are phonologically "unknown."
- Prediction: Production of stops will be more accurate than production of affricates, even though stops were not treated.

11. PREDICTION: *Teaching sounds of which a child has least phonological knowledge ("unknown" aspects of phonology) will result in changes across untreated aspects of the sound system.*

- Example: A child uses optional rules affecting production of stops, has a positional constraint against production of liquids word-initially, and has an inventory constraint against production of fricatives. This child has least phonological knowledge of fricatives.
- Treatment: Teach production of fricatives.
- Prediction: Production of fricatives will improve as well as the other untreated aspects of the sound system, namely, production of stops and liquids.

Elbert and Gierut (1986) indicate that these predictions are "unidirectional." They also warn the reader that such changes in sound production will occur only as stated in the predictions, as they have been supported by documented research. They further suggest that the existing predictions may be revised and new ones may be added as determined by more current research.

Further Discussion of the Selection Variables

After considering several factors offered by many experts, we will explore many of them in greater detail. The clinician should always remember that in the selection of individual target sounds, it is typically a combination of those variables that ultimately guides the final determination. It is also important to consider that once certain sounds have been selected for training, such a decision can be altered according to the client's performance. Ultimately, it is the client's accomplishments that dictate the course of therapy.

Sounds That Are Functional for the Child

The practical clinician always considers the primary goal of therapy to be what is most functional for a particular client. A sound that plays a significant role in the client's phonological system is the most clinically relevant. Sound errors for which the child is teased, that affect social or academic interactions, and that have the highest effect on current or future communicative performance should be considered immediate targets for therapy.

This variable must rise above other factors such as developmental acquisition data. By way of illustration let us consider a 4½-year-old child who misarticulates the /r/ consonant in addition to several other sounds. Normative data may suggest that /r/ is frequently produced incorrectly by children that age and when considered alone, may not seem to be an important initial therapeutic target. However, if this same child's mother indicates that she is concerned that her son cannot make the *r* because his full name is Ryan Roberts and he says it "Wyan Wobots," then the priority for treating that sound changes. It may be extremely important for this child and the child's family that he articulate his name correctly as he gets closer to kindergarten because they are concerned that his peers will tease him and his social interactions will be affected.

Sounds That Are Stimulable

Remember from the previous chapter that stimulability testing is important for two reasons. First, it can serve as a valuable prognostic indicator of the client's progress in therapy. Also, it is one of the variables that clinicians consider when selecting target sounds for treatment. It is commonly agreed that sounds that are produced correctly with auditory, tactile, and visual prompts during stimulability testing will be easier for the client to learn once direct training is initiated.

Clinicians who believe that early success in therapy is imperative to the child's achievement of the established goals and objectives often prefer to teach sounds that are highly stimulable over those that are not as stimulable. This variable should be used with caution, however, since poor stimulability performance during the testing process does not mean that the child will not learn to make the sound once treatment is started. In fact, Sommers et al. (1967) found the opposite to be true. In their study, kindergarten and first-grade children who received poor stimulability scores benefited more from therapy than those who had good stimulability. In essence, good stimulability scores may be indicative of early success in therapy. However, poor stimulability should not preclude the selection of a particular sound if other variables indicate that it is an appropriate therapeutic target.

Sounds That Occur in Key Words or Contextual Testing

As discussed in the Basic Unit of Chapter 6, Eugene McDonald developed a well-known testing instrument called the *Deep Test of Articulation* (McDonald, 1964). This test is used to evaluate the presence of **facilitative phonetic contexts** for the production of a particular phoneme. Clinicians may select possible target sounds and deep test their production. Sounds for which a facilitating context is found may make good initial targets. Van Riper and Emerick (1984) also suggest that the clinician listen carefully to the child's spontaneous speech productions for **key words.** Key words are words in which the misarticulated sound is produced correctly. Sounds that are noted to occur correctly in a key word in connected speech productions may also make good initial targets. If a sound is produced correctly in a particular facilitative context or key word, the treatment process may be accelerated. The clinician may be able to shift therapy to more complex linguistic levels such as phrases and sentences more quickly.

Sounds That Are More Visible

Without a doubt, some sounds are more visible than other sounds. For example, the production of /m/, /p/, and /b/ is much easier to visualize than the production of /ʒ/, /r/, and /ʃ/. Bilabials, labiodentals, linguadentals, and alveolar sounds can be easily seen by closely watching the speaker's mouth. Glides, stridents [s, z, ʃ, ʒ, ʤ, ʧ], and velars, on the other hand, are difficult or nearly impossible to see during their production. Sounds that are more visible may make good initial targets because they are sometimes easier to teach. Very young children often need visual cues to facilitate production of target sounds, and highly visible sounds may be more amenable to this type of teaching strategy. This variable should not preclude the teaching of less visible sounds if they are more appropriate for a particular client.

Sounds That Occur More Frequently

Not all sounds occur with the same level of frequency in the English language. Some are used often, whereas others are used very seldom. For example, the proportional occurrence of /n/ is 11.46% compared to that of /ʒ/ at 0.16% (Edwards, 1997). Errors on frequently occurring sounds may have a greater impact on the child's intelligibility because the errors would occur more often. Because of this, sounds that occur more frequently are more important to overall communicative effectiveness.

If the child exhibits multiple misarticulations, sounds that occur more frequently and have a greater impact on intelligibility make good initial targets. It is important to remember, however, that some sounds that do not occur frequently may make better initial targets than sounds that do occur frequently. For example, even though the proportional occurrence for /ʤ/ is 0.95%, it can be a very important sound target if it has a direct impact on a particular child's life. An example of this is a child named George whose name begins and ends with /ʤ/. The reader is referred to Appendix M for further information on the proportional occurrence of all American English consonants.

Sounds That Affect Intelligibility the Most

The primary goal in articulation therapy is to improve the child's intelligibility. Certain sounds in the English language affect intelligibility more than other sounds. With this in mind, it is clinically sound to select target phonemes that will have the greatest impact on the child's communication by improving his or her intelligibility.

Sounds That Are Inconsistently Mispronounced

Some experts recommend that sounds that are inconsistently mispronounced make good initial therapeutic targets. In essence, if a sound is inconsistently mispronounced, the client can produce the target sound correctly at times. The clinician capitalizes on the child's ability to make the sound at least some of the time and focuses therapy on strengthening correct production of the sound across different phonetic contexts or linguistic levels. The concept of inconsistency is similar to that of stimulability in that those sounds that the child can make at some level during the assessment process may be easier to learn or stabilize. And this may increase the likelihood of early success in therapy.

Sounds That Are Acquired Earlier

Sounds that are acquired earlier in the normal acquisition process are sometimes presumed to be easier to produce and, thus, easier to teach. For example, children in normal development acquire stops and nasals before liquids and sibilants. Furthermore, because many of the early appearing sounds are more visible, they are sometimes easier to teach since visual cues can be readily provided to the client.

However, it should be emphasized that simply because children as a group develop certain sounds before others, it does not guarantee that early developing sounds will be learned more easily in treatment by a particular client. Also, there is no specific research to support this assumption. Therefore, this variable must be used with caution.

Regardless, many clinicians believe that if a child exhibits multiple misarticulations, it is clinically wise to teach sounds that the child "should" be producing at a given age rather than sounds that are still in the acquisition process. We reiterate that these sounds should not be considered over those that are important to the client, those that will increase the client's intelligibility, and those that will have a greater impact on the child's communication.

Sounds That Are Part of the Child's Phonetic Inventory

In the Basic Unit of Chapter 6, we indicated that as part of a thorough assessment, the clinician could perform a **phonetic inventory analysis.** In summary, a phonetic inventory analysis identifies those sounds that the client can make without considering the linguistic targets attempted. It provides some insight into the client's motor abilities for the production of phonemes. This information can assist the clinician's selection of target sounds for training in two ways.

First, the clinician may choose to target sounds that are already part of the client's phonetic **repertoire.** Some clients have the motor ability to make certain sounds but do not always use those sounds in the appropriate linguistic context. An example of this is a client who can produce stop consonants without difficulty in the initial position of words but not in the final position of words. In this case, the problem obviously is not the client's lack of motor skills. Failure to produce consonants in the final position of words is most commonly identified as the phonological process of **final-consonant deletion.**

To further highlight this concept, let us assume that a client failed to produce the following phonemes in the final position of words: [s, z, f, v, t, d, k, g, m, and p]. A phonetic inventory analysis, however, revealed that the client could make [m], [p], and [t] in the medial and final positions with some consistency. The remaining phonemes were not produced in any position. The clinician then may choose to target those sounds for which the client demonstrates some motor readiness before those that are completely absent from the client's repertoire. Doing this may speed up the treatment process because training can focus on facilitating correct production of the sound in appropriate linguistic contexts rather than teaching the motor components of the sound. The clinician may then probe for **generalized productions** of the untaught sounds.

Second, the clinician may choose to target sounds that are not yet part of the child's phonetic inventory. A phonetic inventory analysis in this case may reveal that a child has only a limited number of phonemes within his phonetic repertoire. The use of a limited number of sounds would have a significant impact on the severity of the disorder. The fewer sounds the client makes, the higher the number of errors he or she is likely to manifest. Likewise, the more errors the client demonstrates, the less intelligible his or her speech. With this in mind, the clinician may choose to teach sounds that are not part of the client's repertoire to increase his or her phonetic inventory and thus provide a variety of features from different sound classes. If a phonetic inventory analysis revealed that the client's consonant production was limited to [m], [n], [t], and [p], the clinician might choose to teach the contrastive phonemes [k], [g], [d], and [b]. This may result in a decreased number of errors and improved speech intelligibility.

Exemplars That May Generalize to Others

We previously discussed Elbert and Gierut's (1986) recommendations on the selection of target phonemes according to a set of predictions they developed from the clinical research available at the time. Their predictions capitalize on the behavioral principle of **generalization.** That is, after teaching a specific target behavior, its production may generalize to similar untaught behaviors. This is an important consideration with children who have multiple misarticulations.

The efficient clinician would undoubtedly want to follow a treatment approach that minimizes the amount of time needed to improve the client's overall articulation or phonological skills. Clustering sound errors according to some structural relationship and teaching a few **exemplars** within the group rather than each and every sound can help the clinician accomplish that. After some teaching on the initial targets, the clinician can then probe for **generalized productions** to the untaught sounds. For example, if a child misarticulated [f, v, s, z, θ, ð, ʃ, and ʒ], the clinician might choose to teach each of the unvoiced sounds and then probe for generalized productions to their untaught cognate pairs. If generalized responding indeed occurred, it would eliminate the need to teach eight sounds. This undoubtedly would expedite the clinical process.

We strongly agree with Elbert and Gierut's recommendation that the assumption that teaching one sound will facilitate production of an untaught sound should be made only in cases where research has proven it a clinical reality. Clinicians should be careful not to presume that generalized responding would occur across sounds that have some structural relationships. Simply because sounds share common *structural* relationships (e.g., manner of production, place of articulation, voicing) does not mean that they are part of the same **empirical class.** Behaviors that are part of the same empirical class are *functionally* related and are created by the same or similar **contingencies.** The clinician should always make sure that generalized responding from the taught sound to the untaught sounds has in fact taken place. This is done through additional testing procedures termed **probes.** We will discuss probing procedures in greater detail in an upcoming section of this chapter.

Exemplars That Are Part of a Phonological Process, Rule, or Pattern

As reviewed in previous chapters, in recent years, sound error productions have been described according to phonological processes, patterns, or rules. If a child is diagnosed with a phonological process disorder, often the goal of treatment becomes elimination of the **underlying processes.** In other cases, if specific rules are noted to be missing in the child's phonological system, then the goal of treatment is to teach such rules. Three major pattern classification systems have been advanced in articulation and phonological training: (1) patterns based on place-voicing-manner analysis, (2) patterns based on distinctive features, and (3) patterns based on phonological processes.

Place-Voicing-Manner Patterns. In the place-voicing-manner method, substitution errors are classified according to similarities in their manner of production, place of articulation, and voicing features. Multiple misarticulations are grouped into each of these categories as appropriate, which results in the identification of clusters of errors. Using this type of analysis, the clinician may note that a client misarticulates all of the stops, most of the fricatives, all of the alveolars, or several voiced consonants. The clinician may then select one or more sound exemplar for the classes in error. For example, if a client substitutes stops for fricatives, the clinician may teach a few fricatives and then probe for generalized productions to the untaught sounds within the same sound class. If generalized responding did occur, the clinician would save valuable training time. However, generalized responding should not be presumed, and, if **probing procedures** show that it has not occurred, the clinician should initiate direct training with the remaining **sound exemplars.**

Distinctive Feature Patterns. In the early 1970s the description of sounds according to their distinctive features became extremely popular. Recall that distinctive features are unique characteristics that distinguish a sound from all other sounds. Examples of these are the voice, nasal, posterior, anterior, and sonorant features. This theoretical notion quickly made its way to the assessment and treatment of articulation and phonological disorders.

Using this classification system, children's multiple misarticulations are grouped according to the presence or absence of particular features. For example, analyses of the testing data may reveal that the child's phonological system lacks the posterior, strident, or sonorant feature, resulting in incorrect productions of sounds that have the feature. At other times, the clinician may note that a group of sounds that share a feature (e.g., sonorants, stridents, nasals) are consistently mispronounced or substituted. If this approach were followed, the goal of therapy would become to teach the absent phonological features or the operating rules resulting in sound error productions.

As with the PVM approach, the clinician may choose to teach a few target exemplars from each of the identified feature groups. For example, if the client's phonological system lacked the strident feature so that some or all of the strident sounds [s, z, f, v, ʧ, ʤ, ʃ, ʒ] were either omitted or replaced, the clinician could select a few of the stridents (e.g., /s/, /f/, and /ʃ/) to establish the feature. The clinician would then **probe** for generalized productions to the untaught stridents. As explained under the PVM approach, if generalized responding did take place, the clinician would avoid unnecessary teaching of other sounds. However, we again emphasize that this should not be merely assumed. Rather, the clinician should conduct further testing and if the data reveal that generalized responding has not occurred, direct training with the remaining exemplars should be initiated.

Phonological Processes. One of the most current classification systems to make a dramatic impact on the assessment and treatment of articulation and phonological disorders is the phonological process approach. Clinicians who follow this approach organize a client's misarticulations according to the underlying phonological processes affecting sound production and speech intelligibility. In Chapter 2 we described the phonological processes that have been most frequently defined in the literature according to (a) syllable structure processes (b) substitution processes, and (c) assimilation processes.

In this approach, the goal of therapy is to reduce or eliminate the operating phonological processes affecting a child's speech intelligibility. We previously described some of the recommendations experts have provided for the selection of phonological processes for treatment. However, to reduce or eliminate the underlying processes, a clinician must still select the target phonemes affected by their presence. For example, if the phonological process of stopping affected the fricatives [s, v, f, v, θ, ð, ʃ, ʒ], the clinician could select a few target exemplars for initial training (e.g., /z/, /v/, and /ð/). Reduction or elimination of a phonological process ultimately can be accomplished only by establishing sounds that are incompatible with the presence of the process. In other words, as the clinician teaches production of the sounds or word structural rules affected by the process, its elimination is probable. If training of a few exemplars does not completely eliminate the process, then the clinician can directly teach the remaining exemplars. Probing for generalized responding should be performed as discussed with the PVM and distinctive feature approaches.

Deciding on the Number of Sounds or Patterns To Teach

After considering all of the variables previously discussed and selecting the most appropriate initial target sounds, the clinician must determine the number of sounds that will be taught at one time. If the assessment reveals that only one or two sounds are misarticulated, such a decision can easily be made. This issue becomes a more salient clinical consideration with clients who have multiple misarticulations.

If a clinician strictly adheres to the traditional articulation treatment approach, which will be discussed in greater detail in Chapter 8, no more than two target sounds are taught at once. New target sounds are selected for training only after the client can produce the initial target in sentences. Some clinicians may choose to focus on a single sound, since that can result in more rapid progress. Also, for some clients, simultaneous teaching of multiple targets may become confusing.

Elbert and Gierut (1986) consider the teaching of a restricted set of target sounds in a limited set of stimulus items a **training deep approach.** In this approach a select number of sounds is taught intensively, and other sounds are selected for teaching only after the child has achieved mastery criterion on the initial targets (Roseberry-McKibbin & Hegde, 2000).

Some experts view the restricted teaching of one or two sounds as too narrow and recommend that several sounds be taught simultaneously. Weiss, Gordon, and Lillywhite (1987) provide the following reasons for working on the simultaneous teaching of multiple target sounds:

1. It expedites the rate of progress.

2. It improves intelligibility more readily.

3. It maintains motivation.

4. It reduces the chances of **overgeneralization**.

5. It makes the treatment process more economical, in that the faster the progress, the less cost to the responsible party.

Elbert and Gierut (1986) refer to the simultaneous teaching of multiple target sounds as a **training broad approach.** They state, "The concept behind training broad is limited to practice over a wide range of exemplars. The child is presented with a number of sounds and exemplars, but does not necessarily practice these same items repeatedly" (p. 103). The goal is to expose the child to several target sounds. Introduction of one sound is not precluded by the performance of another sound; the clinician may choose to introduce a sound even if the predetermined mastery criterion has not been reached in the production of a sound already being taught. The **multiple phoneme approach,** which will be described in detail in Chapter 8, is an example of a treatment program that advocates simultaneous teaching of several target sounds (McCabe & Bradley, 1975).

Although both the training deep and the training broad approaches have been found to be effective (Costello & Onstine, 1976; Elbert & McReynolds, 1975, 1978; Hodson & Paden, 1991; McReynolds, 1972; McReynolds & Elbert, 1981b; Weiner, 1981), it is the individual clinician who determines what is appropriate for a particular client. While one client may not benefit from the simultaneous teaching of various sounds, it may prove to be the best therapeutic approach for another client. There are several variables that often help the clinician make the final determination. These include:

- the client's age and readiness to learn;
- the client's intellectual skills and ability to learn;
- the client's language skills;
- the client's motivation to improve;
- the client's level of participation in therapy;
- the client's attention to task;
- the presence of any interfering behaviors; and
- the client's reported history of progress.

In clinical practice, assuming that the client can handle the training of multiple targets, clinicians most often teach four to five target behaviors at the same time. However, this is often influenced by the length of time the clinician expects to have the client on his or her caseload. In the typical university setting, the clinical practicum is often divided into quarters or semesters (approximately a 3-month period), whereas in the public school setting, a student's **individualized education program** is revised once a year. In the medical setting or private practice, it is often the insurance agency or other third-party payers that dictate the amount of therapy time that will be provided. Therefore, clinicians must always be conscious about the number of target behaviors that can realistically be taught in an allotted period of time.

Establishing Baselines

As stated earlier, the assessment data yield important information that can help the clinician select intervention targets. However, that information may not be adequate for establishing a reliable and valid pretreatment performance that will eventually help the clinician evaluate the client's progress over time. Many traditional standardized articulation tests allow minimal opportunities for the occurrence of a specific speech sound or phonological process. For example, single-word tests designed to assess all English consonants typically give three opportunities for the use of a specific sound (in initial-, medial-, and final-word positions). If the child misarticulates the sound during administration of the articulation test, it may be assumed that he or she has not mastered production of the sound. However, this information is limited because it does not reveal the accuracy percentage with which the client produces the sound that was misarticulated during formal testing.

The clinician may counteract this problem by establishing **baselines** of the *potential* treatment targets before starting therapy. Hegde (1998b) defines baselines as measured rates of behaviors in the absence of treatment (p. 114). In essence, baselines provide detailed pretreatment information that can be used to (a) evaluate the child's progress over time, (b) establish treatment effectiveness (or ineffectiveness), and (c) establish clinician accountability. In an era of third-party payers and legal vulnerability, it is extremely important that the clinician establish clinical accountability. It is no longer sufficient to report that a client is "doing very well" or "improving very much." Parents and third-party payers are increasingly demanding detailed documentation of the client's progress. However, it is nearly impossible to reliably measure progress if the child's pretreatment performance is unknown. Therefore, the extra time taken to establish baselines is extremely worthwhile.

Baseline Procedures

Hegde (1998b) suggests four steps that may be used in establishing baselines of various communicative disorders. He emphasizes that although these steps are general enough to be applied across communicative disorders, modifications should be made in the case of specific disorders (p. 115). Taking Hegde's suggestions to heart, his four basic steps will be used to illustrate the establishment of baselines for speech sounds.

Specify the Treatment Targets in Measurable Terms

The first step is to specify the treatment targets. The clinician must have a clear idea of what the intervention targets are before baselines can be established. Also, it is important to state the treatment targets with sufficient detail so that they can be measured. Treatment targets such as "improved articulation" or "decreased use of stopping" are too general and impossible to measure. On the other hand, clearly written target behaviors such as the following can easily be measured:

- production of /s/ in initial-word position at the word level;
- suppression of stopping by teaching /f/, /v/, and /s/ in all word positions;
- production of C-V-C words;
- use of the [+continuant] distinctive feature in CVC words.

Target objectives such as these identify the initial intervention targets and specify the **response topography,** or linguistic level of training. Clinicians can compare the client's performance during baseline measures with the selected treatment targets and decide whether they are indeed appropriate. Many of us have been in clinical situations where we decided to teach a particular phoneme because a child did not produce it correctly on standardized or formal testing only to find out through baseline procedures that he or she can already make it with 90% accuracy. What can account for this discrepancy?

The client may have produced the sound incorrectly in a particular phonetic context or in a particular word during articulation testing. However, baseline trials by definition provide multiple opportunities for the production of a single sound in specific word positions across several words. Therefore, the information obtained during that activity is much more accurate than that obtained during articulation testing. If the clinician had not performed baseline trials in such a situation, he or she may have attributed the client's improved performance to the special intervention provided, when in fact the client could already make the sound with a high accuracy level.

Prepare the Stimulus Items

The second step in establishing baselines is to prepare the stimulus items and design events, questions, and prompts that will evoke the target responses. The stimulus items most frequently used are pictures. With very young children, the clinician may also use real objects to increase the client's participation. At times children respond better to items that can be manipulated. However, it is not always possible to use real objects that represent the word containing the target sound. For example, if the target sound were /l/ in the initial position and one of the selected words were *lost,* an object is not the best choice to prompt that stimulus word. A picture representing the concept of "lost" or a stimulus question (e.g., "When someone can't find their way home, they are . . . ?") may be a better option in this case.

Whatever stimulus items the clinician chooses to use, they should be unambiguous and appropriate for a particular client's age, cultural background, and linguistic abilities. If possible, stimulus items from the client's natural environment should be used during baseline trials and later in treatment. This may help in the eventual maintenance of the target behaviors in the natural setting (to be discussed further in upcoming sections). Hegde (1998b) recommends at least 20 stimulus items for each target behavior.

Prepare a Recording Sheet

The third step is to prepare a sheet on which the child's responses can be recorded. The use of a clearly designed, yet detailed recording sheet helps the clinician document the client's pretreatment performance. The clinician can design a recording sheet that he or she can use routinely. In preparing a recording sheet, it is important to design one that can be used with various treatment targets. Appendix K illustrates a recording sheet that can be used during baseline trials and adapted to various treatment targets.

Administer the Baseline Trials

In the fourth step the clinician is ready to administer the baseline trials. The selected stimulus items are presented in **discrete trials.** Simply stated, a discrete trial is a structured opportunity to produce a given target; in this case the target is the selected speech sound. By definition, discrete trials are separated from one another by a short time interval, typically a few seconds, so that there is a clear beginning and end to each trial.

According to Hegde (1998b) baseline trials can be administered on evoked and modeled trials. During **evoked trials,** the clinician arranges certain stimuli (i.e., pictures, objects, or actions) so that the use of the target response is likely to occur. In **modeled trials,** the clinician also manipulates those stimuli but in addition provides a model of the target response for the child to imitate. The administration of modeled trials can yield important clinical information. If the client can produce the target response with a certain level of accuracy during modeled trials, the clinician can safely assume that treatment can begin at the imitation level. However, if the client's production of the target sound does not improve with modeling, then treatment may have to begin with establishment of the target sound through additional stimulus control such as **phonetic placement, shaping,** or **sound approximation.** Hegde outlines the following steps for administering discrete evoked baseline trials (adapted to illustrate **base rating** of /f/ in the initial position of words):

1. Place the stimulus picture in front of the client, or demonstrate the action or event with objects; for example:

- show the child a picture of *fish* or *fat*;
- lift four fingers to evoke the word *four.*

2. Ask a relevant predetermined question, for example:

- "What do you see in the picture?"
- "What is swimming in the water?"
- "The boy is not skinny, he's . . ."
- "How many fingers do I have up? Let's count them . . . one, two, three . . ."

3. Wait a few seconds for the client to respond. The amount of time needed before presentation of the next stimulus item may vary across children, depending on their individual needs.

4. Record the response on the recording sheet using a +/− system. A correct response would be indicated by a "+" mark, and an incorrect response by a "−" mark. Occasionally, children may not respond after the stimulus item has been presented. This may be recorded by "NR" for no response.

5. Pull the picture toward you, or remove it from the subject's view. This is important to decrease the possibility of the child continuing to respond to a previous stimulus item even after a new stimulus item has been presented. This will decrease confusion on the part of the child and will help avoid competing responses from young children.

6. Return to step 1 to initiate the next trial until all trials are completed.

Modeled baseline trials are conducted in a fashion similar to that of evoked baseline trials with one exception. As the name implies, during modeled trials, the clinician provides a model of the target response for the client to imitate after the stimulus picture has been presented and the predetermined question has been asked.

Determining the Linguistic Level of Training and Preparing Appropriate Stimulus Materials

After reliable baselines have been established, the clinician is one step closer to actually starting therapy. The baseline information helps the clinician determine whether the tentative sounds, processes, or rules selected for training are indeed appropriate **treatment objectives.** This information also helps the clinician identify the level of linguistic complexity that is an adequate starting point for training. For example, if the client's baseline accuracy score for a particular sound was 10% during modeled trials, the client will probably need some initial training at the sound or syllable level. However, if the accuracy score during baseline trials was 50% in evoked word productions, then therapy should start at least at the word level. However, the accepted starting point of therapy sometimes varies according to a particular clinician's treatment philosophy.

In the traditional approach to therapy, the starting point for production training has always been the isolation (sound) or nonsense syllable level. In their explanation of why they start by teaching the sound in isolation, Van Riper and Erickson (1996) indicate that they do so to "avoid the long history of usage that has so strongly reinforced the error. It's easier" (p. 239). They further explain that "we must recognize that the production of that correct sound is our essential target" (p. 239). Van Riper and Erickson speculate that a child who misarticulates a sound has probably received much feedback about his or her incorrect productions from peers, parents, and teachers through such comments as "Don't say wop. Say **rope.**" However, that type of request, which requires a response at the word or sentence level, may be too difficult for the child, and thus he or she continues to "fail." The sound or syllable level can serve as a starting point that may produce some initial success for the child.

In recent years, however, the emphasis of treatment has shifted from a purely phonetic approach to a linguistic approach, since sound misarticulations affect not only the sound but also the internal meaning of the words that contain it. Therefore, the most widely recommended starting point for therapy now is at least the word level. As stated by Lowe (1994), "It is at the word level that sounds make a difference, and it is at the word level that children can perceive the function of sounds in communication" (p. 180). With this in mind, it is extremely important that the clinician devote quality time to the selection of appropriate stimulus words so that the child's communication needs are met in a functional manner. It is fruitless to begin the treatment process by teaching words that the child may or may not use in his or her natural communicative environment.

Lowe (1994) provides a detailed summary of several factors to consider in the selection of stimulus words. These include phonetic context, meaningfulness, communicative potency, syllable shape, and phonetic inventory. He suggests the following as important variables in the selection of stimulus words for treatment of articulation and phonological disorders (summarized presentation of pp. 180–183):

Phonetic Context

• The inventory and arrangement of consonants and vowels within a word or a phonetic context can have a significant influence on production of the word.

• Some contexts will facilitate correct production of target sounds, while others will make production extremely difficult.

• Phonetic context can be used to develop a complexity continuum, with intervention beginning with easier contexts and gradually progressing into more and more difficult contexts.

Meaningfulness

• Meaningfulness implies the degree of familiarity associated with the word by the child.

• The more familiar the child is with the word, the more likely the child is to include it in his or her active vocabulary.

• Familiar words are desirable because they avoid word-recall errors and the added complication of memory demands.

• Children appear to learn sounds at a faster rate when sounds are embedded within meaningful material.

• Words like the child's name or the names of pets, friends, and favorite activities and other words that are frequently used make better stimulus materials.

Communicative Potency

• *Communicative potency* refers to how functional words are in a child's communication system.

• Words like *no, go,* and *stop* are communicatively powerful, as they allow the child to operate on and manipulate the environment.

• Short phrases like *give me, that one,* and *some more* allow the child to control his or her environment and thus demonstrate the value or power of effective communication.

Phonetic and Syllable Inventory

• A child's phonetic and syllable inventory refers to those sounds the child is capable of producing and what syllable forms the child prefers, respectively.

• Phonetic inventory is useful for choosing consonants and vowels that make up the nontarget components of the stimulus words.

• The inclusion of sounds in the child's inventory indicates that the child has the motor ability to produce those sounds (especially if a stringent criterion for inclusion is used).

• The clinician should determine if these sounds can be made upon demand. Their presence in the inventory does not necessarily mean that the sounds are controllable at a conscious level by the child.

• Syllable shape preferences are a further consideration when developing stimulus words.

• If a child consistently reduces CVC words to CV syllables, then the clinician should avoid introducing the target sound in CVC syllable shapes because the child apparently has difficulty producing final consonants. The obvious exception to this would be when final-consonant deletion is the target process for remediation.

• By considering the child's preference for syllable shape, the clinician can choose words that will minimize complexity and thus increase the likelihood of accurate production of new target sounds.

As logical as it is to begin therapy at the word level to increase the functionality of the treatment process, some children are not initially successful at this stage. In our clinical experience, more often than not, children need some initial production training at the isolation or simple syllable level for sound establishment. We agree with Lowe, however, that it is at the word level that sounds make a communication difference. Therefore, we strongly recommend that, if therapy must be initiated at the sound or syllable level, it progress to the word level as quickly as possible. In our opinion, if adequate baseline information is collected, a clinician can easily determine the linguistic level that is most appropriate for a particular client, and the problem of where to begin therapy automatically is solved.

If therapy is initiated at the sound-in-isolation level, no particular stimulus items are used, since the goal at that point is to establish production of the sound through phonetic placement, successive approximation, and so forth. However, after the client's ability to produce the sound stabilizes at that level, the clinician may incorporate the use of stimulus cards containing a grapheme (letter) corresponding to the sound under training. For example, if establishing the *s* sound, the clinician may use a written representation of that sound to evoke its production without additional prompting on the part of the clinician. The clinician may also use verbal analogies such as "the snake sound," "the tiger sound," and "the bee sound" that represent particular phonemes. We have often noted that after some initial training, this type of **verbal prompt** is sufficient to evoke production of the sound, assuming that the client has the motor ability to make the sound.

At the word level, the clinician typically makes use of pictures or objects that contain the target phoneme in a specific word position. If the target phoneme were *s* in word-initial position, for example, the clinician might select pictorial representations of *soap, soup, sock, sick,* and *sun.* There are several commercial stimulus pictures for both articulation and phonological therapy available through companies such as SuperDuper Publications, The Speech Bin, and LinguiSystems. However, a clinician needs to be careful in the use of commercial sources. Remember that these are marketed for the general population and are not tailored to a specific client. At times the stimulus pictures in commercially available resources are not clinically useful or functional for a particular client. Often, the clinician must compile stimulus pictures from an array of sources to meet a client's individual needs. As the sequence of training is shifted to more complex linguistic levels, those pictures can also be used to evoke production of a sound in phrases and sentences.

Developing Measurable Objectives

We have discussed the target behavior selection process in great detail. However, we have not yet addressed what a clinician must do after the individual sounds, phonological processes, or phonological rules for training have been identified. After baselines have been collected and the linguistic level that is most appropriate for training is determined, the clinician must define the target behaviors in measurable or operational terms. The baseline information helps the clinician determine whether the selected target behaviors are indeed appropriate treatment objectives. **Treatment objectives** can be defined as the skills the clinician intends to teach on the way to achieving the selected treatment targets or **long-term goals.** They are frequently referred to as **short-term objectives.**

Initially, *potential* treatment targets may be stated in tentative and unspecific terms. However, it is inappropriate to define specific short-term objectives in such a manner. Although goals like "To improve the client's articulation skills" or "To improve the client's speech intelligibility" can be appropriate long-terms goals, short-term objectives must always specify how a certain goal will be achieved. The clinician must address the specific skills targeted, the anticipated outcomes, the predicted level of accuracy, and the situations in which the client will be expected to use the newly acquired skills.

Hegde (1998b) highlights two important reasons that target behaviors should be written or defined in a precise manner. First, it is imperative that a clinician remain accountable for the services that he or she provides. This can be done only if the target behaviors or short-term objectives are measured before, during, and after treatment. Without precise measurements of the client's performance, the clinician cannot clearly identify the amount of improvement. Also, the assumption that the client improved only after treatment was initiated cannot be made if such documentation is unavailable. Continual measurement of the client's progress is the only solution to this problem. Whether the client reached a specific objective can be determined only if the targets were clearly defined from the beginning.

A second reason that target behaviors should be clear and specific is that it allows external observers to verify the results of the clinical services provided. Many health care agencies, insurance companies, and other third-party payers not only recommend that such documentation be kept but actually demand it for the continuation of services. We are increasingly moving toward a health care era that puts great emphasis on the documentation of progress. No longer are agencies willing to pay for services unless some improvement is noted. We strongly reiterate that such improvement can be documented only if the goals and objectives of therapy are clearly stated from the inception of treatment.

With such considerations, we can now focus on what exactly constitutes a measurable objective or target behavior. A well-written target behavior specifies:

- the *response topography* or actual skill targeted (e.g., production of *s*);
- the *quantitative criterion* of performance (e.g., 90% accuracy);
- the *response mode* (e.g., discrimination versus production training);
- the *response level* (e.g., in sentences);
- the *response setting* (e.g., in the child's home); and
- the *number of speech samples or sessions* in which the target behavior productions are documented (e.g., across three sessions).

The components of a measurable target behavior will vary somewhat depending on the client's skills and treatment needs. The style in which they are written may also need to be suited to a specific clinical setting. The quality of the statement should not suffer by such variations. By asking the following questions, a clinician can usually ensure that all the important components of a measurable objective are included:

- Did I state the skill that I want my client to learn or perform?
- Did I indicate the accuracy criterion or level of performance that I expect my client to reach?
- Did I indicate the mode in which I want my client to respond?
- Did I indicate at what linguistic level I expect my client to use the new skill?
- Did I indicate under what circumstances or situations I expect my client to use the taught skills?

The clinician should keep in mind that the only way a behavior can be measured is if it can be observed in some manner (i.e., seen, heard, touched). Therefore, the selected skills for training must be observable behaviors that can actually be counted, tallied, or identified. Roth and Worthington (1996) wisely advise that in writing behavioral objectives, a clinician needs to use verbs that denote an observable activity.

Examples of observable activities and appropriate verbs include *point, repeat, match, name, tell, ask, count, write, say,* and *lift.* All of these behaviors can be measured. Nonmeasurable activities include *think, believe, discover, feel, appreciate, remember, understand,* and *know.* Although these are certainly action words, their corresponding behaviors cannot be directly observed. We cannot observe a client's thinking, knowledge, feelings, or appreciation. The only way we can assume knowledge, feelings, and the like is through observable behaviors such as crying and test performance. The following is a sampling of measurable short-term objectives for individual sounds, phonological processes, distinctive features, and other behaviors that may contribute to improved articulation and phonological skills:

Treatment Objectives for Individual Sounds

• Train 90% correct production of /s/ and /z/ during evoked single-word productions in the clinical setting.

• At least 90% correct production of /r/ in conversational speech produced at the clinic, at school, and in the child's home across three separate speech samples.

• Production of initial /d/ with 80% accuracy in 10 untrained words during evoked trials in the clinical setting.

• Spontaneous production of /k/ and /g/ in sentences with 90% accuracy over three consecutive sessions in response to the clinician's questions.

• Correct production of /s/ in the initial position of words used in two-word phrases evoked on a set of 20 discrete trials at 90% accuracy.

Treatment Objectives for Phonological Processes

• The reduction of final-consonant deletion by teaching 90% correct production of the following sounds in the word-final position: /p/, /k/, /t/, and /m/.

• The elimination of stopping by teaching 90% correct production of the following fricatives at the conversational level: /s/, /f/, /θ/, and /ʃ/.

• The reduction of syllable deletion by training 20 client-specific multisyllable words in two-word phrases with 90% accuracy.

• To eliminate the presence of velar fronting by training 90% correct production of /k/, /g/, and /ŋ/ in conversational speech across three speech samples gathered in the client's home.

• To establish the contrast between singleton consonants and consonant clusters by training 80% correct production of the following /s/ + stop clusters in the initial position of words: /st/, /sp/, and /sk/.

Treatment Objectives for Distinctive Features

• To establish the nasality feature by training 90% correct production of the following exemplars in words while naming pictured objects in the clinical setting: /m/ and /n/.

• To establish the [+voice/−voice] feature contrast by training 90% correct production of the following cognate pairs in two-word phrases: [p-b], [k-g], [f-v], and [s-z].

• To establish the stridency feature by training at least 90% correct production of /s/, /ʃ/, and /ʧ/ in evoked word trials. Generalized production of the stridency feature to the untrained cognate pairs will be probed when the client reaches the initial training criterion.

• To establish the [continuant-interrupted] feature contrast by training 90% correct production of the following sound exemplars of the [+continuant] feature in single words: /f/, /s/, and /ʃ/. Minimal pairs (e.g., *pan–fan, two–shoe,* and *top–shop*) will be incorporated for contrast training, and generalized productions to the untrained cognate pairs will be assessed.

Other Possible Treatment Objectives

• To eliminate the presence of **homonymous word forms** by training 90% correct production or acceptable approximation of the following words: (*list words affected by homonymy*)

• To increase the client's phonetic repertoire of sounds within his or her inventory by training 90% correct production of the following consonants: /t/, /k/, /s/, and /f/. The client will be expected to produce each sound in a set of 10 untrained words at the sentence level during evoked discrete trials.

• Teach a reduced rate of speech to facilitate precise articulatory contacts in conversational speech. The client will be expected to maintain a rate of 125 words per minute across three 10-minute conversational speech samples in the home situation.

• To increase the client's use of varying **syllable word shapes** by targeting at least 80% correct production of [CVC], [CCVC], and [CVCC] words in sentences in the clinical setting.

• At least 90% accuracy in self-correcting articulation errors of /s/ and /z/ in conversational speech.

The above objectives are not meant to be all inclusive, and they can certainly be tailored to meet a particular child's needs. The response mode, response level, accuracy criterion, and stimulus conditions can and should be altered to fit the client's assessment and baseline performance. The clinician's own treatment philosophy often dictates whether the target behaviors will be written in terms of individual phonemes, phonological processes, distinctive features, or a combination of these.

Planning and Developing a Treatment Program

Before implementing treatment, the clinician often develops a tentative intervention plan by preparing a written document that includes the targeted goals and objectives. The format and style that the clinician uses to prepare the written treatment program is often dictated by his or her employment setting. For example, federal and state laws mandate that school clinicians write and implement an *individualized educational program* (IEP) for clients who receive special education services, which includes speech and language treatment. The exact format of the IEP is usually developed by the *Special Education Local Plan Areas* (SELPAs) in a particular state; however, the content is generally the same. In this case, the clinician has very little flexibility as to how the plan of treatment should be written.

Treatment plans, whatever their form, minimally state the long-term goals and short-term objectives selected to meet the needs of a specific client. A plan may be written in a very simple format, or it may be more comprehensive in nature. As discussed earlier, the clinician's employment setting often dictates with how much detail the plan should be written. A comprehensive treatment program has several components that are typically addressed:

• *The client's identifying information.* This portion of the treatment program provides the client's name, age, address, diagnosis, and so forth. The client's background information, the results of the assessment, and the recommendations for treatment are summarized in a clear and concise manner.

• *The target behaviors selected for training.* The clinician identifies the target behaviors and describes them in measurable terms. The target behaviors must be specific so that the clinician can maintain daily performance data and measure the child's progress.

• *The potential treatment procedures and the tentative sequence of training.* In as much detail as the report format allows, the clinician describes the treatment methods and procedures that will be used to train correct production of the target sound(s). The clinician indicates the training techniques that will be used to establish and stabilize production of the sound and the sequence of training, progressing from isolation to words to phrases, and so forth. The potential reinforcing and response-reducing consequences are also identified. The types of reinforcers that will be used when the client produces the target correctly and the schedule of reinforcement are suggested. The response reduction procedures to be used when incorrect responses are given are identified.

• *The selected maintenance procedures.* The clinician should describe the procedures that he or she will use to promote maintenance of the target behaviors that are taught. The training of family members and caregivers is important so that they appropriately prompt and reinforce the target responses in nonclinical situations.

• *The dismissal criterion.* The dismissal criterion helps the clinician decide when the client will be dismissed from therapy. The child is typically dismissed from therapy when he or she produces the target sound with at least 90% accuracy in conversational speech at home and in other environments. It must be emphasized that this is the ideal dismissal criterion. However, there are many occasions when children are dismissed from therapy even though they do not produce the target sounds with 90% accuracy in conversational speech in natural environments. Lack of progress despite modifications to the treatment program, lack of parent participation, lack of follow-through with home assignments, poor attendance, and inability to arrive to therapy on time are all variables that may warrant early dismissal in particular treatment settings.

• *Follow-up and booster treatment.* Upon dismissal, it is important that the clinician arrange follow-up procedures if possible. Follow-up consists of periodic evaluation of the target responses to ensure their maintenance over time. The initial follow-up session is typically scheduled 3 months after the child's dismissal. Later, these may be done in biannual or annual intervals. If the follow-up assessment at any point indicates a decline in the target response rate, booster treatment can be provided. Booster treatment helps increase the response rate back to the dismissal criterion level; however, it is not as intensive as the original treatment.

The reader may refer to Appendix L for sample treatment plans. The components of the written treatment program will be addressed in greater detail through our discussion of the treatment procedures used in articulation and phonological therapy.

Establishing the Motor Production of Sounds

Although the word level is the recommended beginning point for articulation therapy in most cases, some children may need production training at a more simplistic level because they may not be able produce the sound without very direct instructions. With such children, the clinician may need to first establish the motor production of a target sound through the use of special sound-evoking techniques such as phonetic placement, sound approximation, modeling, verbal instructions, and prompts.

Production training may begin by first establishing the sound in isolation and then progressing to more complex linguistic levels. This is the behavioral process known as **shaping.** For all children, the ultimate goal is the production of a specific sound at the conversational level across various natural communicative environments. However, this process more often than not needs to be broken down into gradual steps to increase the client's likelihood of success. It must be noted that although the sound-evoking techniques under discussion will be individually addressed for simplification, in clinical practice they are frequently used in combination.

Phonetic Placement

Phonetic placement techniques have traditionally been used to teach the position of the articulators during production of a specific sound (Nemoy & Davis, 1937, 1954, 1980; Scripture and Jackson, 1927). It is assumed that the child cannot produce the target sound correctly because, simply stated, he or she does not know how to produce the sound. Therefore, the clinician must employ special facilitative techniques that will help evoke production of the sound. The clinician uses very direct methods to teach clients how to position the articulators for appropriate place of articulation and how to modify the airstream for appropriate manner of production. If necessary, clients are also taught how to voice sounds appropriately.

Weiss, Gordon, and Lillywhite (1987) summarized many instruments and techniques frequently used for phonetic placement, as follows (p. 186):

Instruments

- tongue blades and sticks to manipulate or hold articulators in place;
- breath indicator for mouth and nose;
- graphic records, for example, **spectogram.**

Techniques

- observing diagrams, pictures, or drawings of articulators while producing certain sounds;
- observing **palatograms** or articulators while producing certain sounds;
- observing clinician and self in mirror while producing sounds;
- manipulation of articulators with clinician's fingers;
- verbal description and instruction;
- feeling breath stream with hand or seeing effects of breath stream on a tissue;
- feeling laryngeal vibration.

Hegde (1998b) describes the clinician's physical manipulation of the client's articulators as manual guidance. In **manual guidance,** the clinician physically assists the client in the production of the target sound. For example, in teaching the production of [b], the clinician might have to shape the client's lips for appropriate seal using his or her fingers. This procedure has traditionally been described as **tactile-kinesthetic cueing** or **tactile-kinesthetic stimulation.**

An example of a phonetic placement technique for the production of /l/ includes the following:

1. Touch the client's alveolar ridge with a tongue depressor, cotton swab stick, or gloved finger to indicate the place of articulation for the [l].

2. Touch the client's tongue tip with a cotton swab stick and ask him or her to place the tip of the tongue against the alveolar ridge (the place indicated in step 1).

3. Instruct the client to keep the tip of the tongue against the alveolar ridge, or "bumpy spot," and to say [ə]. The resulting sound is a distorted [l].

4. Now ask the client to continue saying [ə] and drop the tip of his or her tongue at the same time. The resulting production is the syllable sequence [lə].

5. Identify the syllable sequence as the "right" sound and give the client the selected **reinforcer** (e.g., sticker, chip, etc.).

6. Continue the sequence until the sound is well established.

Appendix M provides various facilitative techniques, including phonetic placement procedures, that can be used to establish production of all American English consonants.

Successive Approximation (Shaping)

Successive approximation, or sound shaping, is a facilitative technique that capitalizes on a sound that the client can already make to help him or her learn a new sound (Bankson & Bernthal, 1998; Bleile, 1995; Secord, 1981b, 1989). The sound used to facilitate the production of the target can be a speech sound or another type of sound (e.g., growling noises or "car" noises for the production of /ɝ/) that the client can make without difficulty. Sound approximation is frequently needed in the training of sound production because of the complexity of various sounds. It is not typically sufficient to tell the client, "Say [p]," to evoke the production of the sound. Articulation training often needs to be broken down into gradual steps that lead to accurate production of the target sound.

The goal in successive approximation is to guide the client through a series of graded steps, each progressively closer to the target sound. The clinician begins the process by identifying a sound or initial response that the client can produce. The clinician then arranges instructional steps that help the client move from the initial response (the sound the client can produce) to the terminal response (the target sound). It is important that the initial sound be related in some manner to the terminal response, or the target sound production. For example, if the client cannot produce [b] but can produce [p], the latter would be a likely starting point since these sounds share the same place of articulation and manner of production. It would not make good clinical sense to attempt to shape [b] from [k] since the sounds do not share any articulatory features.

Shriberg (1975) provides an example of a sound-shaping procedure that can be used with a child who misarticulates /ɝ/. In the following example, the [ɝ] is shaped from [l] (p. 104):

1. Stick your tongue out [model provided].
2. Stick your tongue out and touch the tip of your finger [model provided].
3. Put your finger on the bumpy place right behind your top teeth [model provided].
4. Now put the tip of your tongue lightly on that bumpy place [model provided].
5. Now put your tongue tip there again and say [l] [model provided].
6. Say [l] each time I hold up my finger [clinician holds up finger].
7. Now say [l] for as long as I hold my finger up, like this: [model provided for 5 seconds]. Ready. Go.
8. Say a long [l], but this time as you're saying it, drag the tip of your tongue slowly back along the roof of your mouth — so far back that you have to drop it. [Accompany instructions with hand gesture of moving fingertips back slowly, palm up.]

It must be noted that in Shriberg's evocation procedure for /ɝ/, sound approximation is not the sole technique used. You may have noticed that this example illustrates the simultaneous use of phonetic placement, sound approximation, modeling, detailed verbal instructions, and physical prompting.

Modeling

Of all facilitative techniques, **modeling** is probably the least difficult for clinicians to implement (Creaghead et al., 1989). In modeling, the clinician produces (or models) the target response the client is expected to make (Hegde, 1998b; Bankson & Bernthal, 1998; Creaghead et al., 1989; Weiss et al., 1987). The client is then encouraged to repeat the target sound modeled by the clinician. The client's response to the clinician's model is called **imitation** (Hegde, 1998b).

Modeling can be successfully used if the client is able to imitate the selected target response with some level of accuracy. This facilitative technique can be, and is, typically used at all levels of response complexity including the sound in isolation, syllables, words, and sentences. Training should begin at the most complex linguistic level that the client can imitate the target sound. The goal is to shape the response from the most simplistic linguistic level to the ultimate goal of sound production in conversational speech.

While modeling, the clinician asks the client to watch his or her mouth closely and to listen very carefully as the sound is produced. The client is then asked to repeat the target sound. As the client imitates the target sound, the clinician typically draws attention to the kinesthetic properties of the sound by asking the client to focus on how the sound feels (Bankson & Bernthal, 1998). Clinicians may also highlight the sound through the use of **vocal emphasis** (Hegde, 1998b) or **sound amplification** (Bankson & Bernthal, 1998).

In *vocal emphasis* the clinician simply increases his or her vocal intensity on the sound. On sounds that can be prolonged (such as fricatives), the clinician may also increase the length of the production of the target sound. For example, if the target were /s/ in syllables, the clinician would highlight /s/ by modeling it more loudly and by prolonging its production (e.g., "Johnny, say [sssssssi]). In *sound amplification,* the clinician may highlight the target sound by amplifying the model. Bankson and Bernthal (1998) indicate that a sound may be amplified through an auditory trainer. After providing the emphasized model, the clinician asks the client to imitate the target production.

It should be emphasized that in the establishment phase of sound production, modeling is frequently used in conjunction with phonetic placement and successive approximation. For example, in phonetic placement, the client may be asked to imitate the placement of the tip of the tongue against the alveolar ridge. Hegde (1998b) and Hegde and Davis (1995) provide a detailed presentation of how modeling should be implemented and how it should eventually be faded. The reader may consult those sources for more detailed information.

Verbal Instructions and Prompts

Instructions are defined as verbal stimuli that help facilitate a person's actions (Hegde, 1998b). In articulation therapy, verbal instructions may help the clinician gain control over the client's sound productions. Prompts would also help increase the probability of occurrence of a target response. **Prompts** are commonly thought of as "hints" or "cues" used to draw the desired response from a person. Verbal instructions and prompts are invariably used in conjunction with the other facilitative techniques including phonetic placement, successive approximation, and modeling.

In modeling, the clinician demonstrates the action that the client needs to imitate. However, modeling alone may not be a sufficiently strong stimulus to "draw" the response from the client. In that case, detailed verbal instructions preceding the model may be used by the clinician to increase the probability of a correct imitation by the client. Detailed descriptions such as the following may be used by the clinician: "See the back part of my tongue? I'm going to make it go up really high like this. Then the back part of my tongue is going to touch the top part of my mouth way in the back. Can you see? Now I'm going to make our sound like this /kakaka/. Ok, now I want you to try to make the sound. Go ahead. Remember to use the back part of your tongue."

To further increase the likelihood of a correct response, the clinician may use prompts. Prompts can be verbal or nonverbal (Hedge, 1998b). Vocal emphasis is an example of a **verbal prompt** that is frequently used in articulation therapy; it was previously described under modeling. In vocal emphasis the clinician highlights the target response by vocalizing it more loudly or by prolonging its production (e.g., "Bobby, say [zzzzzzu]). Some verbal prompts do not contain any part of the response expected but can still serve to facilitate correct production of the target sound. Examples include the following: "Remember, your tongue needs to stay inside your mouth when you make your sound," "Before you start, I want you to think about where your tongue should be," and "Don't forget to turn on your motor." Verbal prompts are more traditionally known as **verbal cues** or **auditory stimulation.**

Nonverbal or **physical prompts** are often used in articulation therapy. They may be thought of as physical signs and gestures that may help the client visualize correct production of the target sound. Because of this, they have traditionally been referred to as visual cues or visual stimulation.

In nonverbal prompts, the clinician may physically prompt correct production of a target sound by using his or her hand for demonstration. For example, if teaching appropriate articulatory placement for [l], the clinician may demonstrate tongue-tip contact against the alveolar ridge by:

1. placing the right hand under the left hand;

2. identifying the left hand as the alveolar ridge and the right hand as the tongue; and

3. lifting the fingertips of the right hand to make broad contact with the bottom front portion of the left hand.

Clinicians often use this type of physical demonstration without realizing that they are doing so; this type of prompting tends to come naturally for most clinicians. In our experience, it can be a powerful facilitative technique for sound establishment if used appropriately and in conjunction with other methods such as verbal instructions and modeling. Other types of physical or nonverbal prompts include diagrams and written stimuli (Mowrer, 1989).

Hegde (1998b) emphasizes that physical prompts should not be confused with manual guidance. In manual guidance, the clinician actually physically manipulates the client's articulators. When providing physical prompts, however, the clinician merely demonstrates the production of the sound; there is no physical contact with the client.

Increasing and Strengthening Established Behaviors

The goal of any treatment is to teach new behaviors or to strengthen those behaviors occurring with a low frequency. In articulation and phonological therapy the primary goal is to teach sounds that are absent from a client's repertoire or to correct those that are misarticulated. In treating the client's phonological skills, the goal may be to establish certain phonological rules or suppress certain phonological processes so that (a) unstable word forms are eliminated, (b) homonymous word forms are decreased, and (c) phonemic sound contrasts are established (Ingram, 1989b).

The child demonstrates **unstable word forms** when he or she produces a variety of phonetic forms for the same word. For example, the word *dog* may be produced as [ga] on one occasion and [da], [ta], and [gat] on other occasions. This may significantly affect overall speech intelligibility because the listener may be unable to predict or follow the child's productions from one instance to another. A somewhat opposite concept is that of **homonymy.** The child demonstrates homonymous productions when one phonetic word form represents two or more adult words. For example, because of the presence of final-consonant deletion, velar fronting, and stopping in a child's phonological system, [da] may be used in reference to *dog, doll, got, gone, sock,* and *fall.* This may also significantly affect the child's speech intelligibility because homonymous word forms essentially lead to limited word contrasts. If the child produced a sentence like [want da], the adult would not know if the child was requesting a dog, doll, or sock.

The primary goal of articulation and phonological therapy is to improve the client's communication skills and speech intelligibility to facilitate successful communicative interactions in various natural environments. We previously discussed teaching techniques that can be used to establish the *motor production* of sounds (i.e., phonetic placement, modeling, prompting, verbal instruction, and so forth). We will now shift our attention to specific treatment procedures that can be used to increase and strengthen the newly established behaviors as therapy progresses to more complex linguistic levels. These procedures are based on the principles of learning, programmed instruction, and behavior modification. Their efficacy in the treatment of a variety of communication behaviors has been continually demonstrated (see Hegde, 1998b, pp. 122–123, for a review of various studies). Mowrer (1989, p. 186) indicates that a behavior modification program must meet several important criteria:

1. A target behavior must be selected that is operationally defined, has a definite beginning and ending, and can be accurately measured.

2. An attempt must be made to establish a baseline of this behavior before therapy is initiated.

3. The antecedent events (what the clinician is supposed to do and say) must be specified clearly.

4. The target response must be capable of being evaluated objectively as either correct or incorrect.

5. A reinforcement schedule must be specified.

6. A series of tasks organized in a hierarchy from simple to more complex must be identified.

7. The criteria to be met must be established to determine when a task has been mastered and a new task introduced.

8. The exit behavior must be specified and usually consists of a specified performance on a final criterion test.

9. It must be possible to replicate the instructional program; that is, other clinicians should be able to administer the program in exactly the same fashion as the author.

10. The instructional program should be field tested to establish its reliability.

The basic treatment sequence described in this Basic Unit meets all of these criteria. It has been experimentally proven to be effective in the treatment of articulation and phonological disorders (Bailey, Timbers, Phillips, & Wolf, 1971; Baker & Ryan, 1971; Bennett, 1974; Costello & Onstine, 1976; Elbert, Dinnsen, Swartzlander, & Chin, 1990; Elbert & McReynolds, 1975; Fitch, 1973; Gierut, 1989, 1990; Koegel, Koegel, & Ingham, 1986; Koegel, Koegel, Voy, & Ingham, 1988; McReynolds & Elbert, 1981b; Williams & McReynolds, 1975).

Selecting Potential Reinforcers

To increase the production of the target sounds, the clinician must select consequences that will serve as reinforcers. By definition, reinforcers are events that follow behaviors and thereby increase the probability of their recurrence (Hegde, 1998b). So if a response, in this case a target sound, increases when followed by a consequence, then that consequence may be considered a **reinforcer.** It must be noted that technically it is not known whether a selected consequence will indeed serve as a reinforcer until the target behavior has been documented or observed to increase. Therefore, in the initial stages of treatment, clinicians merely select "potential reinforcers" since the reinforcing value of the selected consequences is not known until training of the target sound or phonological skills actually begins.

Two types of consequences may help clients learn, increase, and maintain behaviors: positive reinforcers and negative reinforcers. **Positive reinforcers** are events that, when made contingent upon a response, increase the frequency of that response. Simply stated, consequences that follow a response and increase the occurrence of that response are positive reinforcers. For example, if a child is given a raisin after every correct /s/ production, he or she is more likely to produce /s/ correctly in the future (assuming that raisins are true reinforcers for the child). Raisins in this case would be considered positive reinforcers because they increased the occurrence of the target behavior (i.e., correct /s/ production).

Negative reinforcers are responses or actions that remove, postpone, reduce, or prevent an **aversive stimulus.** Because these actions or events help to prevent or reduce the occurrence of an unpleasant stimulus, they are more likely to recur when the same or a similar aversive event happens in the future. To fully understand negative reinforcement, it is important to consider two very important concepts. First, there is usually an unpleasant event or stimulus that a person wants to avoid or postpone. Second, there is a behavior that in some way reduces, terminates, or postpones that aversive stimulus. Because this behavior somehow reduces or terminates the aversive stimulus, it is likely to occur again when the person is confronted with the same or similar stimulus in the future. Negative reinforcement procedures are not typically used in the treatment of articulation and phonological disorders.

Although there are various types of reinforcers, we will limit our discussion to the most commonly used positive reinforcers in the treatment of articulation and phonological disorders: (a) primary positive reinforcers, (b) secondary reinforcers, and (c) multiple reinforcement contingencies.

Primary Positive Reinforcers

Primary reinforcers are consequences that do not rely on past learning or conditioning. The effects of **primary reinforcers** are not learned but are more biological in nature. Examples of primary reinforcers include sleep, food, water, and other consumables. Food is among the most frequently used primary reinforcer in articulation and phonological therapy. Raisins, candy, M&Ms, cereal, and crackers have been used by clinicians to reinforce children's correct production of the target sounds or phonological skills.

Food can be a powerful reinforcer in establishing new behaviors, especially in children who are very young, nonverbal, or have an associated mental retardation. It can be very effective because it does not depend on past learning. However, even though food is a powerful reinforcer, there are many limitations associated with its use that should be discussed. First, food is not a natural reinforcer for most communicative behaviors, and because of that, it may not promote generalization and maintenance of the intervention targets. Social praise rather than consequences such as candy, raisins, or cereal more likely reinforces speech behaviors. Therefore, when using food as a reinforcer, it is important to pair it with other conditioned reinforcers such as verbal praise. Gradually, food can be withdrawn while the conditioned reinforcers are continued. Again, this is important for the initial generalization and eventual maintenance of the target behaviors over time.

Other problems associated with primary reinforcement are that its effects depend on **deprivation,** it may be susceptible to the satiation effect, and some parents may object to its use. Food may act as a reinforcer only when people are deprived of it. This means not that the child needs to be deprived of all food, but that the child should be motivated for the selected reinforcer. For example, if M&Ms are selected as reinforcers, it is important that the child not be given M&Ms right before the clinic session. This problem may be solved by instructing parents on the appropriate use of food items as reinforcers. Food may also be susceptible to the **satiation effect.** Simply stated, this means that the child may stop working for a specific food item because he or she has had enough. So the child who worked hard for M&Ms at the beginning of the session may stop working after receiving a few M&Ms. The satiation effect may be counteracted by requiring several responses from the child before delivering the reinforcer rather than reinforcing every correct response. Also, the clinician may use various types of food items as reinforcers during a session so that as the child becomes satiated with one, another can be introduced.

If food is used as a reinforcer, it is important to provide parents with a rationale for its use. Some parents may object to the use of primary reinforcement if they do not fully understand why it was selected over other types of reinforcers such as verbal praise and tokens. In addition, parents may object to the use of certain food items because some medical contraindications may exist. For example, it would be inappropriate to use sugar candy with children who are diabetic. Therefore, it is imperative that clinicians always obtain parental permission before using primary reinforcement, to prevent any possible complications.

Secondary Reinforcers

Events or actions that increase the occurrence of a behavior are called **secondary reinforcers.** These types of reinforcers have attained their reinforcing value because of social or cultural benefits. Hegde (1998b) emphasizes that "without the benefits of a social and cultural environment, conditioned or secondary reinforcers are not effective" (p. 86). They depend on past learning or conditioning. Various secondary reinforcers have been used in the treatment of articulation disorders, including social reinforcers (e.g., verbal praise, attention, eye contact, facial expressions), conditioned generalized reinforcers, and informative feedback.

Social Reinforcers. Because of their social benefits, certain words in our language and various actions have attained a reinforcing value. Therefore, these secondary reinforcers can be used to increase and strengthen the production of various behaviors including articulation and phonological skills. Among some of the most frequently used social reinforcers are verbal praise, attention, touch, eye contact, and facial expressions (Hegde, 1998b). The clinician who tells the client, "You did such a good job making your sound that time," is making use of social reinforcement in the form of **verbal praise.** Clinical experience has proven this to be a strong reinforcer in most children who are highly motivated to improve and who have functional language and cognitive skills.

Conditioned Generalized Reinforcers. Conditioned generalized reinforcers, as the name implies, are secondary reinforcers that depend on past experience or conditioning. The term *generalized* implies that they can be used effectively in many situations and with a variety of clients. This type of reinforcement has also been called a token economy system (Mowrer, 1989, p. 164) because of the wide use of tokens as conditioned generalized reinforcers.

Tokens, play money, stickers, points, checkmarks on a piece of paper, beads, and blocks are among the various conditioned generalized reinforcers that clinicians have used. The clinician uses these as immediate reinforcers that can be accumulated and later exchanged by the child for "true" reinforcers such as playtime, a toy car, a pencil, and other material goods. Mowrer (1989) indicated that these "markers or tokens acquire value when the child learns that she can exchange the tokens for material goods or activities that would be of interest to the child" (p. 164). We have certainly seen proof of this in our own clinical practice with children who become sticker or token "hoarders."

Research and our own clinical experience have shown that conditioned generalized reinforcers are an extremely powerful class of reinforcers. Children seem to be inherently motivated to earn something. If the clinician uses this system appropriately, a client will work extremely hard for only a few tokens even during a lengthy session.

Conditioned generalized reinforcers can be incorporated quite easily in articulation and phonological treatment. For example, the clinician may give the child a penny every time he produces the target sound correctly. When the child earns a certain number or pennies, he is allowed to exchange them for a backup reinforcer (e.g., 2 minutes of playtime, a pencil, or a toy car).

Mowrer (1989) described the very interesting concept of a *reinforcement menu* in his discussion of a token economy system. He indicated that the clinician who selects toys as potential reinforcers could mount the toys on a large piece of cardboard paper, each with a price tag. The child is informed that each toy or item costs a certain number of tokens and that he can buy any item on the menu as long as he has enough tokens. A bracelet may cost 50 tokens, a pencil 25 tokens, a whistle 75 tokens, and so on. The clinician needs to be careful to price the items according to the client's performance. If the toys are too expensive, the child may not earn a backup reinforcer for several sessions. With older children, this may not be a problem, but with some young children this can create a frustrating situation that may actually affect overall participation. Also, if using a reinforcement menu, the clinician needs to be careful to select items that appear to have the same reinforcing value. Some clinicians make the mistake of combining some more expensive items with less expensive items. For example, a toy car may be more expensive and thus cost more tokens, whereas a pencil may cost the client fewer tokens because it is a less expensive item. This system may be very effective initially, but as the child purchases all of the more expensive items, he may not be as motivated to purchase the less expensive ones since all he really wanted was the toy car. The clinician would have to replace the expensive items so that the system regains its reinforcing value. Needless to say, this can become expensive for the clinician. It may be more efficient in the long run to select two or three potential backup reinforcers that the client may select from when he or she has acquired enough tokens to buy an item.

In our experience, children typically will work for very inexpensive items if the clinician introduces only those. However, if a clinician starts big and gradually reduces the size, quality, or quantity associated with the backup reinforcer, its effectiveness may diminish. We strongly recommend that the clinician avoid the use of expensive items that for financial reasons cannot be incorporated for an extended period of time.

Informative Feedback. Another important type of conditioned reinforcer is informative feedback. **Informative feedback** serves as a reinforcer by providing the client with specific information about his or her performance. The client who knows that the treatment goal is 90% correct production of /s/ in sentences may benefit from information that he or she is moving in the right direction. This type of feedback informs the client exactly where he or she stands in relation to the treatment goal. Informative feedback can be provided verbally or nonverbally. **Verbal informative feedback** may be provided as follows: "Jimmy, you are doing a very good job on your sound. The last time you were here you made the sound 80% correct. Today you were 90% correct. You are showing very good improvement." Of course, the clinician should spend some time to explain the meaning of the percentages if needed before providing this type of feedback. **Nonverbal informative feedback** may be provided in the form of graphs and charts. The clinician can be as creative as the imagination allows. In our clinical experience, clients from the very young to the very old seem to appreciate the use of charts and graphs. This visual form of documenting progress can be internally motivating for many clients.

Multiple Reinforcement Contingencies

In the treatment of articulation and phonological disorders, the clinician will more likely use a combination of the various reinforcers described. The clinician may combine the use of primary reinforcers with verbal praise so that eventually the use of primary reinforcers can be faded. Also, a token economy system typically is used along with social reinforcers. As the child is given a token, the clinician typically accompanies it with verbal praise such as "Good job" and "That was right." Through **mechanical feedback,** such as commercial computer programs, the child receives instant informative feedback about the accuracy of his or her responses. Some interactive computer programs are also programmed to provide the child with verbal praise such as "That was correct" or "Perfect." In addition to the computer's feedback, the clinician guides the child and provides additional informative feedback.

Schedules of Reinforcement

Schedules of reinforcement refer to the frequency with which the selected reinforcers will be delivered. There are two main types of reinforcement schedules: continuous and intermittent. The reader may consult Hegde (1998b) for a detailed presentation on schedules of reinforcement.

Continuous Reinforcement. When using a **continuous schedule of reinforcement,** the clinician reinforces every one of the client's correct responses. The clinician provides the client with verbal praise, a token, a sticker, or other reinforcer every time the target response is produced correctly. This schedule is often used in the initial stages of treatment. It is helpful in establishing or shaping target behaviors because it can generate a high rate of response. However, since continuously reinforced behaviors may not be sustained when that kind of reinforcement is no longer available, it is imperative that the clinician shift to an intermittent reinforcement schedule in the latter stages of treatment. Also, continuous reinforcement does not match the natural environment very well. At home, at school, on the playground, and so forth the child is likely to have periods of no reinforcement.

Intermittent Schedule. In an **intermittent schedule of reinforcement** some of the client's correct responses go unreinforced. Intermittent schedules are divided into ratio schedules and interval schedules. A **ratio schedule** refers to the *number of responses* that the client must produce before a reinforcer is delivered, while an **interval schedule** relates to the *duration of time* that must elapse before a reinforcer is given to the client. Ratio and interval intermittent schedules are further subdivided into the following categories: fixed-ratio schedule, variable-ratio schedule, fixed-interval schedule, and variable-interval schedule. **Fixed-ratio** and **variable-ratio schedules** are the most commonly used in articulation and phonological therapy due to the more discrete nature of the disorder. Fixed- and variable-interval ratios are used with speech behaviors that can be prolonged over a certain time duration (e.g., speech rate, pitch level, vocal intensity, and fluency). Thus, we will concentrate our discussion on fixed- and interval-ratio schedules of reinforcement.

FIXED-RATIO SCHEDULE. When using a fixed-ratio (FR) schedule, the clinician predetermines the number of responses that the client must produce correctly before a reinforcer is delivered. In articulation and phonological therapy, a child might be required to produce a sound correctly three times before he or she is given a reinforcer. This would mean a fixed ratio of 3. The exact number of responses that must be exhibited varies from child to child and the stage of therapy. Initially, a child may need a reinforcer after every two correct responses. As treatment progresses, perhaps only every 10th or 20th response needs to be reinforced. The goal is that the ratio will gradually grow larger and larger until a minimum number of reinforcers is needed for correct sound productions. A very large ratio can be obtained when using a token economy system by requiring a high number of correct responses before a backup reinforcer can be obtained. In the natural environment, reinforcers will probably occur infrequently. Requiring a large number of correct responses before a reinforcer is delivered more closely matches the client's natural environment.

VARIABLE-RATIO SCHEDULE. A variable ratio (VR) is a powerful schedule of reinforcement. It is most typically used in the latter stages of treatment, at which point the reinforcing contingencies should closely match those encountered in the natural environment. In a VR schedule, the number of responses required for the delivery of a reinforcer varies around an average. Unlike the FR schedule, in which the client knows the exact number of correct responses required for a reinforcer, in a variable-ratio schedule he or she cannot predict when the reinforcer is coming. That is because a VR is based on an average; thus, the actual number of responses required on any given occasion varies. For example, in a VR5 schedule, the clinician reinforces correct production of the target behavior every 5 responses on average. The clinician may reinforce the second response on one occasion, the fourth response on another occasion, and the ninth response on yet another occasion, which results in an average reinforcing value of 5. In the actual clinical setting, clinicians do not necessarily adhere to an exact average when using a VR schedule because of the amount of planning time that it would take to do so. Rather, clinicians make use of a *modified VR schedule,* in which they intermittently and variably reinforce the client's responses. It is used most often at the conversational speech level.

Using Positive Reinforcement Appropriately

Countless research studies have substantiated the principle of positive reinforcement. It is a well-known fact that certain consequences, when made contingent upon a behavior, increase the rate of that behavior. However, many clinicians have found themselves in tough clinical situations that make them doubt whether positive reinforcement really works.

The first author can think back to her first semester of clinical practicum working with a very "challenging" three-year-old diagnosed with a severe phonological disorder. We will call him Bobby. Bobby was definitely a challenge for me as a first-time clinician because I had no idea how to effectively manage his many interfering behaviors. Luckily, I had a wonderful supervisor who guided me through the entire process. As an eager clinician, I spent countless hours preparing activities that I thought would be fun and exciting for Bobby. I remember many times feeling a bit pompous and thinking to myself, "This activity will definitely make him work through the entire 50-minute session." However, just in case, I would prepare a few other activities that I thought would be just as reinforcing for Bobby. I cannot describe the feeling of disappointment when, after having worked on an activity for countless hours, I was unable to interest Bobby in what I had to offer. And I remember thinking, "I knew it. I was right all along. Everything I learned in that treatment procedures class was wrong. Positive reinforcement doesn't work. If it did, Bobby would love every activity that took me hours to prepare, and he would be working on his sounds like crazy." Now, as a more experienced clinician, I can look back at that situation and laugh, knowing that the principle of positive reinforcement does indeed work. As disheartening as this was when I realized it, I now know that it was not the principle that was failing, but I, who was doing almost everything wrong.

When using positive reinforcers to increase a target behavior, there are many things that a clinician should consider so that the procedures are implemented effectively. It is not sufficient to grab a few tokens, give one to the child every time he or she makes a sound correctly, and assume that his responses are being reinforced. To ensure the effective use of positive reinforcement, clinicians should keep the following points in mind:

1. *Do not assume that a consequence is a reinforcer.* Remember that a reinforcing consequence by definition is one that increases the rate of response. It is important that clinicians do not make personal judgments about whether a consequence is or is not a reinforcer. The only way that we know whether a consequence is indeed a reinforcer is if the response rate increases. It is inappropriate to assume

that candy is a reinforcer because a clinician likes that particular candy or that broccoli is not a reinforcer because "no child likes broccoli." The clinician should never include or exclude a stimuli as a possible reinforcer based on what society in general dictates the child will or will not like.

2. *Present the reinforcer immediately after occurrence of the target behavior.* In the early phase of treatment it is imperative that the reinforcing consequences be delivered immediately. There should be no hesitation on the part of the clinician. The clinician should avoid recording the response first and then reinforcing the child for the correct response. This creates a delay in the delivery. One reason it is important to prevent a delay between the response and the delivery of the reinforcer is that it is possible that an intervening behavior will be reinforced instead. Consequences that are not delivered immediately may lose their reinforcing value not because they are inappropriate consequences but because they are being provided inefficiently by the clinician.

3. *Provide the reinforcer in an unambiguous manner.* It is important that the clinician avoid ambiguous statements such as, "I think that sounded okay. I'll go ahead and give you a sticker this time." Statements such as that do not identify whether the client's response was correct or not. At times this happens because clinicians are not certain whether the response was correct. In our opinion, if the clinician has doubts about the accuracy of a response, then the response is probably incorrect. It is important to remember, however, that during the shaping process, responses that are not fully correct may be accepted. The clinician must always be clear about what is acceptable. If the target sound is still being shaped, a statement such as "Good job. You are headed in the right direction, but we still have some work to do" may be used. This reinforces the client's attempt at a correct production but does not give the erroneous impression that the sound produced was fully correct.

4. *Avoid too soft, unsure, or monotonous delivery of verbal reinforcing consequences.* A common mistake is to deliver verbal praise in a monotonous manner. The clinician may say such things as "Good," "I like that," and "That was perfect" without the appropriate affect and facial expression. The clinician may forget that it is perfectly all right to smile. This very mechanical delivery of reinforcement may not be effective. It is important to remember that young children often focus on the clinician's facial expression and tone of voice rather than the actual words used as verbal praise. The child may not perceive the remark "That was not right" as corrective feedback if the clinician accompanies the statement with a big smile, bright eyes, and a high-pitched intonation. Similarly, the statement "That /s/ was perfect" may not act as a reinforcer if the clinician does not use the appropriate affect, facial expression, and vocal intonation.

5. *Ensure that the child knows why he or she is receiving a reinforcer.* In the initial stages of treatment, it is important to be very specific in the use of verbal praise. The child must know exactly why he or she received a reinforcer. For example, saying "Good" after the child accurately produces the /f/ phoneme does not guarantee that the child knows why he or she is being reinforced. The child may assume that "good" relates to his good sitting behavior or good attention to task. Verbal praise such as "Good, you made your /f/ sound perfectly" or "Excellent, you remembered to put your teeth on top of your lips when you made your sound" are more appropriate at the initial stages of therapy. As treatment progresses and the client's accurate responses become more consistent, the detail may be minimized.

6. *Make sure to reinforce the child and not your clipboard or the treatment table.* Eye contact is very important in the delivery of reinforcement, especially ver-

bal praise. It is important to gain the child's attention and emphatically reinforce him or her when the target sound is produced correctly. Often, inexperienced clinicians make the mistake of reinforcing the child in an unsure manner, with little vocal emphasis and no direct eye contact. Again children often respond more to *how* something was said than to *what* was said.

7. *Be consistent with your delivery schedule.* In the initial stages of treatment, it is important to be consistent with the selected schedule of reinforcement. If the clinician tells a child who gets to cross out 1 square after producing a sound correctly that he or she gets to play with bubbles after crossing out 10 squares, it is imperative that the clinician follow through with the implied "promise." The clinician who requires "just a few more" productions after the child has already accomplished the original goal may inadvertently decrease the reinforcing value of the established consequences. Clinicians must be extremely careful not to create such situations, even when it is tempting to require "just a little bit more work" from the child. The schedule of reinforcement may shift from a fixed schedule of reinforcement to a more intermittent schedule when the target sound is produced more consistently. This will be discussed further under our discussion of **maintenance procedures.**

Selecting Response-Reducing Methods

One of the major responsibilities of the clinician is to increase the occurrence of selected speech behaviors. This is accomplished by shaping the target behavior, by using various antecedent stimuli, and by reinforcing occurrence of the target behavior. However, at times the clinician may also need to decrease certain undesirable behaviors. Hegde (1998b) identified two types of behavior that typically need to be decreased: (1) inappropriate communicative behaviors, and (2) behaviors that interfere with the training process. **Inappropriate communicative behaviors** are the client's typical behaviors in place of the appropriate speech–language behaviors. Misarticulated sounds and persistent use of phonological processes are among the many inappropriate communicative behaviors that a clinician may choose to reduce or eliminate.

Interfering behaviors are extraneous behaviors that interrupt the treatment process. In an ideal clinical world, all children would come to therapy ready and willing to learn. However, this is not always the case, especially with very young or severely involved children. Some of the most frequently encountered interfering behaviors are crying, off-seat behavior, and inattention to task. Because these behaviors can make it difficult, if not impossible, for the clinician to teach the target behaviors, sometimes it is necessary to initially concentrate treatment on decreasing the interfering behaviors. As the interfering behaviors occur with less frequency, the clinician can shift the emphasis of treatment to teaching the selected target behaviors.

The presence of interfering behaviors in some children should not necessarily be perceived as an unpleasant clinical situation. Although it does require a lot of patience on the part of the clinician to manage interfering behaviors, it can be personally very gratifying to help a child develop some of the basic skills essential for learning. Our clinicians are often surprised when we tell them that those children who come to the clinic kicking, crying, and screaming can turn out to be some of the most enjoyable and rewarding clinical cases.

Stimulus Presentation

An undesirable behavior can be reduced through *presentation* of a punishing stimulus. In behavior modification terms, the word **punishment** is not socially defined. Rather, a **punisher** is any stimulus that decreases a behavior when it is presented contingent upon that behavior's occurrence. Although a variety of objects and events can serve as punishing stimuli, the most frequently used in reducing inappropriate behaviors in speech–language treatment is **corrective feedback.** Through corrective feedback, the clinician provides the client with specific information about the acceptability of the response immediately after the response is made. Corrective feedback can be verbal, nonverbal, or mechanical.

Verbal corrective feedback is often provided to a client when the clinician judges the response to be inadequate, inappropriate, or unacceptable. Often, the clinician uses phrases like "No, let's try it again," "That was not right," or "You forgot to turn your voice on." This feedback is provided to the client contingent on the occurrence of an inappropriate response and, thus, may decrease the response. For example, if a client said "thop" for *soap,* the clinician would provide some verbal feedback highlighting the error (e.g., "Johnny, you stuck your tongue out too much that time. Remember when you make *s* words, your tongue stays inside your mouth"). Provision of this type of feedback tends to come naturally for clinicians. Most perceive it as information that the client needs in order to learn the selected skills. We have also used verbal corrective feedback in the form of a **clarification request** with some clients. For example, if the client produces the sentence "A *wabbit* is a small animal" for the production of /r/, the clinician may seek clarification of the response by saying "Bobby, this is what I heard . . . 'A *wabbit* is a small animal.' Is that what you meant to say?" Often clients can correct their own productions without the need for additional feedback from the clinician when such clarification requests are used.

Nonverbal corrective feedback can also be used to inform a client when a response is inappropriate or unacceptable. As the name implies, this feedback is provided through nonverbal means such as facial expressions, gestures, and other signals. The clinician may, for example, touch her own teeth with her index finger if the client says "thop" for *soap,* highlighting the inappropriate protrusion of the tongue. It is important to note that nonverbal signals work only when paired with verbal instructions and verbal corrective feedback initially. Otherwise, the child may not decipher the meaning of the signals. In our example, the client may not realize that when the clinician touches her own teeth, it signals an outward protrusion of the tongue. When the meaning of the signal is established, the use of the accompanying verbal instruction may be reduced. This can be important for the maintenance phase of treatment when it is important to provide the client with subtle feedback about his or her performance in the natural environment.

In an era of amazing computer technology, the use of **mechanical feedback** is becoming more and more common in speech–language treatment. Clinicians can use commercial computer software programs for articulation and phonological therapy. These programs often provide the client with immediate feedback about the accuracy of the responses.

Because children are growing up with computers all around them, they are often enthralled by what a computer has to offer. In our own clinical practice, we have witnessed children who are not drawn to the treatment activities prepared by the clinician become immediately enticed when placed in front of a computer screen.

The first author witnessed the magic of computer feedback with her own husband. He bought a commercial software program to learn Spanish and on his first lesson became very engrossed. He reacted very favorably to the computer's feedback of *"muy bien —* very good," *"perfecto —* perfect," and *"maravilloso —* marvelous."

One of the advantages of mechanical feedback is that it is immediate and definitive. If the response is incorrect, the computer or machine will not make tentative statements like "Well, I think that was okay." Rather, it will provide immediate corrective feedback, which is usually in visual or verbal form. The computer may flash statements like "That was not correct. Please try again." If the response is correct, a reinforcer, usually in the form of verbal or visual praise, will be provided. Again, the feedback is conclusive since the computer can make only programmed judgments.

The delivery of precise and immediate feedback is extremely important for learning. However, that alone does not facilitate complete learning of a new behavior on the part of the client. As the computer provides feedback about the inaccuracy of the response, it is assumed that the client has the ability to self-correct the responses. A computer usually cannot expand on the feedback provided. It cannot make follow-up statements like, "Johnny, to make the *s* sound, you need to put the tip of your tongue right behind your teeth. Let's try that." The first author also witnessed this as her husband was using his Spanish computer program. Although he responded favorably to the computer's mechanical reinforcement when his responses were correct, he continually turned to her for help when the computer gave him feedback about an incorrect response that he could not self-correct. As fun and exciting as computers are, ultimately clients need a therapist for the actual learning of new responses.

Stimulus Withdrawal

Inappropriate, incorrect, and unacceptable responses can also be reduced through **stimulus withdrawal.** This is a direct punishment technique by which a specific stimulus is withdrawn every time the incorrect or unacceptable response is made. It is a response-contingent procedure that reduces a behavior through removal of a potential reinforcer. As the reinforcer is removed every time the unacceptable behavior occurs, the client eventually learns that in order to keep the reinforcer he or she must be careful not to make the incorrect response. This procedure is ineffective if the stimulus that is withdrawn is not a reinforcer. There are two types of stimulus withdrawal procedures that can be used in the treatment of articulation and phonological disorders: time-out and response cost.

In **time-out,** there is a period of nonreinforcement, which is imposed when an inappropriate, incorrect, or otherwise unacceptable response occurs and may result in a decreased rate of that response (Hegde, 1998b; Mowrer, 1989). There are several varieties of time-out, including **isolation time-out, exclusion time-out,** and **nonexclusion time-out.** Of the three, the one most frequently used in the treatment of speech–language behaviors is nonexclusion time-out. In *nonexclusion time-out,* an incorrect or undesirable behavior is followed immediately by the cessation of all activity; the child is not removed from the treatment environment. After the incorrect response occurs, the clinician signals the client to stop talking for 5 seconds and avoids eye contact for the entire duration. After the imposed time has passed, the clinician asks the client to resume talking or attempt a new trial. It is presumed that talking or the item the child is given (e.g., a token) after a correct production is reinforcing for the client. In essence, when the client is asked to stop, no reinforcers are forthcoming.

In **response cost,** the clinician withdraws reinforcers on occurrence of the inappropriate behavior, so that the rate of inappropriate responses decreases. In essence, each incorrect response costs the client a previously earned reinforcer. The procedure works only when the client receives or has access to tangible reinforcers that can be accumulated. It is impossible to take back verbal praise or attention. However, marbles, stickers, tokens, and beads can easily be withdrawn.

Two varieties of response cost can be used: (1) the earn-and-lose variety, and (2) the lose-only variety. Procedurally, the **earn-and-lose variety** of response cost must be used in conjunction with a token economy reinforcement system. In essence, the child receives a token for every correct production of the target sound and loses one for every incorrect production. In the **lose-only** variety, the child does not have to earn the tokens. Rather, the clinician gives the child a certain number of tokens at the beginning of the session or treatment activity noncontingently. The clinician then takes a token away every time the client exhibits an incorrect or unacceptable behavior. With this variety, the clinician must be careful to provide sufficient tokens so that they do not run out mid session.

In the treatment of articulation and phonological skills, the earn-and-lose variety of response cost is more efficient. It is likely that a client will have a combination of correct and incorrect responses. Therefore, it is important to reinforce the correct responses to increase the likelihood of their occurrence and punish the incorrect responses to decrease their occurrence. In our own clinical practice, we have witnessed the power of response cost in the treatment of articulation and phonological disorders. Children, especially those with a competitive spirit, appear to dislike losing what they have earned and will work hard to maintain their reinforcers or to re-earn those reinforcers that have been withdrawn. A carefully structured response cost program can be very effective in decreasing incorrect sound productions and increasing the selected target behaviors.

Decreasing the Aversiveness of Response-Reducing Methods

All response-reducing methods have a certain level of aversiveness or unpleasantness. The incorrect behaviors decrease to prevent (a) the presentation of a punishing stimulus or (b) the withdrawal of a reinforcing stimulus. The aversiveness lies in the actual presentation of a negative stimulus or the withdrawal of a positive stimulus. Although there is some associated aversiveness, response-reducing methods can be very beneficial because they facilitate the learning process. Clinicians should always strive, however, to follow a program that uses minimally aversive methods and favors the use of positive reinforcement. As Hegde (1998b) states, "Often, the need for using aversive methods is a strong indication that the treatment targets may be inappropriate, the treatment procedures ineffective, or both" (p. 242). Treatment should never be characterized by a *reinforcement-punishment* ratio that favors punishment. If the clinician finds that response-reducing methods are being used exclusively or in greater quantity than positive reinforcement, he or she should reassess the treatment process by asking the following:

- Am I working at a level that is too difficult for the client?

- Am I using clear instructions, prompts, cues, and so forth?

- Am I using reinforcement contingencies appropriately? Are the contingencies true reinforcers? Am I delivering the reinforcers appropriately? Is the reinforcement schedule appropriate? Have I made appropriate alterations?

- Am I structuring the therapy sessions to fit the client's needs and personality style?

- Are the target behaviors appropriate at this point?

Structuring the Treatment Sessions

The actual treatment sessions may be highly or loosely structured. *Highly structured treatment sessions* are most often associated with "drill" type therapy, while *loosely structured sessions* are often equated with "play therapy" or "incidental learning." In a study designed to evaluate the effectiveness of different ways of structuring treatment, Shriberg and Kwiatkowski (1982b, pp. 246–247) offered the following definitions for different modes of treatment:

- **Drill**—a highly structured and efficient stimulus-response mode.

- **Drill play**—similar to drill, except that a motivational event that is fun for the child is included.

- **Structured play**—the training stimuli are presented as part of play activities; feedback about incorrect responses is optional.

- **Play**—stimulus and response events occur as natural components of play activities.

Shriberg and Kwiatkowski found that drill and drill play were the most effective procedures for obtaining correct production of the target behaviors. These types of intervention strategies are characterized by (a) clearly defined target responses, (b) predetermined response criteria, (c) carefully selected antecedent stimuli to evoke the target production, and (d) appropriate consequent events such as reinforcers and corrective feedback to increase correct production of the target responses. These characteristics are the foundation of the treatment procedures we have addressed in this Basic Unit.

Shriberg and Kwiatkowsi (1982b) noted that while clinicians rated drill play as the most effective, efficient, and personally preferred treatment structure, children preferred play most, then structured play, followed by drill play and, least of all, drill. Of special clinical relevance is the fact that children preferred those treatment structures that were found to be the least effective in teaching the target behaviors. In our minds, two questions arise from these findings:

1. As responsible therapists should we use treatment strategies that are known to be effective in teaching target behaviors?

2. Or do we simply keep our clients entertained by implementing a therapeutic structure that they prefer, albeit ineffective, and compromise their progress in therapy?

We would all probably agree that selecting a treatment structure that has been proven to be effective in treating children's communication behaviors is of prime importance.

Regardless of a person's definition of therapy, the treatment process should never be play for the sake of play. It is unlikely that parents and third-party payers turn to paid experts for therapy that has no defined methods or procedures. If children could learn from playing alone, they probably would not need special clinical services. Articulation and phonological therapy should always be skill oriented, regardless of whether those skills are acquired in highly structured or loosely structured sessions. Sound production is a skill that is acquired through practice. The more the child produces a particular skill, the more likely it will be used in various communicative situations, whether they are highly structured or more natural communicative interactions.

Two variables help the clinician determine how treatment sessions should be structured: the client and the stage of treatment. First, treatment sessions should always be tailored to fit a client's personality style, cognitive and linguistic abilities, attending skills, and other associated behaviors so that his or her therapeutic needs are met. While some children respond very well to loosely structured sessions, others for a variety of reasons require sessions that are highly structured.

Second, clients often need highly structured sessions in the initial stages of treatment. Unless the target behaviors were clearly identified it would be difficult if not impossible to establish a new behavior. Focusing on a very specific objective initially facilitates learning. It is unlikely that a client will learn how to make a particular sound unless the therapy sessions permit multiple opportunities for its occurrence.

All clients will eventually require clinical sessions that are loosely structured as therapy progresses to more complex linguistic levels. The ultimate goal of therapy is the use of the established skills in conversational speech. Therapy at the conversational level should follow a loose format to more closely match natural communication interactions. There is nothing wrong with either style of therapy as long as there is sufficient structure to guarantee that a learning objective is being addressed and that effective procedures are being used.

Administering the Treatment Trials

As indicated earlier, in the initial stages of treatment it is necessary to structure the sessions so that a very specific skill is targeted in training. At that level, the clinician can make use of discrete trials to establish the target sound or phonological skills. A **discrete trial** is an arranged opportunity for the production of a particular behavior. Discrete trials are temporally separated, even if only by a few seconds. There is a definite end to one trial before the next trial is initiated. In articulation and phonological therapy, discrete trials may be conducted at the isolation, syllable, word, phrase, and sentence levels. The sections that follow provide a description of how to conduct discrete trials at those various levels.

Sound in Isolation Level

At the sound in isolation level, a discrete trial may progress as follows. It is important to note that not all sounds can be produced in isolation without an intrusive vowel [ə].

1. The clinician presents an **antecedent stimulus** that helps facilitate production of the target sound. Examples of antecedent stimuli include:

- phonetic placement cues
- visual and verbal prompts
- verbal instructions
- modeling
- combination of facilitative techniques

2. The client is instructed to produce the sound after a specific technique or a variety of facilitative techniques have been provided.

3. The clinician responds to the client's production, as follows:

- a reinforcer is given if the response was acceptable;
- corrective feedback is provided if the response was incorrect or unacceptable.

4. The clinician records the accuracy of the response on a prepared data collection sheet using a +/− system, as follows:

- a correct response is indicated by a "+" mark;
- an incorrect response is indicated by a "−" mark;
- no response is indicated by "NR."

5. The clinician begins another trial after a few seconds.

Sound in Syllable Level

Discrete trials at the syllable level are conducted in a fashion similar to that of the sound in isolation level. Remember that some sounds cannot be produced in isolation; the syllable is thus the most simplistic linguistic level for these. Voiced stop plosives, for example, are impossible to make without an intrusive vowel.

After the sound is made with some consistency at the syllable level and the target sound is clearly identified, the clinician may use a visual stimulus to evoke its production. The clinician can use a **vowel diagram** in which the letter representing the target sound is paired with various pure vowels (e.g., *ba, be, bi, bo, boo*). This can be successful with students who know or have been taught the sound-letter association. This response-evoking method will provide the clinician with an alternative to direct modeling.

Sound at Word, Phrase, Sentence Levels

At the word, phrase, and sentence levels, discrete trials are conducted in a similar fashion. The primary difference is the required length of the response. At the word level, the stimulus items are most often pictures, objects, and events depicting a word that contains the target sound. At the phrase and sentence levels, these same stimuli can be used; however, the client is now instructed to put the word in a phrase or a sentence. This may be difficult for a young child who has not been exposed to the concept of a sentence. He or she may not know exactly what to do when instructed to create a sentence with the target word. Therefore, some initial training is usually necessary to facilitate this task. The clinician may need to provide extensive modeling in sentence production so that eventually a client can create his or her own sentences without the need for modeling. The use of **carrier phrases** (e.g., "I see a . . ." and "I want a . . .") may simplify the task when the initial transition is made from words to sentences. With children who have oral reading skills, the clinician may use written sentences to facilitate production of the target sound at this level if necessary.

A discrete trial at any of these levels may proceed as follows:

1. The clinician places the stimulus picture or object in front of the client or demonstrates the action or event that represents the sound in a word, for example:

- show the child a picture of *rat* or *rain;*
- swiftly move your legs and arms to represent the action *run.*

2. The clinician asks a relevant predetermined question, for example:

- "What do you see in the picture?" or "What is the name of this animal?"
- "What is falling from the sky?" or "What am I pretending to do?"

3. The clinician immediately models the correct response, assuming that modeling is needed, for example:

- "Johnny, say 'rat'."
- "Johnny, say 'rain'."
- "Johnny, say 'run'."

4. The clinician waits a few seconds for the child to respond. The amount of time needed before presentation of the next stimulus item may vary across children, depending on their individual needs. Some children require a longer response time.

5. The clinician responds to the client's production by providing a reinforcer if the response was acceptable or providing corrective feedback if it was incorrect, for example:

- "Johnny, you said your *r* perfectly in the word *run*. Good job."
- "Johnny, that *r* came out just wonderfully."
- "Johnny, that was a perfect *r*. Keep up the good work."
- "Uh-oh, Johnny, that time your tongue was too flat and your *r* sounded like an *a*. We need to try that again."
- "Johnny, stop. Your *r* sounds like an *a* in that word."

6. The clinician records the response on a prepared data collection sheet using a +/− system. A correct response would be indicated by a "+" mark, and an incorrect response would be recorded by a "−" mark. Occasionally, children may not respond after the stimulus item has been presented. This may be recorded by "NR" for no response.

7. The clinician removes the stimulus by pulling it away from the subject's view. This is important to decrease the possibility of the child continuing to respond to a previous stimulus item even after a new stimulus item is presented. This will decrease confusion on the part of the child and will help avoid competing responses from young children.

8. The clinician then returns to step 1 to initiate the next trial until all trials are completed.

Discrete trials should not be equated with "boring" treatment activities. Discrete trials are merely temporally defined opportunities for the occurrence of a response. They are usually incorporated into highly structured tabletop activities; however, they can also be easily infused into structured "play" activities. For example, during a Fishing for Sounds game, the clinician can paper-clip the picture cards used to evoke the sound onto the paper fish. The fish then serve as the stimulus items. A discrete trial incorporated into this generally fun activity may proceed as follows:

1. The clinician places five fish on the floor (the stimulus pictures are attached with paper clips). The client is then instructed to "go fish" with a pole containing a magnet on the end of the fishing line. Hint: You may need to guide the client's "fishing expedition" to make this a time-efficient activity. The child may have a difficult time connecting the magnet with the paper clip on his or her own.
2. After the client "catches" a fish, the clinician asks a relevant predetermined question (e.g., "Johnny, what do you see on the fish?").
3. The clinician immediately models the correct response, assuming that modeling is needed (e.g., "Johnny, say *cat*").
4. The clinician waits a few seconds for the child to respond.
5. The clinician responds to the client's production by providing a reinforcer if the response was acceptable or providing corrective feedback if it was incorrect:

-   "Johnny, you said your *k* perfectly in the word *cat*. Good job"; or
-   "Uh-oh, Johnny, that time your tongue was in the front part of your mouth. You need to try that again. Remember to keep your tongue in the back."

6. The clinician records the response on a prepared data collection sheet using a +/− system.
7. If the sound was produced correctly, the clinician puts the stimulus item aside and instructs the client to "go fish" for another card.
8. If the sound production was incorrect or unacceptable, the clinician instructs the client to "try again" and grants the client permission to "go fish" for another card only after the sound has been produced correctly.

As can be seen, these trials can still be categorized as discrete because they are temporally separated; however, they are not necessarily "stiff" and "unexciting." The clinician should always remember that "play" is not incorporated into therapy for the sake of play. All activities and treatment trials must be production oriented.

Sound in Conversation

At the conversational level, the discrete trial procedure is no longer clinically efficient since natural conversation does not occur in discrete opportunities. Often a conversation is a dialogue; however, at times it is more of a monologue. Frequently, there is conversational overlap between the listener and the speaker.

Instead of discrete trials, at this level the clinician may use **open-ended questions** to evoke free-flowing speech from the client. A myriad of activities can be used to ensure that the client has an opportunity to produce the sound in more natural communicative interactions. Unlike discrete trials, at this point the clinician does not have control over the number of times the sound is produced. Rather, the clinician's responsibility shifts to listening for natural occurrences of the target sound and to delivering intermittent reinforcing contingencies such as verbal praise (e.g., "I've noticed that for the last 15 minutes all of your *s* sounds have been made perfectly. Keep up the good work"). At the conversational level, the clinician should continue to provide corrective feedback for inappropriate responses that the client did not self-monitor and self-correct. The training of self-monitoring skills becomes crucial at this level (we will discuss this at length during our discussion of maintenance procedures).

Moving Through the Treatment Sequence

Soon after treatment is initiated, the clinician will have to make important clinical management decisions. As the client begins to produce the target behaviors more consistently, the clinician will have to ask:

- When do I stop providing modeling or any other special prompting procedures?

- How many target responses do I need to teach before the client has learned the sound or phonological skill?

- When do I move from one linguistic level to the next?

As therapy progresses, the need for special stimuli such as visual prompts, verbal instructions, and modeling will diminish. Although highly necessary in the initial stages of treatment, the use of these stimuli should eventually be faded because they are not part of the client's natural environment. Roth and Worthington (1996, pp. 6–7) indicate that three major factors should be considered in the progression of the therapy sequence: (1) *the type of stimulus provided,* (2) *the mode of production,* and (3) *the response level.* Although there is variation across clients, the sequence of therapy usually progresses in the following order.

Types of Stimuli Provided To Facilitate the Target Production

- physical manipulation or manual guidance
- visual, tactile, auditory, and kinesthetic cues
- modeling
  - exaggerated model with vocal or visual emphasis
  - less conspicuous model
- objects
- pictures
- line drawings
- questions
- oral reading materials
- natural conversational interaction

Expected Mode of Production

- imitated responses after the clinician's model
  - immediate imitation
  - delayed imitation
- cued or prompted responses
- evoked responses upon stimulus presentation
- spontaneous or unprompted productions
- natural conversational interactions

Expected Response Level

- isolation or sound level
- syllable level
- word level
- phrase level
- sentence level
- oral reading level
- conversational level

You will notice that the antecedent stimuli, the expected mode of response, and the expected response level all progress from simple to complex. The most complex level for all three variables is conversational speech. If therapy progresses as expected, natural communicative interactions should be sufficient to evoke the correct production of the target sounds in conversational speech. The goal is to gradually fade modeling or any other special prompting procedures that would not be encountered in the natural environment.

How many target responses does the clinician need to teach before a target behavior is considered learned? To answer this question it is important to differentiate target responses from target behaviors. A **target response,** in the context of articulation and phonological skills, is any word that contains the target phoneme; a **target behavior** is the production of the target sound in varied contexts in conversational speech (Hegde & Davis, 1995). A target response is an exemplar of the target behavior. With this in mind, the answer to the question is usually frustrating for beginning clinicians because of its lack of specificity. The number of target responses that the clinician needs to teach before the target behavior is considered learned varies from one client to another. With one client, 10 target responses may be sufficient, while with another client, 30 responses may have to be taught. **Probe procedures** to assess the level of generalized responding can help the clinician make this determination. Generalization and probe procedures are described in a later section.

Probe procedures may also help the clinician determine when to shift from one linguistic level to the next. In articulation training, the sequence of training typically progresses from the sound in isolation, to syllables, words, sentences, oral reading, and finally conversational speech. The clinician may identify a production criterion that the client needs to reach before a shift is made from one linguistic level to the next. For example, a clinician may decide that training will shift from words to sentences when the client reaches 90% correct production on untaught words during probe trials.

Although we believe that it is important to adhere to a production criterion, this should not preclude the clinician's use of intuition or creativity. In the training process, the clinician often experiments with different linguistic levels of training. In our own clinical practice we frequently "test" the client's readiness to move on to the next level by giving him or her a few practice trials. If the client displays an ability to produce the target sound during these practice trials, he or she may be ready to move on. Remember that the goal of therapy is to progress to conversational speech as quickly as possible. Strictly adhering to a training criterion may slow down the therapeutic process. The clinician needs to find the balance between a level of work that helps the client be successful and one that maximizes the client's performance and progress.

Data Collection

Throughout the entire treatment sequence the clinician should collect data on the client's performance in therapy. This is extremely important to establish the clinician's accountability, to evaluate the effectiveness and efficiency of the chosen intervention program, and to determine the client's progress. Parents, clients, third-party payers, government agencies, and insurance companies invest valuable resources for the provision of therapeutic services. They have the ethical and legal right to know if their time and money are being well spent.

The need for more consistent documentation or periodic assessments by speech–language pathologists is becoming an extremely important issue even in the public schools, where traditionally therapists had to evaluate the client's progress only once a year during a review of the individualized education program (O'Toole, Logemann, & Baum, 1998). The passage of an amendment to the **Individuals with Disabilities Education Act (IDEA)** by Congress in June 1997 shifted the emphasis of special education services in the public schools "from the 'old' IDEA which established the right to an education for students with disabilities, to the 'new' IDEA, which emphasizes the performance of the student and accountability for the students' outcomes" (Amiot, 1998, p. 245). Thus, the reporting or documentation requirements for the student's outcome have increased in frequency and content (Amiot, 1998).

Nearly all employment settings require daily documentation of the client's performance in treatment. It is important that the clinician devise or adapt recording forms that allow for such documentation (see Appendix N for a sample form). In articulation therapy the clinician can judge the client's production of the target sound as correct or incorrect and determine an accuracy percentage. In this manner, the clinician can determine whether the client's skills are improving. The clinician should minimally follow the documentation guidelines dictated by his or her employment agency.

We have found that documentation of the client's performance during every treatment session can easily be incorporated into the treatment of articulation and phonological disorders when the treatment targets or target objectives are clearly identified. If the clinician is certain about what he or she is teaching and what the client is expected to do, charting becomes an easy task. It is when the clinician has not taken the time to clearly identify what will be taught that the documentation process becomes a tedious chore. Incidentally, we have frequently found that documenting the accuracy of responses in front of the child, especially upper elementary and adolescent clients, can be highly reinforcing. In our own clinical practice we have often heard children make such comments as, "I don't want any more minuses," "How many pluses did I get today?" and "Tomorrow I'm gonna get them all right."

Probing for Generalized Responses

Hegde (1998b) describes **generalization** as the intermediate target of clinical intervention. We previously described the initial target as the establishment and strengthening of new behaviors, while the final target is the maintenance of those behaviors across time and across varied situations. In clinical terms, generalization refers to "either a temporary production of a recently learned response in different contexts and situations, or the production of new (untrained) responses based on recent or remote learning" (p. 179). For example, after learning the production of /f/ at the word level in the clinical setting, the client may show generalized responses of this sound in words produced at home or school (in a new context or situation). Or, the client may demonstrate production of /v/ (new, untaught response) after establishing the production of /f/. In either case, the generalized responses occur in the absence of current reinforcement.

If the behaviors that initially appeared as generalized responses continue to be produced in the absence of reinforcement, they will begin to decrease and eventually disappear. For this reason, Hegde (1998b) describes generalization as a temporary operation that should not be the goal of treatment. If these behaviors are to be maintained over time, the clinician cannot simply ignore them and assume that they will continue. Rather, special procedures must be implemented that will guarantee their maintenance over time. These will be addressed under our discussion of response maintenance procedures.

Several types of generalization have been described in the literature. We have opted to address those that are most relevant to articulation and phonological disorders. The occurrence of generalized responses can enhance the client's progress, and they are a welcomed component of the therapy process.

Types of Generalization

Generalization to Untaught Stimulus Items

In behavioral terms, generalization to untaught items is described as **physical stimulus generalization** (Hegde, 1998b). This type of generalized responding occurs when a learned response is evoked by *stimuli* that were not used in teaching the response (untrained items). It occurs because of the similarity of the trained and untrained stimulus items.

Physical stimulus generalization has been documented in the treatment of articulation and phonological disorders (Arndt, Elbert, & Shelton, 1971; Elbert & McReynolds, 1975, 1978; Hoffman, 1983; McReynolds, 1972; McReynolds & Elbert, 1981b; Mowrer, 1971; Powell & Elbert, 1984; Shelton, Elbert, & Arndt, 1967). Various research studies have documented that children produce the target sounds not only in the words in which they were treated, but also in other, untreated words. This type of generalization has important clinical implications. If a child generalizes the production of the target sounds to untrained stimuli, the time needed for training may be minimized and the maintenance process may be initiated sooner.

Generalization Across Word Positions

Elbert and Gierut (1986) describe the generalization of accurate sound production across word positions. This type of generalized responding refers to the production of a sound taught in one position to untreated word positions. According to Elbert and Gierut's review of the literature, studies have not conclusively demonstrated that teaching a sound in a particular word position promotes greater generalization than teaching the sound in any other word position (p. 123). Therefore, Elbert and Gierut conclude that teaching sounds in any position can facilitate generalized responses in untrained word positions. This type of generalized responding also has important clinical implications. If the clinician can expect some level of generalization across word positions, it seems more clinically fruitful to teach various sounds in one specific position than to teach one sound across all word positions to a certain criterion. Of course, the clinician should always assess for such generalized responses to verify their occurrence and directly teach in other positions if the child continues to misarticulate the sound in those positions.

Generalization Across Response Topographies

The production of the trained sound in linguistic units or response topographies (e.g., syllables, words, phrases, sentences) that were not directly taught exemplifies generalized productions across linguistic units (Elbert & Gierut, 1986). An example of this type of generalization is illustrated by the child who uses /p/ in phrases and sentences despite having been trained to use it only in single words. Hegde (1998b) refers to this form of generalization as **intraverbal generalization** or **generalized expansion of response topography.**

Generalized responding across linguistic units has been documented in the treatment of articulation disorders (McReynolds, 1972; Powell & McReynolds, 1969; Elbert, Dinnsen, Swartzlander, & Chin, 1990). If that type of generalization can be expected, the clinician may focus training on one linguistic level and assess for generalized production to more complex response topographies. If that occurs, then training may progress to a level at which the child cannot produce the sound. It is important to move through the various linguistic levels as soon as possible since the ultimate goal is the production of the target sound in conversational speech. The more quickly the child progresses to the conversational speech level, the more quickly the clinician can focus on the maintenance of the learned responses and behaviors.

Generalization Within Sound Classes

Traditionally, sounds have been described according to various features. This has led to the description of phonemes according to sound classes. A **sound class** can be defined as a group (or class) of sounds that share certain characteristics or features. For example, /s/, /z/, /f/, /v/, /ʃ/, /ʒ/, /θ/, /ð/ are categorized under the fricatives sound class because they all share the phonetic feature of frication. Many frameworks have been used to establish sound classes. These include (a) cognate sound pairs; (b) manner, place, and voice features; (c) distinctive features; and (d) phonological processes.

The concept of sound classes is important in the description of generalized responding because studies have reported generalization *within* sound classes (see Elbert & Gierut, 1986). This type of generalization has been reported for sound classes as related to (a) manner, place, and voice features (McNutt, 1994; Shelton et al., 1967); (b) distinctive features (Costello & Onstine, 1976; McReynolds & Bennett, 1972); and (c) phonological processes (McReynolds & Elbert, 1981b; Elbert & McReynolds, 1978; Powell & Elbert, 1984; Weiner, 1981).

Although generalized responding has been documented within sound classes in various studies, clinicians should never presume that such generalized responding would take place in the phonological system of a particular child. Clinicians can use this information to systematically select the initial treatment target; however, the clinician should always verify the reality of generalized responding and not merely assume that it has occurred. For example, the clinician should never conclude that by training /s/ and /f/, other fricatives affected by the phonological process of *stopping* will be suppressed unless special testing confirms this is a clinical reality in a particular child.

Generalization Across Sound Classes

A more complex form of generalization is generalization *across* sound classes. This type of generalization implies that sounds that are seemingly unrelated according to their many phonetic features (e.g., manner, place, voicing) could actually affect each other when treated. Improvement of untreated sounds following treatment of presumably unrelated sounds has been reported in the literature (Gierut, 1985; Weiner, 1981). Gierut (1985) found that teaching production of the voiceless fricative [s] resulted in the accurate production of the voiced [l]. Weiner (1981) reported improved production of final fricative consonants after teaching final stop consonants. He also found that when stopping of fricatives was eliminated, fronting of stops was also eliminated. Although this type of generalization may initially seem unlikely, Elbert and Gierut's (1986) suggestion that generalization across sound classes has been observed only in cases in which the errors were analyzed according to phonological processes or rules may help explain it. It could be that a child does not produce a sound because of an operating phonological pattern (e.g., deletion of final consonants), and when a sound within that pattern is taught, other sounds that are part of the pattern may also improve. For example, if a child deleted [d], [t], [k], [g], [b], and [p] in the final position because of the process of final-consonant deletion, and of these only [b] and [p] were trained, then maybe generalized productions of [d], [t], [k], and [g] could be observed. So sounds that according to traditional definitions seemed unrelated are actually related because of underlying phonological patterns. Further research is needed in this area. Are all phonological processes or phonological patterns susceptible to this type of generalization, or are there only specific patterns in which it can be expected?

Generalization Across Situations

Generalization *across situations* refers to the generalized production of behaviors taught in a clinical or specific setting to various other locations and audiences. This type of generalization is also described as **stimulus generalization,** and even more specifically as **physical-setting generalization** and **audience generalization** (Hegde, 1998b). Physical-setting generalization occurs when responses taught in one physical setting are produced in other settings in which teaching did not take place. Audience generalization takes place when responses taught by a given audience (e.g., a clinician) are evoked by audiences or other people not involved in the teaching (e.g., the child's grandmother).

In articulation and phonological therapy, initial teaching of the target behaviors generally takes place in the clinical environment and is conducted by the speech–language pathologist. Research has shown that children may extend accurate production of the target sounds to other environments such as the child's home, classroom, or playground (Carrier, 1970; Bankson & Byrne, 1972; Costello & Bosler, 1976; Olswang & Bain, 1985). Researchers have also reported generalized responding of the target sound to untrained audiences such as teachers and peers (Conley, 1966; Engel, Brandriet, Erickson, Gronhoud, & Gunderson, 1966).

Generalization across environments and audiences is an integral part of the treatment process. It is functionally irrelevant if the client produces the target behaviors only in the clinical room and in the presence of the clinician; the clinical setting plays a minute role in the client's life. Unfortunately, this type of generalized responding is not evident in all children. Therefore, the clinician often needs to incorporate special techniques that may facilitate audience and physical-setting generalization and the eventual maintenance of those behaviors across time in various situations. We will address this further in an upcoming section focusing on maintenance procedures.

Assessing Generalized Responses

The occurrence of generalized responses can be determined through special assessment procedures called **probes.** After a certain number of target responses (words) have been taught to a predetermined criterion, the clinician can assess for generalized responses to untaught words, untaught phonemes, untaught positions, and untaught linguistic levels. For example, the clinician can teach the target sound /f/ in a certain number of words (e.g., *fat, four, five, farm, fix,* and *fight*). After those words have been taught to a predetermined criterion (e.g., 10 consecutive correct evoked productions), the clinician can *probe* for generalized productions to:

- untrained words: *fun, feet, fox, fan,* and *phone*
- untrained phonemes (cognate pair): *vine, vest, vote, valentine, vegetable*
- untrained word position: *leaf, half, life, safe, beef*
- untrained linguistic level (sentences): *The boy is fat; I am four years old; The farm is big; I like to fix things; I fight with my brother.*

As indicated earlier, a **probe** is a procedure used to assess the generalized production of a trained target behavior. Probes can be conducted through discrete trials or a conversational speech sample, depending on the linguistic level of training at the time of probing (Hegde, 1998b). **Discrete trial probes** are conducted similarly to baseline trials. The clinician selects stimulus items that have not been taught, presents them to the client, and records the client's response. An important distinction between baseline trials and probe trials is that the clinician does not model the target production in the latter. The clinician simply shows a picture, asks a predetermined question, and records the client's response. The client is reinforced for adequate participation (see Appendix O for a sample probe recording sheet). The clinician then calculates the percentage of correct untaught response productions. This helps to identify the extent of generalized responding by the client.

During a **conversational probe,** the clinician collects one or several conversational speech samples and then analyzes them for generalized responding of the taught target behaviors. No reinforcing or punishing contingencies are provided during the conversational speech sample. At this point, the clinician assesses the client's production of the target sound in untaught words and situations and at untaught linguistic levels and so forth in the absence of any special prompting.

Implementing a Maintenance Program

As stated earlier, the ultimate goal is production of the target objectives in the client's natural environment over time. This behavioral process is known as **maintenance.** To ensure that the client maintains the production of the target sounds or phonological skills over time in various natural communicative environments, the clinician must identify strategies that will help promote that.

Traditionally, maintenance was seen as a step in therapy that began in the latter stages of treatment when the client produced the target behavior with a high level of accuracy in spontaneous speech. However, Hegde (1998b) emphasizes that some maintenance strategies can and should be planned even before direct intervention is started, not only after the behaviors have been established (p. 191). A carefully planned maintenance program increases the chances not only that the client will use the target sounds or phonological skills during spontaneous speech, but also that he or she will maintain those skills over time.

There are many factors that the clinician should consider in regard to (a) the selection and manipulation of antecedent stimuli, (b) the selection of responses for training, and (c) the manipulation of treatment contingencies in an effort to enhance maintenance of the newly learned articulation and phonological skills. It must be noted that these can apply to various communicative disorders, but for our purposes they will be tailored to fit articulation and phonological disorders.

Selection and Manipulation of Stimuli

The selection of appropriate stimulus items may help promote maintenance of the target sound or phonological skills selected for training. On the other hand, the use of inappropriate or randomly selected stimuli may hinder the maintenance process. Therefore, it is very important that the clinician spend quality time in the selection of stimulus items in the treatment of articulation and phonological skills.

Select Standard Stimuli from the Client's Natural Environments

When possible, it is imperative that clinicians select stimulus items from the client's natural environments to teach the production of target sounds and phonological skills. This is important because those stimuli will help promote maintenance of the behaviors by serving as antecedent stimuli in various environments. If stimulus items that are part of the child's natural environment are used in the clinical setting, he or she more likely will produce the target sounds when faced by those stimuli outside of the clinical setting. Although it may be more time efficient to select stimulus items from commercially available resources, that may not be the most clinically efficient method in relation to response generalization and maintenance. The words or pictures selected from commercial materials may or may not be stimuli that the client encounters in his or her natural environment. And although those words or pictures may help evoke production of the target sound in the clinical setting, they may not do so in the client's home, school, and so forth. Therefore, it is extremely important that clinicians incorporate the use of naturally occurring stimuli as much as possible.

The clinician may ask the client's parents to bring pictures, objects, toys, and other items that can be easily transported to the clinical environment. We acknowledge that this cannot always be done for various reasons; however, if there is even a remote possibility of integrating such items into the client's treatment sessions without creating an excessive burden, the clinician should approach parents with such an idea. When working with a school-age child, the clinician should try to collaborate with the classroom teacher to incorporate vocabulary words, spelling word lists, homework assignments, textbooks, and other curriculum materials into the child's articulation-phonological treatment sessions. As stated earlier, this may aid in initial generalization and eventual maintenance of the target behaviors.

Select Common Verbal Antecedents

The use of common **verbal antecedents** during the training process is just as important as the selection of stimuli from the child's natural environments. Verbal antecedents refer to words or phrases used to evoke production of the target sound. Verbal antecedents can be very specific, such as prompts and instructions used during the establishment phase (e.g., "Put your tongue between your teeth and blow"). These types of specific verbal antecedents are more appropriate in the beginning stages of therapy when the child cannot consistently produce the treatment target. In the later stages, it is more clinically appropriate to use verbal antecedents that the child will encounter in everyday settings and situations. So, after the sound has been established, it is important that clinicians begin to use more common verbal antecedents to evoke the target sound. This may begin as soon as the child can produce the sound at the word level. Verbal antecedents that parallel the natural environment include the following:

▶ Antecedent: "Tell me what you're playing with."
  Expected response: "My *ball*"—[b] is the target sound.

▶ Antecedent: "What are you eating?"
  Expected response: "I'm eating *cookies*"—[k] is the target sound.

▶ Antecedent: "Name your body parts."
  Expected response: *"Eyes, nose, ears, legs, fingers . . ."*—[z] is the target sound.

▶ Antecedent: "What's the title of the book you are reading?"
  Expected response: *"Jack and the Beanstalk"*—[ʤ] is the target sound.

These are examples of verbal antecedents that may frequently occur in the child's natural home and classroom environments during interaction with parents and significant others and with the classroom teacher. Because the verbal antecedents are used by the clinician in the clinical setting, they will more likely evoke production of the target sound when they occur in the home or school environment.

Vary the Audience

Because of the clinician's primary role in the therapy process, he or she becomes a strong antecedent stimulus for the production of the target behavior. This is exemplified by the child who articulates a perfect /s/ in the presence of the clinician but continues to demonstrate a frontal lisp with his or her parents, friends, teachers, and others. In that case, the target sound is under strict stimulus control because it occurs only in the presence of the clinician. To promote the use of the target sound in the presence of various people, the clinician must vary the audience-antecedent controls by involving parents, siblings, friends, and teachers in treatment. This is extremely important because the clinician is not the typical audience of the child's sound productions. We will review this with greater detail in an upcoming section of this unit.

Vary the Physical Setting

Without a doubt the goal of therapy should be the child's production of the target sounds in various natural environments such as home and school. Use of the trained behaviors solely in the therapy environment is not clinically efficient. In our experience, however, the child's production of the target sounds in extraclinical environments does not happen automatically unless special strategies are incorporated in therapy. To promote extraclinical production of the target behaviors the clinician needs to make a concerted effort to hold treatment sessions in the child's various communication environments such as the library, school playground, regular classroom, cafeteria, and so forth. In the public schools, these environments are literally just around the corner from the therapy room.

Important Response Considerations

There are some important variables that the clinician should consider in regard to the responses under training. Selection of client-specific responses, training of multiple exemplars, and reinforcement of the target behavior at complex response topographies help ensure their maintenance in natural settings.

Select Client-Specific Objectives

One of the maintenance strategies that can be considered even before direct training is started is the selection of client-specific objectives. Without a doubt, certain objectives will be more functional. Those objectives that meet the client's individual needs are more likely to be generalized and maintained over time. Also, those behaviors are more likely to be reinforced by the client's significant others in various natural environments.

Select Multiple Exemplars

It is important that the clinician train as many exemplars of a target behavior as needed to achieve initial generalization and maintenance over time. Obviously, a target sound occurs in many words, and each such word is simply an example of it. Some children may generalize the target sound to untrained words after only a few exemplars have been trained. However, other children may need training on many words before initial generalization to untrained words occurs.

Reinforce Complex Response Topographies

Clinicians should move through the various topographic levels as quickly as possible. It is important that clinicians not spend too much time training production of a target sound or phonological skill at a level that is too simple. Inexperienced clinicians should be especially careful of this. It is not unusual for clinicians who feel uncertain about their own skills to continue to train a skill at a manageable level. The client's successful production of the target behavior at a certain level is often reinforcing for the clinician. If therapy is shifted to a level at which the client may show some initial difficulty, the clinician may feel at a loss about what to do. Therefore, therapy is shifted back to the level at which the client was known to be successful. It is imperative that clinicians proceed to more complex levels so that the target behaviors are reinforced in natural conversational interactions. This is necessary if the target responses are to be generalized and maintained.

Manipulation of Response Contingencies

The manipulation of response contingencies is probably the most important aspect of maintenance. The clinician should constantly reevaluate the programmed contingencies for their effectiveness. The clinician should also ensure that the schedules of reinforcement are appropriate for a particular stage of treatment. The contingencies used to initially establish the target behavior are different from those used to maintain the behaviors over time.

Use Intermittent Schedules of Reinforcement

In the natural environment, it is unlikely that the child will be reinforced every time he or she produces a target sound correctly. Reinforcers from parents, friends, and teachers are more likely to come sporadically. The child may be reinforced for a few responses, while many others may go unreinforced. Therefore, it is important that the clinician move the training sequence from a continuous schedule of reinforcement to an intermittent schedule. This will decrease the likelihood that the child will discriminate between the treatment and nontreatment conditions. *It is also important to use an intermittent schedule of reinforcement because that schedule will help maintain the target responses over longer periods of time than behaviors that are reinforced continuously.*

The clinician can start with a continuous schedule of reinforcement when establishing the sound. However, as the response becomes more consistent, an intermittent schedule may be used. The intermittent schedule may gradually progress from a relatively high level of reinforcement (e.g., an FR2 schedule) to one that requires greater numbers of responses (e.g., FR10). In an FR10 schedule and beyond many responses will go unreinforced. It is important that the clinician stretch the reinforcement schedule in a gradual manner to decrease the possibility of response extinction. In the final stages of treatment, the clinician should reinforce the target behaviors only occasionally to parallel the natural environment.

Use Conditioned or Naturally Occurring Reinforcers

It is important that the clinician use conditioned reinforcers in the clinical setting, since verbal praise, attention, approval, and eye contact most often reinforce verbal behaviors in natural environments. Although it is necessary to use primary reinforcers with some children, the clinician should be careful to fade their use as treatment progresses. It is important to fade the use of primary reinforcers since their continued use may not support generalized responses and maintenance of the target behaviors. When using a token economy system, it is imperative that the schedule of reinforcement be stretched to a point where the child is required to provide several responses before a reinforcer is delivered.

Delay Reinforcement

In the early stages of treatment when target sounds are shaped and established, reinforcers should be delivered immediately and promptly. Immediate reinforcement helps increase the response level of the selected target behaviors. However, when the target behaviors begin to occur consistently, it is important to deliver the reinforcers on a delayed basis for maintenance purposes. In the natural environment, children will not always receive immediate reinforcement for the use of the target sounds. Reinforcement at home, in school, and in other natural communicative environments most often is provided on a delayed basis. Therefore, to prevent discrimination between the clinical and the home environment, the clinician should program the delivery of reinforcing contingencies so that they more closely match the client's natural environments.

Train Parents and Significant Others in Contingency Management

Maintenance of the target sound over the course of time is highly dependent on the delivery of reinforcing contingencies in the client's natural environments. Because clients spend most of their time with significant others, it is important to train significant others to appropriately respond to the client's sound productions. Clinicians cannot assume that parents possess the skills to appropriately reinforce the child's responses. Also, parents may not know what type of corrective feedback should be provided. Therefore, clinicians should take the time to directly establish such skills in parents and significant others. We will describe the family's involvement in therapy in an upcoming section of this Basic Unit.

Reinforce Generalized Responses

It is important that the clinician pay close attention to the client's production of the target sounds. Occasionally, a client will begin to use the target response in more complex response topographies. For example, if production of /s/ at the word level is being taught, the child may begin to use /s/ in short sentences. If the clinician observes such generalized responses, it is important that they be strongly reinforced to ensure that they continue.

Teach Self-Control Procedures (Self-Monitoring and Self-Correcting)

The issue of **self-control,** more commonly termed **self-monitoring,** has become increasingly popular in recent years (Dunn, 1983; Koegel, Koegel, & Ingham, 1986; Koegel, Koegel, Voy, & Ingham, 1988; Shriberg & Kwiatkowski, 1990). In the context of articulation and phonological treatment, self-control refers to the child's ability to *monitor* and *correct* his own sound productions without constant cueing or prompting from the clinician, parents, or others involved in treatment. Since a client will not have a person instructing him at all times, it is important to establish the client's ability to monitor and correct his own errors. The client's level of self-monitoring and self-correcting will have a direct impact on maintenance of the speech skills acquired in therapy.

The clinician can teach **self-monitoring** and **self-correcting** skills by having the client identify his own correct and incorrect productions. The clinician may ask the client to chart his own productions. We have found it useful to audiotape or videotape portions of clinical sessions for self-control training. Some clients may not be able to identify their errors until they literally "see" or "hear" them with their own eyes and ears from audio- or videotaped samples. Clients can also be trained to stop themselves as soon as they notice they have made an error. Some clients may always have to carefully monitor themselves. Therefore, it is imperative that the clinician consider self-monitoring and self-correcting skills as important target behaviors for training. In our own clinical practice, we often write short-term objectives that reflect such training (e.g., "Marissa will self-monitor and self-correct incorrect productions of /s/ and /z/ with at least 90% accuracy in conversational speech in therapy, at home, and in the classroom").

Teach Contingency Priming

Hegde (1998b) describes **contingency priming** as the client's ability to prompt others for reinforcement. Since parents, teachers, peers, and others may sometimes fail to notice the production of target behaviors, the client may be taught to prime them to reinforce such productions. We all use contingency priming in everyday situations. A wife who asks her husband, "What do you think of my hair now?" after he fails to notice her new haircut is demonstrating contingency priming. Of course, the wife is assuming that her husband indeed likes her new hairstyle. The child who asks, "Mom, did you notice I got an A on my report card?" is also likely prompting his mother for some form of verbal praise (or possibly a token like a $5 bill). Clients with articulation-phonological problems can be trained to ask parents, teachers, and peers similar questions for reinforcement of their sound productions. The client can make use of such questions as:

- "Mrs. Rodriguez, have you noticed I make my *s* sound really well now?"
- "Mom, have you noticed I've been talking really nice and slow for the last few minutes?"
- "Hey, Jim, what do you think of my *r* sounds? Don't they sound good?"
- "Dad, can you listen to me while I make some *th* words?"

Involving Family and Significant Others

It is imperative that clinicians involve family members, significant others, teachers, and peers in the treatment of articulation disorders. This will facilitate production of the target sounds to other situations and will promote their maintenance over time. Family members and others can be trained to teach communicative behaviors and to maintain behaviors taught by the clinician. In the treatment of children with articulation disorders, the most relevant people to involve in the treatment process are the child's parents, teachers, and peers.

Working with Peers

The notion that peers influence each other's behaviors is a well-established fact. At one time or another, we have all experienced the effects of "peer pressure" on our own behaviors. Peer influences can be both negative and positive. In the treatment of articulation-phonological disorders, we can capitalize on the positive effects of peer influences by making the child's peers part of the treatment process. Training the child's friends or peers to help teach and maintain the selected target behaviors can be extremely beneficial for the long-term effects of therapy.

In training peers to teach target sound production, it is important that the clinician teach them to (a) evoke and model the target responses, (b) reinforce correct production of the target responses, (c) provide corrective feedback for incorrect responses, and (d) allow general opportunities for communication. The child's peers may also be taught to document the occurrence of specific behaviors and to tally incorrect and correct responses. In our experience, young children highly enjoy assuming the role of "teacher" and take their responsibility of helping in therapy very seriously. It is amazing to see well-trained young peers at work.

In the treatment setting, peers are usually selected from a child's articulation treatment group. This can be easily done in the public school setting, where therapy is usually delivered in a group format. From our experience, it is not unusual for children who are placed in a specific group because they make the same type of errors to master production of the target sound(s) at a varied pace. One child may be at the word level, another at the sentence level, and yet another at the conversational level. Children can provide each other with corrective feedback and reinforcement during therapy sessions. In our own clinical practicum, we train children to monitor and chart each other's productions as correct or incorrect. We have found that this serves several purposes:

1. It helps build a child's awareness skills.

2. It shifts the delivery of treatment contingencies solely from the clinician to other children, which aids in initial generalization and maintenance.

3. It expands the treatment setting to include other environments, as the children encounter one another at the library, in assemblies, on the playground, and so forth, which also helps promote generalization and maintenance.

We have found that children take the role of teacher seriously. They enjoy playing the part of the clinician. It is amazing how accurate children can be in identifying correct and incorrect productions. The time spent in developing peer trainers is invaluable for the long-term success of speech therapy services.

Working with Teachers

Without a doubt, classroom teachers play a significant role in children's lives. Children are in school an average of 7 hours a day. The majority of that time is spent interacting with the classroom teacher. The child with an articulation disorder is no exception. Therefore, if the articulation-phonological skills trained by a speech–language pathologist are to be maintained in the client's natural environments, it is important that the classroom teacher become an integral part of the therapy process. We have found that most classroom teachers are willing to help "in some way."

The first author has frequently encountered teachers who have a strong desire to learn what they can do to help a child reach his or her goals and objectives.

In our delivery of articulation and phonological treatment, we have found that the teacher's role is most significant in the maintenance phase of therapy. After a sound has been well established and the child can produce it consistently at least at the sentence level, it is wise to train the classroom teacher to provide corrective feedback and reinforcement for the child's productions. Teachers can also be asked to give the child specific cues to help improve the production of the target sound in the classroom. For example, the teacher may be trained to instruct the child, "Emily, remember to put your tongue behind your teeth when you make your *s* sound." Nonverbal cues such as hand signals may also be used in the classroom. If the speech–language pathologist has taken the time to develop a healthy working relationship with the classroom teacher, these types of assistance will usually not be considered a burden.

Working with Parents and Significant Others

For obvious reasons, parents and significant others play an extremely important role in children's lives. Parents are expected to teach their children how to ride a bike; they are expected to help their school-age children with classroom homework assignments; and they are expected to teach their children how to play sports and games. Speech–language pathologists should expect parents to become involved in their children's speech therapy.

As with that of classroom teachers, we have found that the parent's role has the greatest impact during the strengthening and maintenance phase of therapy. After the sound has been well established and the child can produce it consistently at least at the word level, parents can be trained to:

- identify the desirable and undesirable sound productions;

- evoke the target sounds by modeling and providing verbal and visual instructions at the level of training (i.e., words, sentences, oral reading, conversation);

- provide subtle prompts to facilitate correct production of the target behaviors (e.g., subtle hand signals);

- reinforce the child's correct productions of the target sounds;

- provide corrective feedback for incorrect productions of the target sounds through subtle signals (The parents should be trained to be supportive and nonjudgmental in their delivery of corrective feedback. Parents should also be trained to reinforce more than correct.);

- stop reinforcing incorrect sound productions (Some parents may inadvertently reinforce their children's incorrect productions by making such comments as "He sounds so cute when he says his *r*s that way.");

- conduct home treatment programs after adequate training by the speech–language pathologist.

The extent to which parents participate in therapy varies widely. Some parents take a keen interest in their children's treatment and are willing and ready to do anything possible to help. Other parents may not be quite as interested. We should emphasize, however, that parents who appear uninterested often do not realize that they have a role in therapy until the clinician makes them aware of such. The clinician should never assume that parents are uninterested until all attempts have been made to involve them in therapy. If a parent continues to refuse to extend therapy into the home environment by evoking target productions, by conducting speech therapy sessions at home, and by reinforcing and providing corrective feedback, the clinician should candidly disclose the fact that this will likely limit the client's overall progress in therapy.

Dismissing the Client from Therapy, Performing Follow-Up Assessments, and Providing Booster Therapy

In an ideal world, a client would always be dismissed from therapy when he or she reached all of the set goals and objectives. Unfortunately, it is not always that simple. Many variables affect a clinician's determination to dismiss a client. The most obvious is the client's achievement of his or her goals and objectives and maintenance of the skills acquired in therapy. However, not all clients reach the maintenance phase before they are dismissed.

Some clients are dismissed after a certain period of therapy. For example, if clinical services are funded by a third-party payer, the clinician must discontinue therapy when the allotted number of sessions is reached. The clinician may also decide to dismiss a client from therapy because a plateau in his or her ability to make progress has been reached, which is not atypical in clients whose articulation or phonological problems are due to a neurological, structural, or other organic variable. The structural or neurological problems may interfere with the overall progress that can be realistically expected.

Other clients may be dismissed because of their poor motivation to improve. It is the client who is ultimately responsible for following through with assignments, monitoring his or her productions, and practicing correct sound productions as often as possible. The clinician unfortunately cannot force a client to "want to improve." If the clinician has done everything within his or her control to increase the client's participation in therapy and a lack of motivation continues to interfere with the client's progress, dismissal from therapy should be highly considered. Clinicians often have a difficult time dismissing clients whose progress is limited by poor motivation or poor follow-through. The clinician may question whether he or she has done everything possible to "motivate" the client—perhaps if the treatment approach were changed, the client would participate more. However, motivation is a very real factor that may limit a client's progress, and clinicians should be willing and ready to dismiss a client if progress is limited by that variable. Clinicians may need to consider the financial effectiveness of delivering services to a client who apparently does not want to improve.

If the client has been dismissed from therapy under ideal and positive circumstances, it is important that the clinician follow-up with the client to ensure that the progress made in therapy has been maintained. A **follow-up assessment** is a quick procedure that helps the clinician make such a determination. If the clinician finds that the client's skills have diminished or regressed, a short period of intervention may be warranted. Hegde (1998b) refers to this as **booster therapy.**

Using Specific Treatment Activities

Clinicians working with children frequently use fun and exciting treatment activities in hopes that they will increase the child's interest and cooperation in therapy. The activities are presented in a game format so that the child feels like he is playing rather than working. The child's cooperation can be increased if the activities are structured appropriately. However, clinicians must remember that the primary goal of therapy is not to keep the child entertained, but to improve production of the target sounds.

Even though fun and exciting treatment activities do have a place in articulation therapy, they must be structured in such a way that maximize the child's sound production training. The target sounds will not improve if the child spends most of his or her time cutting, pasting, and playing in the absence of sound production training. Clinicians should always keep in mind that the target sound will improve only with continual practice.

It is important that clinicians select treatment activities that will not only increase the child's participation in therapy, but also allow many opportunities for production practice. Also, clinical activities should be preplanned and very organized so that treatment time is not devoted to deciding what to do next. Treatment activities should not take more than a few seconds to introduce and initiate. If a treatment activity is so complex that it takes 5 minutes to explain, it is clinically inefficient. Clinical time is precious and should not be wasted in lengthy explanations. The following is a compilation of widely used treatment activities that are judged to be simple and clinically efficient:

Let's Go Fishing for Sounds

- Cut fish out of poster board using a fish pattern. Ten fish are usually sufficient.

- Attach a paper clip through each fish.

- Write a target sound or a target word containing the sound on each fish.

- Create a fishing pole from a string and magnet (some clinicians purchase a play-size fishing pole that is relatively inexpensive to which they attach a magnet).

- Place the stimulus items (fish) on the floor and instruct the child to "go fish" for a word.

- After the child selects a fish, instruct him or her to say the target sound on that fish a given number of times.

- The child cannot "fish" for another word until he or she successfully produces the sound or target word for the selected number of times.

Variations and Suggestions

- The clinician can photocopy the stimulus words and paste them on one side of the fish so that the fish itself serves as the stimulus item and possible reinforcer.

- The clinician needs to be careful not to give the client too many choices that will actually take time away from production training. Remember that the goal of therapy is to stabilize the production of the target sound, not to catch fish. The activity should serve only as a facilitating technique and should not become the target of therapy. One way of preventing this from happening is to lay out one or two fish at a time, rather than all the fish at once. This structures the client's decision making.

Let's Uncover the Picture

- Put a picture of an object such as an animal, superhero character, or cartoon character on a piece of poster board covered with contact paper or laminated.

- Cut up pieces of construction paper and tape them over the picture to conceal it.

- Ask the child to say his sound or word a given number of times.

- If the child says the word correctly the predetermined number of times, he or she is allowed to remove a piece of paper to reveal a part of the picture.

- The activity continues until the entire picture is revealed.

Put a Smile on the Face

- On a sheet of paper draw 10 round faces with eyes and nose. Do not put on the mouth.

- Have the child say the sound or target word a given number of times.

- After the client correctly produces the target word correctly a predetermined number of times, he or she can draw a smile on a face.

Variations and Suggestions

- Follow each single sound with a smile for a correct sound or a frown for an error.

- These activities can also be used with words.

Let's Toss Some Eggs

- Number the spaces in an egg carton.

- Have the child toss a paper clip into the carton.

- He must say a sound, word, or sentence the number of times indicated.

- A picture card can be used to evoke the target word or sentence.

Let's Hunt for Eggs

- Photocopy the stimulus pictures selected for training.

- Fold the photocopied stimulus items and place them inside several (approximately 10) plastic eggs.

- Hide the eggs around the clinical room area.

- Make sure to "hide" the eggs in a visible manner so that the child does not have any difficulty finding them. This will ensure that treatment time is not wasted by the activity.

- After the client finds an egg, instruct him or her to say its target word a selected number of times (e.g., 5 times).

- The client must say the target sound correctly the number of times indicated before he or she can find another egg.

- When the client finds all of the eggs hidden, he or she can be given some playtime or other tangible reinforcer.

Caution: Not all children celebrate Easter; it is important that the clinician ensure that this activity does not violate the child's cultural or religious beliefs.

Let's Paste an Apple on a Tree

- Draw a ditto of a tree.

- Every time the child says five correct syllables or words, he or she may paste an apple on the tree. Apples can be made out of red construction paper.

Variations and Suggestions

- Paste spots on a cow, petals on a flower, light bulbs on a Christmas tree, body parts on a person, etc.

Let's Find the Sound

- Create 12 flashcards or pictures of objects whose names contain the target sound.

- First, the child is asked to name the object shown.

- Then the clinician displays the cards.

- If the target were /s/, the clinician might say, "I'm going to pretend this piece of paper [a blank card] is soap. You close your eyes. I'll hide the soap under one of these cards. You must guess which card the soap is under. Say, 'Is the soap under the pencil?' "

- The child must ask the carrier question until he finds the soap. He looks under the cards himself.

Variation and Suggestions

- With a group, have the children each take one turn looking for the target. The one who finds it gets to hide it next, though the clinician supplies the carrier phrase.

Let's Feed the Hungry Bear

- Create a bear from a medium-sized, brown paper bag.

- Decorate the bag so that it has eyes, a nose, and a mouth.

- Create the mouth by making a slit on the paper bag big enough for the stimulus cards to slip through.

- Ask the child to select a stimulus card and produce its target word a given number of times. When the client correctly produces the target word the determined number of times, he or she can "feed" the bear.

- The child is then instructed to select another card, and the process is continued until the child has fed all of the cards to the bear. When all of the stimulus cards are in the paper bag, the child can be given playtime or other tangible reinforcer.

Let's Make a Bracelet

- Select medium-sized, plastic paper clips of various colors (e.g., blue, yellow, red, white, and so forth).

- Attach a paper clip to each stimulus card (approximately 10).

- Instruct the child to select a stimulus card and say the target word a given number of times.

- When the child produces the target word correctly the determined number of times, he or she can keep the paper clip.

- As the child "earns" each paper clip, he or she is instructed to connect them, working toward making a bracelet.

- When the child produces all of the stimulus items selected for practice, he or she should have collected 10 paper clips. The clinician can assist the child in connecting the paper clip bracelet around his or her wrist.

Let's Play a Memory Game

- Make a photocopied matching set of the selected stimulus pictures containing the target sound (approximately five sets).

- Place the pictures face down.

- Instruct the child to pick a card and then to turn over another card in hopes of matching the one picked. The object is to get as many matches as possible. If the second card turned over doesn't match the first card, it is turned back over and left in place. Then the child tries again.

- Instruct the child to say the target word or the carrier phrase, "I picked the ____" every time a picture is turned over.

- When the child gets all five matches, he or she earns playtime or other tangible reinforcer.

Variation and Suggestions

- The client and the clinician take turns picking pictures to match. This may make the game more competitive for older children.

Let's Play Basketball

- The clinician can use a trash can or any other container with a large diameter to serve as the basketball "hoop" and several small balls (e.g., 10 balls) to play basketball with the child.

- Instruct the child to select a stimulus picture card and say the target word a given number of times.

- After the child correctly produces the target word the predetermined number of times, he or she is allowed to toss the ball into the "basket."

- When the child tosses every ball into the basket, he or she can be given playtime or other tangible reinforcer. The clinician should make sure that the ball does not have too much bounce to prevent it from bouncing out of the basket. A foam ball works well.

These activities are only some among many activities used by clinicians in articulation therapy. Many clinicians are extremely creative and develop their own activities. For those whose creativity is not a forte, there are several commercially available resources that can be purchased and tailored to individual clients.

Assessing and Treating Phonological Awareness Skills in School-Age Children: A Basic Introduction to the Topic

As indicated in the Basic Unit of Chapter 3, within the last several years, speech–language pathologists, among other professionals (e.g., reading specialists and resource specialists), have placed a strong focus on the concept of **phonological awareness.** Experts have defined phonological awareness, which is also termed **phonemic awareness,** as "the knowledge of meaningful sounds, or phonemes, in our language and how those sounds blend together to form syllables, words, phrases, and sentences" (Robertson & Salter, 1997, p. 5). Please see Chapter 3 for a more detailed definition of phonological awareness.

In recent years researchers have theorized that there may be a link between severe speech and phonological disorders and poor phonological awareness in young children (e.g., Bird & Bishop, 1992; Hodson, 1994; Hodson, 1997; Domnick, Hodson, Coffman, & Wynne, 1993; Marion, Sussman, & Marquardt, 1993; Stackhouse, 1992; Webster & Plante, 1992). Experts have further speculated that poor phonological awareness skills in young children are linked with or serve as strong predictors of later problems in reading and spelling (e.g., Ball, 1993; Catts, 1991; Clarke-Klein & Hodson, 1995; Goldsworthy, 1996; Pratt & Brady, 1988; Stackhouse, 1997; Swank & Catts, 1994; Williams, 1984). Thus, it has been suggested that young children with severe phonological disorders may lack age-appropriate phonological awareness skills, and that that puts them at risk for reading and spelling problems later in childhood (Bird, Bishop, & Freeman, 1995; Roseberry-McKibbin & Hegde, 2000). The reader is referred to Stackhouse (1997) for a thorough review of the connection among phonological disorders, phonological awareness, and literacy problems.

In the Basic Unit of Chapter 3 we highlighted some skills that have been attributed to a child's phonological awareness. Examples of these are identifying words that sound alike (rhyming), identifying the number of sounds or syllables in a word, segmenting words into their individual sounds or syllables, manipulating phonemes to create words, identifying the position of a phoneme within a word, using invented spellings, and so forth. Speech–language pathologists involved in the clinical intervention of children with moderate to severe articulation, phonological, and language disorders often include phonological awareness activities in their intervention programs (Stackhouse, 1997, p. 191).

Stackhouse (1997) further indicates that "it is now expected that the work of speech–language therapists will promote and support literacy skills as an integral part of speech–language intervention programmes" (p. 190). Snowling and Stackhouse (1996) carefully clarify, though, that the role of the speech–language pathologist is not to teach reading and spelling but to identify problems with and train the foundational skills that may contribute to literacy development (p. 240). The first author's clinical experience in the public school setting would support Stackhouse's claim that speech–language pathologists are increasingly expected by administrators, program coordinators, and other education support staff to play a key role in the training of phonological awareness skills to promote improved literacy. In that speech–language pathologists are becoming more and more involved in assessing and training phonological awareness skills in children with and without articulation or phonological disorders, we will address some basic assessment and treatment considerations on that topic.

Assessment of Phonological Awareness Skills

Formal instruments for testing phonological awareness of children include the *Test of Phonological Awareness* (Torgesen & Bryant, 1994), *Phonological Awareness Profile* (Robertson & Salter, 1995b), and *Assessment of Sound Awareness and Production* (Mattes, 1998). Another formal assessment, the *Lindamood Auditory Conceptualization Test* (Lindamood & Lindamood, 1971), although not originally designed as a phonological awareness testing instrument, provides some information on such skills, particularly phoneme discrimination and sound segmentation.

The clinician can also design various informal measures that can provide some information on the child's phonological awareness skills. The results can then be related to the child's reading and spelling. The clinician should always consult with other professionals involved in the child's academic program such as reading specialists, resource specialists, and the regular education teacher. The following list includes various phonological awareness skills and specific tasks the clinician can ask the child to perform to evaluate their development:

• **Rhyming**—the ability to identify words that sound alike or rhyme; the ability to provide a word that rhymes with a presented word; the ability to sort rhyming from non-rhyming words.

  • Do these words rhyme or sound alike: *cat–hat*?

  • Which word does not rhyme with the other words: *dog, hog, hat, log*?

  • Tell me three words that rhyme with *hot*.

  • [The clinician selects pictures of words that rhyme and words that do not rhyme and places them in front of the child to sort.] Put all the pictures whose names rhyme in one pile. Put the ones whose names don't rhyme in another pile.

• **Alliteration**—the ability to identify words that begin or end with a certain sound.

  • Which word(s) end with the *f* sound?
  • Which word(s) start with the *sh* sound?
  • Does *bus* start with a *b*?
  • Tell me three words that start with *p*.

• **Phoneme isolation**—the ability to identify whether a specific sound occurs in the beginning, end, or middle of a word.

  • Tell me if the *b* is in the beginning, middle, or end of the word *bus*.
  • What is the last sound in the word *pan*?

• **Phoneme manipulation**—the ability to delete, add, or substitute a sound in a word to create other words.

  • What do you get if you take *h* away from *hat*?
  • Say the word *man* without the *m*.

- Say *hit* without the last sound.
- Say *fat*. Now say *at*—what sound was left out on the second word?
- Say *hat*. Now say it with a *b* instead of an *h* at the beginning.

- **Sound and syllable blending**—the ability to blend two or more sounds that are temporally separated by a few seconds into a word.

  - Listen carefully. What does *tea – cher* say?
  - Listen to me carefully. What does *h – a – t* say?

- **Syllable and sound identification**—the ability to identify the number of syllables or sounds in a word through clapping, finger tapping, or verbally stating the number of syllables.

  - Tell me how many beats (syllables) there are in the word *hotdog*.
  - Tell me how many sounds there are in the word *cat*.

- **Sound segmentation**—the ability to break down a word into its individual sound components.

  - What are the three sounds in the word *dog*?
  - What are the sounds in the word *house*?

As with all informal measures, clinicians need to have adequate knowledge of what can be expected in normally developing children at specific ages before drawing any conclusions. A kindergarten child, for example, who may have very limited exposure to the written word cannot be expected to have the same phonological awareness skills as a third grader who has already had some formal training in reading. Kindergarten children can be expected to do well in rhyming words, identifying the number of syllables in words, blending syllables into words, and segmenting words into syllables (Robertson & Salter, 1995a). First-grade children who have mastered the above skills are increasingly successful with segmenting simple words into phonemes, isolating the position of a sound within a word, identifying the number of sounds in simple words, and manipulating phonemes within a word to create other words (Robertson & Salter, 1995a). The reader is referred to Stackhouse (1997) for a review of a stage model of literacy development (pp. 162–164).

Robertson and Salter (1995a, p. 5) list several signs of weakness in phonological awareness, or what they term *phonological processing,* in children. They indicate that these children may have difficulty in:

- recognizing and producing rhyming words or patterns of alliteration;
- orally breaking words into syllables or sounds;
- identifying whether a specific sound occurs at the beginning, end, or middle of a word;
- identifying the number of sounds in a word;
- blending sounds to make a word; and
- repeating multisyllabic words.

Treatment of Phonological Awareness Skills

Robertson and Salter (1995a, 1997) indicate that approximately 20–25% of children do not develop adequate phonological awareness skills to make the connection between sounds and the letters that represent them (phoneme-grapheme relation). They further emphasize that although this relatively high percentage of children may be at risk for literacy problems, most instructional programs do not address foundational phonological awareness skills since the majority of children already have them (Robertson & Salter, 1995a, p. 5). Again, speech–language pathologists are increasingly becoming involved in the remediation of children with poor phonological awareness skills, especially with those who also receive clinical intervention for articulation, phonological, and language disorders.

The detailed activities that can be used to train children who are diagnosed with poor phonological awareness and are thought to be at risk for reading and spelling problems are too vast to summarize in this chapter. In general, clinicians design or use activities that help promote development of the phonological awareness skills needed prior to formal reading instruction, including rhyming, alliteration, sound and syllable blending, sound and syllable segmentation, phoneme isolation, phoneme identification, phoneme manipulation, and so forth. Parents can easily be trained to facilitate basic phonological awareness skills such as rhyming, syllable identification, and phoneme isolation in the home environment.

The procedures discussed for teaching articulation and phonological skills can be used to establish phonological awareness skills. One important difference is that the target behaviors become the rhyming, blending, segmenting, phoneme identification, and phoneme manipulation skills that are either absent or limited in a particular child. The clinician still needs to use stimulus materials to evoke the target skills, clearly identify the skills that the client is expected to learn, provide reinforcing contingencies and corrective feedback, and arrange the sequence of training so that it progresses from simple to complex.

There are an increasing number of commercially available phonological awareness programs and activity workbooks that can simplify the clinician's workload in the preparation of stimulus materials. Among these are the *Phonological Awareness Kit* (Robertson & Salter, 1995a), the *Phonological Awareness Kit–Intermediate* (Robertson & Salter, 1997), the *Phonological Awareness Training for Reading* (Torgesen & Bryant, 1993), and the *Lindamood Phoneme Sequencing Program for Reading, Spelling, and Speech–Third Edition* (Lindamood & Lindamood, 1998).

An increasingly popular computer software program designed to teach auditory processing and phonemic awareness skills is Earobics Pro Plus: Step 1 (4–7 years), which was released in May 1998. A few months later, in November 1998, Earobics Pro Plus: Step 2 (7–10 years) was released to meet the needs of older children. This program, available through Cognitive Concepts, Inc., is extensive and systematic and provides repeated practice. Children must reach the mastery criterion of one skill before progressing to a more complex skill. In our own use of Earobics Pro Plus: Step 1, we have found that most children react favorably to the program and appear to enjoy the skill-oriented tasks. The speech signal is very good, and the programmed reinforcing and corrective feedback contingencies are delivered immediately and with appropriate verbal animation. It should be noted that some of the underlying conceptual premises of two earlier versions of Earobics have been recently questioned (see Diehl, 1999), but those versions are no longer available for consumer purchase. The reader is referred to Diehl (1999) for an excellent critical review of the technical aspects of and conceptual framework supporting each of the six games that make up the Earobics program.

Roseberry-McKibbin and Hegde (2000) indicate that more research is needed to conclusively demonstrate the causal relation between decreased phonological awareness and later reading and spelling and the efficacy of phonological awareness treatment in preventing literacy problems in later childhood. Diehl (1999) indicates that there is still much research to be done in the area of phonological awareness, particularly regarding the relation between word recognition and reading comprehension. Stackhouse (1997) has identified the following specific areas as necessary future developments in the subfield of phonological awareness (adapted from pp. 190–191):

• The development of appropriate phonological awareness assessment materials, with an increase in data collection from normally developing children across a wide range of ages primarily for comparison purposes. Without such data it is difficult to identify a delay in phonological awareness skills and the need for intervention.

• A comparison of phonological awareness and literacy development of children with phonological impairments over time through longitudinal studies. This can help identify to what extent an expressive phonological impairment interferes with phonological awareness and literacy development.

• An increased knowledge base of what phonological awareness training materials work well, with whom, and why. Evaluating the efficacy of various programs should be of high priority.

Summary of the Basic Unit

• Once the assessment has been completed and a child is diagnosed with either an articulation or a phonological disorder, therapy can be initiated.

• The clinician selects potential **target behaviors,** which are typically outlined as **short-term objectives** and **long-term goals.**

• Target behaviors should be functional, useful, and ethnoculturally appropriate.

• Several guidelines have been advanced for the selection of phonological processes and individual sounds for training.

• The clinician should consider teaching phonological processes that have the greatest impact on speech intelligibility, that result in early success, and that are crucial for a particular client (e.g., idiosyncratic or unusual processes).

• In selecting individual sounds the clinician should consider those that are functional for a particular child, are **stimulable,** occur in **key words** or particular **facilitative phonetic contexts,** are more visible, occur more frequently, will have a greater impact on intelligibility, and may **generalize** other sounds, among other variables.

• The clinician needs to determine the number of sounds that will be trained at the same time. This consideration is most important with clients who have multiple misarticulations. The clinician can take a **training-deep approach,** in which only one or two sounds are taught to criterion at the same time before introducing others. Some clinicians prefer a **training-broad approach,** in which several sounds are taught at the same time.

- Before starting therapy, clinicians should collect **baseline data** to determine the rate of response for each target sound. The clinician identifies the potential treatment target, prepares stimulus items to evoke its production, prepares a recording sheet to document the client's performance, and administers the baseline **discrete trials.**

- The clinician needs to determine the linguistic level that will be initially trained. Baseline data can help the clinician make such a determination. A clinician's own treatment philosophy may also dictate the linguistic level at which treatment is initiated.

- The clinician should develop measurable objectives that clearly identify the response topography or skill targeted, the quantitative mastery criterion, the response mode, the response level, the response setting, and the number of speech samples or sessions in which the target behaviors will be documented.

- In most clinical settings, the clinician must develop a **treatment program** delineating what will be targeted in therapy and the procedures that will be used. Treatment programs can be written in varied styles and forms. They can be simple, comprehensive, or a specific format (e.g., **individualized education program**).

- With some clients, the clinician may need to establish the motor production of the target sounds. Various techniques can be used including **phonetic placement, successive approximation, modeling,** and **verbal instructions and prompts.**

- After the sounds have been established, the clinician needs to increase and strengthen the target sound or target behaviors. **Positive reinforcers, negative reinforcers, primary reinforcers, social reinforcers,** and **conditioned generalized reinforcers** can be used.

- The reinforcers are delivered on a continuous schedule in the initial stages of treatment and are gradually faded to an intermittent fixed or variable schedule.

- **Interfering** or **inappropriate behaviors** can be reduced by the use of various response-reducing methods, including **time-out, response cost, verbal corrective feedback, nonverbal corrective feedback,** and **mechanical feedback.**

- **Treatment sessions** can be loosely or highly structured. This often depends on the client, the stage of therapy, and the clinician's treatment philosophy. Loosely structured treatment sessions should be skill oriented rather than "play"-oriented.

- **Treatment trials** can be administered as **discrete trials** in the beginning stages of therapy, then progress to more spontaneous conversational interactions as the client moves through the various linguistic levels.

- The clinician should be systematic in the collection of treatment data to help assess the effectiveness and efficiency of treatment and to assess the client's progress.

- After the target behaviors have reached a predetermined criterion, the clinician can **probe** for **generalized responses** to untrained response modes, untrained words, untrained settings, untrained audiences, and so forth.

• To ensure that the client will use the trained target behaviors in varied settings and with varied audiences across time, the clinician needs to implement various **maintenance procedures.**

• The clinician will need to determine when the client is ready for **dismissal.** Various factors play a part in that decision. **Follow-up** assessments can be conducted after the client is dismissed, and **booster therapy** can be provided as needed.

• In recent years, speech–language pathologists have taken a more direct role in the assessment and treatment of **phonological awareness skills.** The lack of such skills is considered a significant variable in poor literacy skills in some children. Poor phonological awareness skills have been documented in children with severe phonological disorders.

Advanced Unit

♦ ♦ ♦ ♦ ♦ ♦ ♦ ♦ ♦ ♦ ♦ ♦ ♦ ♦ ♦ ♦ ♦ ♦ ♦ ♦

Treatment of Various Organic and Neurogenic Speech Disorders

The Basic Unit of this chapter addressed the many treatment principles and procedures that can be used with children with articulation and phonological disorders. In essence, all clients need various stimulus manipulations, specification of acceptable and unacceptable responses, modeling of correct responses and shaping as needed, reinforcing contingencies for correct responses, and corrective feedback for incorrect responses. Furthermore, the clinician assesses for generalized responses and implements various techniques that can help promote maintenance of the trained skills (Hegde, 1998b).

Although such principles are known to be effective in the treatment of a variety of communication disorders, in this Advanced Unit we will address some other procedures that may be especially efficacious in treating the speech difficulties associated with specific disorders: apraxia of speech, developmental apraxia of speech, dysarthria, cerebral palsy, cleft palate, and hearing impairment. We previously addressed the characteristics and etiologies of these disorders in the Advanced Unit of Chapter 6. Thus, we will not repeat such information in this Advanced Unit (the reader is referred to Chapter 6 for a review). The information addressed in this Advanced Unit is meant to be a basic introduction to the treatment of those organic and neurogenic-based speech disorders. It is likely that students will have specific courses that focus on the assessment and treatment of these disorders at both the undergraduate and the graduate levels.

Apraxia of Speech

As reviewed in Chapter 6, apraxia of speech is a motor programming disorder of neurogenic origin. The primary etiology for the neurological damage leading to apraxia of speech (AOS) is a left hemisphere stroke in the frontal lobe, although several other causes have also been identified. The onset of the disorder is acute rather than progressive, and it is most common in adults. The severity of apraxia of speech can range from mild to profound depending on the extent of damage. This often manifests in varied speech characteristics from one client to another.

Since there are no widely used medical or surgical treatments for AOS (Bloom, 1997; Duffy, 1995), the treatment for this neuromotor speech disorder is primarily behavioral (Duffy, 1995; Hegde, 1996b). The focus of therapy is primarily on articulation and prosody since those are the speech parameters that are most often affected (Bloom, 1997). Intervention for resonance, phonation, and respiration is rarely needed, except in some cases of severe apraxia (Duffy, 1995). Duffy indicates that the goal of therapy in clients with AOS is to "maximize the effectiveness, efficiency, and naturalness of communication" (p. 417). The goal also is to restore or compensate for impaired functions and to modify the need for normal speech (Duffy, 1995, p. 417). Counseling in the form of providing information about why certain aspects of speech are no longer normal or why they may never be normal is an important component of treatment. The clinician should also thoroughly inform the client and his or her significant others about what will be done to remediate or compensate for the problem, what types of efforts it will take on their part, and the likely outcome of treatment.

Duffy (1995) distinguishes *communication-oriented* from *speaker-oriented* treatment approaches in the management of apraxia of speech and dysarthria. In a communication-oriented approach, the goal is to improve communication even if the speech skills affected by the disorder do not improve. Duffy (p. 378) identifies the following modifications to improve the client's overall communication effectiveness:

- altering the number of listeners;

- altering the amount of interfering noise;

- altering the speaker-listener distance and eye contact;

- informing new listeners about the speech problem and its cause;

- informing new listeners about the client's preferred method of communicating; and

- identifying the most effective strategies for repairing communication breakdowns (e.g., repeating utterances as needed, rephrasing, spelling, writing, and answering clarifying questions).

Speaker-oriented treatment activities focus on increasing the client's speech intelligibility and improving the efficiency, naturalness, and quality of communication (Duffy, 1995, p. 377). The client's motor production becomes the primary target. Speech drills have an important role in the treatment of apraxia of speech since the client's skills are likely to improve only with continued practice. Therapy often follows a sequential organization from simple to complex tasks; the clinician should consider the following sequence in training:

1. Automatic speech tasks (e.g., counting, reciting the alphabet, singing, saying the days of the week) should be trained before spontaneous speech tasks (naming pictures, producing sentences, and so forth).

2. Sounds that have a higher frequency of occurrence should be trained before less frequently occurring sounds unless dictated by other variables (e.g., the client's name contains a sound that does not occur very often). Training high-frequency sounds will likely have a greater impact on the client's speech intelligibility than training low-frequency sounds.

3. Sounds that are stimulable should be trained before those that are less stimulable. The client with apraxia of speech will probably experience much communication failure. It is important to structure therapy so that success is likely.

4. Treat sounds in word-initial position before sounds in other positions. Clients with apraxia of speech tend to have the most difficulty with word-initial sounds. If the client can successfully produce the initial sound in a word, then the

remaining sounds tend to be produced correctly. It is important to train the client to successfully manage production of the initial sounds in words to increase the likelihood that the rest of the word will be produced correctly.

5. Visible sounds should be trained before nonvisible sounds or those that are difficult to see. Clients with apraxia of speech tend to benefit from visual placement cues for the production of sounds. For obvious reasons, visual cues are more successful in evoking the correct production of sounds that are visible than of those that are difficult to see.

6. The clinician should consider the following hierarchy by manner of production (listed from easiest sound class to most difficult): vowels, plosives, nasals, laterals, fricatives, and affricates. In relation to place of articulation, bilabials and alveolars should be trained before back sounds. These are generally more visible. Voiceless sounds will probably be easier for the client to produce than voiceless sounds. Also, singleton consonants should be trained before clusters. Creating this hierarchy of easy to more difficult will probably result in greater success for the client.

7. In keeping with the sequential organization of treatment for apraxia of speech, single-syllable words should be trained before multisyllable words and single words should be taught before phrases.

8. High-frequency words should be trained before low-frequency words. If the client has difficulty with the production of high-frequency words, the number of errors will probably be high. It is important to train correct production of such words to decrease the possibility of errors in the client's productions.

9. In selecting words and phrases for training, the clinician should choose those that are meaningful for the client. It is important to establish functional communication as quickly as possible; therefore, the clinician should teach words and phrases that have an impact on the client's life before those that are less meaningful. Thus, production of the client's name, address, wife's name, children's names, and so forth should be taught before other words.

The stimuli used to evoke correct production of the treatment targets can be auditory, visual, and tactile. Initially, the client may need all three types of stimulation. The clinician typically provides auditory stimulation by providing a verbal model of the target production and using specific verbal instructions. Visual feedback is provided by asking the client to watch the clinician's productions or by having the client produce the target in front of a mirror. Tactile cues are most often given through phonetic placement training with tongue blades, cotton swab sticks, and physical manipulation of the articulators. The clinician should be prepared to be versatile with the use of special stimuli, as some may work better than others with specific clients. Rosenbek (1985) warns that the use of the mirror may be distracting for some patients and may also be upsetting for those who have a facial paresis. The clinician should use the mirror only if it proves helpful with a particular client.

The use of auditory, visual, and tactile stimulation by the clinician should be reduced and eventually eliminated as therapy progresses and the client displays some improvement. Also, clients may be trained to self-cue as special evoking procedures provided by the clinician are faded. We can recall a patient who was trained to self-prompt the production of *enchilada* (a Mexican dish pronounced /ɛn·ʧə·la·də/) by placing her own hands around her waist and thinking "inch-a-lot-a." This proved to be particularly helpful for this client, who adored Mexican food and often ordered enchiladas when dining at a restaurant.

Eight-Step Continuum

Rosenbek (1985, pp. 289–290) describes an eight-step treatment continuum relating to the level of modeling and prompting that is provided to the client during articulation practice. The continuum progresses from maximal to minimal stimulation.

Step 1: The client is asked to carefully watch and listen to the clinician; the client is instructed to make the target production in unison with the clinician. This is termed **integral stimulation.**

Step 2: The clinician provides the client with a visual and auditory model of the target production — the cues "listen to me" and "watch me" are used. The client is instructed to listen carefully. The clinician then mouths the production without voice so that only the visual cue is provided. The client is then asked to imitate the clinician's production aloud.

Step 3: The clinician provides a model for the client to imitate. The cues "listen to me" and "watch me" are withdrawn. Only the verbal antecedent stimulus "I'll say it first and you say it after me" accompanied by the model is used at this point.

Step 4: The clinician provides a model for the client to imitate, as in step 3. However, during this step, the client is instructed to consecutively repeat the target production several times.

Step 5: The clinician writes the word corresponding to the target production on a piece of paper or other writing area and asks the client to read the word aloud.

Step 6: The clinician presents the written word corresponding to the target production. However, the client is asked to produce the word aloud only after the written stimulus has been removed or hidden.

Step 7: The clinician uses a question to prompt the target production. Modeling cues are abandoned, and the clinician arranges verbal antecedents to evoke "volitional" speech from the client (e.g., "What is your son's name?").

Step 8: Target verbal productions are facilitated through role-playing situations.

This continuum provides a basic prototype that clinicians can follow in the sequential presentation of *antecedent stimuli*. However, it should be modified as necessary to meet the needs of individual clients. Some clients, for example, may not have adequate literacy skills to benefit from steps 5 and 6. Others may have some visual problems that interfere with their ability to read written stimuli. In such cases, steps 5 and 6 should be bypassed.

PROMPT

Another program that capitalizes on the use of specific cues to facilitate the production of speech is the Prompts for Restructuring Oral Muscular Phonetic Targets (PROMPT) approach. This program was originally developed for treating the communication needs of children with developmental apraxia of speech (Chumpelik, 1984). It was subsequently applied to adults with AOS (Square, Chumpelik, & Adams, 1985). This program uses touch pressure, kinesthetic, and **proprioceptive** cues to facilitate speech production (Duffy, 1995). This approach trains finger placements on the client's face and neck to prompt the place of articulation and manner of production (features) for the articulatory target. The finger placements also provide information about the degree of jaw movement needed and the appropriate duration of the syllable or segment. The prompts may be used initially in isolation to facilitate the production of individual sounds. However, they may eventually be chained to facilitate articulatory movements between sounds to create words. Duffy (1995) indicates that this program is probably most appropriate with chronic, severe clients with apraxia of speech whose spontaneous verbal output is very limited and for whom other approaches have failed.

Other specific techniques that can be used in the treatment of apraxia of speech include progressive assimilation, phonetic placement, melodic intonation therapy (MIT), gestural reorganization, and contrastive stress drills.

Progressive Assimilation

The clinician attempts to reestablish production of the target sounds from sounds that are not affected or from other nonspeech gestures. This method is similar to the **successive approximation** or **shaping method** described in the Basic Unit of Chapter 6. For example, the client may be asked to lightly bite his lower lip with his upper teeth and then exhale, which may yield /f/. The client may be asked to tightly pucker his lips and then say /ə/ to derive the production of /u/. The voiceless palatal /ʃ/ may be shaped from /s/ as the client is asked to protrude his or her lips while making /s/. This method is appropriate for patients with severe apraxia of speech, since they often must relearn to produce single sounds and syllables (Rosenbek, 1985).

Phonetic Placement

The use of phonetic placement techniques was also discussed in the Basic Unit of Chapter 6. These techniques have been used extensively with children and adults with functional articulation disorders. Phonetic placement includes giving the client detailed descriptions of the position of the articulators during the production of specific sounds and using diagrams and pictures to supplement the clinician's verbal descriptions. If necessary, the clinician physically manipulates the client's articulators to evoke appropriate placement for the production of the sound. The clinician can also provide tactile feedback through the use of a tongue blade and cotton swab sticks. Phonetic placement cues are often needed with severe clients who may have difficulty producing sounds at the isolation or syllable level.

Melodic Intonation Therapy

Melodic intonation therapy (MIT) is a formal treatment program originally developed for the treatment of adults with severe nonfluent aphasia (Albert, Sparks, & Helm, 1973; Helm-Estabrooks, Nicholas, & Morgan, 1989). The use of this approach eventually made its way to the treatment of clients with apraxia of speech. The heart of the program is the use of musical intonation, continuous voicing, and rhythmic tapping to teach or reestablish verbal expression. This program is systematic, and it is hierarchically organized, progressing from simpler to more complex tasks.

Duffy (1995) indicates that adequate candidates for this approach are clients with good verbal comprehension, preserved self-criticism, a paucity of spontaneous verbal output, and nonfluent speech characteristics. He further states that this approach may be most appropriate for clients who fail to respond to more traditional programs such as the eight-step continuum.

Hegde (1996b) summarizes the general procedures and hierarchical organization of MIT as follows (pp. 19–20):

General Procedures

• High-probability words, phrases, and sentences are selected for training.

• Pictures or other environmental cues are used to evoke each target utterance.

• Each word, phrase, or sentence is intoned slowly and with constant voicing.

• Normal speech pitch and stress variations are maintained.

• The client's left hand is tapped once for each intoned syllable.

• A signal is provided by the clinician's left hand prompting the client when to listen and when to intone.

• Treatment is moved to the preceding step when the client fails a step.

Level 1

• *Humming:* The clinician shows a picture, hums the target item, and taps the corresponding number of syllables on the client's left hand. *No response is required from the client.*

• *Unison singing:* The client is instructed to intone in unison with the clinician, while the clinician taps the client's left hand.

• *Unison with fading:* The client is instructed to intone in unison with the clinician while the clinician taps the client's left hand. The clinician fades the model halfway through the phrase.

• *Immediate repetition:* The clinician instructs the client to listen while he or she intones the phrase and taps the corresponding number of syllables on the client's hand. The clinician then asks the client to imitate the target production.

• *Response to a probe question:* Following a correct immediate imitation, the clinician intones a probe question (e.g., "What did you say?").

Level 2

• *Introduction of item:* The clinician intones the target phrase twice and taps the corresponding number of syllables on the client's hand. *No response is required from the client.*

• *Unison with fading:* In unison with the clinician, the client intones the utterance, while the clinician taps the corresponding number of syllables on the client's hand. The clinician fades halfway through the phrase.

• *Delayed repetition:* The clinician intones and taps and, after 6 seconds of delay, lets the client tap with assistance. The clinician then asks the client to intone without assistance.

• *Response to a probe question:* Six seconds after the client's response, the clinician intones the probe question but does not tap the client's hand. The client is then instructed to intone the phrase.

Level 3

• *Delayed repetition:* The clinician taps the client's hand and intones the target phrase. Six seconds later, the client is asked to intone the phrase. The clinician provides tapping assistance.

• *Introducing* sprechgesang *(speech song):* The clinician presents the target phrase twice slowly, without singing, but with exaggerated rhythm and stress. No tapping is provided, and *no response is required from the client.*

• *Delayed spoken repetition:* The clinician presents the phrase with normal prosody, without hand tapping. After 6 seconds, the client is asked to imitate the target production with normal prosody.

• *Response to a probe question:* The clinician asks a probe question with normal prosody. After a 6-second delay, the client is asked to respond to the probe question with normal prosody.

Gestural Reorganization

Gestural reorganization refers to a treatment approach that uses hand gestures to facilitate correct verbal productions in clients (Wertz, LaPointe, & Rosenbek, 1991). Like MIT, this treatment approach has been used in clients with aphasia in addition to clients with AOS. This approach has been used in two ways: (1) to provide clients who have severe apraxia of speech with an alternative mode of communication, and (2) to facilitate or reestablish speech production. Manual language systems such as American Indian sign language (Amerind) and American Sign Language (ASL) have been used successfully in gestural reorganization programs. These manual systems are usually modified in some way for simplification. Rosenbek (1985) considers Amerind, ASL, and other systematic manual systems as *symbolic gestures* as opposed to *timing gestures* (e.g., hand tapping, finger tapping, or other repetitive gestures). We will further address timing gestures in the treatment of AOS.

When using symbolic gestures, the clinician pairs target utterances with gestures that may help facilitate their production. The clinician begins by selecting the words, phrases, or sentences for training and then selects gestures that mean the same thing as those target expressions. The symbolic gestures for those words or phrases can be selected from already established manual systems such as Amerind and ASL, or the clinician can invent gestures that are appropriate for the expressions. The clinician then devotes the time needed to explain the meaning of the gestures and the premise of the treatment approach to the client.

The next step is to establish the use of the gestures by the client. The client can be asked to match the clinician's gestures while modeling the target hand shape or movement. The clinician can also use pictures to evoke the use of a particular gesture. Shaping procedures and manual guidance are used as necessary. Once the client can shape the hand gesture to match the clinician's gesture or the picture stimulus, treatment progresses to facilitating the spontaneous use of the target gestures. The use of the trained gestures can serve as a functional and alternative mode of communication for clients who are essentially mute or have very limited verbal productions.

After the gestures have been well established, the clinician pairs them with target verbal expressions. Therapy generally progresses from the simultaneous production of the gesture and the target utterance to the separate use of each. This often requires the intensive training of several small steps. Eventually, the gestures can be faded if appropriate, while the verbal expressions continue to be practiced and reinforced.

Timing gestures have also been used in the treatment of apraxia of speech. Rosenbek (1985) describes these as "simple repetitive gestures, such as hand tapping, that can be made to accompany appropriate speech units" (p. 294). Tapping of the client's hand by the clinician was previously described as an essential component of melodic intonation therapy. Clients can also be trained to self-prompt by using their own timing gestures to facilitate speech production. These can be used with patients at all severity levels. Some patients discover such timing gestures on their own (Rosenbek, 1985).

The establishment of timing gestures should begin with frequently used and simples gestures such as tapping with a finger, drumming with one or more fingers, simultaneous squeezing of the thumb and index finger, tapping with one foot, and tapping the side of one leg with one or more fingers. The rationale for the use of such prompts should be clearly explained to the client. As the client learns to perform such timing gestures in a predictable manner, they are paired with the production of target words, phrases, or sentences. Initially, the client uses the established gestures while producing the utterance in unison with the clinician. Once this is established, the clinician provides a model of the gesture and the target utterance and asks the client to imitate both. Phrases and sentences systematically become longer and more complex. The clinician fades his or her own tapping, and then fades the verbal model as therapy progresses to more spontaneous productions and conversational speech. The client's gestures may be faded if appropriate as he or she becomes verbally more proficient. Some clients may always require the use of such gestures as a self-prompting technique. A more subtle form of the gestures may need to be taught so that they are less obvious to the listener.

Contrastive Stress Drills

Contrastive stress drills are a treatment method that can be used to promote articulatory proficiency and natural prosody, particularly the stress and rhythm of spoken language, in clients with apraxia of speech. This method has also been used in the treatment of clients with dysarthria. In this approach, different phrases and sentences are used to train stress placement on different words. In articulation training, the clinician constructs phrases and sentences with a single target sound in them (e.g., "My name is Bob" for /b/; "Terry is her name" for /t/). The clinician then asks a series of questions structured so that the client responds with the target phrase while placing extra stress on the target word or sound (e.g., the clinician asks, "Is her name Mary?" and the client responds, "No, her name is *Terry*."). The client is likely to stress the target word and thus improve the articulatory proficiency of the target sound. The client is reinforced for the precision of the target sound. A similar procedure is used to teach appropriate stress and rhythm in words. The process may progress as follows:

- The clinician creates a series of phrases and sentences (e.g., "Terry likes steak.").

- The clinician then asks a question that will force stress to fall on different words in the target phrases or sentences (e.g., "Does Mary like steak?" may evoke "No, *Terry* likes steak"; "Does Terry like pork chops?" may evoke "No, Terry likes *steak*.").

- The clinician reinforces the use of appropriate stress on varying words.

Because a discussion of all of the possible treatment approaches for AOS is beyond the scope of this chapter, the reader is referred to Duffy (1995), Wertz, LaPointe, and Rosenbek (1991), and Rosenbek (1985) for more detailed information.

Developmental Apraxia of Speech

Developmental apraxia of speech is a childhood disorder that shares features with apraxia of speech in adults. The neuropathology for developmental apraxia of speech has not been documented, thus creating some controversy about the legitimacy of the disorder. Many clinicians reserve the label of developmental apraxia of speech for children with severe articulation disorders that display many characteristics typically associated with apraxia of speech in adults. Developmental apraxia of speech (DAS) is primarily a sensorimotor disorder affecting the articulatory and prosodic parameters of speech production. The child with DAS exhibits particular difficulty with programming the sequences of movement involved in the production of words and sentences.

Haynes (1985) indicates that "information regarding specific therapeutic techniques for the person with developmental apraxia of speech can be gleaned not only from direct references to the disorder itself, but also from a study of literature on acquired apraxia of speech as well as many of the general principles included in articulation therapy" (p. 262). Thus, some of the treatment approaches discussed under acquired apraxia of speech can be modified to meet the needs of children with developmental apraxia of speech.

In general, the treatment for DAS, as for its adult counterpart, tends to follow a sequential organization, progressing from simple to complex speech tasks. The vowels and consonants targeted for remediation should be clearly outlined. Also, the clinician should determine the linguistic level that is the most appropriate starting point for therapy. For some children it may be the syllable level, while other kids may be ready to start at the word or sentence level.

Velleman and Strand (1994, p. 131) emphasize that treatment at the isolation level does not correspond to the nature of the disorder and does not address the underlying motor programming problem. They further offer the following basic principles of a speech production treatment program for children with developmental apraxia of speech:

1. The primary focus of treatment should be the control and organization of syllable structures within a variety of linguistic contexts.

2. Treatment should facilitate correct production of varying syllable shapes and the organization of such shapes into longer and more complex phonotactic patterns (combinations of syllables).

3. A sound-by-sound approach emphasizing phoneme production in isolation before progressing to words and phrases *does not* address the hierarchical dynamic movement problems associated with developmental apraxia of speech.

4. Treatment should not focus on auditory discrimination training since that does not address the production problem.

5. Treatment should be structured so that frequent short breaks are offered. System fatigue may be prevented in this manner since that is typically a problem in developmental apraxia of speech.

6. Treatment sessions should be divided into short parts:

   (a) imitation of body and/or oral motor sequences (assuming those are a problem);

   (b) syllable sequence drill activities (e.g., [gʌdʌbʌ] or *go to bed;* [bʌdʌgʌ] or *buttercup*);

   (c) meaningful single-word activities including a core group of words that will help increase the client's speech intelligibility;

   (d) short-sentence activities starting with a key carrier phrase and changing one word (e.g., "I like the . . ." or "I see the . . ."); the complexity and length are gradually increased.

Hegde (1996b) and Haynes (1985) indicate that extensive speech drills may be used in which the sequencing of movements involved in speech production is emphasized. As with apraxia of speech in adults, the clinician can use auditory, visual, and tactile cues to facilitate correct production of the target sounds, words, or phrases. Children with DAS often benefit from a multimodality approach, especially when new sounds are introduced. Some children with DAS have been found to benefit from touch cues for the production of specific sounds since they provide both visual and tactile information. For example, the clinician places her finger on the client's lips while modeling the target production of /b/. The tactile cues are given simultaneously with auditory and visual cues initially and gradually faded. The reader is referred to Bashir, Grahamjones, and Bostwick (1984) for a detailed description of this approach. In our discussion of apraxia of speech in adults, we described the use of the PROMPT approach (Chumpelik, 1984), a tactile, kinesthetic, and visual cueing system originally developed for the treatment of developmental apraxia of speech.

Velleman and Strand (1994) also suggest the use of "key word pictures" in a flip book accompanied by the target syllable productions for children who have difficulty producing nonsense syllables. For example, the clinician may place a picture of a sheep paired with the syllable [ba] and the picture of a ghost paired with the syllable [bu]) in the child's flip book to facilitate production of these syllables. At the short-sentence level, the clinician can use "predictable books" or books that repeat routinized verbal patterns (Velleman & Strand, 1994). Haynes (1985) stresses the importance of a *core vocabulary* or *keyword vocabulary,* which has proved beneficial for clients with severe developmental apraxia of speech. This may facilitate an increase in intelligible verbal communications. Like Velleman and Strand, Haynes suggests the use of *carrier phrases* such as "I want a . . ." or "I see . . ." to extend the client's sequencing efforts. According to Haynes, these may provide the client with a basis for the production of many appropriate utterances that can be incorporated into functional and meaningful sentences.

Speech rate reduction is often helpful for children with DAS during connected speech productions. Often reducing the rate of speech provides the client with the time needed to appropriately sequence the movements necessary for words and sentences. Haynes (1985) also recommends the use of rhythm, intonation, and stress paired with a motor movement such as foot tapping to facilitate improved speech productions. These approaches were previously addressed in the treatment of apraxia of speech in adults. Furthermore, training self-monitoring skills in the child is extremely important for the use of verbal productions in extraclinical settings and their maintenance over time.

With children who have severe developmental apraxia of speech, nonverbal communication systems may be used to facilitate functional communication. The child may be taught sign language or an augmentative communication system. The success of nonverbal communication systems is highly dependent on the child's intellectual abilities and receptive language skills. See Velleman and Strand (1994) and Hall et al. (1993) for a detailed presentation on the characteristics, assessment, and treatment of developmental apraxia of speech.

Dysarthria

Dysarthria is a group of motor speech disorders resulting from neurological damage that can affect all speech parameters: articulation, resonance, phonation, respiration, and prosody. At least seven types of dysarthrias have been identified: flaccid dysarthria, spastic dysarthria, hypokinetic dysarthria, hyperkinetic dysarthria, ataxic dysarthria, unilateral upper motor neuron dysarthria, and mixed dysarthria. The etiology of the neurological damage leading to each type of dysarthria is varied including stroke, progressive neurological disorders, metabolic disorders, and inherited disorders. We discussed several of these in the Advanced Unit of Chapter 6.

Unlike apraxia of speech, medical interventions along with behavioral therapy are available to clients with dysarthria. Many are appropriate only for specific dysarthrias. For example, **laryngoplasty** can be done in patients with vocal fold paralysis. Laryngoplasty refers to a surgical procedure in which the paralyzed vocal fold is displaced medially with the help of implant materials. This helps promote better approximation of the vocal folds during phonation, which helps improve vocal quality. This surgical procedure is reversible; the implant materials may be removed if necessary. Duffy (1995) indicates that laryngoplasty in people with unilateral vocal fold paralysis may result in improved pitch, loudness, and intonation; however, breathiness, harshness, and vocal fatigue may persist (p. 392). Other surgical techniques that can help patients with vocal fold paralysis are *teflon or collagen injection* and *recurrent laryngeal nerve resection*. *Botulinum toxin (Botox) injection* has been successfully used with patients with **spasmodic dysphonia** (see Duffy, 1995, pp. 392–393 for details on various surgical procedures for improved phonation). Pharyngeal flap surgery, described under the section on cleft palate, can help decrease hypernasality in some dysarthric speakers. Also, prescription of specific medications has proven helpful in patients with movement disorders such as Parkinson's disease and Huntington's chorea. Such medications may also help the patient's concomitant speech problems. Furthermore, prosthetic devices such as a **palatal lift** have been used with some dysarthric speakers. A palatal lift prothesis has a palatal portion that attaches to the teeth and a lift portion that extends posteriorly to lift the soft palate. This device can help patients with velopharyngeal insufficiency achieve adequate velopharyngeal closure for improved resonance. This device can help decrease hypernasality in some clients.

Because medical intervention does not meet the needs of all dysarthric speakers or all the needs of an individual speaker, behavioral intervention plays a key role in improving the client's speech production. The primary goal of behavioral management is increased efficiency, effectiveness, and naturalness of communication (Duffy, 1995). In our discussion of apraxia of speech we addressed Duffy's distinction between communication-oriented tasks and speaker-oriented tasks. Communication-oriented tasks are as important in intervention with dysarthric clients as in intervention with those who have apraxia of speech. The clinician often counsels the client and significant others about the goals of therapy, their own role and involvement in the therapy process, and the likely outcome of treatment. The client and significant others can be trained to use the following techniques during communicative interactions:

• The client should inform the listener at the outset of an interaction how to effectively communicate with him or her (e.g., by demonstrating use of a **communication board**). In essence, the client is trained to take active responsibility for successful communications.

• The client should set the context and topic of conversation before beginning interactions with the listener. Knowing the topic of conversation often aids the listener to predict or guess what the client might say.

• The client should modify the content and length of utterances. Decreasing the length of utterances helps the listener keep pace with the client. If the client talks too rapidly, speech intelligibility may be significantly compromised.

• Significant others should modify the physical environment. There should always be adequate lighting so that the listener receives nonverbal information from the client (e.g., facial expressions, visible movement of some sounds, and so forth). Also, excessive ambient noise should be reduced.

• The client and significant others should maintain eye contact during communication interactions, establish effective communication strategies, and agree on the methods of feedback that will be provided in varied settings. For example, the client and his or her spouse may agree that while at home verbal cues to slow down may be used, but in other social settings a tap on the shoulder may be provided.

Speaker-oriented tasks can be used in the treatment of all speech parameters: respiration, phonation, resonance, articulation, and prosody. We will concentrate our discussion on the tasks that can be used to improve the client's articulation skills. As with apraxia of speech, treatment activities are highly structured and repetitive; speech drills for continued practice play an important role in the treatment of dysarthric speakers. Proper head, trunk, and body positioning are crucial for articulation training. It is difficult to address improved articulatory proficiency if the client is slumped forward in his wheelchair, for example.

As with other speech disorders, the clinician determines the error patterns in a particular client. The behavioral methods discussed in the Basic Unit of Chapter 6 can be used to treat the articulation difficulties in dysarthric speakers. The client is provided instructions and demonstrations to facilitate appropriate placement of the articulators. Phonetic placement and shaping procedures are used as needed. The clinician models the target productions, and the client is expected to imitate them. The following strategies can be used to evoke improved articulation of sounds in words and sentences:

• The client is trained to use a reduced rate of speech to improve speech intelligibility (this may be accomplished through finger tapping, use of a **pacing board,** metronome, or **delayed auditory feedback** device). A reduced rate of speech may allow time for full range of movement, increased coordination, and improved linguistic phrasing (Duffy, 1995).

• The client is trained to exaggerate or overarticulate the production of consonants, particularly in the medial and final positions. This helps improve the precision of their production.

• The client is trained to use an increased open-mouth posture to promote better oral projection of sounds.

The client is given immediate feedback about his or her production of the target sounds, words, or phrases. Tasks are arranged in a hierarchy from simpler to more complex. **Contrastive stress drills,** as discussed under apraxia of speech, can be used to improve articulatory precision and prosody in dysarthric speakers.

Some clients may need to be trained to use compensatory articulatory movements. For example, the tongue blade may be used instead of the tongue tip when the tongue is markedly weak. Also, linguadental contact for nasals may be used when the lips are too weak to achieve adequate seal. Some clinicians also teach strengthening, relaxation, and stretching exercises prior to or in conjunction with articulation treatment. However, their effectiveness has been questioned (Duffy, 1995). The reader is referred to Duffy (1995), Dworkin (1991), Rosenbek and LaPointe (1985), and Yorkston, Beukelman, and Bell (1988) for further information on the medical and behavioral management of patients with dysarthria.

Cerebral Palsy

Cerebral palsy is a congenital disorder resulting from brain damage before birth, during birth, or after birth. Thus, it is generally considered a childhood neurological disorder. Cerebral palsy has been classified into several types (e.g., athetoid, spastic, ataxic, mixed) according to the physical manifestations of the disorder. Children with cerebral palsy may have accompanying speech disorders, which can affect all parameters of speech production including articulation.

The treatment of children with cerebral palsy is multidisciplinary because of the varied physical, communicative, emotional, intellectual, and social problems that may accompany the disorder. Speech–language pathologists are generally members of a team that typically includes a nurse, doctor, physical therapist, occupational therapist, audiologist, social worker, and psychologist. The speech–language pathologist should always work closely with the team of specialists involved in the child's medical or rehabilitative care. Clinicians should also work closely with the child's parents and thoroughly explain their role in the treatment process.

Therapy for children with cerebral palsy usually begins in infancy. At that point, the speech–language pathologist's role is primarily to facilitate adequate prespeech motor movements and adequate motor functioning for swallowing and feeding. Air et al. (1989) indicate that in working with infants with cerebral palsy, clinicians have three priorities: (1) parent education, (2) communication and language stimulation, and (3) facilitation of prespeech skills.

Assuming that the child with cerebral palsy obtains sufficient sensorimotor functions to support verbal communication, the clinician may or may not need to treat the client's articulation skills. Some children acquire fairly normal articulation, while others require special intervention. In the treatment of articulation disorders in children with cerebral palsy, the clinician often follows the procedures used with functional articulation disorders. The child's skills are thoroughly assessed, and the clinician identifies any sound errors or error patterns. Clinicians may also need to assess the use of any compensatory articulatory postures by the child or the presence of abnormal reflexes (e.g., tongue thrust). Furthermore, the presence of a concomitant neuromotor programming disorder such as apraxia of speech should be investigated.

Air et al. (1989) indicate that the goals of articulation therapy are to increase the speed, range, and accuracy of the child's lingual, labial, and mandibular movements. Articulation training should always be provided with consideration of respiration, phonation, and resonation issues. Those parameters need to be sufficiently stabilized so that they support articulation development and articulation training. Articulation therapy may be divided into three processes: (1) the ability to move the articulators in isolation from other body parts — *differentiation;* (2) the ability to make specific movements — *praxis;* and (3) the ability to speed up those movements — *diadochokinesis* (Mysak, 1980).

Once the clinician has established independent movement of the articulators (without accompanying body movements), the training of specific movements needed for speech can be initiated. The bilabial, linguavelar, linguapalatal, linguaalveolar, and linguadental articulatory contacts required for the production of various speech sounds become the direct treatment targets. Auditory, tactile, and visual cues will probably be needed to facilitate those movements initially. Other phonetic placement cues, shaping procedures, physical manipulation of the articulators, and modeling should be used as much as needed. These will be gradually faded.

Increasing the speed of the child's articulatory movements once they have been established becomes the next goal of therapy. Air et al. (1989) indicate that this can be done by serial production of voiced and voiceless and nasal and nonnasal sounds. The clinician selects syllable combinations that contain sounds that the child can produce (e.g., /nɑ/, /dɑ/, /kɑ/, and /gɑ/). The client then practices repetitive productions of the chosen syllables in two-, three-, and four-syllable sets to increase the speed of the articulatory movements (e.g., /nɑ-tɑ/, /nɑ-dɑ/, /nɑ-nɑ/, /nɑ-kɑ/, and /nɑ-gɑ/). This is done in succession from two-syllable sets to three-syllable sets to four-syllable sets. Eventually, two-word combinations can be introduced.

If the assessment reveals specific errors (i.e., substitutions, omissions, distortions) or error patterns (i.e., phonological processes), the clinician can incorporate the use of the basic principles discussed in the Basic Unit of this chapter to address the articulation treatment needs of children with cerebral palsy.

In some children, speech does not become a functional mode of communication. Speech may be so severely impaired that the child's intelligibility is significantly compromised. For those children alternative or augmentative modes of communication (AAC) are most appropriate to facilitate functional communication. Examples of AAC systems include gestural communication, simple communication boards containing words and pictures, and sophisticated electronic or computer devices. (Discussion of the use and training of AAC systems in children with cerebral palsy is beyond the scope of this chapter.) Some children may need language therapy in addition to articulation treatment (see Long, 1994).

Cleft Palate

Because cleft lip and palate is a congenital disorder present at birth, special intervention in children with such structural anomalies can begin in infancy. As discussed in the Advanced Unit of Chapter 6, clefting results from the lack of fusion of the upper lip, the hard palate, the soft palate, and/or the uvula early in the embryonic stage of human development. An opening in the palatal regions connects the nasal and oral cavities, which can have a significant effect on speech production.

In the United States, surgical management of cleft lip and palate is common practice and begins early in infancy. Unfortunately, this is not the case in third world countries, where people do not always have access to adequate medical care. Medical specialists use varied surgical methods to fuse cleft lip and palate in infants. The technical aspects of such surgeries are beyond the scope of this chapter. Cleft lip is repaired at about 3 months of age. It is desirable that the infant be at least 10 weeks old and weigh 10 pounds prior to the initial surgery (Golding-Kushner, 1997). Cosmetic revisions of the nose and lip are done at later ages. Surgical repair of the palate is typically done between 12 and 18 months of age. The primary reason for repair of cleft palate is to separate the oral from the nasal cavity, which has a significant positive effect on speech production and eating. Surgical repair of cleft palate when the child is between 12 and 18 months of age results in better speech and language development and less maladaptive behaviors (e.g., compensatory articulation errors). Golding-Kushner (1997) indicates that if surgery is delayed until after 2 years of age, children are at higher risk for severe maladaptive compensatory articulation disorders that can be difficult to treat (p. 211).

In approximately 16–20% of cases, hypernasality due to **velopharyngeal insufficiency** occurs even after surgical closure of the cleft palate (Golding-Kushner, 1997). In those cases, further surgical intervention may be required in the form of **pharyngeal flap surgery.** This is a secondary surgical procedure in which a muscular flap is cut from the posterior pharyngeal wall, raised, and attached to the velum. The flap is open on either side to allow for nasal breathing, nasal drainage, and production of nasal speech sounds. A pharyngeal flap helps close the velopharyngeal port during the production of nonnasal consonants and thus reduces hypernasality. Construction of a flap that is unnecessarily too wide must be avoided since that increases the risk of airway obstruction, snoring, and hyponasality.

The child with cleft lip and palate often requires several other surgical or medical interventions. Repair of a **fistula,** which is an opening that remains or appears after surgery, may be needed. An unrepaired fistula may have negative effects on both speech production and eating, depending on its size and location along the palate. The child may also need consistent dental care to promote an adequate oral hygiene program that will help prevent the premature loss of teeth. Also, because orthodontic problems are common in children with cleft lip and palate, orthodontic care may be crucial. Orthodontic problems include malocclusion, crossbite, rotated or jumbled teeth, and extra teeth. These may or may not affect articulation, depending on the severity and level of orthodontic care. A prosthodontist, dentist, or orthodontist with a specialty in the construction of artificial teeth and prosthetic oral devices may also be involved in the client's care. Some children may need the construction of artificial teeth if their permanent teeth are missing or require other devices such as a **speech bulb.** This device is designed to eliminate hypernasality in children with velopharyngeal insufficiency. A speech bulb contains a palatal retainer and pharyngeal extension that terminates in a bulb usually made of acrylic. The speech bulb serves the same purpose as the pharyngeal flap, in that it helps with velopharyngeal closure by reducing the amount of space in the pharyngeal area. For more detailed information on the medical treatment of children with cleft palate, see Golding-Kushner (1997) and McWilliams, Morris, and Shelton (1990).

Speech–language pathologists who work in children's hospitals are often involved in the treatment of children with cleft lip and palate in the neonatal intensive care unit or critical care unit if the child requires further hospitalization after birth. Therapy at that point focuses primarily on parent education, counseling, and feeding issues. The SLP consults and collaborates with other specialists (e.g., nurses, occupational therapists, audiologists, and doctors).

Many children's hospitals also have craniofacial clinics in which a team of specialists assesses the child's needs after being released for home. The child is followed up every 6 to 12 months in the early years to ensure that his or her surgical, dental, cosmetic, communication, and educational needs are adequately addressed. The frequency with which the child is assessed diminishes as he or she grows older. The speech–language pathologist is an integral member of the craniofacial team.

Although surgical repair of cleft lip and palate is now done at a very early age in this country, that does not guarantee that normal articulation and speech production will develop in a particular child. Therefore, any child with cleft lip and palate is considered to be at high risk for speech and language disorders. If problems with phonation, articulation, and respiration occur despite all preventative efforts, the clinician may need to provide direct intervention.

In the treatment of articulation or phonological disorders in children with cleft lip and/or palate, the clinician can use the general principles for the treatment of functional articulation and phonological disorders. After the assessment, the clinician identifies the specific sound errors or error patterns and decides on the most relevant treatment target for a particular client. The general behavioral treatment principles discussed in the Basic Unit of this chapter can be successfully used to meet the articulation needs of children with cleft palate speech. The clinician should consider the following suggestions, which may be unique to children with repaired clefts (adapted from Hegde, 1996b, pp. 75–76):

• The clinician should educate the parents about the speech mechanism and the possible reason for persisting articulation errors despite surgical repair of the cleft.

• The clinician should teach more visible sounds before less visible sounds except for the linguadentals.

• The clinician should teach stops and fricatives before other classes of sounds since those are most often affected in children with repaired clefts.

• The clinician should avoid or postpone training on /k/ and /g/ if the child's velopharyngeal functioning is inadequate.

• The clinician should teach fricatives, affricates, or both if they are stimulable or after stops are mastered.

• The clinician should teach linguapalatal sounds, lingua-alveolars, and linguadentals, in that order.

• The clinician should structure therapy so that it progresses from syllables to words, phrases, and sentences.

• The clinician should use visual, auditory, and tactile cues as needed. Phonetic placement, successive approximation, and modeling should be used frequently at first and gradually faded.

• The clinician should teach the client to direct the breath stream orally. Visual and tactile feedback can be provided to increase the client's success. The client can be instructed to feel the flow of air on the back of his hand or to see it when a tissue is placed in front of his or her mouth.

• The clinician should teach the child to articulate with less effort and facial grimacing.

• The clinician should train compensatory articulatory productions if structural distortions are present that prevent normal articulation (e.g., a stiff and short upper lip may affect an adequate seal for bilabials; the client may be taught to make an upper teeth–lower lip contact instead).

If the child exhibits resonance problems in addition to articulatory difficulties, that speech parameter may also have to be treated directly. The clinician should not address resonance problems through behavioral interventions if they are a result of **velopharyngeal incompetence** (structural or physiological inability to achieve velopharyngeal closure). If the child does not have the ability to achieve velopharyngeal closure, the clinician's efforts to decrease hypernasality will be unsuccessful. In such cases, the child may need medical intervention through a pharyngeal flap procedure or prosthetic device (e.g., a speech bulb) before speech therapy can be initiated. Air et al. (1989) indicate that a trial period of behavioral speech therapy may be provided in cases where specialists are uncertain whether the child can achieve velopharyngeal closure. A trial period of 3 months is often sufficient to determine whether the resonance issues will need further medical intervention.

Assuming that the child can achieve velopharyngeal closure, speech therapy has a key role in reducing the child's hypernasality. The clinician can start by strengthening the speech articulators through direct methods such as articulation therapy or semidirect methods such as blowing and sucking exercises. In the initial stages of treatment, discrimination training may be warranted in some clients who have a difficult time distinguishing oral and nasal resonance. Oral resonance may be achieved by occluding the client's nares while he or she makes the target production (i.e., an oral sound or a word with only oral sounds). Initially, the nares may need to be occluded during the entire production. As therapy progresses, the clinician may need to occlude the client's nares only as he or she begins the production and then suddenly release as the client is instructed to continue the production. Eventually, the clinician may need only to lightly touch the client's nares to prompt adequate oral resonance. Enhanced loudness or sudden bursts of loudness may also facilitate improved oral resonance since more articulatory effort is needed as the intensity of speech increases. Increased mouth opening may also promote improved oral resonance.

Because there is a high incidence of vocal nodules in children with cleft palate, often due to compensatory efforts or vocal hyperfunction, the clinician may need to address problems of phonation in addition to articulation and resonance. The clinician should clearly identify abusive vocal behaviors (e.g., yelling, screaming, throat clearing, and coughing) and provide systematic voice therapy. Because of our emphasis on articulation disorders, the treatment of abusive vocal behaviors is beyond the scope of this chapter. The reader may consult Boone and McFarlane (1988), McWilliams, Morris, and Shelton (1990), and Wilson (1972) for more information.

Hearing Impairment

Hearing impairment refers to a reduced hearing acuity in children and adults. The degree of loss can range from mild to profound. The terms *hard of hearing* and *deaf* are often differentiated. Deaf individuals have a profound hearing loss of at least 90 dB HL. The degree of loss in hard of hearing individuals can range from mild to severe (but the loss is less than 90 dB HL). People who are hard of hearing typically have some residual hearing that can be maximized through amplification devices such as a hearing aid. The articulatory proficiency of people with decreased hearing acuity often varies according to the degree of loss.

The treatment of deaf and hard of hearing individuals is multifaceted. Articulation difficulties are often only one of the problems associated with hearing loss and deafness. Language disorders, learning disabilities, and reading difficulties may also accompany a hearing loss. Treatment is provided by a team of specialists or professionals, including medical specialists, nurses, audiologists, regular education teachers, special education teachers, interpreters, and vocational counselors. The speech–language pathologist is only one member of the treatment team and must be willing and ready to consult and collaborate with other specialists. Audiologists can provide invaluable information about the type and extent of the hearing loss and the amount of residual hearing. It is the audiologist who fits the client with a hearing aid or other amplification device. However, all specialists involved in the client's care must be familiar with the intricacies of the amplification device (e.g., how it is turned on and off, how the battery is replaced, how to turn the volume up and down).

Although various aspects of communication can be affected in deaf and hard of hearing individuals, because of the nature of this text, we will concentrate on the treatment of articulation skills. Speech therapy should be started as early as possible. The younger the child, the better the prognosis for improved articulation skills and natural-sounding speech. The child's family should be involved in treatment from the very beginning to facilitate the use of trained behaviors in the home environment. The family can be specifically trained to conduct therapy sessions at home that parallel the clinician's treatment targets, objectives, and activities.

The use of visual, tactile, and kinesthetic cues is especially important in teaching speech sound production in hard of hearing and deaf individuals. Some clinicians familiar with the program use the Ling system for speech training (Ling, 1976). In this program, sounds are taught through audition first, with the addition of visual and tactile cues as necessary. The clinician may also include speech perception or auditory training activities to supplement articulation and phonological training if the client has some residual hearing or functional audition. This may help clarify "auditory confusions" or contrasts between sounds and words (Paterson, 1994).

The general principles and procedures described in the Basic Unit of Chapter 7 are certainly appropriate to meet the articulation and phonological needs of deaf and hard of hearing clients. However, the clinician may need to more heavily rely on visual, tactile, and kinesthetic cues to facilitate correct production of sounds in isolation, syllables, and words. The clinician should pay special attention to stops, fricatives, and affricates since these are especially difficult for children with hearing loss. Also, voiced-voiceless sound distinctions may need to be directly trained. Paterson (1994) offers a specific treatment for voiceless fricatives that underscores the need for a multimodality treatment approach (e.g., including audition, vision, touch, and orosensory modalities). Treatment of fricatives progresses from simple to complex tasks. The client's productions are gradually shaped to match or approximate the target fricatives (see Paterson, 1994, pp. 216–221) for the details of this approach.

The clinician should be systematic in the use of antecedent stimuli, the selection of target responses, and the provision of feedback. The effectiveness of articulation treatment with deaf and hard of hearing children should be constantly reevaluated to ensure that speech is an appropriate and realistic communication choice.

Summary of the Advanced Unit

• Treatment for apraxia of speech (AOS) is primarily behavioral. It is hierarchical, systematic, and repetitive. Speech drills are often used. Specific treatment approaches include an **eight-step continuum, PROMPT, progressive assimilation, phonetic placement, melodic intonation therapy (MIT), gestural reorganization,** and **contrastive stress drills.**

• Treatment for developmental apraxia of speech (DAS) is also systematic and hierarchical, moving from simple to complex tasks. Tactile, kinesthetic, and visual cueing systems such as **Touch Cue** and **PROMPT** methods have also been used with DAS.

• Although the treatment of AOS is primarily behavioral, the treatment of dysarthria can include medical, prosthetic, and behavioral interventions. Behavioral treatment can include **communication-oriented** and **speaker-oriented tasks.** Treatment of dysarthria is systematic and repetitive.

• **Cerebral palsy,** a congenital neurological disorder, is often classified into various types according to the physical manifestations of the disorder. Treatment for clients with cerebral palsy typically begins in infancy. Therapy is multidisciplinary, and the speech–language pathologist is only one of several professionals involved in the client's care. Articulation therapy focuses on establishing accurate articulatory movements for speech and increasing the speech of such movements in gradually more complex syllable units. **Augmentative or alternative modes of communication** (AAC) are appropriate for children with cerebral palsy who do not acquire functional speech.

• Children with **cleft lip and palate** require surgical medical intervention for the fusing of clefts. Primary surgeries of the palate are done quite early, between 12 and 18 months of age. Secondary surgical intervention may be needed in some patients for improved **velopharyngeal competence,** closure of **fistulas,** or cosmetic purposes. Traditional methods for articulation therapy can be successfully used to meet the articulation or phonological problems of children with cleft palate.

• **Hearing impairment** can range from mild to profound, which may yield varying communication disorders across children with hearing loss or deafness. The treatment of deaf and hard of hearing children is multidisciplinary. Traditional treatment approaches can be used successfully with hard of hearing children. The clinician may need to use visual, tactile, and kinesthetic cueing at a greater level in the articulation treatment of deaf and hard of hearing children.

Chapter 8

◆ ◆ ◆ ◆ ◆ ◆ ◆ ◆ ◆ ◆ ◆ ◆ ◆ ◆ ◆ ◆ ◆ ◆

Specific Treatment Programs and Approaches

Nothing is more useful to man than to speak correctly.
—PHAEDRUS, *FABLES*

In the Basic Unit of Chapter 7 we described the general sequence of treatment for articulation and phonological disorders. In the Advanced Unit of the same chapter we described some treatment techniques that can be used with specific disorders (e.g., dysarthria and apraxia of speech). In essence, the treatment sequence begins with the selection of goals and objectives that will help improve the client's communication skills. While the entire process typically necessitates several short-term objectives, the ultimate goal of treatment is the client's use and maintenance of the newly acquired skills in his or her linguistic community across varied situations, settings, and audiences.

The general treatment sequence described in the Basic Unit of Chapter 7 can be successfully used with varied populations and can easily be adapted to meet the needs of individual clients. It incorporates treatment principles that have been thoroughly investigated and repeatedly found to be efficacious. It is safe to say that the learning principles that are the heart of the general sequence we presented have made their way to almost every program that claims to "teach" any behavior, articulation and phonological skills included.

As in any profession that wishes to move forward, over the last few decades many researchers and clinicians in speech–language pathology have attempted to develop specific treatment programs or approaches to help meet the needs of children with articulation and phonological disorders. Some of the programs are based on years of empirical research, while others have evolved primarily from uncontrolled clinical data. Bankson and Bernthal (1998) have divided these treatment programs into two general categories: **motor-based** and **linguistic-based approaches.**

Motor-based approaches are those that primarily focus on teaching the motor behaviors associated with the production of a particular speech sound. These are often considered "traditional" approaches since they focus on the motor aspect of sound production, as did many of the pioneering articulation treatment programs.

In more recent years, several linguistic-based approaches have emerged. The underlying philosophy of these programs is that some children produce sound errors not because they are unable to articulate sounds but because they have not yet learned certain phonological rules of the adult system. In other words, the child's motor production of sounds is affected by the underlying phonological rules that he or she has not yet acquired. Logically then, treatment would focus on teaching the absent rules.

Although this dichotomy serves as a valid organization device, Bankson and Bernthal (1998) carefully emphasize that most treatment programs have both motor and linguistic elements. For example, Hodson and Paden's Cycles Approach, to be described later in this chapter, is generally perceived as a linguistic-based approach since its focus is to decrease or eliminate phonological processes that affect a child's intelligibility. However, when examined closely, it quickly becomes evident that this program has a strong motor component in the establishment of specific sound exemplars affected by the active phonological processes. Most programs that claim to improve a child's speech intelligibility through the reduction of active phonological processes make use of sound production training to some extent.

Many distinctive feature programs are also considered linguistic-based approaches since the goal of treatment is to establish linguistic sound and sound class contrasts by teaching distinctive features. As the **continuancy** feature is established, for example, a linguistic contrast is created in words like *shoe* and *two*. If the continuancy feature were lacking in a child's repertoire, sound substitutions such as [p/f] and [t/s] might occur. Therefore, the goal of therapy is to teach the continuancy feature and consequently decrease such phonological errors. However, to accomplish that the clinician must select and teach sound exemplars containing the feature. At this point this "linguistic-based" approach obviously incorporates a motor production element (this approach will also be addressed later in detail).

Although on the surface and by their titles most treatment programs sound unique, when carefully examined, many of them actually share several features. They all advocate the selection of particular target behaviors, make use of certain antecedent stimuli (e.g., pictures, objects, written words), expect a response from the client, and provide consequences according to the client's responses (e.g., verbal praise, tokens, playtime, verbal corrective feedback). Through an examination of the many programs, one of the major differences we have observed is that some provide the user with very specific details about the actual **treatment procedures,** while others are a bit more obscure. Another difference is the focus on particular target behaviors or the skill that should be taught. While some programs choose to teach one sound a time, others focus on establishing several sounds at the same time, and yet others focus on developing certain linguistic rules or contrasts. Such an emphasis has led to titles like Multiple-Phoneme Approach, Distinctive Feature Approach, and Minimal Pair Contrast Method.

In this chapter we will describe some of the most popular and well-known treatment approaches that have emerged throughout the years. We will not, however, embrace a motor-based versus linguistic-based dichotomy since in our opinion all of the programs under discussion have elements of both. Although such a division may be very important in the diagnostic process for descriptive purposes, we have a difficult time conceptualizing that any linguistic sound system rule identified in the assessment process could be taught without direct teaching of the sounds or sound classes affected by the rule. For example, it would be difficult to eliminate the phonological process of stopping without directly teaching some or all of the fricatives affected by that process. We believe that the most significant difference between such approaches lies not in *how* something is taught, but in *what* is taught and how the chosen target behaviors are grouped. Because of this, we will discuss the selected programs in the chronological order of their inception as much as possible.

Traditional Approach

The **traditional approach** to articulation therapy has gained its name primarily by the length of its existence. This is the best-known approach, and its foundation was laid early in the 1900s by several pioneers in the field of speech–language pathology (Scripture & Jackson, 1927; Stinchfield & Young, 1938; Van Riper, 1939).

Although many researchers and professionals helped guide the development of the traditional approach, Charles Van Riper is the person primarily credited for its existence. During the late 1930s, Van Riper consolidated the most current treatment techniques available at the time and developed a comprehensive and structured treatment approach. That approach was transferred to paper in 1939 in Van

Riper's classic text *Speech Correction: Principles and Methods.* Since 1939, Van Riper has revised his treatment approach to include new and updated information from various sources (i.e., Backus & Beasley, 1951; Gerber, 1973; McDonald, 1964; Milisen, 1954; Mysak, 1959; Winitz, 1969, 1975).

The hallmark of the traditional approach is its progression from sensory-perceptual training to maintenance of the newly acquired speech sound. It is composed of five major phases: (1) sensory-perceptual or ear training, (2) production training for sound establishment, (3) production training for sound stabilization, (4) transfer and carryover training, and (5) maintenance of the learned behaviors across time. Van Riper and Erickson (1996) depict this progression as a staircase, delineating precise steps the client must surmount on the way to correct sound production.

Although the word *traditional* may sometimes connote something old, outdated, and not very useful, that is not the case for the traditional approach to articulation therapy. Those of us who have been involved in the treatment of articulation disorders for some time will likely acknowledge that we often make use of many of the principles outlined by Charles Van Riper in 1939 in his text *Speech Correction.*

Some of those principles have continued to prove their efficacy. Although some aspects of the traditional approach are now controversial (e.g., sensory-perceptual training), several other aspects continue to provide many clinicians with adequate tools in the training of articulation skills. With that in mind, the following outlines the traditional approach, beginning with sensory-perceptual training and progressing to the ultimate goal of maintenance of the target sound (see Secord, 1989, for an excellent overview of this approach).

Sensory-Perceptual Training (Ear Training)

Sensory-perceptual training is the first goal of therapy. At this stage a standard for the target sound is identified and defined. The client is not involved in production of the target sound; rather, the emphasis of training is on the development of an auditory standard from which the client can make comparisons.

The essence of **sensory-perceptual training** is that through auditory stimulation practice, the client will become aware of his own sound errors. In other words, the client's ability to identify the sound and perceive his own errors provides a foundation for production training. Sensory-perceptual training, also known as **ear training,** consists of the following phases: identification, isolation, stimulation, and discrimination. The complexity of the skills trained increases as the client progresses from one phase to the other.

Phase 1: Identification

The goal of this phase is to teach the client the auditory, visual, and tactile-kinesthetic properties of the target sound (sound, look, and feel). The client learns to recognize the target sound from among several possible sounds composed of similar and dissimilar properties.

The clinician describes the target sound according to its acoustic, visual, and tactile-kinesthetic properties and gives it a label. With young children, sounds may be labeled as follows:

- /t/ "ticking sound"
- /s/ "snake sound"
- /ʃ/ "quiet sound"
- /r/ "lion sound"

- /z/ "bee sound"
- /l/ "singing sound"
- /k/ "coughing sound"
- /tʃ/ "sneezing (achoo!) sound"
- /θ/ "tongue sound"
- /f/ "angry cat sound"

Secord (1989) appropriately cautions that with older children and adults, anatomical descriptions may be more appropriate. Also, more sophisticated terms can be used to describe the sound's auditory, visual, and tactile-kinesthetic properties. For example, if the target sound is /f/, the clinician may tell the client, "This sound is made by putting your upper teeth lightly against your bottom lip and blowing air slowly. As you blow, you can feel a cool sensation on the top portion of your bottom lip."

At the end of this phase, the client should demonstrate the ability to recognize the sound in isolation and perceive many of its important characteristics. Some clients may also show the capacity to describe the target sound's salient features.

Phase 2: Isolation

At this point, the client is expected to use his or her newly acquired recognition skills to isolate the target sound when it is produced against a background of other speech sounds. In essence, the client must be able to identify words, phrases, and sentences that contain the target sound as the clinician produces them. The clinician may ask a child to point to the "happy face" or other appropriate symbol if the word or phrase contains the target sound or to the "sad face" if it does not have the target sound. The complexity of the task is gradually increased.

During this phase, the client may also be instructed to identify the position of the target sound within the stimulus word: initial (beginning), medial (middle), or final (end). For example, if the target sound is [r], the client must be able to identify whether it occurs at the beginning, middle, or end of the word [rʌn]. Instructions such as "Bobby, tell me if your sound is in the beginning, middle or end of the word" may be provided. It may be necessary for the clinician to do some initial training to facilitate the client's understanding of the activity. This may be especially important with very young children, who may not understand the concept of beginning, middle, and end.

Phase 3: Stimulation

The clinician presents the target sound by varying its loudness and duration. Sentences loaded with various uses of the target sound, as well as tongue twisters, are presented. In essence, the client is bombarded with productions of the target sound.

The client is asked to identify the target sound as it occurs in the various stimulation activities presented. The goal of this phase is to increase the client's sensitivity to the occurrence of the sound and to develop an internalized auditory model of the sound.

Phase 4: Discrimination

At this point, the client is asked to make an external comparison with his or her internal auditory image of the sound. Simply stated, the client judges the clinician's productions of the target sound as correct or incorrect. Van Riper and Emerick (1984) described two major tasks in discrimination testing: (1) error detection and (2) error correction. In *error detection,* the child is instructed to identify sound errors purposely made by the clinician; and in *error correction,* the child must explain how the sound was in error and how it can be corrected. The paucity of data supporting the effectiveness of auditory discrimination training for improvement of sound production has raised questions about the need for this phase of therapy. This topic was discussed in detail in the Basic and Advanced Units of Chapter 4.

Production Training—Sound Establishment

After the client has learned to identify the most important acoustic features of the target sound and can make correct judgments about whether a sound is produced correctly, the second stage of treatment is initiated. In the production training stage, the goal is to evoke and establish a new sound pattern that will replace the client's error pattern.

The sound can be evoked using several methods, such as imitation; auditory stimulation; phonetic placement; contextual cues; **moto-kinesthetic cues;** and sound approximation (see Secord, 1989, for details). Many of these methods were reviewed in the Basic Unit of Chapter 7. Specific techniques for teaching sounds are also provided in Appendix M.

Again, the goal is to evoke a new sound pattern from the client so that his or her error pattern is replaced. To accomplish this, the clinician uses any combination of sound establishment techniques. Production training for sound establishment can be difficult, especially with particular sounds such as /r/ and /s/. However, this stage can also be fun and exciting. Getting a client to produce a sound that he or she was not able to make before training can be very rewarding for the clinician. Also, the clinician's creativity can flourish at this stage of articulation therapy.

Production Training—Sound Stabilization

After the target sound has been established, the clinician shifts the focus of therapy to stabilizing the client's production of the sound at all linguistic levels. In the traditional approach as originally outlined, stabilization training is initiated at the simplest level of production—isolation—and progresses to the most complex level—conversation.

In his discussion of the traditional approach, Secord (1989) outlined the progression of therapy as follows: isolation, nonsense syllables, words, phrases, sentences, and conversation. However, he emphasized that not all clinicians begin at the isolation level. Some believe that the syllable level is the most appropriate because in natural speech, sounds do not occur in isolation. These clinicians insist that the syllable is the basic element of speech since many sounds cannot be produced in isolation. For example, if one tries to produce [b] in isolation, it quickly becomes evident that it cannot be produced without an intrusive schwa [ə].

While some believe that the syllable level is the most appropriate starting point for therapy, others advocate the word level as the entry point of stabilization training. Proponents of this view argue that words are more meaningful since by definition phonemes are units that signal changes in meaning. We previously addressed this topic in the Basic Unit of Chapter 7.

Recently, it has come to be generally believed that training should begin at the linguistic level that is appropriate for the individual client. If a client can produce the phoneme in isolation and syllables, it is clinically efficient to begin training at the word level. As Secord indicates, "No matter what stabilization level is chosen as the beginning point, as the client enters the level, ability to produce the sound is weak and generally unstable. As the client leaves the level, however, production should be consistently accurate and fluent" (p. 142). In other words, the goal of training is to stabilize the client's production of the target sound at the lowest level of difficulty and gradually progress to more complex linguistic levels. In the traditional approach, stabilization at one level is considered a prerequisite for entry to the next level. This maximizes the client's chances for success as he or she progresses from one level to the next. We will describe the steps in detail, assuming that each serves as a prerequisite for the next.

Stage 1: Isolation

The goal at this stage is to develop a stronger and more consistent correct production of the target sound through various practice activities. Some of the visual cues used in the establishment phase are also used at this stage. Secord (1989, p. 142) outlined some common tasks that are typically used for sound stabilization at the isolation level:

- practicing prolonging the target;
- varying the number of productions emitted at any one time;
- varying the intensity with which the sound is produced;
- whispering the new sound;
- starting and stopping production in response to the clinician's signal;
- simultaneously talking and writing the new sound;
- responding to large and small letters that represent the target by using loud or soft sounds depending on the size of the letter cues;
- playing "speech games" in which the child responds by producing the target sound a certain number of times when it is his or her turn;
- playing with a deck of cards with different numbers used to indicate to the child the number of times to produce the sound;
- switching from one sound to another and then back to the target so that the target is said immediately after the client has repositioned the articulators.

Stage 2: Nonsense Syllables

The goal at this point is to help the client develop a stronger and more consistently correct production of the target sound in a variety of nonsense syllable contexts. The target sound may be practiced in a variety of syllable shape contexts and word positions. For example (adapted from Secord, 1989, p. 143):

Syllable	Shape	Word Position
/bu/	CV	initial (prevocalic)
/ub/	VC	final (postvocalic)
/ubu/	VCV	medial (intervocalic)
/bum/	CVC	initial (prevocalic)
/mub/	CVC	final (postvocalic)

The vowel can be replaced by any of the stressed vowels to create more nonsense syllables, and the target can be practiced in clusters. Training can shift from nonsense syllables to nonsense words by giving familiar objects funny or silly names.

Stage 3: Words

Stabilization training shifts to true words when the client can produce the target sound easily and consistently in nonsense syllables. The target sound is practiced in words using a series of substages, moving from simple monosyllable to complex multisyllable exemplars. The substages may include the following (adapted from Secord, 1989, Table 5.2, p. 145):

Substage	# of Syllables	Examples for /p/
Initial (prevocalic) words	1	pot, pig, pen
Final (postvocalic) words	1	up, mop, lap
Medial (intervocalic) words	2	open, upon, epic
Initial clusters	1	play, plate, plump
Final clusters	1	apple, zipper, opal
Medial clusters	2	applause, apply, oppress
All word positions	1–2	[any appropriate word]
All word positions	any	application, prime, stop
All word positions; multiple targets	any	paper, popping, proper

The goal is to teach the client to produce the target sound in a variety of contexts, from simple to very complex words. Word training begins with the use of a core group, typically consisting of meaningful words such as the client's name, family names, social words, academic curriculum words, and so forth. When the client produces the target sound consistently in the core group, the clinician expands the group to a larger set of training words.

Stage 4: Phrases

At this stage, training shifts from single words to two- to four-word phrases. This serves as an in-between stage from words to sentences. Bankson and Bernthal (1998) indicate that the phrase level is an in-between stage especially if carrier phrases are used.

Carrier phrases are simpler than assorted phrases and sentences since only a single word is changed as the target words are practiced in sequence (e.g., I see the *boat;* I see the *bear;* I see the *balloon;* I see the *baby;* I see the *basket*). Some clinicians skip the phrase stage altogether and begin the sentence level with short sentences.

Stage 5: Sentences

Whether the clinician skips the phrase level or not, the next stage in stabilization training is sentences. The goal is to stabilize production of the target sound in sentences of varying length and complexity. Secord (1989) recommends the following substages of sentence-level stabilization training (examples for /b/):

- Simple short sentences with one instance of the target sound—My dog is *big;* I want the *ball;* My name is *Brenda.*
- Sentences of various lengths with one instance of the target sound—Yesterday I *bought* a doll at the store; Why did you *bring* your dog here? My mommy made *bean* soup for dinner.
- Simple short sentences with two or more instances of the target sound— My *baby* sister likes *bubbles;* She *bought* a *blue* dress; Daddy made a *big bench.*
- Sentences of various lengths with two or more instances of the target sound—My daddy made a *big bench* for the *backyard;* She *broke* Mom's *brown* lamp; I like to play with *bubbles,* and I like to play dodge *ball.*

The clinician can use several techniques (Van Riper, 1978) to help establish production of sentences: slow-motion speech, echo speech or shadowing, unison speaking, the corrective set, and role-playing. In **slow-motion speech** the clinician and the client say the target sentence at the same time using a very slow rate of speech. In **shadowing,** or echo speech, the clinician says the target sentence and then gives the client a signal indicating that it his or her turn. The client repeats the sentence as quickly and automatically as possible.

The clinician can also use **unison speech,** in which hand tapping or other signals of rhythm are employed in sentence production. The client follows the clinician's physical movements and prosody as he or she repeats the sentence in unison with the clinician. The **corrective set** capitalizes on an activity that most children enjoy: correcting the clinician. In this activity the clinician purposely misarticulates the target sound and asks the child to correct it. On occasions children who are not able to produce a sentence correctly when instructed to do so are able to model it appropriately when "teaching" the clinician.

Finally, **role-playing** can be used with children who cannot produce the target sound in a normal training situation. Children are instructed to take on a dramatic theatrical role to facilitate correct production of the target sentences.

Stage 6: Conversation

The conversation level is the last stage of production stabilization training before therapy progresses to the transfer and carryover phase. When the client produces the target sound consistently in sentences of varying length and complexity, the clinician typically shifts production training to conversation tasks. Conversation practice in the treatment room lays the foundation for training in various extraclinical settings such as home, the playground, and the classroom.

Production training at this level usually progresses from structured tasks (planned conversation) to unstructured tasks (everyday conversational speech). In structured conversation tasks, the clinician controls the treatment activities so that only words containing the target sound are practiced. For example, the client may be asked to tell a story about several pictured objects that contain the target sound. Another example is the use of a city map on which all of the locations and street names contain the target sound (Secord, 1989). Some published materials such as "sound posters" are also available. The posters contain a variety of pictured objects, all containing a specific target sound in their names.

Once the client can successfully produce the target sound in structured conversation tasks, the clinician shifts the focus of therapy to natural conversation, in which no restrictions are placed on the client. Open-ended prompts such as, "Tell me about your friends at school" and "Tell me about your last birthday party" can be used to evoke conversation.

Transfer and Carryover

One of the most important aspects of articulation training is the client's use of the newly acquired skills in extraclinical situations. It is not uncommon for children who are 100% accurate in the clinical setting to revert to old speech patterns at home, on the playground, in the classroom, and in other natural environments. Because clients do not live in an isolated environment such as the clinical room and have only limited interaction with the speech–language pathologist, it is imperative that the treatment environment be extended to include other settings, other people, and other situations.

Secord (1989) defines **transfer** as the extension of newly learned behaviors from the original setting to various other settings. He differentiates transfer from **carryover** and identifies the latter as the child's ability to use the newly acquired sound in conversation. He summarizes various strategies offered by Van Riper and Emerick (1984) to promote the client's transfer and carryover of the newly acquired speech skills. We discussed these and several other factors in the Basic Unit of Chapter 7.

Speech Assignments

The clinician provides the client with speech assignments that can be completed at home, in school, in the office, and so forth. The speech assignments are prepared so that they meet each client's individual needs. The clinician should ensure that the speech assignments are not so complicated that they are too difficult for the client and his or her parents to complete at home independently.

Self and Peer Monitoring

The clinician instructs the client or a significant other (e.g., sibling, classmate, friend) to monitor the client's speech and document his or her errors. When using classmates or friends as peer evaluators, the clinician should always ensure that school regulations are being followed and that the peer's newfound role does not create emotional conflicts between him or her and the client.

Practice in Other Situations

The clinician designs treatment activities so that the client has the opportunity to practice the sound in various natural-speaking situations. Secord indicates that the "client must be able to use the new sound in sending messages, in interacting socially, in thinking, in expressing emotions" (p. 151). The clinician should ensure that the client has the foundational skills to be successful in more complicated speaking situations.

Proprioceptive Awareness Exercises

According to Secord (1989), the client should possess adequate proprioceptive skills to monitor his or her own speech. In other words, the client should not only be able to hear his or her speech productions but must also be able to "feel" them. Various exercises can be used to enhance the client's proprioceptive awareness, including: speaking with earplugs, speaking while wearing earphones that supply a masking noise, whispering, and speaking in pantomime.

Varying the Audience and Setting

The clinician varies the client's audience to promote production of the target sound with people other than the speech–language pathologist. Speaking situations with the classroom teacher, parents, and other professionals can be arranged outside the clinical setting.

Maintenance

The ultimate goal in articulation therapy is maintenance of the newly learned skills in various natural environments across time. It is important not only that the client transfer and carry over the skills learned in the clinical setting to extraclinical situations, but also that he or she maintains those skills over time. To promote maintenance of the newly acquired skills, the clinician may arrange follow-up sessions with the client. The client may be seen on a decreasing basis, once a week initially, then once a month for a few months, once every 3 months, once every 6 months, and so forth until he or she is ready for final dismissal from therapy.

Summary of the Traditional Approach

• The traditional approach was developed by various researchers but is primarily associated with **Charles Van Riper,** who originally published it in 1939 in his text *Speech Correction: Principles and Methods.*

• The approach has **five phases:** (1) sensory-perceptual training, (2) production training (sound establishment), (3) production training (sound stabilization), (4) transfer and carryover training, (5) maintenance.

• Training focuses on **one sound** at a time (when one sound is corrected, then another sound is trained until all of the target sounds are treated).

• **Sensory-perceptual training** includes identification, isolation, auditory stimulation, and discrimination.

• **Production training** for sound **establishment** may include auditory stimulation (imitation) and the use of contextual cues, phonetic placement, moto-kinesthetic training, and sound approximation.

• **Production training** for sound **stabilization** progresses in the following order: isolation, nonsense syllables, words, phrases, sentences, and conversation.

• **Transfer** and **carryover** can be promoted by assigning speech homework, arranging peer evaluations, varying the speaking situations, varying the audience, and teaching self-monitoring skills.

• **Maintenance** of the newly acquired skills is ensured by conducting treatment sessions on a gradually decreasing basis. The clinician can conduct sessions with the client once a week for a month, and then once a month for a few months, once every 3 months, once every 6 months, and so forth until the client is ready for final dismissal.

• Most clinicians today vary one or several aspects of the traditional approach in their clinical use. For example, clinicians may opt to teach three or four sounds at a time rather than one at a time. Also, clinicians may choose to begin with production training and skip sensory-perceptual training altogether if the client's perceptual skills are adequate.

Sensorimotor Approach

McDonald's Approach

The **sensorimotor approach** to articulation treatment was first developed by McDonald in 1964. Thus, this approach is frequently referred to as **McDonald's sensorimotor approach.** McDonald's approach is based on the assumption that the syllable is the basic unit of training and that certain phonetic contexts can be used to facilitate correct production of an error sound. Auditory discrimination training is not included in this program, and production training is initiated at the syllable level rather than isolation. This differentiates the sensorimotor approach from the previously discussed traditional approach. The primary goal of the program is to increase the child's auditory, tactile, and proprioceptive awareness of the motor patterns involved in speech sound production through motor production–oriented tasks.

When using this approach, it is important that the clinician identify a phonetic context or contexts in which the child produces the target sound correctly. When a phonetic context is found, it can be incorporated into the sound production tasks to facilitate the child's correct responses of the target sound. Facilitative phonetic contexts may be found by administration of *The Deep Test of Articulation* (McDonald, 1964). McDonald's sensorimotor approach is composed of three primary objectives: (1) heightening the child's responsiveness to the patterns of "ballistic" speech movements, (2) reinforcing the child's correct production of the error sound, and (3) facilitating the child's correct production of the error sound in systematically varied phonetic contexts.

Heightening the Child's Responsiveness

The first phase of training is production practice with sounds that the child can produce correctly (nonerror sounds). The sounds are practiced in bisyllable (CVCV) reduplicated productions, combined with each of the most commonly used vowels (e.g., [kiki], [kɪkɪ], [keke], [kækæ], [kʌkʌ], [kuku], [koko], and [kɑkɑ]).

The clinician selects a sound that the client can produce correctly and combines it with a vowel to create reduplicated syllable combinations (e.g., [kiki]). The clinician begins treatment by asking the client to imitate the modeled production of bisyllables with equal stress on both syllables (e.g., [kiki]). Next, the clinician asks the client to imitate the modeled bisyllables with primary stress on the first syllable (e.g., [kiˈki]).

The clinician then instructs the client to imitate the modeled production of bisyllables with primary stress on the second syllable (e.g., [kikiˈ]). The clinician also asks the child to describe the placement of the articulators and the direction of the articulatory movements. This is done to heighten the child's awareness of the speech motor patterns.

The clinician selects another vowel for bisyllable production practice with the same consonant (e.g., shift training from [kiki] to [koko]). After the child produces one consonant in CVCV combinations with various vowels, the clinician gives similar training with other nonerror consonants. Next, the clinician initiates training on trisyllable (CVCVCV) combinations, following the same general procedures used with bisyllables. Training of bisyllables and trisyllables can also be done with sounds that the client produces in error, but the clinician should make no effort to remediate those sounds at this point.

Reinforcing Correct Articulation of the Target Sound

In the second phase, the clinician initiates training on the sounds that are typically misarticulated, using the facilitative phonetic context (i.e., the phonetic context that evokes a correct production of the error sound). The theoretical assumption behind the sensorimotor approach is that all sounds can be produced correctly in at least one phonetic context. Phonetic contexts can be found by analyzing the client's connected speech or by deep testing. Again, deep testing can be performed with McDonald's *Deep Test of Articulation* (1964).

McDonald provided an example of a child who produced /s/ correctly in the facilitative context *watch–sun* (a deep-test item). The facilitative context may differ for each child. Using the facilitative context that evokes a correct production of the target sound, the clinician asks the child to say the two-word combination in the following sequence (using McDonald's example of *watch–sun*):

1. The child practices the facilitative context (*watch–sun*) in slow-motion speech, deliberately using a slower rate to articulate each sound in the sequence.
2. The child practices *watch–sun* placing equal stress on both syllables.
3. The child produces *watch–sun* placing primary stress on the first syllable.
4. The child produces *watch–sun* placing primary stress on the second syllable.
5. The child prolongs the target sound until a signal is given to complete the whole word (i.e., the child says *watchsssss* until the clinician gives a signal to complete the disyllable by saying *watchsssss-un*).
6. The child practices *watch–sun* in short sentences such as "Watch sun will burn you" and "Watch sun is out"). Initially, the sentences are practiced without any specific instructions on rate or stress. Then the clinician instructs the child to practice the sentences by saying them with a variety of stress patterns.

CLINICIAN: Did you say, "*Look,* sun will burn you?"

CHILD: No, I said, "*Watch,* sun will burn you."

CLINICIAN: Did you say, "Watch, *fire* will burn you?"

CHILD: No, I said, "Watch, *sun* will burn you."

CLINICIAN: Did you say, "Watch, sun *might* burn you?"

CHILD: No, I said, "Watch, sun *will* burn you."

CLINICIAN: Did you say, "Watch, sun will *tan* you?"

CHILD: No, I said, "Watch, sun will *burn* you." (McDonald, 1964, p. 145)

It must be noted that the sentences used for production practice are not always meaningful. According to McDonald, meaningful sentences are not requisite since the primary goal is the practice of movement sequences.

Facilitating Correct Articulation of the Target Sound in Varied Contexts

The third general phase of the sensorimotor approach is correct production of the client's target sounds using the facilitative context in which the sound is produced correctly in a variety of phonetic contexts. The following describes the steps in this phase of training, continuing to use *watch–sun* for illustration.

The clinician trains correct production of the target sound in varied phonetic contexts by changing the words in which the target sound appears. For example, the initial phonetic context of *watch–sun* is varied to *watch–sea, watch–sit, watch–send, watch–sat,* and so forth.

The clinician then shifts training to production practice in the context of different first and second words. For example, *watch–sun* changes to *teach–sit, reach–sun, pitch–sat,* and so forth. The varied word combinations are practiced with different rate and stress patterns and in sentence contexts.

Last, the clinician instructs the child to practice the target sound in totally different phonetic contexts. For example, the training sequence may change from *watch–sun* to *mop–sun, book–sun, bear–sun,* and so forth. The same general procedures are followed at this point, and the clinician implements generalization and maintenance procedures.

Shine and Proust's Sensorimotor Approach

In 1982, Shine and Proust offered an adaptation of McDonald's original sensorimotor treatment program. Like McDonald's, their program is based on the principles of coarticulation. However, Shine and Proust extended the number of phases included in the program to six and outlined various steps within each phase. Compared to McDonald's original program, Shine and Proust's adaptation is much more comprehensive and structured. The phases of the program are: (1) evaluation, (2) awareness, (3) establishment, (4) intratherapy generalization, (5) transfer/extratherapy generalization, and (6) maintenance. The reader is referred to Shine (1989) for a comprehensive review of this approach.

Evaluation Phase

Shine (1989) recommends a comprehensive evaluation that will help the clinician differentially diagnose the problem and aid in the identification "of appropriate antecedent stimuli at new levels of language and coarticulatory complexity" (p. 338).

The following testing activities may be completed for a comprehensive assessment. Shine and Proust indicate that not all tests are necessary for all clients.

1. Administer a standardized articulation test such as the *Goldman-Fristoe Test of Articulation, Arizona Articulation Proficiency Scale,* or

Photo Articulation Test. The goal is to assess all English sounds in single-word contexts.

2. Sample varied phonetic contexts by administration of the *Screening Deep Test of Articulation* (McDonald, 1968).

3. Obtain a representative connected speech sample.

4. Conduct a phonological process analysis to determine patterns of misarticulations.

5. Administer other assessment procedures as deemed necessary to comprehensively assess the client's communicative deviancies.

After the clinician administers all of the appropriate testing instruments and activities, the data should be analyzed. The clinician (a) compiles a list of mispronounced phones, (b) completes a phonetic inventory, and (c) identifies phonetic contexts that facilitate correct production for the mispronounced phones. The clinician may also complete additional testing of varied contexts if necessary by administering the *Deep Test of Articulation* (McDonald, 1964) or *Clinical Probes of Articulation Consistency* (Secord, 1981a). The final step in the evaluation phase is the selection of target phones for treatment and phonetic contexts that help facilitate their correct production.

Awareness Phase

In the awareness phase the client is oriented to the speech mechanism and the specific articulators that aid in the production of sounds. The primary goal is to "heighten" the client's awareness of the auditory, tactile, proprioceptive, and kinesthetic sensations associated with the correct articulatory movements for particular sounds.

Orientation to Speech Helpers. The terminal objective for this step is the client's spontaneous naming or identification of 8 of 10 "speech helpers" following imitative articulation of a variety of phones, speech movements, or other vocal behaviors. The criterion is approximately 30 to 40 minutes of training. Shine (1989) indicates that this step under the awareness phase is optional depending on the individual needs of the client.

The speech helpers include the lips, teeth, tongue, gum ridge, alveolar ridge, hard palate, soft palate, voice box (larynx), nose, ears, and expired breathstream. The clinician allows the client to "self discover" his or her own speech helpers during production of speech movements or other vocal behaviors with minimal cueing. Examples of cues include: (a) the client's lips touching while saying *mama,* (b) the client's breathstream moving a small piece of paper during production of /p/, and (c) stimulation of the back of his or her hand during production of /f/. The client's awareness of the speech helpers is presumed when he directly points to his own articulators or identifies them in a mirror or line drawing.

Taylor and Shine (1978) developed the use of a *shadow-gram profile* to help with the identification of speech helpers. A sagittal representation of the client's speech helpers is made on a poster board or paper. The clinician can use a bright light to reflect a shadow of the patient's profile and trace an outline. The shadow-gram is then incorporated into therapy or can be sent home with the client for home practice.

The next step, heightening awareness training, is initiated with clients who continue to experience difficulties in spontaneous identification of the speech helpers.

However, this step can be skipped with clients demonstrating good awareness skills. With such clients, the clinician progresses to the establishment phase.

Heightening Awareness of Auditory, Tactile, and Proprioceptive/Kinesthetic Sensations. The terminal objective for this step is the client's correct imitation of consonants within his or her phonetic inventory in (a) CVCV bisyllable and disyllable contexts, (b) CVCVCV trisyllable contexts, and (c) VCCV abutting consonant contexts in variable stress patterns. The training criterion is 20 consecutive correct responses for each context or level of production.

This procedure is optional but is generally recommended for clients with multiple misarticulations (i.e., seven or more error phones), a severe articulation deviancy, or poor intelligibility. Shine (1989) indicates that this phase may also be beneficial for clients exhibiting minimal motor speech involvement or apraxia of speech.

All sounds in the child's phonetic inventory are used for training during this phase, especially those phonemes that are produced correctly spontaneously or with stimulation in at least a CV or VC context. Training progresses from productions that require minimal coarticulatory skills (e.g., /bibi/) to those that are much more complex (e.g., /malijæ/). The client is also trained to produce varied stress patterns by imitating the clinician's primary stress pattern on the first or second syllable with bisyllables and on the first, second, or third syllables with trisyllables. After a correct imitation, the client may also be asked to identify which articulators touched and where they touched and the direction of the movement of the articulators (e.g., front to back, back to front, back-front-back).

Establishment Phase

The terminal objective in the establishment phase is the client's correct articulation of the target sound(s) in prevocalic or postvocalic abutting bisyllable contexts (e.g., CVC-CVC [*duck–sun*]). The training criterion is 20 consecutive correct responses in short phrases and sentences following auditory modeling, prompting, or visual stimulation.

Training is initiated using only the facilitative context in which the sound is produced correctly. The establishment phase consists of seven steps in which the target sound is practiced in a variety of contexts and prosodic speaking patterns. Shine (1989) offers an example of the facilitative context *duck–sun* for correct production of /s/ to illustrate the seven steps.

Step 1. The client produces *duck–sun* (facilitative context) with near equal stress. Firm coarticulation is encouraged without a pause between the syllables. In other words, the CVC-CVC production *duck–sun* should be produced as one "silly" or "funny" word. The clinician may use contrastive training tasks (e.g., pictorial representation of *duck–sun* versus *duck–thun*) to increase the client's awareness of correct versus incorrect productions.

Step 2. The client produces the facilitative context *duck–sun* at a slow rate to provide extended duration of tactile, auditory, and proprioceptive/kinesthetic feedback. The clinician draws the client's attention to the movement of the articulators and the sound's manner of production. Shine (1989) indicates that the clinician should "teach the patients as much as possible about correct production" (p. 349).

Step 3. The client produces the facilitative context while prolonging the target sound (e.g., *duck–sssssssun*). The clinician may use his or her index finger to indicate how long the target sound should be prolonged. Auditory, tactile, and other forms of feedback are provided to increase the client's "cognitive awareness." Because not all sounds can be prolonged, this step is done only with continuants.

Steps 4 and 5. The clinician models the facilitative context stressing the syllable that contains the target sound (*duck–**sun***). The criterion is 20 consecutive correct responses. The clinician repeats this procedure but now stresses the syllable that does not contain the target sound (***duck**–sun*).

Steps 6 and 7. The clinician models the facilitative context in phrases and short sentences and instructs the client to imitate them. Sentences such as "I have a *duck–sun*," "I want my *duck–sun*," and "*Duck–sun* can go" may be used as practice stimuli. The clinician should use sounds that are part of the client's phonetic inventory to construct phrases and sentences as much as possible. At this point, the clinician may also use contrastive stress patterns for practice with different intonation patterns. For example, the clinician asks, "Do you have a duck–moon?" and the client responds, "No, I have a *duck–SUN*."

Generalization Phase (Intratherapy Generalization)

In the generalization phase the terminal objective becomes the correct articulation of the target sound in a wide variety of bisyllable contexts progressing to spontaneous production in connected speech in response to visual, auditory, and conversational interactive stimulation. The training criterion at this point is 20 consecutive correct responses in structured communicative interactions and at least 80% accuracy in conversational speech. This phase also has various steps that are followed sequentially.

Step 1. The facilitative context used during the establishment phase is also used to initiate the intratherapy generalization phase. To demonstrate the steps in the generalization phase, we will continue to use Shine and Proust's example of *duck–sun* [dʌk–sʌn] and the target sound /s/. In step 1, the clinician *systematically* varies the consonant and vowel in the syllable *not containing* the target sound (*duck*). That is, the [dʌ] component is varied, while the abutting (adjacent) /k/ and the second syllable (*sun*) remain constant. For example, the clinician may systematically vary the productions in the following order: [dʌk–sʌn], [tæk–sʌn], [pɛk–sʌn], [beɪk–sʌn], [fɪk–sʌn], [vɪk–sʌn], [mik–sʌn], [dʌk–sʌn], [tɑk–sʌn], [loʊk–sʌn], [joʊk–sʌn], [hʊk–sʌn], and so forth. The order of vowel variation is done in such a manner that it minimally changes the tongue hump and height. Consonants are also shifted as minimally as possible.

Step 2. The procedures followed in step 2 are similar to those in step 1. However, at this point, the clinician *randomly* rather than systematically varies the consonant and vowel within the syllable *not containing* the target sound. Random variations promote maximal changes between stimulus presentations. When this step is completed, the clinician introduces a homework assignment.

Step 3. The clinician *systematically* varies the consonant and the vowel in the syllable *containing* the target sound. The /ʌn/ in *sun* is systematically changed, while the *duck* component and the /s/ remain constant. For example, the clinician may vary the productions in the following manner: [dʌk–sʌn], [dʌk–sɑd], [dʌk–soʊp], [dʌk–sum], [dʌk–sup], [dʌk–soʊf], and so forth. Again, the level of vowel and consonant variations between stimulus presentations should be minimal at this point.

Step 4. The procedures in this step are similar to those in step 3. However, the clinician now *randomly* varies the consonant and vowel in the syllable *containing* the target sound. Homework assignments are provided.

Step 5. The clinician *randomly* varies the consonant and vowel in *both* syllables (i.e., [dʌ] in *duck* and [ʌn] in *sun*), while the abutting /k/ and the target sound /s/ remain constant. Stimulus presentations may include [dʌk–sʌn], [mik–sʌm], [fɪk–seiv], [tɑk–sæm], and so forth.

Step 6. The clinician *systematically* varies the *consonant abutting* (next to) the target sound to develop word pairs with a minimal shift in movement. The following sequence may be followed: [dʌk–sʌn], [dʌg–sʌn], [dʌd–sʌn], [dʌn–sʌn], [dʌt–sʌn], [dʌp–sʌn], [dʌb–sʌn], [dʌm–sʌn], [dʌf–sʌn], [dʌv–sʌn], and so forth.

Step 7. The clinician *randomly* varies the *consonant abutting* the target sound. At this point, the stress patterns may also be varied.

Step 8. The clinician *randomly* modifies the contexts from steps 1 through 7 to develop variable word pairs. The client is encouraged to form his or her own word pairs.

Step 9. Shine (1989) indicates that this step is optional. The clinician uses the previously assigned homework activities for production practice in the clinical situation.

Step 10. The clinician creates sentences using any and all contexts practiced in steps 1 through 9. Contrastive stress tasks may also be used (described in step 7 of the establishment phase).

Step 11. The client is given the opportunity to create sentences using the modified contexts practiced in steps 1 through 10. When step 11 is completed, the clinician assesses facilitative contexts for the postvocalic /s/ by administering *The Deep Test of Articulation* (picture form or sentence form). The clinician initiates training if necessary.

Intratherapy generalization may be expanded by including reading materials, stories, action or sequence pictures, and conversation in therapy. These activities can serve as probes to determine whether additional treatment is necessary.

Transfer Phase (Extratherapy Generalization)

When the client reaches the established criterion under the generalization phase, the next phase is initiated. In the transfer phase, the terminal objective is the client's correct articulation of the target sound in prevocalic and postvocalic positions during spontaneous conversation. The training criterion during this phase is the client's production of the target sound with at least 80–90% accuracy in a wide variety of environments and speaking conditions or situations.

When appropriate, the clinician and the client independently collect data using paper and pencil or a hand counter. They also calculate and chart the data. The clinician determines the level of extratherapy generalization (i.e., child's accuracy of target sound production) in a variety of everyday speaking situations through observation or tape recordings.

Maintenance Phase

Maintenance of the target sound in extraclinical situations is promoted through periodic follow-up sessions. Shine (1989) suggests conversational samples of 2 to 5 minutes of "talking time" once per week initially, once weekly for 1 month, twice monthly for 2 months, and finally once monthly for 2 to 3 months. Termination from speech therapy is determined based on the client's performance during follow-up sessions.

Management of Antecedent and Consequent Stimuli

Shine and Proust (1982) recommend a strict stimulus-response-stimulus (S-R-S) treatment paradigm in the initial stages of the program. The clinician provides one stimulus to evoke the desired response, and the client is then expected to respond. There is a possibility that the client's response will be correct, incorrect, or absent. Regardless, the clinician should avoid multiple stimulations for a single response. If the frequency of incorrect or no responses is too high, the clinician should evaluate the antecedent stimuli—in this case, the facilitating phonetic context—for the probable reasons for such a pattern. The clinician should select antecedent stimuli that consistently evoke the target response. The authors further recommend consequent stimuli in two forms: (1) token reinforcement, and (2) verbal feedback.

Summary of the Sensorimotor Approach

• The sensorimotor approach was developed by McDonald (1964); thus, it is also referred to as **McDonald's sensorimotor approach.**

• This approach is based on the assumption that the **syllable** is the **basic unit of training** and that certain **phonetic contexts** can be used to facilitate production of an error sound.

• **Auditory discrimination** is not included in this program, and **production training** begins at the syllable level.

• The goal is to increase the child's **auditory, tactile,** and **proprioceptive awareness** of the motor patterns involved in speech sound production through motor-oriented tasks.

• Phonetic contexts that evoke a correct production of the target sound are known as **facilitative phonetic contexts.**

• Facilitative phonetic contexts can be determined by administration of *The Deep Test of Articulation* (McDonald, 1964).

• McDonald's sensorimotor approach is composed of three major objectives: (1) heightening the child's responsiveness to the patterns of "ballistic" speech movements, (2) reinforcing the child's correct production of the error sound, and (3) facilitating the child's correct production of the error sound in systematically varied phonetic contexts.

• Shine and Proust (1982) adapted McDonald's sensorimotor approach to include more detailed training objectives and accuracy criteria. They also incorporated more recent approaches to articulation and phonological remediation into the sensori-motor paradigm.

• Shine and Proust's program includes an awareness phase, an establishment phase, a generalization phase (intratherapy generalization), a transfer phase (extratherapy generalization), and a maintenance phase.

• The awareness phase helps the child become oriented to the "speech helpers" and helps heighten the child's awareness of auditory, tactile, and proprioceptive/kinesthetic sensations associated with correct articulatory movements.

• The establishment phase facilitates correct articulation of the target sound either prevocalically or postvocalically in abutting bisyllable facilitative contexts.

• The generalization phase promotes correct articulation of the target sound in a wide variety of bisyllable contexts progressing to spontaneous production in connected speech in response to visual, auditory, and conversational interactive stimulation.

• The transfer phase is designed to promote correct articulation of the target sound in prevocalic and postvocalic positions during spontaneous conversation.

• Maintenance of the target sound in extraclinical situations is promoted through periodic follow-up sessions

• The establishment, generalization, and transfer phases have various steps that help accomplish the terminal objective for the phase.

Multiple-Phoneme Approach

The **multiple-phoneme approach** was developed by McCabe and Bradley in 1969 at the University of North Carolina (Bradley, 1989). It was primarily advanced to meet the needs of children with multiple articulation errors. Thus, this approach is considered to be most appropriate for individuals exhibiting six or more articulation errors (McCabe & Bradley, 1973, 1975). The multiple-phoneme approach is a highly structured program whose primary features include (a) the simultaneous teaching of multiple phonemes, (b) a systematic application of behavioral principles, and (c) an analysis of sound production in conversational speech.

According to Bradley (1989), the multiple-phoneme approach maintains many of the steps included in the traditional approach but uses them with some modification. For example, it deemphasizes auditory discrimination training as a first step in therapy. Rather, it undertakes auditory discrimination training after the client achieves a certain level of accuracy in sound production. According to Bradley, this modification is based on research evidence suggesting that production training also teaches discrimination.

Because the program follows well-established behavioral principles, it clearly outlines a sequence of training progressing from simple to more complex behaviors. McCabe and Bradley outline criteria for mastery at each step, and various record-keeping forms are used to document the client's performance. Documentation is performed during each session.

The program also uses a pre- and post-therapy assessment to document the client's progress. A 150-word conversational sample is collected from the client and analyzed according to whole-word accuracy (WWA). The examiner listens to the tape-recorded sample and marks on the written transcript each word that contains at least one articulation error. After the transcript has been completed, the examiner calculates a WWA score by calculating the percentage of words spoken correctly. Dividing the number of words spoken with at least one articulation error by the total number of words (i.e., 150 words) produces a WWA score. For example, if a client produces 90 words in error, his WWA score would be 60 (i.e., $90 \div 150 = 60$). Bradley (1989) indicates that the WWA can be used to supplement the information obtained from single-word articulation tests.

The multiple-phoneme approach is divided into three phases, with many steps under each phase. The three phases are: (1) establishment, (2) transfer, and (3) maintenance. The steps under each phase lead toward achievement of the goal by outlining the specific stimuli, response description, reinforcement schedule, and criterion level (Bradley, 1989). The following outlines the three phases and various steps of the multiple-phoneme approach as discussed by Bradley.

Phase I—Establishment

The goal of phase I is that the client should produce each consonant sound of English correctly when presented with a grapheme or phonetic symbol representing it. This phase is made up of various steps.

Step 1: Establishment of Accurate Sound Production

Phase I, step 1 is designed to evoke correct production of each target sound when the client is presented a grapheme (printed letter) or phonetic symbol representing it. Correct sound production is facilitated initially by maximal stimulation through *visual + auditory + tactile* (phonetic placement) cueing. This is referred to as level C cueing. The level of stimulation is then reduced to *visual + auditory* cueing (level B), and finally to *visual* cueing only (level A).

The clinician may use the sound production sheet (SPS) as a recording system for each stimulus modality used to achieve accurate production of each sound in isolation. The following is a brief example of how the SPS is arranged (Denham, McCabe, & Bradley, 1979):

[p]	**[b]**	**[m]**
A–1 2 3 4 5	A–1 2 3 4 5	A–1 2 3 4 5
B–1 2 3 4 5	B–1 2 3 4 5	B–1 2 3 4 5
C–1 2 3 4 5	C–1 2 3 4 5	C–1 2 3 4 5
[w]	**[t]**	**[d]**
A–1 2 3 4 5	A–1 2 3 4 5	A–1 2 3 4 5
B–1 2 3 4 5	B–1 2 3 4 5	B–1 2 3 4 5
C–1 2 3 4 5	C–1 2 3 4 5	C–1 2 3 4 5

The same arrangement is used for each consonant sound of English. The letter A refers to *visual* stimulation only, B refers to *auditory-visual* stimulation, and C refers to *auditory-visual-tactile* stimulation. The numbers 12345 refer to the total opportunities given for production of the sound at each cueing level during one session.

Level A, #1: Visual Cueing Only. The clinician presents the client with an upper- or lower-case letter (grapheme) representing the target sound and asks, "Do you know what sound this letter makes?" If the client responds "yes," then he or she is instructed to produce the sound in isolation on five successive trials. The clinician records the accuracy of the responses on the SPS using / (slash) for correct and − (minus) for incorrect. If the client responds "no" (indicating that he or she does not know what sound the symbol represents), the clinician shifts treatment to level C, which offers maximal stimulation through visual + auditory + tactile cueing.

Level C: Visual + Auditory + Tactile Cueing. The clinician uses verbal instructions along with auditory and tactile stimulation to evoke correct production of the target sound. The clinician may use any other effective method(s) to achieve sound production accuracy. This type of assistance is provided before each opportunity until four out of five correct responses are recorded. Only five trials are provided for each sound during an individual session since several other sounds are also targeted. If the client fails to reach the criterion in three sessions, a branching activity should be initiated for that sound. If the client is successful, then the clinician shifts therapy to the next modality level.

Level B: Auditory + Visual Cueing. The clinician shows the letter representing the sound and models the sound for the child to imitate (auditory + visual stimulation). The auditory-visual stimulus is modeled only once, and the child is asked to produce the sound on five consecutive trials. The accuracy criterion is five consecutive accurate responses during one session or four of five correct responses for two consecutive sessions.

Level A, #2: Visual Cueing Only. When the criterion is reached for level B, the clinician shifts treatment to level A. Only visual cueing is provided at that level through presentation of the grapheme representing the sound. The authors indicate that that level may be skipped for children under 5 years of age since most children at that age would not have established sound-symbol associations. The clinician reinforces the client's correct responses by providing verbal praise and tokens as needed.

The SPS is used with all English consonants (whether they are produced accurately or inaccurately) during the first therapy session. The procedures previously outlined are followed for training. Nonerror sounds are included in training to promote experience with the procedures and to ensure initial success. Sounds produced correctly typically reach criterion in one or two sessions, and their training is omitted in subsequent steps.

Step 2: Holding Procedure

Phase I, step 2 is known as the holding procedure. This step is appropriate for sounds that reach criterion on the sound production sheet but are not ready to progress to the syllable or word level for several sessions because of time constraints. It helps maintain the correct production of the sounds by requiring that the client provide one accurate response in modality A during every treatment session until the sound is ready for advancement to the next level.

Phase II—Transfer

The ultimate goal of phase II is that the client should use all of the error sounds accurately in conversational speech. This phase includes five steps of therapy progressing from syllables to conversational speech. The primary difference between the multiple-phoneme approach and the traditional approach is that in this approach five or more sounds are worked on during each therapy session. Also, each sound may be worked on at different linguistic levels of complexity.

Step 1: Syllable

This step is used only if the client fails to produce the word correctly in 6 out of 10 monosyllabic probe words. The probe consists of 5 words with the target sound in the initial position and 5 words with the sound in the final position. If the client passes the word probe, the syllable step is skipped and training proceeds to the word level until the client achieves the 90% accuracy criterion.

At the syllable level, the client practices the target sound with a variety of vowels including a high-front vowel /i/, a low-front vowel /æ/, a neutral vowel /ʌ/, a high-back vowel /u/, and a low-back vowel /ɑ/. McCabe and Bradley (1973, 1975) recommend using line drawings of tongue positions for each vowel accompanied by the standard spelling for that vowel.

Each target sound is practiced in both initial and final positions of syllables. The client produces the syllable 5 times after the clinician provides one auditory-visual model or one visual stimulus. The clinician aims for 25 or more responses in a 1- to 2-minute syllable task. The criterion for this step is 80% accuracy across two consecutive sessions or 90% accuracy in a single session.

Step 2: Words

After the client achieves the mastery criterion in step 1 (syllable practice), the word step is initiated. The objective at this step is accurate production of the target sound in selected words. McCabe and Bradley (1973, 1975) recommend 25 to 30 varied words (i.e., verbs, nouns, modifiers, and prepositions) that may be used later in phrases and sentences.

The client is presented with printed words or pictured stimuli representing the target word. The client is then asked to produce the target word. At this point, the clinician may accept incorrect production of nontarget phonemes.

The clinician shifts training from words to phrases and sentences when the client produces the target sound in a given position (i.e., initial, medial, or final) with 80% accuracy over two sessions or 90% accuracy in one session. If the client does not produce the target sound according to the accuracy criterion in one position, training continues at the word level for that position.

However, if the client reaches the accuracy criterion in a given position, training for the target sound in that position progresses to the next step. This may occur in children who reach accuracy criterion in the initial position but not in the final position because of the phonological process of final-consonant deletion. In that case, the clinician may abandon the multiple-phoneme approach for a more linguistic-based approach such as minimal contrast therapy or phonological process therapy (Bradley, 1989). These approaches will be discussed later in the chapter.

Step 3: Phrases and Sentences

The objective at this level is accurate word production and improved self-monitoring skills. At this point the response unit is the entire word instead of the target sound (i.e., all sounds in the word should be produced correctly). The client is asked to construct practice sentences by incorporating words taught in step 2 and adding new words as needed to complete the sentence.

For children who have a difficult time formulating phrases and sentences on their own, the clinician may model a target phrase or sentence and ask the client to repeat it. For children who can read, reading may be used to facilitate production of phrases and sentences. The clinician can use rebus symbols, Bliss symbols, or pictures to assist production in children who cannot read.

A variety of sentences (imperative, declarative, and interrogative) are practiced as a foundation for conversation in upcoming steps. If the clinician notes errors resulting from coarticulation, he or she should try to retain the same phonetic environments that facilitate correct production for additional practice sentences. As in the previous two steps, the accuracy criterion for exiting the phrase-sentence level is 80% accuracy across two consecutive sessions or 90% for one session.

Step 4: Reading/Story

The objective at this step is accurate production of the target sounds in connected utterances containing four- to six-word units. To make the task clinically efficient, it is important that the clinician select reading materials that are age-appropriate and at a comfortable reading level for the child.

For clients who are nonreaders, other activities must be used to evoke connected utterances containing four- to six-word units. McCabe and Bradley recommend the use of comic books, picture books, and sequence cards for children who are nonreaders. Also, the clinician may tell a story and ask the client to repeat it. Recently, many excellent wordless books have been published, and those may also make appropriate materials for children in this situation.

At this step, whole-word accuracy of every word spoken is expected. The criterion for moving to the next step is 80% accuracy across two consecutive sessions or 90% in one session.

Step 5: Conversation

The conversation level is the last step in the establishment phase of training. The objective at this step is accurate production of all sounds used in conversational speech. The clinician encourages discussions, descriptions, comments, questions, fact statements, identification of cause-effect relations, and talks about emotions and desires to evoke conversational output from the client. The clinician should avoid the sole use of questions and answers.

In cases in which the clinician monitors only one or two sounds that have moved to the conversation level, only those words containing the target sounds are counted as responses. When multiple target sounds need to be monitored (e.g., 10 to 12) simultaneously, the clinician may group sounds according to manner of production or place of articulation and monitor the sounds in a particular group for 3 to 5 minutes. Each group is monitored in turn for the same amount of time.

When most sounds are being monitored at the conversational level, every word spoken is counted as a response and the clinician can calculate the whole-word accuracy level as previously described. At this level, certain errors may occur because of phonetic context. It is important that the clinician note the context in which the errors occur so that the associated phrases or sentences can be used as material for additional practice. These phrases or sentences may be entered on a documentation sheet as "trouble" phrases.

The criterion at the conversational step varies a bit from the previous steps because of a necessary adjustment for younger children. For children 6 years and older, the criterion for completion of this step is 80% accuracy on all words spoken during the entire session over two consecutive sessions or 90% for one entire session. For children younger than 6 years, the authors suggest adjusting the criterion level for age according to Schmidt, Howard, and Schmidt's (1983) data on whole-word accuracy in children developing speech normally. Bradley (1989) gives an example of 69% as the accuracy criterion for 3-year-old children based on Schmidt et al.'s data.

Phase III—Maintenance

The goal of phase III is maintenance of 90% whole-word accuracy in conversational speech across various speaking situations without direct treatment or external monitoring. Bradley (1989) indicates that a 5% accuracy loss is typical for most speakers within 3 months after initial dismissal from therapy. Because of this, the accuracy criterion at this phase moves to approximately 95%. Maintenance may be accomplished by the following: (a) return clinic visits, (b) clinician visits to classrooms, (c) telephone conversations, and (d) reports from others who associate with the client (Bradley, 1989). The client's skills should be monitored for 3 months (i.e., the time span studied by McCabe and Bradley, 1975).

Summary of the Multiple-Phoneme Approach

- The multiple-phoneme approach was designed by **McCabe and Bradley** in 1975 and was based on **behavioral principles.** It was originally developed to meet the needs of clients exhibiting multiple articulation errors associated with cleft palate.

- This approach facilitates instruction on **several error** sounds during each treatment session.

- It uses a traditional training sequence but provides specific suggestions for data collection, goals and objectives, and training criteria.

- The approach is divided into **three phases:** establishment, transfer, and maintenance.

- The **establishment phase** consists of two steps, one focusing on accurate sound production and the second incorporating a holding procedure.

- The **transfer phase** has five steps that resemble the sequence of training used in the traditional approach: syllables, words, phrases and sentences, reading and storytelling, and conversation.

- The **maintenance phase** can be accomplished by (a) return clinic visits, (b) clinician visits to the classroom, (c) telephone conversations, and (d) reports from others who associate with the client.

- The client's skills should be **monitored** for **3 months** (i.e., the time span studied by McCabe and Bradley, 1975).

Paired-Stimuli Approach

The **paired-stimuli approach** to articulation therapy was first developed by Weston and Irwin in 1971. In subsequent years, Irwin and Weston (1971–1975) published a commercially available program entitled the *Paired Stimuli Kit*. This approach is highly structured and carefully sequenced to progress from words to sentences to conversation. This method of articulation training depends on the identification of a **key word** to teach correct production of a target sound in other contexts. It capitalizes on operant principles and is organized so that a single speech sound is the target at any one time. Because this program teaches one sound at a time, it is most suited for children who have sound distortions or a few articulation errors.

Step I: Word Level

At this level, a target sound is selected for remediation. The clinician must then identify four key words, two containing the target sound in the **initial position** and two containing it in the **final position** to be used in the initial stages of training. A word is considered a **key word** when the child can correctly produce the target sound in the word in at least 9 out of 10 trials. The key word should contain the target sound only once.

When key words cannot be found in the client's repertoire that meet the selection criterion (i.e., correct production of the target sound in the word in at least 9 out of 10 trials), the clinician can create key words by directly teaching them until the criterion is met. Administration of the *The Deep Test of Articulation* (McDonald, 1968) may help the clinician identify key words that facilitate correct production of the target sound.

The next step is the selection of **training words,** in which the target sound is misarticulated. The target sound should occur only once in the training words in either the initial or the final position. To qualify as a training word, the target sound should be misarticulated in two out of three productions. At least 10 training words should be found for both the initial and the final positions. (If remediation were needed in only one position, training words would be selected only for the sound in that position.)

The clinician must then select pictured stimuli that will help evoke the target productions. Because pictures serve as the stimuli, both the key words and the training words must be items that can be illustrated. The clinician fastens the **first** key word (picture) with the target sound in the **initial position** to the center of a picture board and arranges the 10 training words (pictures) around it (see Figure 8.1).

Once the picture board is arranged, the actual treatment sequence is initiated. The clinician places the picture stimuli in front of the client, points to the key word, and asks him or her to name the key word. The clinician reinforces the client's response if it is produced correctly. The likelihood that the client will produce the key word correctly is high since it must be correct in 9 of 10 probe trials to qualify as a key word.

Training Word 9	Training Word 10	Training Word 1
Training Word 8	**KEY WORD** Client: _____ Phoneme: / / Position: Initial Final	Training Word 2
Training Word 7		Training Word 3
Training Word 6	Training Word 5	Training Word 4

Figure 8.1. Paired-stimuli training sheet sample (without pictures).

At this point, the clinician points to the first training word and asks the client to name it. After the client produces the first training word, the clinician instructs the client to name the key word again. The clinician then asks the client to name another training word. Such alternation between a training word and the key word continues until a **training string** is complete. A training string is the successful pairing of the key word with each of the 10 training words.

The clinician reinforces the client's accurate productions of both the key word and training words by giving him or her a token. Misarticulations of nontarget sounds are ignored. Irwin and Weston recommend that a clinician aim for at least three training strings in a 30-minute session. The training criterion is 80% (8 out of 10) correct productions of the training words in two consecutive training strings. The clinician follows the same stimuli arrangement and training sequence for the **second** key word, but now the target is in the **final position.**

In the next stage of training, the **third** key word is taught. This is done as previously described for key words one and two; however, there is one modification. At this point, the child is instructed to say the third key word (with the target sound in the **initial position**) and a training word as a **response unit.** That is, the key word and training word are said with only a very brief pause between the two, such as *fan–five* and *fan–fist.* The clinician reinforces the client by giving him or her one token following each correct **response unit** (i.e., the target sound must be produced correctly in both the key word and the training word). The training criterion at this point is 80% (8 out of 10) **correct response units** over two successive training strings.

The **fourth** key word (with the target sound in the final position) is taught as described for key word three; however, the delivery of the reinforcement is modified. The clinician reinforces the client by giving him or her one token following **two** correct **response units** in succession. This is an FR2 schedule of reinforcement. The target sound should be produced correctly in four words (twice in the key word and once in each of the two training words). The training criterion remains the same.

When the client reaches the training criterion for the fourth key word, the next step is to conduct a probe. Probes measure the client's production accuracy in a conversational speech sample under conditions of no reinforcement. The probe criterion is at least 80% accuracy of the target sounds in conversation, with a minimum of 15 to 20 occurrences.

Step II: Sentence Level

During step II, the clinician pairs the **first** key word (target sound in initial position) with the 10 selected training words as before. At this stage, however, the clinician points to a training word and asks a question that evokes the target response in a **sentence.** For example, the clinician asks, "Did the *fan* blow the *flowers?*" and the client responds, "Yes, the *fan* blew the *flowers.*" In this example, *fan* is the selected key word, and *flowers* is 1 of the 10 training words.

The clinician reinforces correct productions with a token using an FR3 schedule of reinforcement. A single token is provided only after three **consecutive** correct sentences. A sentence is considered correct when the target sound is produced correctly in **both** the key word and the training word in the sentence. Thus, at this point the client must produce the target sound correctly in six words before receiving a reinforcer (three times in the key word and one time in each of the three training words).

The clinician continues this sequence until a **training string** is completed. At the sentence level, a training string consists of 10 questions by the clinician that help evoke the target sound in sentences and 10 sentence-level responses by the client. The clinician should adhere to the training criterion of 80% (8 out of 10) correct sentence productions over two successive training strings.

Next, the clinician uses the **second** (target sound in final position) and **third** (target sound in initial position) key words and their 10 training words to evoke sentence-level productions. At this point, the clinician asks two questions alternately, one using the **second** key word and one using the **third** key word. The client is reinforced on an FR3 schedule, as previously described. Again, the clinician should adhere to the training criterion of 8 out of 10 correct sentences over two training strings.

In the next step, the clinician asks four questions, alternately using the **first** (target sound in initial position) and **fourth** (target sound in final position) key words and their 10 training words. The schedule of reinforcement and the training criterion remain as previously described. It should be noted that Weston and Irwin's *Paired Stimuli Kit* provides appropriate questions for specific key words.

Step III: Conversation Level

In step III, the clinician performs activities that engage the child in conversation (e.g., open-ended questions about specific topics). The clinician stops the conversation when (a) the child correctly produces a target sound in four words or (b) the child incorrectly produces a target sound in any word. If the child produces the target sound incorrectly, the clinician models the correct production and asks the child to repeat it. The clinician reinforces the child verbally and through informative feedback by showing the client the scoring of correct responses.

As the child achieves the initial criterion at the conversation level, the clinician then requires the correct production of a target sound in seven words. Probes are performed when the child meets this more stringent criterion. In subsequent stages, the clinician requires the correct production of a target sound in 10 and 13 words. Again, the clinician probes at each stage as the child meets the criterion.

At this point, the clinician provides verbal praise and informative visual feedback of scoring only when all productions are correct. For all probes, the clinician takes a conversational sample. The clinician should not provide any feedback during probes. The clinician terminates training on the target sound when the child produces it correctly on 15 consecutive opportunities in conversation held on two successive treatment sessions separated by at least one day.

Summary of the Paired-Stimuli Approach

• The paired-stimuli approach was developed by Irwin and Weston (1971–1975).

• The original concept was later expanded to a commercially available program, the *Paired Stimuli Kit* (Irwin & Weston, 1971–1975).

- This approach is used to teach one speech sound at a time through the use of a **key word.**

- It is based on the principle of stimulus-response generalization.

- The approach is composed of three major steps, each consisting of various substeps.

- Step 1 consists of production practice at the word level, step 2 at the sentence level, and step 3 in conversation.

- The steps and substeps provide specific goals and objectives, training criteria, and treatment tasks and procedures.

Programmed Conditioning for Articulation: A Behavioral Approach

The principles of behavior modification have made their way to nearly every training program involving learning. In articulation treatment, the behavioral contingencies of stimulus-response-consequences can be used to shape new behaviors and teach sound productions at all levels of linguistic complexity. According to Hegde (1996b), "Elements of behavioral approaches are found in almost all programs of articulation and phonological treatment including those that are not typically described as behavioral" (p. 35).

Clinicians who are well versed in the principles of behavior modification can typically develop their own training programs for articulation treatment. However, to facilitate the training process, Baker and Ryan (1971) developed a commercially available program based on behavioral principles and programmed learning concepts. Their program, available through Monterey Learning Systems, is known as the *Programmed Conditioning for Articulation*. The general sequence of training is based on the traditional approach (discussed earlier); however, Baker and Ryan adhere very closely to the principles of programmed instruction.

The following will highlight the primary instructional phases and training steps of *Programmed Conditioning for Articulation* (PCA). The reader may refer to the original source for specific information and detailed training instructions.

General Procedures

The PCA makes use of a basic instructional pattern for all phases of the program. The clinician shows the client a stimulus item (e.g., a picture) and models the target behavior; the client provides a response; and the clinician reinforces the client's accurate production. In behavioral terms, this is well known as the stimulus-response-consequence contingency paradigm. The clinician models the target response, and the client is expected to imitate the clinician's model. Pictures, graphemes, and storytelling are also used to evoke the target responses.

Baker and Ryan recommend an average response rate of 300 productions per hour of instruction. Reinforcers are initially delivered on a continuous schedule of reinforcement (crf). The schedule of reinforcement is shifted to an intermittent schedule (50% and 10%) as the client's productions improve. The criterion for advancing from one step to another is 10 consecutive correct responses. If the client consistently produces the target response incorrectly, the clinician incorporates the use of branching activities. Branching activities are sound production tasks designed to strengthen production of the target sound at a simpler level. The criteria for shifting training to branching activities is 10 errors in a row or three consecutive sessions with an accuracy response rate of less than 80%.

Sound Evocation Programs

Sound evocation programs are provided for /s/, /r/, /l/, /θ/, /ʃ/, and /ʧ/. The clinician can use those programs to teach target sounds that are not in the client's phonetic repertoire at even the most simplistic level. General instructional suggestions for evoking other phonemes are also provided.

Establishment Phase

This first phase of training is the establishment phase. The major steps under the establishment phase are: isolation, nonsense syllables, words, phrases, sentences, contextual reading, story narration/picture description, and conversational speech. Each of these 8 steps contains a series of substeps. This phase also includes the previously described sound evocation programs and 91 branching steps.

Sound in Isolation

The goal at this point is the production of the sound at the isolation level. The client practices the sound in isolation, and his or her responses are reinforced on a continuous schedule (100% of correct responses are reinforced).

Nonsense-Syllable Level

The goal during this phase is the correct production of the target sound in nonsense syllables. The client's responses are still reinforced on a continuous schedule (100% of correct responses are reinforced). This phase contains the following substeps:

- **Substep 1** is the production of the sound in nonsense syllables with the target sound (X) in the initial position. The short vowels (a, e, i, o, u) are presented randomly—(Xa, Xe, Xi, Xo, Xu).

- **Substep 2** is the production of the sound in nonsense syllables with the target sound (X) in the final position. The short vowels (a, e, i, o, u) are presented randomly—(aX, eX, iX, oX, uX).

- **Substep 3** is the production of the sound in nonsense syllables with the target sound (X) in the medial position. The short vowels (a, e, i, o, u) are presented randomly—(aXa, eXe, iXi, oXo, uXu).

Word Level

The goal at the word level is the correct production of the target sound in words. The client's responses are reinforced on an intermittent schedule (50% of correct responses are reinforced—5 out of 10 responses). This phase also has various substeps that are followed in sequence:

- **Substep 1** is the production of the target word with X (the target sound) in the initial position.

- **Substep 2** is the production of the target word with X (the target sound) in the final position.

- **Substep 3** is the production of the target word with X (the target sound) in the medial position.

Phrase Level

The goal at this level is the correct production of the target sound in phrases (simple connected speech). The client's responses are reinforced on an intermittent schedule (50% of correct responses are reinforced). This phase has three substeps that are followed in sequence:

- **Substep 1** is the production of the word containing X (the target sound) in the initial position in 2- to 3-word phrases.

- **Substep 2** is the production of the word containing X (the target sound) in the final position in 2- to 3-word phrases.

- **Substep 3** is the production of the word containing X (the target sound) in the medial position in 2- to 3-word phrases.

Sentence Level

The goal at the sentence level is the correct production of the target sound in sentences (simple connected speech). The client's responses are still reinforced on an intermittent schedule (50% of correct responses are reinforced). This phase also contains three substeps:

- **Substep 1** is the production of the word containing X (the target sound) in the initial position in 4- to 6-word sentences.

- **Substep 2** is the production of the word containing X (the target sound) in the final position in 4- to 6-word sentences.

- **Substep 3** is the production of the word containing X (the target sound) in the medial position in 4- to 6-word sentences.

Contextual Reading Level

The goal during the contextual reading level is the correct production of the target sound in contextual reading tasks (complex connected speech). The client practices the sound in contextual reading tasks. If the client is a nonreader, the clinician goes to the story narration level, substep 2. The client's responses are reinforced on a continuous schedule (100% of correct responses are reinforced).

Story Narration/Picture Description Level

The goal of therapy at this point is the correct production of the target sound during story narration (complex connected speech). This level has two steps, which are taught in sequence:

• **Substep 1** involves the production of the target sound in story narration. The clinician instructs the client to read a story silently and then tell about what he or she just read in phrases and or complete sentences. This substep is skipped if the client is a nonreader, and therapy progresses to substep 2.

• **Substep 2** is the production of the target sound in stories upon picture presentation. The clinician presents a picture stimulus, and the client is instructed to tell a story about the picture using complete sentences. The client's responses are reinforced on a continuous schedule (50% of correct responses are reinforced).

Conversation Level

The goal at the conversation level is the correct production of the target sound in conversation or naturally occurring connected speech. Like the story narration level, the conversation level has two sequential substeps:

• **Substep 1** is the production of the target sound in naturally occurring conversation. The client's responses are again reinforced continuously (100% of correct responses are reinforced).

• **Substep 2** also involves the production of the target sound in naturally occurring speech. However, at this point the client is reinforced on an intermittent basis (only 10% of correct responses are reinforced—1 in 10 responses).

When the client reaches the set criterion for conversation level, substep 2, the clinician stops therapy and administers the criterion test. If the client is successful, the clinician shifts therapy to the transfer phase. The establishment phase may be initiated again with a new target sound or sounds.

Transfer Phase

The transfer phase is the second phase of training. It is designed to facilitate the client's production of the target sound in natural environments such as home, playground, classroom, and so forth. The first step of the transfer phase (described below) is actually initiated during the establishment phase through the provision of word lists, phrases, and sentences for home practice with a parent. Parents are instructed to work with the client at home for 5 minutes and record his or her responses for documentation.

Training at Home with Parent

At this point the goal of training is the correct production of the target sound in home activities with the client's parents. The client is reinforced on a continuous schedule (100% of correct responses are reinforced). This phase has the following five substeps:

• **Substep 1** is the production of single words containing X (the target sound). The parent provides a model for the child to imitate.

• **Substep 2** is the production of phrases containing a word with the target sound. The parent provides a model for the client to imitate.

- **Substep 3** is the production of sentences containing a word with the target sound. The parent provides a model for the client to imitate.

- **Substep 4** is production of the target sound during reading tasks or picture story narration. The client reads a story or tells a story after picture presentation.

- **Substep 5** is production of the target sound in naturally occurring conversation.

Clinician Training in Different Environments

The goal of therapy at this point is the correct production of the target sound in different physical settings with the clinician. The client's responses are reinforced on a continuous schedule (100% of correct responses are reinforced). The criterion at each step is 90% accuracy in at least 10 target responses recorded by the clinician. This phase also contains five substeps:

- **Substep 1** is the production of the target sound in conversation with the clinician outside the clinical room (outside the door).

- **Substep 2** is the production of the target sound in conversation with the clinician outside the clinical room (down the hall).

- **Substep 3** is the production of the target sound in conversation with the clinician outside the clinical room (outside the building or in another room).

- **Substep 4** is the production of the target sound in conversation with the clinician in the playground, cafeteria, or away from the school or clinic grounds.

- **Substep 5** is the production of the target sound in conversation with the clinician outside the classroom.

Training in the Classroom with Clinician and Others

The goal of therapy at this point is the correct production of the target sound in conversation with varied audiences such as the clinician, teacher, and classmates in the classroom. The client's responses are reinforced on a continuous schedule (100% of correct responses are reinforced). The criterion at each step is 90% accuracy in at least 10 target responses recorded by the clinician. This phase also contains five substeps:

- **Substep 1** is production of the target sound in conversation with the clinician in the classroom.

- **Substep 2** is production of the target sound in conversation with the clinician and the classroom teacher in the classroom.

- **Substep 3** is production of the target sound in conversation during small-group activities.

- **Substep 4** is production of the target sound in conversation during large-group activities.

- **Substep 5** is production of the target sound in conversation or monologues (e.g., "show and tell" activities in front of the class).

The client then takes a transfer criterion test. If he or she is successful, treatment progresses to the maintenance phase.

Maintenance Phase

The final phase, maintenance, is a 2-month component of the training program. The goal at this point is the correct production of the target sound in varied settings and situations and with different audiences across time. The maintenance phase has five substeps. **Substeps 1, 2, 3,** and **4** involve the production of the target sound in conversation with the clinician in once-a-week meetings during the first month. **Substep 5** is the production of the target sound in conversation with the clinician in a single meeting during the second month. The criterion for each step at this phase is 10 consecutive correct responses. The client's responses are reinforced on a continuous schedule (100% of correct responses are reinforced).

Summary of the *Programmed Conditioning for Articulation* Approach

- *Programmed Conditioning for Articulation* is a commercially available program based on the principles of behavior modification.

- This approach was developed by Baker and Ryan (1971) and is available through Monterey Learning Systems.

- It is based on the traditional approach's general sequence of training. However, Baker and Ryan adhere very closely to the principles of programmed instruction.

- General procedures used in all phases of the program follow a stimulus-response-consequence contingency paradigm. A stimulus is presented (e.g., a model or picture), the client provides a response, and the clinician reinforces the client's response.

- The program provides goals and objectives for each phase of training and specific training criteria and schedules of reinforcement.

- Baker and Ryan recommend an average response rate of 300 productions per hour for instruction.

- The level of reinforcement progresses from a continuous schedule in the initial stages of treatment to an intermittent schedule in the later stages.

- Sound evocation programs are provided for /s/, /r/, /l/, /θ/, /ʃ/, and /tʃ/ and may be used with clients who do not have those sounds in their phonetic repertoire.

- The program includes an establishment phase, a transfer phase, and a maintenance phase.

- The **establishment phase** includes the following steps: isolation, nonsense syllable, word, phrase, sentence, contextual reading, story narration, and conversation. Each step in the establishment phase includes various substeps.

- The **transfer phase** is designed to facilitate the client's production of the target sound in natural environments such as home, playground, classroom, and so forth. The major components include (a) training at home with parents, (b) training in different environments with the clinician, and (c) training in the classroom with the clinician and others.

• The **maintenance phase** is a 2-month component of the training program, which facilitates correct production of the target sound in varied settings and situations and with different audiences across time.

Distinctive Feature Approach

The distinctive feature approach is best described as an articulation treatment approach based on the distinctive features of sounds (i.e., phonemic characteristics that create linguistic contrasts between sounds and sound classes). The component parts of each phoneme (i.e., place of production, manner of articulation, voicing features, and so forth) make up its distinctive features.

The assumption behind this approach is that the child with a phonological disorder is missing distinctive features, and, thus, the goal of treatment should be to establish those missing features by teaching relevant sounds (Hegde, 1996b). Advocates of this approach theorize that as a distinctive feature is established, it will generalize from the trained exemplar to other untrained members of the sound class in which the features may be absent (Bankson & Bernthal, 1998). For example, the [**+continuant**] feature established by direct training of /f/ may generalize to /θ/, /s/, and /ʃ/. Hegde (1996b) emphasizes that more research is needed to support this theoretical assumption; it is not uncommon for something that seems logically valid to be empirically invalid.

The distinctive feature approach is most appropriate with children who exhibit multiple misarticulations that can be grouped on the basis of distinctive feature patterns. This approach is not appropriate for children whose sound distortions or errors mostly lack a definite pattern. Unlike the traditional approach or multiple phoneme approach that is credited primarily to one person, the distinctive feature approach was developed and researched by multiple investigators and thus is attributed to various people. However, some specific programs based on the concept of distinctive features have been developed, and five of those will be discussed according to their primary developers. The reader will quickly note that all of these distinctive feature programs share some characteristics. Most were developed from the early to late 1970s, with the exception of Blache's program.

McReynolds and Colleagues Program

McReynolds and Bennett (1972) developed one of the original distinctive feature programs. They developed this instructional program while investigating the nature of feature generalization. Their program consists of the following two teaching phases:

Phase 1: Nonsense syllables (initial position). Production training in this phase focuses on nonsense syllables containing the target feature in the initial position of words (e.g., the syllable /sɑ/ for the +continuant distinctive feature).

• Step 1. The child is instructed to produce a consonant in which the feature is lacking.

- Step 2. The child is instructed to contrastively produce two consonant sounds in syllables, the sound segment learned in step 1, and a second consonant selected to contrast with the first.

Phase 2: Nonsense syllables (final position). Phase 2 is similar to phase 1; however, it focuses on the production of nonsense syllables containing the distinctive feature in the final position (e.g., /ɑs/).

McReynolds and Engmann (1975) recommended that distinctive feature training be initially limited to sound units that reflect only one contrast (e.g., [s] vs. [z]). In subsequent stages of training the clinician could incorporate sound units that vary by two or more distinctive features (e.g., [s] vs. [k]).

Costello and Onstine's Program

Costello and Onstine (1976) extended McReynolds and Bennett's (1972) original program. They developed a distinctive feature program based on motor programming principles. In other words, they added a motor component to a program that was originally intended to be purely linguistic in nature. Costello and Onstine's program uses a cognitive-linguistic model for error analysis but bases intervention on a motor production approach. They selected distinctive features for training based on (a) the developmental order for the feature, (b) whether the feature is completely omitted or misused, and (c) the number of phonemes affected by the feature.

It must be noted that Costello and Onstine's program was originally a study designed to teach young children /t/ versus /θ/ and /t/ versus /s/ because the [**+continuant**] feature was not well established in their subjects. This resulted in the substitution of stops for continuants. The program was divided into nine phases:

Phase 1: Sound establishment (isolation). In phase 1 the production of /t/ versus /θ/ and /t/ versus /s/ was established.

Phase 2: Production practice in CV syllables. Phase 2 involved production of the target sound in CV contexts.

Phase 3: Production practice in VC syllables. Phase 3 was similar to phase 2, but production of the target was practiced in VC contexts.

Phases 4 & 5: Production practice in words. Phase 4 included imitation of /θ/, /t/, and /s/ in the releasing, or initial position of words. In phase 5, the sounds were imitated in the arresting or final position of words.

Phases 6 & 7: Production practice in phrases and sentences. Phase 6 included imitation of /θ/, /t/, and /s/ in releasing and arresting (initial and final) positions in words embedded in phrases and sentences. In phase 7, the sounds were practiced in sentences that were not imitated by the clinician.

Phases 8 & 9: Production in connected speech. Phase 8 involved production of /θ/, /t/, and /s/ in releasing and arresting positions in stories and conversational speech. In the final phase — phase 9 — the sound contrasts were produced in utterances used outside the clinical environment.

Weiner and Bankson's Program

Weiner and Bankson (1978) developed a program designed to teach the [**+frication**] distinctive feature in a child who substituted stops for fricatives (i.e., the child did not have the [+frication] feature in his repertoire). Their program was rather unusual in that it focused on the presence of frication only, instead of the correct production of a particular sound segment.

Unlike other researchers using the distinctive approach to therapy (e.g., McReynolds and Bennett, 1972), Weiner and Bankson did not focus training on one particular phoneme representing the distinctive feature, expecting it to generalize to other untrained sound segments. Rather, their training centered on the presence of the distinctive feature regardless of the correctness of the remaining features in the sound segments. In other words, if the child produced the target sound in error but maintained the [+frication] feature, his response was considered correct and reinforced. The program consists of three primary phases: identification, imitative production, and probing.

Identification

The first step in the training program was to develop the child's awareness of [+frication] in a number of contexts. This was done initially by introducing the concept of "dripping" sounds (stops) and "flowing" sounds (fricatives). The child was then asked to identify words that began with dripping sounds versus flowing sounds.

Imitative Production

The second step involved production training. The child was instructed to imitate fricative sounds and was reinforced for the production of [+frication] regardless of the correctness of the remaining features in the segments. In other words, the [+frication] production was considered correct and reinforced even if the target sound was not completely correct according to all of its features. For example, if the target sound was /f/, a [+frication] sound, and the child produced /h/ instead, also a [+frication sound], the child's production was reinforced. However, if the target sound was /f/ and the child produced /p/ instead, a [−frication] sound, the response was considered incorrect. This task was accomplished by having the child imitate words containing fricatives in the initial position, with such fricatives emphasized through increased duration of the initial sound (e.g., *f-f-f-ish*). Next, the child was required to judge whether the word he produced began with a dripping sound or a flowing sound. Feedback was provided for both production and identification. This step was then repeated without exaggeration of the word-initial fricative.

Probing

The last step was to present a 20-item picture-naming task in which each item began with a fricative sound. The task assessed the child's ability to produce words with the [+frication] feature appropriately regardless of the correctness of the remaining features in the sound segments. Weiner and Bankson reported that the client they followed throughout the study was able to successfully produce the [+frication] on a 20-item picture-naming task.

Blache's Approach

Blache (1989) presented a very thorough and structured approach using distinctive feature training. Discussion of Blache's complete program is beyond the scope of this section. However, the reader may refer to Blache's chapter on a distinctive feature approach to therapy in Creaghead, Newman, and Secord (1989, pp. 361–382) for more detailed information. In essence, Blache utilizes the minimal word-pairs teaching approach in four basic steps.

Step 1: Discussion of Words

Once the clinician identifies a potential word-pair contrast for a particular distinctive feature, he or she must then determine whether the child comprehends the meaning of the two words. The clinician can check for comprehension by selecting stimulus pictures that represent each of the words and asking the child to point to the corresponding picture when the word is said. For example, if the word pair selected is the letter *t* and the word *key,* the child might be asked: "Which one opens the door? Which one is a letter of the alphabet? Which one goes into a lock? Which one do you write?"

Step 2: Discrimination Testing and Training

After the clinician ensures that the client knows the meaning of the selected contrast words, the clinician tests the client's ability to perceive the feature contrast. To do this, the clinician presents one word of the selected minimal pair (e.g., *fan–pan* or *bear–pear*). The child is instructed to point to the picture that corresponds to the word the clinician has named. A criterion of seven consecutive correct responses is used to establish perception of the contrasting word pairs. Blache (1989) indicates that the probability of guessing is very low when such a stringent criterion is used.

Step 3: Production Training

After the clinician ascertains that the client can discriminate between the selected minimal pair words, therapy is shifted to the production of the features contrast. In this step, the child is instructed to say the word. The clinician then points to the picture of the word corresponding to the child's production (e.g., if the child says "pan," the clinician points to the picture of a pan; if the child says "fan," the clinician points to the picture of a fan). Since the minimal pair words include the child's typical error production and the target production, he or she should always be able to correctly pronounce one word of the pair. The child may or may not produce the other word in the pair.

Step 4: Carryover Training

When the child can pronounce the target word, the word is included in longer and more complex linguistic environments. Initially, the word may be paired with the indefinite article *a* in varied phonetic contexts and then in two-word phrases. When the child produces the target word in two-word utterances, utterances are gradually made longer and longer. The carrier phrases "Touch the . . ." and "Point to the . . ." may be used to facilitate meaningful productions while the target feature is practiced. The final phase is the use of the word in meaningful situations, social situations, and in the school and home.

The child is given a word book containing all the target words that have been taught. Parents are encouraged to practice the productions of such words with their child in the home setting. While they are encouraged to praise the child for good productions, at no moment are they instructed to correct the child's speech. If the child's parents do not appear motivated to practice the target productions at home, "an educational counseling program is instituted to develop better motivational reinforcement for the child and improve monitoring behavior on the part of the parent" (Blache, 1989, p. 369).

Summary of the Distinctive Feature Approach

* The distinctive feature approach is an articulation treatment approach based on a distinctive feature analysis.

* It was designed to teach a child the missing distinctive features that may be leading to his articulation or phonological disorder.

* Distinctive features are established by teaching the relevant sounds.

* The theory is that as a distinctive feature is established, it will generalize from the trained exemplar to untrained members of the sound class in which that feature is absent. Further research is needed to substantiate that theoretical assumption.

* The distinctive feature approach is most appropriate with children exhibiting multiple misarticulations that can be grouped on the basis of distinctive feature patterns.

* The approach is not appropriate for children who primarily display sound distortions or errors lacking a definite pattern.

* The approach was developed and researched by several investigators.

* Specific programs based on the concept of distinctive features include McReynolds and colleagues' program, Costello and Onstine's program, Weiner and Bankson's program, and Blache's program. Although each program has unique features, they all share many concepts.

Cycles Approach

Hodson and Paden (1983, 1991) advanced an articulation treatment approach that combines linguistic and motor-oriented approaches to remediation. Their approach, commonly known as the **cycles approach,** was designed for severely unintelligible children who exhibited the use of several phonological processes. The cycles approach targets for instruction certain phonological patterns that are lacking in the client's repertoire. The reader may consult Hodson (1989) or Hodson and Paden's text *Targeting Intelligible Speech: A Phonological Approach to Remediation* (second edition, 1991) for extensive details on the cycles remediation approach to articulation therapy.

   The general procedures included in the cycles treatment approach are as follows (Hodson & Paden, 1983, 1991; Hodson, 1989):

   1. **Stimulation**—Use of auditory, tactile, and visual stimulation cues to facilitate awareness of the target patterns. The child is made aware of the auditory, tactile, and visual characteristics of the target sound.

2. **Production training**—Participation in production training, also referred to as kinesthetic stimulation, to evoke sound productions that are incompatible with occurrence of the phonological process selected for remediation, so that the operation of the process is reduced in the child's speech.

3. **Semantic awareness contrasts**—Minimal pair training is used to increase the client's awareness of the semantic contrast between his or her typical (incorrect) production and the target production.

The remediation program is planned around cycles, thus the name *cycles approach*. Hodson (1986a) defined a **cycle** as a "period of time during which all phonological patterns in need of remediation are facilitated in succession" (p. 41). A cycle is also defined as the "time period required for the child to successfully focus for 2 to 6 hr on each of his or her basic deficient patterns" (Hodson & Paden, 1991, p. 96). *Patterns* refer to the phonological processes or phonological skills targeted for remediation or reduction (e.g., final-consonant deletion, syllable deletion, stopping, velar fronting). Hodson (1989) emphasized that treatment cycles can range from 5 or 6 weeks to 15 or 16 weeks, depending on the client's number of deficient patterns and the number of stimulable phonemes within each pattern.

Hodson and Paden offer a very detailed and elaborate treatment program. The following sections highlight their remediation approach; however, the reader is referred to Hodson and Paden (1991) and Hodson (1989) for further information.

Identification of Target Patterns

The first step is to assess the client's phonological performance to identify the patterns affecting his or her intelligibility. This may be done by administering the *Assessment of Phonological Processes–Revised* (APP–R) (Hodson, 1986a). The APP–R incorporates the use of objects and questions to evoke 50 spontaneous naming responses and continuous speech. A percentage of occurrence for several phonological processes is calculated and used to derive phonological deviancy scores and severity ratings. These scores may help the clinician develop a plan of therapy.

Selection of Target Patterns and Phonemes

Hodson and Paden (1991) believe that the primary concern of remediation should be to facilitate the "broad" elements the child is missing that are fundamental for making his or her speech more intelligible (pp. 97–98). Therefore, the clinician should arrange a hierarchy of phonological patterns that the child demonstrated at least 40% of the time on the *Assessment of Phonological Processes–Revised*. The phonological pattern that is the most stimulable is considered the optimal remediation target so that the child can achieve immediate success. Remediation then shifts to the next most stimulable pattern until all priority patterns are stimulated during one cycle.

Hodson (1989) and Hodson and Paden (1991) identify the following as *potential* **primary target patterns or phonemes:**

- **early developing phonological patterns**—word-initial and word-final singletons (stops, nasals, glides), utterances containing two or three syllables, CVC and VCV word structures;

- **posterior/anterior contrasts**—velar stops (/k/ and /g/), alveolar stops (/t/ and /d/), glottal fricative (/h/);

- **/s/ clusters**—word-initial /s/ clusters (/sp/, /st/, /sm/, /sn/, /sk/) and word-final /s/ clusters (/ts/, /ps/, /ks/);

- **liquids**—/l/ and /r/ phonemes, velar-liquid clusters (/kl/, /gl/, /kr/, /gr/), alveolar-liquid clusters (/tr/, /dr, /sl/), labial-liquid clusters (/pl/, /bl/, /fl/, /pr/, /br/, /fr/), and postvocalic /ɚ/.

Hodson and Paden (1991) also designate some secondary target patterns. These are targeted after the client demonstrates: (a) acquisition of all early developing phoneme classes (nasal, stops, and glides), basic word structures, and posterior or anterior contrasts; (b) suppression of the gliding process for production-practice words that contain liquids; and (c) emergence of stridency and some consonant clusters in spontaneous speech. Secondary target patterns may include **voicing contrasts, vowel contrasts, singleton stridents,** other **consonant clusters,** and **residual context-related processes** such as assimilation, metathesis, reduplication, and idiosyncratic rules.

In addition to primary and secondary target patterns, Hodson and Paden identify some **advanced target patterns.** They indicate that these are usually appropriate for upper-elementary school-age children experiencing problems with **multisyllabic words** and **complex consonant sequences.**

It should be emphasized that although Hodson and Paden provide potential primary, secondary, and advanced remediation targets, actual target patterns will vary according to each child's individual performance and unique needs. However, they do emphasize that certain patterns are inappropriate as primary targets for unintelligible children (e.g., voiced-final obstruents, final /ŋ/, weak-syllable deletion, and *th* phonemes) since phonologically normal children also demonstrate alterations of these patterns.

Structure of Remediation Cycles

Once the clinician selects target patterns appropriate for the client, the actual remediation process is initiated. Again, the remediation process is organized around cycles. Target patterns are facilitated via stimulation (auditory, tactile, visual) and production training of phonemes and the use of minimal pairs at the appropriate stage of therapy. Hodson (1989) offered the following suggestions for treating target patterns during cycles:

1. Each phoneme exemplar within a target pattern should be trained for approximately 60 minutes per cycle before shifting to the next phoneme in that pattern and then on to other phonological patterns. A cycle can be a single 60-minute session, two 30-minute sessions, or three 20-minute sessions.

2. Desirably, stimulation should be provided for two or more target phonemes (in successive weeks) within a pattern before changing to the next target pattern. In essence, each deficient phonological pattern is stimulated for 2 hours or more within each cycle.

3. Only one phonological pattern should be targeted during any one session so that the client has an opportunity to focus. Also, patterns should not be intermingled initially in the target words.

4. A cycle is complete when all target phonological patterns have been taught.

5. After one cycle has been completed, a second cycle is initiated that will cover those patterns that have not yet emerged or are in need of further instruction.

6. At least three to six cycles of phonological remediation, involving 30 to 40 hours of instruction (40 to 60 minutes per week), are usually required for a client to become intelligible.

Instructional Sequence for Remediation Sessions

Hodson and Paden's (1991) remediation approach is organized around cycles, as already described. The individual sessions also follow a specific instructional sequence. Hodson and Paden have used this instructional sequence in their university phonology program, but they emphasize that it can be adapted for use in schools, clinics, and hospitals (depending on the frequency and length of treatment sessions). The sequence is as follows:

1. **Review of previous session.** At the beginning of each session, the prior week's production practice word cards are reviewed, unless a new pattern is initiated during the cycle. If the target patterns are changed, the previous session's cards are set aside for a later cycle.

2. **Auditory bombardment.** Auditory bombardment is provided through slight amplification, usually with an auditory trainer, for about 2 minutes. The child, who is wearing headphones, simply listens while the clinician slowly reads approximately 12 words containing the target sound. The clinician may demonstrate the child's error and contrast it with the target. The list of words is repeated twice if the client remains attentive. At no point during this activity is the child allowed to repeat the target words. At the end of the auditory bombardment activity, the child is allowed to repeat one or two words into the microphone from a different list containing possible production practice words.

3. **Target word cards.** The client draws, colors, or pastes pictures of three to five target words on large index cards. The name of the picture is written on each card. The picture cards are controlled for phonetic environment.

4. **Production practice.** The client participates in production practice activities through game-based activities. The client is expected to have a very high success rate in terms of correct production. Shifting experiential-play activities every 5 to 7 minutes helps to maintain a child's interest in repetition of the target words. The client is also given the opportunity to use target words in conversation.

Production practice includes auditory, tactile, and visual stimulation for correct production at the word level. Usually five words per target sound are used in a single session, and the client is instructed to produce the words. A variety of games are used in each session. These activities are the heart of an instructional session.

5. **Stimulability probing.** Prior to ending the session, the target phoneme for a specific pattern to be addressed during the next session is selected. The selection of the phoneme is based on the child's performance on stimulability testing. Modeling, slight amplification, and cueing may be provided during such testing.

6. **Auditory bombardment.** Auditory bombardment is repeated using the 12-item word list from the beginning of the session. Again, slight amplification is provided, and the child is not allowed to repeat the listed words.

7. **Home program.** Parents or significant others are instructed to read the 12-item word list used in the auditory bombardment task once a day. The child is also instructed to review the target word list by naming the picture cards for the week at least once daily. The time devoted to this activity each day may be as minimal as 2 minutes. Involvement of the parents or significant others in the home is viewed as an extremely important component of the program for carryover of the learned skills.

Selection of Production Practice Words

It is important to select practice words that will maximize the client's performance, especially in the early stages of treatment. If practice words are not selected with care, the client may experience significant failure and associated frustration that could have been easily prevented. For example, if the remediation target is elimination of final-consonant deletion, it is wise to initially select practice words that are CVC in structure versus more complex, multisyllabic words such as *telephone*. As treatment progresses and the client's skills improve, the practice words may increase in complexity. Hodson (1989) suggests the following in selecting practice words:

• Select words versus nonsense syllables for production practice.

• If possible, use monosyllabic words with facilitative phonetic contexts during the initial cycles.

• Avoid words containing phonemes produced at the same place of articulation as the substitute phoneme during early cycles. For example, *cat, can, kiss, kite, goat,* and *gun* would be inappropriate practice words for remediation of velar fronting.

• It is desirable to use words for which actual objects can be incorporated, especially for preschool children.

• Production practice words should be appropriate for each child's vocabulary level.

Remediation Activities

Hodson and Paden (1991) recommend the use of experiential-play activities, minimal contrasting pairs, and confrontation activities as part of the remediation sessions. **Experiential-play activities** are structured so that they are reinforcing for the child. Examples of such activities are the *flashlight game* (finding picture cards with a flashlight and naming each card), *fishing, bowling,* and *tic-tac-toe.* Clinicians may use their own knowledge and creativity to develop activities that are age-appropriate and reinforcing for each child. Hodson (1989) emphasizes that activities should be pragmatically oriented and provides an example of a student clinician who used a camera to evoke the target cluster /sm/ in the word *smile.*

Minimal contrasting pairs (details of which will be discussed later in the chapter) can be incorporated into therapy when the child has "sufficient skills to experience success and not be frustrated" (Hodson, 1986a, p. 51). Minimal pairs may help the child recognize the semantic difference between the target word production and his or her typical production.

Summary of the Cycles Approach

- The cycles approach was developed by Hodson and Paden (1983).

- It is a linguistic and motor-oriented approach.

- This approach was designed for severely unintelligible children and uses several phonological processes.

- The general procedure consists of sound awareness **stimulation** through auditory, tactile, and visual cues; **production training;** and **semantic awareness** contrast training.

- A remediation program is planned around cycles—periods of time during which all phonological patterns in need of remediation are facilitated in succession.

- Treatment cycles range from 5 or 6 weeks to 15 or 16 weeks, depending on the client's number of deficient patterns and the number of stimulable phonemes within each pattern.

- Target patterns for remediation may be identified via administration of the *Assessment of Phonological Processes–Revised* (Hodson, 1986a).

- **Primary** potential target patterns include (a) early developing phonological patterns, (b) posterior/anterior contrasts, (c) /s/ clusters, and (d) liquids.

- **Secondary** patterns include voicing contrasts, vowel contrasts, singleton stridents, other consonant clusters, and other residual context-related processes.

- Each **remediation session** includes a review period, auditory bombardment, color and paste activity with target word cards, production practice, stimulability probing, a second period of auditory bombardment, and home activities.

- Hodson and Paden emphasize the importance of remediation activities such as experiential-play activities, the use of minimal contrasting pairs, and confrontation activities.

Phonological Knowledge Approach

The **phonological knowledge approach** assumes that children's *knowledge* of the phonological rules of the adult system is reflected in their productions. This approach was developed by Elbert and Gierut and presented in their text *Handbook of Clinical Phonology: Approaches to Assessment and Treatment* (1986). The reader may consult Elbert and Gierut's book for more detailed information.

In essence, the authors propose that the greater the consistency of correct productions in varied contexts, the higher the level of phonological knowledge. Likewise, the lower the consistency of correct productions, the lower the level of phonological knowledge. Unlike many approaches that begin treatment with the most stimulable sounds, the phonological knowledge approach begins treatment with sounds that reflect the least knowledge and ends with those that reflect the greatest degrees of knowledge. The following reflects the major components of the phonological knowledge approach.

Obtain a Representative Sample

The first step in deciding which sounds are appropriate intervention targets is to obtain a representative speech sample that will permit analysis of the child's use of sounds in context. The strategies discussed in the assessment chapters may be used to evoke a connected speech sample from the child. Elbert and Gierut recommend tape-recording the sample so that the child's utterances can be phonetically transcribed at a later time. The child's utterances may also be "glossed" or repeated so that the target productions are known during later analysis.

The spontaneous speech sample may be supplemented with story retelling activities, standard articulation tests, and contextual testing. In essence, these combined activities should: (a) sample all of the sounds of English, (b) sample the sounds in all word positions, (c) sample the sounds in different words to determine the consistency of production, and (d) sample each word more than once to determine the variability in production.

In addition to the connected speech sample and single-word productions, the clinician should sample **potential minimal word pairs** to determine if the child is using sounds contrastively (e.g., *boat–bow, fat–pat,* and *key–tea*). Furthermore, **morphophonemic alterations** (e.g., *pig–piggie, dog–dogs, run–running, stop–stopped*) should be evoked to determine if such rules are operating or affecting the child's sound productions.

Analyze the Sample

The clinician's next step is to analyze the sample obtained from the child. Several components should be carefully examined.

Determine the Distribution of Sounds

The sample is analyzed so that the child's **phonetic inventory** is identified. A phonetic inventory refers to all of the sounds the child can make regardless of their linguistic correctness in relation to the target sound. The clinician also identifies the child's **phonemic inventory.** A phonemic inventory includes only those sounds that the child uses contrastively or those that signal a difference in meaning. The use of minimal word-pair productions (e.g., *mop* and *hop*) can help the clinician establish a phonemic inventory. The clinician then determines the **distribution of sounds** that are part of the child's phonemic inventory. The clinician notes whether sounds are used contrastively in all word positions and for all target morphemes.

Determine the Use of Phonological Rules

The clinician identifies the child's use of **static phonological rules** (also known as **phonotactic constraints**). Linguistically, phonotactic constraints restrict the occurrence of certain sounds (in some word positions) and sound sequences. Elbert and Gierut identified three phonotactic constraints that may operate in a child's sound system: (a) positional constraint—production of a sound only in specific contexts or positions); (b) inventory constraint—restriction of certain sounds in the child's sound system; and (c) sequence constraint—restriction of certain sound sequence combinations.

The child's **dynamic phonological rules** are also determined. "Dynamic rules alter the production of sounds by either adding, deleting, or changing segments in specific contexts or environments" (Elbert & Gierut, 1986, p. 56). Two types of dynamic rules include **allophonic rules** and **neutralization rules.** Allophonic rules refer to the phonetic variations in the production of a particular sound. A child who has operating allophonic rules can produce one phoneme in several different ways (allophonic variations). Neutralization rules describe the child's merging of two phonemes into a single phonetic production. In other words, the child can produce two sounds correctly in one position but collapses the phonemes into one phonetic production in a specific context. Elbert and Gierut offer an example of a child who can produce the velar sounds [k] and [g] correctly in prevocalic positions (e.g., *cut, goat,* or *comb*) but collapses the two into one production in postvocalic positions (e.g., [dʌk] for both *duck* and *dug* and [pɪk] for both *pig* and *pick*).

Determine the Nature of the Child's Lexical Representations

During this step, the goal is to determine whether the child's "lexical representation is similar to . . . [or] different from the adult target" (Elbert & Gierut, 1986, p. 58). The child's lexical representations, or actual productions, are considered adultlike if they correspond to the adult target. The child's productions must be phonemic as adult productions are. That can be determined by the production of minimal-pair words or morphophonemic alterations, which reveal sounds as contrastive elements.

The child's productions are considered nonadultlike when they are unlike the adult target. In essence, the child's productions are not phonemic if there is no evidence that they are being used contrastively.

Rank the Child's Productive Phonological Knowledge

The clinician creates a **hierarchical arrangement** of sound productions that reflect least knowledge (misarticulations in all word positions and in all morphemes) to most knowledge (no misarticulations). Elbert and Gierut (1986) illustrate this arrangement in figure form as a "decision tree." The reader is referred to Elbert and Gierut (1986, pp. 61–63) for a detailed description of their hierarchical arrangement.

Select Treatment Sounds and Order of Treatment

Target sounds for treatment are chosen based on the child's productive phonological knowledge. The clinician can begin treatment by targeting sounds that reflect the least knowledge first and moving up through the hierarchy to sounds that reflect the most knowledge, or vice versa. Unlike most treatment programs that advocate the selection of sounds that are the most stimulable, Elbert and Gierut (1986) recommend that therapy begin with sounds that demonstrate the least phonological knowledge and progress to sounds that reflect the most knowledge. They highlight the benefits of generalization "across the entire sound system" if such an approach is taken (p. 64).

Treatment Procedures

Elbert and Gierut recommend the use of **minimal- or maximal-pair contrast training** to teach the selected target sounds. In contrast training, the clinician selects pairs of words consisting of a target sound and a contrast sound. The target sound is the adult model while the contrast sound is typically the child's error production. When minimal pairs (word pairs that differ by only one phoneme) cannot be found, the clinician may use *near minimal pairs* (word pairs that differ by more than one sound). The details of minimal-pair and maximal-pair training are described later in this chapter.

The sequence of training in Elbert and Gierut's approach progresses from imitative to spontaneous productions. During the imitation phase, the clinician primarily makes use of drill to train the target sound; the clinician presents a model of the contrast word pair for the child to imitate. To evoke spontaneous productions, the clinician may use drill, sorting, and matching activities. In drill, the client is asked to name minimal-picture pairs upon confrontation. In sorting, the child is first instructed to name both pictures in the minimal pair and then is asked to place each picture in its representative target or contrast sound pile. The clinician may also ask the child to match one picture with its minimal pair; the child is presented with several pictures and is then instructed to select one, name it, and find its minimal-pair match.

To promote generalization and maintenance, it is important for the clinician to vary the context of sound productions, select child-specific stimulus items, and loosely structure the treatment environment in later stages. In addition, the clinician needs to monitor the client's daily progress and progress over time.

Summary of the Phonological Knowledge Approach

- The phonological knowledge approach was developed by Elbert and Gierut (1986).

- Elbert and Gierut proposed that the greater the consistency of correct productions in varied contexts, the higher the level of phonological knowledge by the child. Likewise the greater the inconsistency of correct productions in varied contexts, the lower the level of phonological knowledge.

- A representative sample is collected that permits an analysis of the child's use of sounds in contexts.

- The spontaneous speech sample is supplemented with spontaneous single-word productions evoked through picture- and object-naming activities. Single-word productions should: (a) sample all target English sounds, (b) sample target sounds in all word positions, (c) sample the sound in different words to determine the consistency of production, and (d) sample each word more than once to determine the variability in production.

- The collected language sample is analyzed to: (a) determine the distribution of sound, (b) determine the child's use of phonological rules, and (c) determine the nature of the child's lexical representations.

- A hierarchical arrangement of the sound productions that reflect the least phonological knowledge to the most phonological knowledge is made.

• Target sounds with the least degree of phonological knowledge are selected as initial targets. Treatment then progresses to sounds that reflect the most knowledge.

• Elbert and Gierut recommend the use of minimal-pair training to teach the selected target sounds.

• The sequence of training progresses from imitative to spontaneous productions through drill, sorting, and matching activities.

• Generalization and maintenance are promoted by varying the context of sound production, selecting child-specific stimulus items, and loosely structuring the treatment environment in later stages. The clinician also monitors the client's daily progress and progress across time.

Contrast Therapy Approach

The **contrast approach** is a "cognitive-linguistic" approach to the treatment of articulation and phonological disorders. It has been incorporated into many treatment programs, including Blache's distinctive feature approach, Hodson and Paden's cycles approach, and Elbert and Gierut's phonological knowledge approach. This approach is most frequently used in remediating phonological processes, but it may be integrated into any treatment in which a contrast can be made between the target production and the child's typical (error) production. The goal is to increase the child's awareness of the semantic difference between his or her error production and the adult model.

Other names associated with this approach include **minimal-pair contrast therapy, minimal-pair therapy, minimal-pair approach, meaningful word contrastive pairs, near minimal-pair approach,** and **maximal contrast approach.** Regardless of the name used, the major concept behind this approach is the use of word pairs to form a linguistically meaningful contrast between the target sound(s) and the child's error productions. Because many researchers have investigated and contributed to this approach, a specific person's name is not usually associated with it.

The contrast therapy approach can be subdivided into two major categories: (a) **minimal contrast training,** and (b) **maximal contrast training.** Although similar, the approaches differ primarily in the level of phonemic contrast between the words in the selected pair(s). As the name implies, in minimal-pair training the contrast between the words in a pair is minimal, in that the phonemes typically differ by only one or two features (e.g., *bat–pat, four–pour,* and *tea–key*). On the other hand, in maximal-pair training the word pairs have multiple phonemic feature contrasts or maximal opposition (e.g., *chain–lane, can–fan,* and *gear–shear*). They usually vary by at least two features. Although the two systems are similar in concept, minimal-pair training is more commonly used. Investigators have reported positive changes in children's phonological skills through the use of this approach (Weiner, 1981; Elbert & Gierut, 1986; Gierut, 1989, 1990). The following will describe the general procedures in the use of minimal pairs; the procedures can be extended to maximal-pair training with some modifications.

Although a variety of minimal word pairs can be formed randomly, most clinicians use word pairs for training that contrast the child's typical (error) production and the target production. For example, if the child fronts velar consonants, substitutions such as *tea* for *key* and *date* for *gate* may result. The clinician would then select pictures that represent the minimal word pair as stimulus items (e.g., a picture illustrating *tea* and *key*). The child's typical production does not always result in a meaningful word, however. For example, a child who fronts velar consonants may produce [tau] for *cow,* and obviously [tau] does not have meaning in the English language. Because minimal contrast training is linguistic in nature, it is important to use productions that are semantically meaningful. In such cases, the clinician can use his or her creativity and grant such "nonsense" words meaning (e.g., the child may be told that [tau] is the name of a selected animal). It is recommended that the clinician select 8 to 10 word pairs representing the contrasts.

Recently, Goldstein and Gierut (1998) questioned the common practice of pairing the target sound with its corresponding error production as previously described. They question the logic in a treatment approach that places emphasis on the incorrect substitute when the goal of treatment is to eliminate such error productions. Other recent investigations (Gierut, 1989, 1990, 1991, 1992; Gierut & Neumann, 1991) have shown that an alternate form of minimal-pair treatment can be even more effective than the conventional method. In the alternative method, the target sound is paired with a correct sound from the child's repertoire rather than the corresponding error substitute. Through such practice the primary goal of this approach of teaching meaningful contrasts is maintained while the continual "practice" of the error production is eliminated. Which way this approach will go will greatly depend on the continuation of such research.

Perceptual Training

Minimal-pair training can focus on the child's perception of the linguistic contrasts or the production of the contrasts, or both. In perceptual training, the clinician begins by selecting the word pairs that represent the target contrast. The clinician then places both pictures in the word pair in front of the client and asks him or her to "point to the _____." For example, if the target contrast is open syllables versus closed syllables with a child who deletes final consonants, word pairs such as *bee–beat, see–seat,* and *bow–boat* can be used. The clinician tells the child, "I want you to show me the *bow.* Point to the bow. Perfect. Now I want you to show me the *boat.* Point to the boat please. That was great."

Perceptual training is most appropriate with children who actually display difficulties identifying the difference between the words in the pair. It should not precede production training if the clinician has clear evidence that the child can perceive the difference between the words, except as a quick introductory activity to production training.

Production Training

In production training, the child is required to verbally produce the selected minimal pairs. The clinician analyzes the client's misarticulations and selects word pairs that reflect the contrast between the substituted or deleted sound and the target sound. The word pairs are selected for remediation of the child's phonological processes or error patterns. In the previous example of final-consonant deletion, the clinician may select word pairs such as *bow–boat, bee–beet, toe–toad, pie–pine,* and so forth. The same approach may be used with a child who substitutes one sound for another as in [θ/s]. Word pairs such as *so–though, sick–thick,* and *sought–thought* may be appropriate in that case. The clinician then obtains pictures that illustrate the words in the selected pairs. Typically, 8 to 10 word pairs depicting the contrast are recommended. The training sequence may be structured as follows:

1. The clinician places the word pairs in front of the child, models both the target and the contrast words, and asks the child to imitate them.

2. The clinician provides several opportunities for the production of the target and contrast words during imitative trials.

3. The clinician reinforces the client for correct production of the target and the contrast words.

4. The clinician then asks the client to spontaneously name the pictures. To introduce the activity, the following sequence may be used (assuming that the child can perceive the contrast):

CLINICIAN:	"Joey, we're gonna play a little game. I'm gonna show you these two pictures, and then I want you to name the one that you want to take from me. Let me show you first. I'll give you these, and then I'll ask you for one. Joey, give me the picture of *bee*."
CHILD:	"Here you go"—hands clinician the picture of *bee*.
CLINICIAN:	"Good. Now give me the picture of *beet*."
CHILD:	"Here it is"—hands clinician the picture of *beet*.
CLINICIAN:	"Thank you. You're doing perfect. Now I want you to give me the picture that I point to as I say it. Okay, let's try it again. Joey, give me the picture of *bee*"—while pointing to the picture of bee.
CHILD:	"Here you go"—hands clinician picture of *bee*.
CLINICIAN:	"Now I want the picture of *bee*"—while purposely pointing to the picture of *beet*.
CHILD:	[with look of confusion] "No, you did it wrong."
CLINICIAN:	"Oh, silly me, did I say that wrong? Let me try it again. Joey, give me the picture of *beet*"—while pointing to the picture of *beet*.
CHILD:	"Here you go"—hands clinician picture of *beet*. "You did it right now."
CLINICIAN:	"Thank you. I'm glad I got it right this time. I remembered to put the *t* at the end, didn't I?"

5. At this point the clinician instructs the client, "Say the name of the picture that <u>you</u> want and point to it at the same time. Do it just like I showed you." The client is given the picture of the word that he verbalizes. For example, if he verbalizes *bee* but points to *beet,* the clinician gives him the picture of *bee*. The client may indicate that he did not want that picture by saying, "No, not that one." The clinician provides the child with appropriate corrective feedback such as, "Oh, you

meant to say *beet,* but it came out *bee.* If you want to say *beet,* you need to put the *t* sound at the end. Try it again: *beet, beet, beet.*" If the client says *beet* correctly, he is given the picture of *beet* and, if necessary, a tangible reinforcer such as a token.

The clinician may be extremely creative in the way minimal-pair production training is sequenced. In our experience, sometimes the client's responses dictate the clinician's reaction and sometimes vice versa. The training session should be well planned, but the clinician should allow for some flexibility. It must also be noted that the above sequence presumed that the client had the motor ability to produce [t] in the final position to contrast the words *bee* and *beet.* The clinician should always ensure that the client is able to produce the target sound in the selected words, or minimal-pair training activities may be counterproductive and extremely frustrating for the child (and the clinician). This is based on our own clinical experience with minimal-pair training.

As indicated earlier, a second category of contrast therapy is **maximal-pair** training. In maximal-pair training the word pairs have multiple (maximal) phonemic contrasts. The clinician may use the treatment procedures previously described; however, the target word pairs differ by several features.

Summary of the Contrast Therapy Approach

• The contrast therapy approach is a "cognitive-linguistic" approach to the treatment of articulation and phonological disorders.

• This approach has been incorporated into many treatment programs including Blache's distinctive feature approach, Hodson and Paden's cycles approach, and Elbert and Gierut's phonological knowledge approach.

• This approach is used most frequently in remediating phonological processes, but it can be integrated into any treatment in which a contrast can be made between the target production and the child's error production.

• The goal of the contrast approach is to increase the child's awareness of the semantic difference between his or her error productions and the adult model. Recent investigations have questioned the common practice of contrasting the target production with the child's error production.

• The contrast approach can be subdivided into two major categories: (a) minimal contrast training, and (b) maximal contrast training.

• Contrast training can focus on the child's perception of the linguistic contrasts or the child's production of the contrasts, or both.

Research Support and Further Research Needs

There is a paucity of empirical research to support the effectiveness of the many treatment approaches discussed in this chapter. Some of the more popular and widely used programs offer extensive anecdotal data but no conclusive evidence demonstrating their efficacy. The **traditional approach** is generally considered an effective approach because it has withstood the test of time and has helped clinicians meet the needs of many clients with articulation disorders. However, despite its longevity, the many components of that program have not been evaluated. In recent years, the need for auditory discrimination training has been challenged, and the emphasis of starting therapy at the isolation level in all clients has been questioned. Likewise, no controlled studies have been conducted to evaluate the effectiveness of **sensorimotor approaches** to articulation treatment. Shine and Proust's (1982) sensorimotor articulation program does recommend the use of a strict stimulus-response-stimulus (S-R-S) treatment paradigm based on the principles of learning and programmed instruction. Such principles have repeatedly been proven effective in the treatment of articulation disorders. However, the underlying basis for the program of using facilitative phonetic contexts in gradually more complex syllables has not been evaluated.

The **multiple-phoneme approach** does offer some limited research support. McCabe and Bradley (1975), developers of the program, found statistically significant gains in the articulatory proficiency of 44 clients aged 5 to 14 on the *Arizona Articulation Proficiency Scale* and a specially designed articulation protocol. Further support for the program was offered by Black (1972). Black reported an 80% dismissal rate of a public school caseload during the first year the multiple-phoneme approach was used, in comparison to a 20% dismissal rate the previous year when the program was not used. However, these data, although supportive of the program, lacked adequate controls and are not conclusive evidence for the effectiveness of the multiple-phoneme approach.

A few studies report that teaching sounds with specific features may result in generalized production of untreated sounds that share the same features (Costello & Onstine, 1976; McReynolds & Bennett, 1972; Weiner & Bankson, 1978). Generalized responding is the underlying assumption of many **distinctive feature approaches.** Other studies have failed to obtain significant generalization, however, and generalized productions have often been variable across subjects. The number of subjects in these treatment studies have been few, and only a few features have been clinically established. Therefore, it is difficult to make a comprehensive evaluation of the clinical usefulness of the distinctive feature approach to treatment. Additional data are needed to evaluate its effectiveness.

Hodson and Paden's **cycles approach,** although widely used, also lacks experimental research supporting its effectiveness. The data offered by the authors are primarily anecdotal and based on uncontrolled clinical interventions. This approach is essentially a package of various components. Which components make the most change in the child's articulatory and phonological skills cannot be determined until controlled comparative evaluations are made.

Of all the treatment approaches addressed, the **contrast therapy approach** enjoys the most research support of its effectiveness (Ferrier & Davis, 1973; Weiner, 1981; Elbert & Gierut, 1986; Gierut, 1989, 1990, 1991, 1992; Gierut & Neumann, 1991).

In essence, there is a need for more and better controlled treatment studies, in which treatment is compared with no treatment either in group designs or single-subject designs. As indicated earlier, most available studies are case studies. A few experimental studies are available, but they often use inadequate controls. There is a strong need for treatment efficacy studies that establish the independent effects of different treatment procedures. In the next stage of research, comparative evaluations of treatment approaches should be conducted. In the group design approach, multiple treatments with multiple groups may be evaluated. In the single-subject approach, alternating treatment designs may be used to compare the relative effects of different treatments. We already have more than a few therapies. But because we do not know the comparative effectiveness of treatment procedures, we do not have an empirical basis on which to select treatments. In the absence of such data, clinicians select treatment procedures based on extraneous factors (e.g., the method in which he or she was trained, the clinician's own treatment philosophy, the practicality of the approach). Clinicians should minimally strive to keep up with the latest research documenting the effectiveness or ineffectiveness of the treatment programs they incorporate into their own practice.

References

Acevedo, M. (1991, November). *Spanish consonants among groups of Head Start children*. Paper presented at the annual convention of the American Speech-Language-Hearing Association, Atlanta, GA.

Air, H., Wood, A. S., & Neils, J. R. (1989). Considerations for organic disorders. In N. A. Creaghead, P. W., Newman, & W. A. Secord (Eds.), *Assessment and remediation of articulatory and phonological disorders* (2nd ed.). Columbus, OH: Merrill.

Albert, M., Sparks, R., & Helm, N. (1973). Melodic intonation therapy for aphasia. *Archives of Neurology, 29,* 130–131.

Allen, G. (1984). Some tips on tape recording speech–language samples. *Journal of the National Student Speech-Language-Hearing Association, 12,* 10–17.

Amayreh, M. M., & Dyson, A. T. (1998). The acquisition of Arabic consonants. *Journal of Speech, Language, and Hearing Research, 41,* 642–653.

American Speech-Language-Hearing Association. (1983). *Social dialects: A position paper.* Rockville, MD: American Speech-Language-Hearing Association.

American Speech-Language-Hearing Association. (1989). Report of ad hoc committee on labial-lingual posturing function. *Asha, 31,* 92–94. Rockville, MD: American Speech-Language-Hearing Association.

American Speech-Language-Hearing Association. (1991). The role of the speech–language pathologist in management of oral myofunctional disorders. *Asha, 33* (Suppl. 5), 7. Rockville, MD: American Speech-Language-Hearing Association.

American Speech-Language-Hearing Association. (1994, March). Code of ethics. *Asha, 36* (Suppl. 13), 1–2.

Amiot, A. (1998). Policy, politics, and the power of information: The critical need for outcomes and clinical trials data in policy-making in the schools. *Language, Speech, and Hearing Services in Schools, 29,* 245.

Andrews, N., & Fey, M. (1986). Analysis of the speech of phonologically impaired children in two sampling conditions. *Language, Speech, and Hearing Services in Schools, 17,* 187–197.

Arlt, P. B., & Goodban, M. T. (1976). A comparative study of articulation acquisition as based on a study of 240 normals, aged three to six. *Language, Speech, and Hearing Services in Schools, 7,* 173–180.

Arndt, W. B., Elbert, M., & Shelton, R. L. (1970). Standardization of a test of oral stereognosis. In J. Bosman (Ed.), *Second symposium on oral sensation and perception.* Springfield, IL: Charles C. Thomas.

Arndt, W. B., Elbert, M., & Shelton, R. L. (1971). Prediction of articulation improvement with therapy from early lesson sound production task scores. *Journal of Speech and Hearing Research, 14,* 149–153.

Backus, O., & Beasley, J. (1951). *Speech therapy with children.* Boston: Houghton Mifflin.

Bailey, J. S., Timbers, G. D., Phillips, E. L., & Wolf, M. M. (1971). Modification of articulation errors of predelinquents by their peers. *Journal of Applied Behavioral Analysis, 4,* 266–281.

Baker, R. D., & Ryan, B. P. (1971). *Programmed conditioning for articulation.* Monterey, CA: Monterey Learning Systems.

Ball, E. W. (1993). Assessing phoneme awareness. *Language, Speech, and Hearing Services in Schools, 24,* 130–139.

Ball, M. J., & Kent, R. D. (1998). *The new phonologies.* San Diego, CA: Singular Publishing Group.

Bankson, N. W., & Bernthal, J. E. (1990a). *Bankson-Bernthal test of phonology.* Chicago: Riverside Press.

Bankson, N. W., & Bernthal, J. E. (1990b). *Quick screen of phonology.* Chicago: Riverside Press.

Bankson, N. W., & Bernthal, J. E. (1998). Phonological assessment procedures. In J. E. Bernthal & N. W. Bankson (Eds.), *Articulation and phonological disorders* (4th ed., pp. 233–269). Boston: Allyn & Bacon.

Bankson, N., & Byrne, M. (1962). The relationship ability and consistency of articulation of /r/. *Journal of Speech and Hearing Disorders, 24,* 341–348.

Bankson, N., & Byrne, M. (1972). The effect of a timed correct sound production task on carryover. *Journal of Speech and Hearing Research, 15,* 160–168.

Barr, M. L., & Kiernan, J. A. (1988). *The human nervous system: An anatomical viewpoint* (5th ed.). Philadelphia: J. B. Lippincott.

Bartoshuk, A. (1964). Human neonatal cardiac responses to sound: A power function. *Psychonomic Science, 1,* 151–152.

Baru, A. V. (1975). Discrimination of synthesized vowels [a] and [ɪ] with varying parameters in dog. In G. Fant & M. A. Tatham (Eds.), *Auditory analysis and the perception of speech.* London: Academic.

Bashir, A., Grahamjones, F., & Bostwick, R. (1984). A touch-cue method of therapy for developmental verbal apraxia. *Seminars in Speech and Language, 5,* 127–137.

Bassi, C. (1983). Development at 4 years. In J. V. Irwin & S. P. Wong, (Eds.)., *Phonological development in children 18 to 72 months.* Carbondale, IL: Southern Illinois University Press.

Battle, D. E. (1998). *Communication disorders in multicultural populations* (2nd ed.). Boston: Butterworth-Heinemann.

Bauman-Waengler, J. (1994). Normal phonological development. In R. J. Lowe (Ed.), *Phonology: Assessment and intervention applications in speech pathology.* Baltimore: Williams & Wilkins.

Bayles, K., & Harris, G. (1982). Evaluating speech and language skills in Papago Indian children. *Journal of American Indian Education, 21*(2), 11–20.

Bench, J. (1969). Audio-frequency and audio-intensity discrimination in the human neonate. *International Audiology, 8,* 615–625.

Bennett, C. W. (1974). Articulation training in two hearing impaired girls. *Journal of Applied Behavioral Analysis, 7,* 439–445.

Berko Gleason, J. (1993). *The development of language* (3rd ed.). New York: Macmillan.

Bernhardt, G. (1994). The prosodic tier and phonological disorders. In M. Yavas (Ed.), *First and second language phonology.* San Diego, CA: Singular Publishing Group.

Bernthal, J. E., & Bankson, N. W. (1998). *Articulation and phonological disorders* (4th ed.). Boston: Allyn & Bacon.

Bhatnagar, S. C., & Andy, O. J. (1995). *Neuroscience for the study of communicative disorders.* Baltimore: Williams & Wilkins.

Bird, J., & Bishop, D. V. M. (1992). Perception and awareness of phonemes in phonologically impaired children. *European Journal of Disorders of Communication, 27,* 289–311.

Bird, J., Bishop, D. V. M., & Freeman, N. H. (1995). Phonological awareness and literacy development in children with expressive phonological impairments. *Journal of Speech and Hearing Research, 38,* 446–462.

Birnholz, J. C, & Benacerraf, B. R. (1983). The development of human fetal hearing. *Science, 22,* 516–518.

Blache, S. E. (1982). Minimal word pairs and distinctive feature training. In M. A. Crary (Ed.), *Phonological intervention: Concepts and procedures.* San Diego, CA: College-Hill Press.

Blache, S. E. (1989). A distinctive feature approach. In N. A. Creaghead, P. W. Newman, W. A. Secord (Eds.), *Assessment and remediation of articulatory and phonological disorders* (2nd ed.). Columbus, OH: Merrill.

Black, L. (1972). *So you want to dismiss 80 percent of your caseload.* Paper presented at the North Carolina Special Education Conference, Raleigh, NC.

Blakeley, R. W. (1980). *Screening test for developmental apraxia of speech.* Austin, TX: PRO-ED.

Bleile, K. M. (1995). *Manual of articulation and phonological disorders: Infancy through adulthood.* San Diego, CA: Singular Publishing Group.

Bleile, K. M. (1996). *Articulation and phonological disorders: A book of exercises* (2nd ed.). San Diego, CA: Singular Publishing Group.

Bloom, R. L. (1997). Communication disorders following focal brain damage. In C. T. Ferrand & R. L. Bloom (Eds.), *Introduction to organic and neurogenic disorders of communication* (pp. 166–190). Boston: Allyn & Bacon.

Bloomer, H., & Hawk, A. (1973). Speech considerations: Speech disorders associated with ablative surgery of the face, mouth and pharynx—Ablative approaches to learning. In *Asha Report #8: Orofacial Anomalies.* Washington, DC: American-Speech-Language Hearing Association.

Boone, D. R., & McFarlane, S. C. (1988). *The voice and voice therapy* (4th ed.). Englewood Cliffs, NJ: Prentice-Hall.

Bradley, D. P. (1989). A systematic multiple-phoneme approach. In N. A. Creaghead, P. W. Newman, W. A. Secord (Eds.), *Assessment and remediation of articulatory and phonological disorders* (2nd ed.). Columbus, OH: Merrill.

Branigan, G. (1977). *Some early constraints on word combinations.* Unpublished doctoral dissertation, Boston University.

Bridger, W. (1961). Sensory habituation and discrimination in the human neonate. *American Journal of Psychiatry, 117,* 991–996.

Burdick, C. K., & Miller, J. D. (1973). New procedures for training chinchillas for psychoacoustic experiments. *Journal of the Acoustical Society of America, 54,* 789–792.

Burdick, C. K., & Miller, J. D. (1975). Speech perception in the chinchilla: Discrimination of sustained /a/ and /i/. *Journal of the Acoustical Society of America, 58,* 415–427.

Bzoch, K. R. (Ed.). (1997). *Communicative disorders related to cleft lip and palate* (4th ed.). Austin, TX: PRO-ED.

Calvert, D. (1982). Articulation and hearing impairments. In L. Lass, J. Northern, D. Yoder, & L. McReynolds (Eds.), *Speech, language and hearing* (Vol. 2). Philadelphia: Saunders.

Carrier, J. K. (1970). A program of articulation therapy administered by mothers. *Journal of Speech and Hearing Disorders, 35,* 344–353.

Carrow, E. (1974). *Austin Spanish articulation test.* Austin, TX: Learning Concepts.

Carter, A. (1974). *The development of communication in the sensorimotor period: A case study.* Unpublished doctoral dissertation, University of California, Berkeley.

Carter, A. (1979). Prespeech meaning relations: An outline of one infant's sensorimotor morpheme development. In P. Fletcher & M. Garman (Eds.), *Language acquisition* (pp. 71–92). Cambridge, MA: Cambridge University Press.

Carter, E. T., & Buck, M. W. (1958). Prognostic testing for functional articulation disorders among children in the first grade. *Journal of Speech and Hearing Disorders, 23,* 124–133.

Catts, H. (1991). Facilitating phonological awareness: Role of speech–language pathologists. *Language, Speech, and Hearing Services in Schools, 22,* 196–203.

Cheng, L. L. (1991). *Assessing Asian language performance: Guidelines for evaluating limited-English-proficient students.* Oceanside, CA: Academic Communication Associates.

Cheng, L. L. (Ed.). (1995). *Integrating language and learning for inclusion: An Asian-Pacific focus.* San Diego, CA: Singular Publishing Group.

Cheng, L. L. (1998). Asian- and Pacific American cultures. In D. E. Battle (Ed.), *Communication disorders in multicultural populations* (2nd ed., pp. 73–116). Boston: Butterworth-Heinemann.

Chomsky, N. (1981). *Lectures on government and binding.* New York: Foris Publications.

Chomsky, N., & Halle, M. (1968). *The sound pattern of English.* New York: Harper & Row.

Chumpelik, D. (1984). The PROMPT system of therapy: Theoretical framework and applications for developmental apraxia of speech. *Seminars in Speech and Language, 5,* 139–153.

Clarke-Klein, S., & Hodson, B. (1995). A phonologically based analysis of misspellings by third graders with disordered-phonology histories. *Journal of Speech and Hearing Research, 38,* 839–849.

Clements, G. N., & Keyser, S. (1983). *CV phonology: A generative theory of the syllable.* Cambridge, MA: MIT Press.

Comrie, B. (Ed.). (1990). *The world's major languages*. New York: Oxford University Press.

Conley, D. (1966). *The effects of using standardized instructions to evaluate speech correction procedures.* Unpublished master's thesis, Arizona State University, Tempe.

Costello, J., & Bosler, C. (1976). Generalization and articulation instruction. *Journal of Speech and Hearing Disorders, 41,* 359–373.

Costello, J., & Onstine, J. (1976). The modification of multiple articulation errors based on distinctive feature theory. *Journal of Speech and Hearing Disorders, 41,* 199–215.

Crawford, J. (1996). *Endangered Native American languages: What is to be done and why?* [Article]. Washington, DC: National Clearinghouse for Bilingual Education. Retrieved December 20, 1999, from the World Wide Web: http://www.ncbe.gwu.edu/miscpubs/crawford/endangered.htm

Creaghead, N. A. (1989). Development of phonology, articulation, and speech perception. In N. A. Creaghead, P. W. Newman, & W. A. Secord (Eds.), *Assessment and remediation of articulatory and phonological disorders* (2nd ed.). Columbus, OH: Merrill.

Creaghead, N. A., Newman, P. W., & Secord, W. A. (1989). *Assessment and remediation of articulatory and phonological disorders* (2nd ed.). Columbus, OH: Merrill.

Crystal, D. (1987). *The Cambridge encyclopedia of language.* Cambridge, UK: Cambridge University Press.

Curtis, J. F., & Hardy, J. C. (1959). A phonetic study of misarticulation of /r/. *Journal of Speech and Hearing Research, 2,* 244–257.

Dabul, B. (1986). *Apraxia battery for adults.* Austin, TX: PRO-ED.

Dalbor, J. (1980). *Spanish pronunciation: Theory and practice* (2nd ed.). New York: Holt, Rinehart and Winston.

Darley, F., Aronson, A., & Brown, J. (1969a). Clusters of deviant speech dimensions in the dysarthrias. *Journal of Speech and Hearing Research, 12,* 462.

Darley, F., Aronson, A., & Brown, J. (1969b). Differential diagnostic patterns of dysarthria. *Journal of Speech and Hearing Research, 12,* 246.

Darley, F., Aronson, A., & Brown, J. (1975). *Motor speech disorders.* Philadelphia: Saunders.

Davis, B. L., & MacNeilage, P. F. (1995). The articulatory basis of babbling. *Journal of Speech and Hearing Research, 38,* 1199–1211.

Dean, E., Howell, J., Hill, A., & Waters, D. (1990). *Metaphon resource pack.* Windsor, UK: NFER-Nelson.

DeCasper, A., & Fifer, W. (1980). Of human bonding: Newborns prefer their mothers' voices. *Science, 208,* 1174–1176.

DeCasper, A., & Spence, M. (1986). Prenatal maternal speech influences newborns' perception of speech sounds. *Infant Behavior and Development, 9,* 133–150.

De la Fuente, M. T. (1985). *The order of acquisition of Spanish consonant phonemes by monolingual Spanish speaking children between the ages of 2.0 and 6.5.* Unpublished doctoral dissertation, Georgetown University, Washington, DC.

Delattre, P. (1965). *Comparing the phonetic features of English, German, Spanish, and French* (pp. 95–97). Heidelberg: Verlog.

Denham, C. D., McCabe, R. B., & Bradley, D. P. (1979). *Multiple phoneme articulation approach.* Tempe, AZ: Ideas.

Diehl, S. F. (1999). Listen and learn? A software review of Earobics. *Language, Speech, and Hearing Services in Schools, 30,* 108–116.

Dillard, J. L. (1972). *Black English: Its history and usage in the United States.* New York: Random House.

Dirckx, J. H. (Ed.). (1997). *Stedman's concise medical dictionary for the health professions* (3rd ed.). Baltimore: Williams & Wilkins.

DiSimoni, F. G. (1989). *Comprehensive apraxia test.* Dalton, PA: Praxis House.

Domnick, M., Hodson, B., Coffman, G., & Wynne, M. (1993, November). *Metaphonological awareness performance and training: Highly unintelligible prereaders.* Poster presented at the annual meeting of the American Speech-Language-Hearing Association, Anaheim, CA.

Donegan, P. J., & Stampe, D. (1979). The study of natural phonology. In D. A. Dinnsen (Ed.), *Current approaches to phonological theory* (pp. 126–173). Bloomington: Indiana University Press.

Dore, J., Franklin, M. B., Miller, R. T., & Ramer, A. L. (1976). Transitional phenomena in early language acquisition. *Journal of Child Language, 3,* 13–28.

Drummond, S. (1993). *Dysarthria examination battery.* Tucson, AZ: Communication Skill Builders.

Drumwright, A. (1971). *The Denver articulation examination.* Denver: Ladoca Project and Publishing Foundation.

Dubois, E. M., & Bernthal, J. E. (1978). A comparison of three methods of obtaining articulatory responses. *Journal of Speech and Hearing Disorders, 43,* 295–305.

Duffy, J. R. (1995). *Motor speech disorders: Substrates, differential diagnosis, and management.* St. Louis, MO: Mosby.

Dunn, C. (1983). A framework for generalization in disordered phonology. *Journal of Childhood Communication Disorders, 7,* 46–58.

Dunn, C., & Newton, L. (1986). A comprehensive model for speech development in hearing-impaired children. *Topics in Language Disorders, 6*(3), 25–46.

Dworkin, J. P. (1984). Specific characteristics and treatment of the dysarthrias. In H. Winitz (Ed.), *Treating articulation disorders: For clinicians by clinicians.* Baltimore: University Park Press.

Dworkin, J. P. (1991). *Motor speech disorders: A treatment guide.* St. Louis, MO: Mosby.

Dyson, A. T. (1986). Development of velar consonants among normal two-year-olds. *Journal of Speech and Hearing Research, 29,* 493–498.

Dyson, A. T., & Paden, E. P. (1983). Some phonological acquisition strategies used by two-year-olds. *Journal of Childhood Communication Disorders, 7,* 6–18.

Earobics Pro Plus Step 1: Auditory development and phonics programs [Computer software]. (1998). Cambridge, MA: Cognitive Concepts.

Earobics Pro Plus Step 2: Auditory development and phonics programs [Computer software]. (1998). Cambridge, MA: Cognitive Concepts.

Edwards, H. T. (1997). *Applied phonetics: The sounds of American English* (2nd ed.). San Diego, CA: Singular Publishing Group.

Edwards, M. L. (1983). Selection criteria for developing therapy goals. *Journal of Childhood Communication Disorders, 7,* 36–45.

Edwards, M. L., & Bernhardt, B. (1973). *Phonological analyses of the speech of children with language disorders.* Unpublished paper, Stanford University, Palo Alto.

Edwards, M. L., & Shriberg, L. D. (1983). *Phonology: Applications in communicative disorders.* San Diego, CA: College-Hill Press.

Eilers, R. E. (1980). Infant speech perception: History and mystery. In G. Yeni-Komshian, J. Kavanagh, and C. A. Ferguson (Eds.), *Child phonology:* Vol. 2. *Perception.* New York: Academic Press.

Eilers, R. E., & Minifie, F. (1975). Fricative discrimination in early infancy. *Journal of Speech and Hearing Research, 18,* 158–167.

Eilers, R. E., & Oller, D. K. (1976). The role of speech discrimination in developmental sound substitutions. *Journal of Child Language, 3,* 319–329.

Eilers, R. E., Wilson, W., & Moore, J. (1977). Developmental changes in speech discrimination in infants. *Journal of Speech and Hearing Research, 20,* 766–780.

Eimas, P. (1974). Auditory and linguistic processing of cues for places of articulation by infants. *Perception Psychophysiology, 16,* 513–521.

Eimas, P., Siqueland, E., Jusczyk, P., & Vigorito, J. (1971). Speech perception in infants. *Science, 146,* 668–670.

Eisenberg, R. (1976). *Auditory competence in early life: The roots of communicative-behavior.* Baltimore: University Park Press.

Elbert, M., Dinnsen, D. A., Swartzlander, P., & Chin, S. B. (1990). Generalization to conversational speech. *Journal of Speech and Hearing Disorders, 55,* 694–699.

Elbert, M., & Gierut, J. (1986). *Handbook of clinical phonology: Approaches to assessment and treatment.* Austin, TX: PRO-ED.

Elbert, M., & McReynolds, L. V. (1975). Transfer of /r/ across contexts. *Journal of Speech and Hearing Disorders, 40,* 380–387.

Elbert, M., & McReynolds, L. V. (1978). An experimental analysis of misarticulating children's generalization. *Journal of Speech and Hearing Disorders, 44,* 459–471.

Elfenbein, J. L. (1994). Children who are hard of hearing. In J. B. Tomblin, H. L. Morris, & D. C. Spriestersbach (Eds.), *Diagnosis in speech–language pathology.* San Diego, CA: Singular Publishing Group.

Elliot, G. B., & Elliot, K. A. (1964). Some pathological, radiological and clinical implications of the precocious development of the human ear. *Laryngoscope, 74,* 1160–1171.

Emerick, L. L., & Haynes, W. O. (1986). *Diagnosis and evaluation in speech pathology* (3rd ed.). Englewood Cliffs, NJ: Prentice-Hall.

Enderby, P. M. (1983). *Frenchay dysarthria assessment.* Austin, TX: PRO-ED.

Engel, D. C., Brandriet, S. E., Erickson, K. M., Gronhoud, K. D., & Gunderson, G. D. (1966). Carryover. *Journal of Speech and Hearing Disorders, 31,* 227–233.

Fairbanks, G., & Green, E. (1950). A study of minor organic deviations in "functional" disorders of articulation; 2. Dimension and relationship of the lips. *Journal of Speech and Hearing Disorders, 15,* 165–168.

Fairbanks, G., & Lintner, M. (1951). A study of minor organic deviations in functional disorders of articulation. *Journal of Speech and Hearing Disorders, 16,* 273–279.

Faircloth, M. A., & Faircloth, S. R. (1970). An analysis of the articulatory behavior of a speech-defective child in connected speech. *Journal of Speech and Hearing Disorders, 35,* 51–61.

Felsenfeld, S., McGue, M., & Broen, P. A. (1995). Familial aggregation of phonological disorders: Results from a 28-year follow-up. *Journal of Speech and Hearing Research, 38,* 1091–1107.

Ferguson, C. A. (1978). Learning to pronounce: The earliest stages of phonological development in the child. In F. D. Minifie & L. L. Lloyd (Eds.), *Communicative and cognitive abilities — Early behavioral assessment.* Baltimore: University Park Press.

Ferguson, C. A. (1986). Discovering sound units and constructing sound systems: It's child's play. In J. S. Perkell & D. H. Klatt (Eds.), *Invariance and variability of speech processes.* Hillsdale, NJ: Erlbaum.

Ferguson, C. A., & Farwell, C. B. (1975). Words and sounds in early language acquisition. *Language, 51,* 419–439.

Ferguson, C. A., Menn, L., & Stoel-Gammon, C. (1992). *Phonological development: Models, research, implications.* Parkton, MD: York Press.

Ferrier, E., & Davis, M. (1973). A lexical approach to the remediation of final sound omissions. *Journal of Speech and Hearing Disorders, 38,* 126–130.

Fey, M. E., Cleave, P. L., Ravida, A. I., Long, H. S., Dejmal, A. E., & Easton, E. L. (1994). Effects of grammar facilitation on the phonological performance of children with speech and language impairments. *Journal of Speech and Hearing Research, 37,* 594–607.

Fisher, H., & Logemann, J. (1971). *The Fisher-Logemann test of articulation competence.* Boston: Houghton Mifflin.

Fisichelli, R. M. (1950). *An experimental study of the prelinguistic speech development of institutionalized infants.* Unpublished doctoral dissertation, Fordham University, New York.

Fitch, J. L. (1973). Voice and articulation. In B. B. Lahey (Ed.), *The modification of language behavior* (pp. 130–177). Springfield, IL: Charles C. Thomas.

Fletcher, S. G. (1972). Time-by-count measurement of diadochokinetic syllable rate. *Journal of Speech and Hearing Research, 15,* 763–770.

Fletcher, S. G. (1978). *Time-by-count measurement of diadochokinetic syllable rate.* Austin, TX: PRO-ED.

Flexer, C., Gillette, Y., & Wray, D. (1997). Communicative management of persons with multiple disabilities. In C. T. Ferrand & R. L. Bloom (Eds.), *Introduction to organic and neurogenic disorders of communication: Current scope and practice* (pp. 319–344). Needham Heights, MA: Allyn & Bacon.

Fluharty, N. (1978). *Fluharty preschool speech and language screening test.* Boston, MA: Teaching Resources Corporation.

Fry, D. B. (1965). The dependence of stress judgments on vowel formant structure. In E. Zwirner & W. Bethge (Eds.), *Proceedings of the Sixth International Congress of Phonetic Sciences* (pp. 306–311). Basel, Switzerland: Karger.

Fudala, J. B., & Reynolds, W. M. (1986). *Arizona articulation proficiency scale* (2nd ed.). Los Angeles: Western Psychological Press.

Gallagher, T. M., & Shriner, T. H. (1975a). Articulatory inconsistencies in the speech of normal children. *Journal of Speech and Hearing Research, 18,* 168–175.

Gallagher, T. M., & Shriner, T. H. (1975b). Contextual variables related to inconsistent /s/ and /z/ production in the spontaneous speech of children. *Journal of Speech and Hearing Research, 18,* 623–633.

Gammon, S., Smith, P., Daniloff, R., & Kim, C. (1971). Articulation and stress juncture production under oral anesthetization and masking. *Journal of Speech and Hearing Research, 14,* 271–282.

Garbutt, C. W., & Anderson, J. O. (1980). *Effective methods for correcting articulatory defects.* Danville, IL: Interstate Printers & Publishers.

Gerber, A. (1973). *Goal: Carryover.* Philadelphia: Temple University Press.

Gierut, J. (1985). *On the relationship between phonological knowledge and generalization learning in misarticulating children.* Doctoral dissertation, Indiana University, Bloomington.

Gierut, J. (1989). Maximal opposition approach to phonological treatment. *Journal of Speech and Hearing Disorders, 54,* 9–19.

Gierut, J. (1990). A functional analysis of phonological contrast treatment. In L. B. Olswang, C. K. Thompson, S. F. Warren, & N. J. Minghetti (Eds.). *Treatment efficacy research in communication disorders* (p. 252). Washington, DC: American Speech-Language-Hearing Foundation.

Gierut, J. (1991). Homonymy in phonological change. *Clinical Linguistics and Phonetics, 5,* 119–137.

Gierut, J. (1992). The conditions and course of clinically induced phonological change. *Journal of Speech and Hearing Research, 35,* 1049–1063.

Gierut, J., & Neumann, H. J. (1991). Teaching and learning /θ/: A nonconfound. *Clinical Linguistics and Phonetics, 6,* 191–200.

Gildersleeve, C., Davis, B., & Stubble, E. (1996, November). *When monolingual rules do not apply: Speech development in a bilingual environment.* Paper presented at the annual convention of the American Speech-Language-Hearing Association, Seattle, WA.

Golding-Kushner, K. J. (1997). Cleft lip and palate, craniofacial anomalies, and velopharyngeal insufficiency. In C. T. Ferrand & R. L. Bloom (Eds.), *Introduction to organic and neurogenic disorders of communication: Current scope and practice* (pp. 193–228).

Goldman, R., & Fristoe, M. (1969, 1986). *The Goldman-Fristoe test of articulation.* Circle Pines, MN: American Guidance Service.

Goldsmith, J. A. (1990). *Autosegmental and metrical phonology.* Oxford, UK: Basil Blackwell.

Goldstein, B. (1988). *The evidence of phonological processes of 3- and 4-year-old Spanish speakers.* Unpublished master's thesis, Temple University, Philadelphia, PA.

Goldstein, B. (1993). *Phonological patterns in speech-disordered Puerto Rican Spanish-speaking children.* Unpublished doctoral dissertation, Temple University, Philadelphia, PA.

Goldstein, B. (1995). Spanish phonological development. In H. Kayser (Ed.), *Bilingual speech–language pathology: An Hispanic focus* (pp. 17–38). San Diego, CA: Singular Publishing Group.

Goldstein, B., & Iglesias, A. (1996). Phonological patterns in normally developing 4-year-old Spanish-speaking preschoolers of Puerto Rican descent. *Language, Speech, and Hearing Services in the Schools, 27*(1), 82–90.

Goldstein, H., & Gierut, H. (1998). Outcomes measurement in child language and phonological disorders. In C. M. Frattali (Ed.), *Measuring outcomes in speech–language pathology.* New York: Thieme Medical Publishers.

Goldsworthy, C. (1996). *Developmental reading disabilities: A language-based treatment approach.* San Diego, CA: Singular Publishing Group.

Gonzalez, A. (1981). *A descriptive study of phonological development in normal speaking Puerto Rican preschoolers.* Unpublished doctoral dissertation, Pennsylvania State University, State College, PA.

Gordon-Brannan, M. (1994). Assessing intelligibility: Children's expressive phonologies. *Topics in Language Disorders, 14,* 17–25.

Goswami, U., & Bryant, P. E. (1990). *Phonological skills and learning to read.* Hillsdale, NJ: Erlbaum.

Greenlee, M. (1974). Interacting processes in the child's acquisition of stop-liquid clusters. *Papers and reports on child language development, 7,* 85–100.

Grunwell, P. (1982). *Clinical phonology.* London: Croom Helm

Grunwell, P. (1985). *Phonological assessment of child speech (PACS).* Windsor, UK: NFER-Nelson.

Grunwell, P. (1987). *Clinical phonology* (2nd ed.). London: Croom Helm.

Grunwell, P. (1997a). Developmental phonological disability: Order or disorder. In B. W. Hodson & M. L. Edwards (Eds.), *Perspectives in applied phonology.* Gaithersburg, MD: Aspen Publications.

Grunwell, P. (1997b). Natural phonology. In M. J. Ball & R. D. Kent (Eds.), *The new phonologies: Developments in clinical linguistics.* San Diego, CA: Singular Publishing Group.

Haelsig, P. C., & Madison, C. L. (1986). A study of phonological processes exhibited by 3-, 4-, and 5-year-old children. *Language, Speech, and Hearing Services in the Schools, 17,* 107–114.

Hall, P. K. (1994). The oral mechanism. In J. B. Tomblin, H. L. Morris, & D. C. Spriestersbach (Eds.), *Diagnosis in speech–language pathology.* San Diego, CA: Singular Publishing Group.

Hall, P. K., Jordan, L. S., & Robin, D. A. (1993). *Developmental apraxia of speech: Theory and clinical practice.* Austin, TX: PRO-ED.

Halle, M. (1992). Phonological features. In *International encyclopedia of linguistics* (Vol. 3, pp. 207–212). Oxford: Oxford University Press.

Halliday, M. A. K. (1975). *Learning how to mean — Explorations in the development of language.* London: Edwards Arnold.

Hare, G. (1983). Development at 2 years. In J. V. Irwin & S. P. Wong (Eds.), *Phonological development in children 18 to 72 months.* Carbondale, IL: Southern Illinois University Press.

Harris, G. A. (1998). American Indian cultures: A lesson in diversity. In D. E. Battle (Ed.), *Communication disorders in multicultural populations* (2nd ed., pp. 117–156). Boston: Butterworth-Heinemann.

Hayes, B. (1988). Metrics and phonological theory. In F. Newmeyer (Ed.), *Linguistics: The Cambridge Survey. II. Linguistic theory: Extensions and implications* (pp. 220–240). Cambridge, UK: Cambridge University Press.

Haynes, S. (1985). Developmental apraxia of speech: Symptoms and treatment. In D. F. Johns (Ed.), *Clinical management of neurogenic communicative disorders* (2nd ed., pp. 259–266). Boston: College-Hill Press.

Haynes, W., & Moran, M. (1989). A cross-sectional developmental study of final consonant production in southern black children from preschool through third grade. *Language, Speech, and Hearing Services in Schools, 20*(4), 400–406.

Haynes, W. O., & Pindzola, R. H. (1998). *Diagnosis and evaluation in speech pathology* (5th ed.). Needham Heights, MA: Allyn & Bacon.

Haynes, W. O., Pindzola, R. H., & Emerick, L. L. (1992). *Diagnosis and evaluation in speech pathology* (4th ed.). Englewood Cliffs, NJ: Prentice-Hall.

Healy, T., & Madison, C. (1987). Articulation error migration: A comparison of single word and connected speech samples. *Journal of Communication Disorders, 20,* 129–136.

Hecht, M., Collier, M., & Ribeau, S. (1993). *African American communication*. Newbury Park, CA: Sage Publications.

Hegde, M. N. (1996a). *PocketGuide to assessment in speech–language pathology*. San Diego, CA: Singular Publishing Group.

Hegde, M. N. (1996b). *PocketGuide to treatment in speech–language pathology*. San Diego, CA: Singular Publishing Group.

Hegde, M. N. (1998a). *A coursebook on scientific and professional writing for speech–language pathology* (2nd ed.). San Diego, CA: Singular Publishing Group.

Hegde, M. N. (1998b). *Treatment procedures in communicative disorders* (3rd ed.). Austin, TX: PRO-ED.

Hegde, M. N., & Davis, D. (1995). *Clinical methods and practicum in speech–language pathology* (2nd ed.). San Diego, CA: Singular Publishing Group.

Helm-Estabrooks, N. (1992). *Test of oral and limb apraxia*. Chicago: Riverside Publishing.

Helm-Estabrooks, N., Nicholas, M., & Morgan, A. (1989). *Melodic intonation therapy program*. San Antonio, TX: Special Press.

Hetzron, R. (1990). Semitic languages. In B. Comrie (Ed.), *The world's major languages* (pp. 654–663). New York: Oxford University Press.

Highwater, J. (1975). *Indian America*. New York: David McKay.

Hodson, B. W. (1980). *The assessment of phonological processes*. Danville, IL: PhonoComp.

Hodson, B. W. (1985). *Computer analysis of phonological processes*. Stonington, IL: PhonoComp.

Hodson, B. W. (1986a). *The assessment of phonological processes–revised*. Austin, TX: PRO-ED.

Hodson, B. W. (1986b). *Assessment of phonological processes–Spanish*. San Diego, CA: Los Amigos Association.

Hodson, B. W. (1989). Phonological remediation: A cycles approach. In N. A. Creaghead, P. W. Newman, & W. A. Secord (Eds.), *Assessment and remediation of articulatory and phonological disorders* (2nd ed.). Columbus, OH: Merrill.

Hodson, B. W. (1994). Helping children become intelligible and literate: The role of phonology. *Topics in Language Disorders, 14,* 1–6.

Hodson, B. W. (1997). Disordered phonologies: What we have learned about assessment and treatment. In B. W. Hodson & M. L. Edwards (Eds.), *Perspectives in applied phonology* (pp. 197–224). Gaithersburg, MD: Aspen Publishers.

Hodson, B. W., & Paden, E. P. (1981). Phonological processes which characterize unintelligible and intelligible speech in early childhood. *Journal of Speech and Hearing Disorders, 46,* 369–373.

Hodson, B. W., & Paden, E. P. (1983). *Targeting intelligible speech: A phonological approach to remediation*. San Diego, CA: College-Hill Press.

Hodson, B. W., & Paden, E. P. (1991). *Targeting intelligible speech: A phonological approach to remediation* (2nd ed.). Austin, TX: PRO-ED.

Hoffman, P. R. (1983). Interallophonic generalization or /r/ training. *Journal of Speech and Hearing Disorders, 48,* 215–221.

Hoffman, P. R., Norris, J. A., & Monjure, J. (1990). Comparison of process targeting and whole language treatment for phonologically delayed preschool children. *Language, Speech, and Hearing Services in Schools, 21,* 102–109.

Hoffman, P. R., Schuckers, G. H., & Ratusnik, D. L. (1977). Contextual-coarticulatory inconsistency of /r/ misarticulation. *Journal of Speech and Hearing Research, 20,* 631–643.

Holmgren, K., Lindblom, B., Aurelius, G., Jalling, B., & Zetterstrom, R. (1986). On the phonetics of infant vocalization. In B. Lindblom & R. Zetterstrom (Eds.), *Precursors of early speech*. New York: Stockton Press.

Hudak, T. J. (1990). Thai. In B. Comrie (Ed.), *The world's major languages* (pp. 757–777). New York: Oxford University Press.

Hulitt, L. M., & Howard, M. R. (1997). *Born to talk: An introduction to speech and language development* (2nd ed.). Boston: Allyn & Bacon.

Iglesias, A. (1978). *Assessment of phonological disabilities*. Unpublished assessment tool, Ohio State University, Columbus.

Ingram, D. (1976). *Phonological disability in children*. New York: American Elsevier.

Ingram, D. (1981). *Procedures for the phonological analysis of children's language*. Baltimore: University Park Press.

Ingram, D. (1989a). *First language acquisition: Method, description, and explanation*. New York: Cambridge University Press.

Ingram, D. (1989b). *Phonological disability in children* (2nd ed.). London: Whurr.

Irwin, J. V., & Weston, A. J. (1971–1975). *Paired stimuli kit*. Milwaukee, WI: Fox Point.

Irwin, J. W., & Wong, S. P. (Eds.). (1983). *Phonological development in children 18 to 72 months*. Carbondale, IL: Southern Illinois University Press.

Irwin, O. C. (1947a). Infant speech: Consonant sounds according to manner of articulation. *Journal of Speech and Hearing Disorders, 12,* 402–404.

Irwin, O. C. (1947b). Infant speech: Consonant sounds according to place of articulation. *Journal of Speech and Hearing Disorders, 12,* 397–401.

Irwin, O. C. (1948). Infant speech: Development of vowel sounds. *Journal of Speech and Hearing Disorders, 13,* 31–34.

Irwin, O. C. (1952). Speech development in the young child: Some factors related to the speech development of the infant and young child. *Journal of Speech and Hearing Disorders, 17,* 269–279.

Irwin, O. C., & Chen, H. P. (1946). Infant speech: Vowel and consonant frequency. *Journal of Speech and Hearing Disorders, 11,* 123–125.

Jakobson, R. (1941). Kindersprache, aphasie und allgemeine lautgesetze. Uppsala, Sweden: Almquist & Wiksell.

Jakobson, R. (1968). *Child language, aphasia and phonological universals* (A. R. Keiler, Trans.). The Hague: Mouton.

Jakobson, R., Fant, G., & Halle, M. (1952). *Preliminaries to speech analysis: The distinctive features and their correlates*. Cambridge, MA: MIT Press.

Jakobson, R., & Halle, M. (1956). *Fundamentals of language*. The Hague: Mouton.

Jensen, P., Williams, W., & Bzoch, K. (1975, November). *Preference of young infants for speech vs. nonspeech stimuli*. Paper presented to the annual American Speech and Hearing Association Convention, Washington, DC.

Jimenez, B. C. (1987). Acquisition of Spanish consonants in children aged 3–5 years, 7 months. *Language, Speech, and Hearing Services in the Schools, 18*(4), 357–363.

Johansson, B., Wedenburg, E., & Westin, B. (1964). Measurement of tone response by the human fetus. *Acta Otolaryngology of Stockholm, 57,* 188–192.

Johnson, J., Winney, B., & Pederson, O. (1980). Single word versus connected speech articulation testing. *Language, Speech, and Hearing Services in the Schools, 11,* 175–179.

Jusczyk, P., Rosner, B., Cutting, J., Foard, C., & Smith, L. (1977). Categorical perception of nonspeech sounds by 2-month-old infants. *Perceptual Psychophysics, 21,* 50–54.

Kamhi, A. G., Pollock, K. E., & Harris, J. L. (1996). *Communication development and disorders in African American children.* Baltimore: Paul H. Brookes.

Kaye, A. (1990). Arabic. In B. Comrie (Ed.), *The world's major languages* (pp. 664–685). New York: Oxford University Press.

Kayser, H. (1995). *Bilingual speech–language pathology: An Hispanic focus.* San Diego, CA: Singular Publishing Group.

Kayser, H. (1998). Hispanic cultures and language. In D. E. Battle (Ed.), *Communication disorders in multicultural populations* (pp. 157–195). Boston: Butterworth-Heinemann.

Kenney, K. W., & Prather, E. M. (1986). Articulation development in preschool children: Consistency of productions. *Journal of Speech and Hearing Research, 29,* 29–36.

Kent, R. (1998). Normal aspects of articulation. In J. E. Bernthal & N. W. Bankson (Eds.), *Articulation and phonological disorders* (4th ed., pp. 1–62). Boston: Allyn & Bacon.

Kent, R. D., & Bauer, H. R. (1985). Vocalizations of one-year-olds. *Journal of Child Language, 13,* 491–526.

Khan, L., & Lewis, N. (1986). *Khan-Lewis phonological analysis.* Circle Pines, MN: American Guidance Service.

Kim, N. (1990). Korean. In B. Comrie (Ed.), *The world's major languages* (pp. 881–898). New York: Oxford University Press.

Koch, H. (1956). Sibling influence on children's speech. *Journal of Speech and Hearing Disorders, 21,* 322–329.

Koegel, R. L., Koegel, L. K., & Ingham, J. C. (1986). Programming rapid generalization of correct articulation through self-monitoring procedures. *Journal of Speech and Hearing Disorders, 51,* 24–32.

Koegel, R. L., Koegel, L. K., Voy, K. V., & Ingham, J. C. (1988). Within-clinic versus outside-of-clinic self monitoring of articulation to promote generalization. *Journal of Speech and Hearing Disorders, 53,* 392–399.

Krauss, M. (1992). The world's languages in crisis. *Language, 68*(1), 4–10.

Kresheck, J. D., & Socolofsky, G. (1972). Imitative and spontaneous articulatory assessment of four-year-old children. *Journal of Speech and Hearing Research, 15,* 729–733.

Kuczwara, L. A., Birnholz, J. C., & Klodd, D. A. (1984). Auditory responsiveness in the fetus. *National Student Speech-Language-Hearing Association Journal, 14,* 12–20.

Kuehn, D. P., Lemme, M. L., & Baumgartner, J. M. (Eds.). (1989). *Neural bases of speech, hearing, and language.* Boston: College-Hill Press.

Kuhl, P. K. (1979). Speech perception in early infancy: Perceptual constancy for spectrally dissimilar vowel change. *Journal of the Acoustical Society of America, 66*(6), 1668–1679.

Kuhl, P. K. (1987). Perception of speech sounds in early infancy. In C. Salapatek & L. Kohen (Eds.), *Handbook of infant perception:* Vol. 2. *From perception to cognition.* New York: Academic Press.

Kuhl, P. K., & Miller, J. D. (1975). Speech perception by the chinchilla: Voiced-voiceless distinction in alveolar plosive consonants. *Science, 190,* 69–72.

Kuhl, P. K., & Miller, J. D. (1978). Speech perception by the chinchilla: Identification functions for synthetic VOT stimuli. *Journal of the Acoustical Society of America, 63,* 905–917.

Langdon, H. W., & Cheng, L. L. (Eds.). (1992). *Hispanic children and adults with communication disorders.* Gaithersburg, MD: Aspen Publishers.

Leman, W. (1998). *The Cheyenne language.* [Article]. Retrieved December 20, 1999, from the World Wide Web: http://www.mcn.net/~wleman/cheyenne.htm

Leonard, L. B. (1985). Unusual and subtle phonological behavior in the speech of phonologically disordered children. *Journal of Speech and Hearing Disorders, 50,* 4–13.

Leonard, R. J. (1994). Characteristics of speech in speakers with oral/oralpharyngeal ablation. In J. Bernthal & N. Bankson (Eds.), *Child phonology: Characteristics, assessment, and intervention with special populations* (pp. 54–78). New York: Thieme Medical Publishers.

Leopold, W. F. (1947). *Speech development of a bilingual child: A linguist's record. Vol. II: Sound-learning in the first two years.* Evanston, IL: Northwestern University Press.

Levitt, H., & Stromberg, H. (1983). Segmental characteristics of speech of hearing-impaired children: Factors affecting intelligibility. In I. Hochberg, H. Levitt, & M. Osberger (Eds.), *Speech of the Hearing Impaired* (pp. 53–73). Baltimore: University Park Press.

Lewis, B., Ekelman, B., & Aram, D. (1989). A familial study of severe phonological disorders. *Journal of Speech and Hearing Research, 32,* 713–724.

Lewis, B., & Freebairn-Farr, L. (1991). *Preschool phonology disorders at school age, adolescence, and adulthood.* Paper presented at the convention of the American Speech-Language-Hearing Association, Atlanta, GA.

Liberman, A. M. (1970). The grammar of speech and language. *Cognitive Psychology, 1,* 301–323.

Linares, T. A. (1981). Articulation skills in Spanish-speaking children. In R. V. Padilla (Ed.), *Ethnoperspectives in bilingual education series. Vol. III. Ethnoperspectives in bilingual education research: Bilingual education technology* (pp. 363–367). Ypsilanti: Michigan State University.

Lindamood, C., & Lindamood, P. (1971). *Lindamood auditory conceptualization test.* Austin, TX: PRO-ED.

Lindamood, C., & Lindamood, P. (1998). *The Lindamood phoneme sequencing program for reading, spelling, and speech* (3rd ed.). Austin, TX: PRO-ED.

Ling, D. (1976). *Speech and the hearing-impaired child: Theory and practice.* Washington, DC: AG Bell Association.

Lippke, B. A., Dickey, S. E., Selmar, J. W., & Soder, A. L. (1997). *Photo articulation test* (3rd ed.). Austin, TX: PRO-ED.

Locke, J. L. (1980a). The inference of speech perception in the phonologically disordered child. I. A rationale, some criteria, the conventional tests. *Journal of Speech and Hearing Disorders, 45,* 431–444.

Locke, J. L. (1980b). The inference of speech perception in the phonologically disordered child. II. Some clinically novel procedures, their use, some findings. *Journal of Speech and Hearing Disorders, 45,* 445–468.

Locke, J. L. (1983). *Phonological acquisition and change.* New York: Academic Press.

Long, S. H. (1994). Language and other special populations of children. In V. Reed, *An introduction to children with language disorders* (2nd ed.). New York: Merrill.

Love, R. J., & Webb, W. G. (1996). *Neurology for the speech–language pathologist* (3rd ed.). Boston: Butterworth-Heinemann.

Lowe, R. J. (1986). *Assessment link between phonology and articulation: ALPHA.* Moline, IL: LinguiSystems.

Lowe, R. J. (1994). *Phonology: Assessment and intervention applications in speech pathology.* Baltimore: Williams & Wilkins.

Lowe, R. J. (1996). *Workbook for the identification of phonological processes* (2nd ed.). Austin, TX: PRO-ED.

Lowe, R. J., Knutson, P. J., & Monson, M. A. (1985). Incidence of fronting in preschool children. *Language, Speech, and Hearing Services in the Schools, 16,* 119–123.

Lundeen, C. (1991). Prevalence of hearing impairment among school children. *Language, Speech, and Hearing Services in the Schools, 32,* 87–96.

Macken, M. A., & Barton, D. P. (1980). A longitudinal study of the acquisition of the voicing contrasts in American-English word-initial stops, as measured by voice onset time. *Journal of Child Language, 7,* 41–74.

Macken, M. A., & Ferguson, C. A. (1983). Cognitive aspects of phonological development: Model, evidence, and issues. In K. E. Nelson (Ed.), *Children's language* (Vol. 4). Hillsdale, NJ: Erlbaum.

Marion, M. J., Sussman, M. H., & Marquardt, T. P. (1993). The perception and production of rhyme in normal and developmentally apraxic children. *Journal of Communication Disorders, 17,* 52–59.

Martin, F. N. (1986). *Introduction to audiology* (3rd ed.). Englewood Cliffs, NJ: Prentice-Hall.

Mason, M., Smith, M., & Hinshaw, M. (1976). *Medida Española de articulacion.* San Ysidro, CA: San Ysidro School District.

Mason, R. M. (1988). Orthodontic perspectives on orofacial myofunctional therapy. *International Journal of Orofacial Myology, 14,* 49–55.

Mason, R., & Proffitt, W. (1974). The tongue-thrust controversy: Background and recommendations. *Journal of Speech and Hearing Disorders, 39,* 115–132.

Matheny, A., & Panagos, J. (1978). Comparing the effects of articulation and syntax programs on syntax and articulation improvement. *Language, Speech, and Hearing Services in Schools, 9,* 57–61.

Mattes, L. J. (1998). *Assessment of sound awareness and production.* Oceanside, CA: Academic Communication Associates.

McCabe, R. B., & Bradley, D. P. (1973). *The systematic multiphonemic approach to articulation therapy.* Short course presented at American Speech and Hearing Association South Eastern Regional Conference, Atlanta, GA.

McCabe, R. B., & Bradley, D. P. (1975). Systemic multiple phonemic approach to articulation therapy. *Acta Symbolica, 6,* 2–18.

McDonald, E. (1964). *Deep test of articulation.* Pittsburgh, PA: Stanwix House.

McDonald, E. (1968). *Screening deep test of articulation.* Pittsburgh, PA: Stanwix House.

McDonald, E. T., & Aungst, L. (1970). Apparent impedence of oral sensory functions and articulatory proficiency. In J. Bosma (Ed.), *Second symposium on oral sensation and perception.* Springfield, IL: Charles C. Thomas.

McLaughlin, S. (1998). *Introduction to language development.* San Diego, CA: Singular Publishing Group.

McNutt, J. (1994). Generalization of /s/ from English to French as a result of phonological remediation. *Journal of Speech–Language Pathology and Audiology / Revue d'orthophonic et d'audiologie, 18,* 109–114.

McReynolds, L. (1972). Articulation generalization during articulation training. *Language and Speech, 15,* 149–155.

McReynolds, L., & Bennett, S. (1972). Distinctive feature generalization in articulation training. *Journal of Speech and Hearing Disorders, 37,* 462–470.

McReynolds, L., & Elbert, M. (1981a). Criteria for phonological process analysis. *Journal of Speech and Hearing Disorders, 46,* 197–204.

McReynolds, L., & Elbert, M. (1981b). Generalization of correct articulation in clusters. *Applied Psycholinguistics, 2,* 119–132.

McReynolds, L., & Engmann, D. (1975). *Distinctive feature analysis of misarticulations.* Baltimore: University Park Press.

McWilliams, B. J., Morris, H. L., & Shelton, R. L. (1990). *Cleft palate speech* (2nd ed.). Philadelphia: B. C. Decker.

Medlin, V. L. (1975). *Handbook for speech therapy.* Austin, TX: PRO-ED.

Mehler, J., Jusczyk, P., Lambertz, G., Halsted, N., Bertoncini, J., & Amiel-Tison, C. (1988). A precursor of language acquisition in young infants. *Cognition, 29,* 143–178.

Menn, L. (1975). Evidence for an interactionist-discovery theory of child phonology. *Papers and Reports on Child Language Development, 12,* 169–177, Stanford University.

Menn, L. (1983). Development of articulatory, phonetic, and phonological capabilities. In B. Butterworth (Ed.), *Language production* (Vol. 2). London: Academic Press.

Menyuk, P. (1968). The role of distinctive features in children's acquisition of phonology. *Journal of Speech and Hearing Research, 11,* 138–146.

Meza, P. (1983). *Phonological analysis of Spanish utterances of highly unintelligible Mexican-American children.* Unpublished master's thesis, San Diego State University, San Diego, CA.

Milisen, R. (1954). The disorder of articulation: A systematic and clinical and experimental approach. *Journal of Speech and Hearing Research, 17,* 352–366.

Miller, J. D., & Kuhl, P. K. (1976). Speech perception by the chinchilla: A progress report on syllable initial voiced-plosive consonants. *Journal of the Acoustical Society of America, 59,* S54(A).

Mitchell, P. R., & Kent, R. (1990). Phonetic variation in multisyllable babbling. *Journal of Child Language, 17,* 247–265.

Moerk, E. L. (1992). *A first language taught and learned.* Baltimore: Paul H. Brookes.

Morris, S. E. (1975). Pre-speech assessment. In S. E. Morris (Ed.), *Pre-speech and language programming for the young child with cerebral palsy.* Wauwatosa, WI: Curative Rehabilitation Center.

Morrison, J., & Shriberg, L. (1992). Articulation testing versus conversational speech sampling. *Journal of Speech and Hearing Research, 35,* 259–273.

Morse, P. A. (1972). The discrimination of speech and non-speech stimuli in early infancy. *Journal of Exceptional Child Psychology, 14,* 477–492.

Moskowitz, A. (1973). Acquisition of phonology and syntax: A preliminary study. In G. Hinitikka, J. Moravcsik, & P. Suppes (Eds.), *Approaches to natural language.* Dordrecht, Holland: Reidel.

Mowrer, D. E. (1971). Transfer of training in articulation therapy. *Journal of Speech and Hearing Disorders, 36,* 427–445.

Mowrer, D. E. (1989). *The behavioral approach to treatment.* In N. A. Creaghead, P. W. Newman, & W. A. Secord (Eds.), *Assessment and remediation of articulatory and phonological disorders* (2nd ed.). Columbus, OH: Merrill.

Mowrer, O. (1960). *Learning theory and symbolic processes.* New York: Wiley.

Muir, D., & Field, J. (1979). Newborn infants orient to sounds. *Child Development, 50,* 431–436.

Mysak, E. D. (1959). A servomodel for speech therapy. *Journal of Speech and Hearing Disorders, 24,* 144–149.

Mysak, E. D. (1980). *Neurospeech therapy for the cerebral palsied.* New York: Teachers College Press, Columbia University.

Nemoy, E., & Davis, S. (1937). *The correction of defective consonant sounds.* Boston: Expression.

Nemoy, E., & Davis, S. (1954). *The correction of defective consonant sounds* (rev. ed.). Boston: Expression.

Nemoy, E., & Davis, S. (1980). *The correction of defective consonant sounds* (16th printing). Londonderry, NH: Expression.

Newman, P. W., & Creaghead, N. A. (1989). Assessment of articulatory and phonological disorders. In N. A. Creaghead, P. W. Newman, & W. A. Secord (Eds.), *Assessment and remediation of articulatory and phonological disorders* (2nd ed). Columbus, OH: Merrill.

Newport, E., Gleitman, A., & Gleitman, L. (1977). Mother I'd rather do it myself: Some effects and non-effects of maternal speech style. In C. Snow & C. Ferguson (Eds.), *Talking to children: Language input and acquisition.* New York: Cambridge University Press.

Netsell, R. A. (1986). *A neurobiologic view of speech production and the dysarthrias.* Boston: College-Hill Press.

Nicolosi, L., Harryman, E., & Kresheck, J. (1996). *Terminology of communication disorders: Speech-language-hearing* (4th ed.). Baltimore: Williams & Wilkins.

Ohde, R. N., & Sharf, D. J. (1992). *Phonetic analysis of normal and abnormal speech.* New York: Merrill.

Oller, D. K. (1980). The emergence of the sounds of speech in infancy. In G. Yeni-Komshian, J. Kavanagh, & C. A. Ferguson (Eds.), *Child phonology. Vol I: Production.* New York: Academic Press.

Oller, D. K., Wieman, L. A., Doyle, W. J., & Ross, C. (1975). Infant babbling and speech. *Journal of Child Language, 2,* 1–11.

Olmsted, D. (1971). *Out of the mouth of babes.* The Hague: Mouton.

Olswang, L. B., & Bain, B. A. (1985). The natural occurrence of generalization during articulation treatment. *Journal of Communication Disorders, 18,* 109–129.

O'Toole, T., Logemann, J. A., Baum, H. M. (1998). Conducting clinical trials in the public schools. *Language, Speech, and Hearing Services in Schools, 29,* 257–262.

Owens, R. E. (1996). *Language development: An introduction* (4th ed.). Boston: Allyn & Bacon.

Paden, E. P., Matthies, M. L., & Novak, M. A. (1989). Recovery from OME-related phonologic delay following tube placement. *Journal of Speech and Hearing Disorders, 54,* 94–100.

Palmer, J. M. (1993). *Anatomy for speech and hearing* (4th ed.). Baltimore: Williams & Wilkins.

Panagos, J., & Prelock, P. (1982). Phonological constraints on the sentence productions of language disordered children. *Journal of Speech and Hearing Research, 25,* 171–176.

Panagos, J., Quine, M., & Klich, R. (1979). Syntactic and phonological influences on children's articulation. *Journal of Speech and Hearing Research, 22,* 841–848.

Paterson, M. M. (1994). Articulation and phonological disorders in hearing-impaired school-aged children with severe and profound sensorineural losses. In J. E. Bernthal & N. W. Bankson (Eds.), *Child phonology: Characteristics, assessment, and intervention with special populations* (pp. 199–224). New York: Thieme Medical Publishers.

Patkowski, M. S. (1994). The critical age hypothesis and interlanguage phonology. In M. Yavas (Ed.), *First and second language phonology* (pp. 205–221). San Diego, CA: Singular Publishing Group.

Paynter, E. T., & Bumpas, T. C. (1977). Imitative and spontaneous articulatory assessment of three-year-old children. *Journal of Speech and Hearing Disorders, 42,* 119–125.

Pendergast, K., Dickey, S., Selmar, J., & Soder, A. (1969). *Photo articulation test.* Danville, IL: Interstate.

Perez, E. (1994). Phonological differences among speakers of Spanish-influenced English. In J. E. Bernthal & N. W. Bankson (Eds.), *Child phonology: Characteristics, assessment, and intervention with special populations* (pp. 245–254). New York: Thieme Medical Publishers.

Perkins, W. H., & Kent, R. D. (1986). *Functional anatomy of speech, language, and hearing: A primer.* San Diego, CA: College-Hill Press.

Peterson, H. A., & Marquardt, T. P. (1994). *Appraisal and diagnosis of speech and language disorders* (3rd ed.). Englewood Cliffs, NJ: Prentice-Hall.

Pierce, J. R., & Hanna, I. V. (1974). *The development of a phonological system in English speaking American children.* Portland, OR: HaPi Press.

Poole, E. (1934). Genetic development of articulation of consonant sounds in speech. *Elementary English Review, 11,* 159–161.

Powell, J., & McReynolds, L. V. (1969). A procedure for testing position generalization from articulation training. *Journal of Speech and Hearing Disorders, 12,* 629–645.

Powell, T. W., & Elbert, M. (1984). Generalization following the remediation of early- and late-developing consonant clusters. *Journal of Speech and Hearing Disorders, 49,* 211–218.

Prather, E., Hedrick, D., & Kern, C. (1975). Articulation development in children aged two to four years. *Journal of Speech and Hearing Research, 40,* 55–63.

Pratt, A., & Brady, S. (1988). Relation of phonological awareness to reading disability in children and adults. *Journal of Educational Psychology, 80,* 319–323.

Preisser, D. A., Hodson, B. W., & Paden, E. P. (1988). Developmental phonology. *Journal of Speech and Hearing Disorders, 53,* 125–130.

Prosek, R., & House, A. (1975). Intraoral air pressure as a feedback cue in consonant production. *Journal of Speech and Hearing Research, 18,* 133–147.

Ringel, R., House, A., Burk, K., Dolinsky, J., & Scott, C. (1970). Some relations between orosensory discrimination and articulatory aspects of speech production. *Journal of Speech and Hearing Disorders, 35,* 3–11.

Roberts, J., Burchinal, M., & Foote, M. (1990). Phonological process decline from 2½ to 8 years. *Journal of Communication Disorders, 23,* 205–217.

Robertson, D., & Salter, W. (1995a). *The phonological awareness kit*. East Moline, IL: LinguiSystems.

Robertson, D., & Salter, W. (1995b). *The phonological awareness profile*. East Moline, IL: LinguiSystems.

Robertson, D., & Salter, W. (1997). *The phonological awareness kit: Intermediate*. East Moline, IL: LinguiSystems.

Roseberry-McKibbin, C. (1995). *Multicultural students with special needs*. Oceanside, CA: Academic Communication Associates.

Roseberry-McKibbin, C., & Hegde, M. N. (2000). *An advanced review of speech–language pathology: Preparation for NESPA and comprehensive examination*. Austin, TX: PRO-ED.

Rosenbek, J. C. (1985). Treating apraxia of speech. In D. F. Johns (Ed.), *Clinical management of neurogenic communicative disorders* (2nd ed., pp. 267–312). Boston: College-Hill Press.

Rosenbek, J. C., & LaPointe, L. L. (1985). The dysarthrias: Description, diagnosis, and treatment. In D. F. Johns (Ed.), *Clinical management of neurogenic communicative disorders* (2nd ed., pp. 97–152). Boston: College-Hill Press.

Rosenbek, J. C., & Wertz, R. T. (1972). A review of fifty cases of developmental apraxia of speech. *Language, Speech, and Hearing Services in Schools, 5,* 23–33.

Roth, F. P., & Worthington, C. K. (1996). *Treatment resource manual for speech-language pathology*. San Diego, CA: Singular Publishing Group.

Rvachew, S. (1994). Speech perception training can facilitate sound production learning. *Journal of Speech and Hearing Research, 37,* 347–357.

Sander, E. (1972). When are speech sounds learned? *Journal of Speech and Hearing Disorders, 37,* 55–63.

Schmauch, V., Panagos, J., & Klich, R. (1978). Syntax influences on the accuracy of consonant production in language-disordered children. *Journal of Communication Disorders, 11,* 315–323.

Schmidt, L. S., Howard, B. H., & Schmidt, J. F. (1983). Conversational speech sampling in the assessment of articulation proficiency. *Language, Speech, and Hearing Services in Schools, 14,* 210–214.

Scripture, M., & Jackson, E. (1927). *A manual of exercises for the correction of speech disorders*. Philadelphia: F. A. Davis

Secord, W. (1981a). *C-PAC: Clinical probes of articulation consistency*. San Antonio, TX: Psychological Corporation.

Secord, W. (1981b). *Eliciting sounds: Techniques for clinicians*. San Antonio, TX: Psychological Corporation.

Secord, W. (1981c). *T-MAC: Test of minimal articulation competence*. San Antonio, TX: Psychological Corporation.

Secord, W. (1989). The traditional approach to therapy. In N. A. Creaghead, P. W. Newman, W. A. Secord (Eds.), *Assessment and remediation of articulatory and phonological disorders* (2nd ed.). Columbus, OH: Merrill.

Seikel, J. A., King, D. W., & Drumright, D. G. (1997). *Anatomy and physiology for speech, language, and hearing* (expanded edition). Pacific Grove, CA: Delmar.

Seymour, C. M., & Nober, E. H. (1998). *Introduction to communication disorders: A multicultural approach*. Boston: Butterworth-Heinemann.

Seymour, H., & Seymour, C. (1981). Black English and Standard American English contrasts in consonantal development for four- and five-year-old children. *Journal of Speech and Hearing Disorders, 46,* 276–280.

Shekar, C., & Hegde, M. N. (1995). India: Its people, culture, and languages. In L. L. Cheng (Ed.), *Integrating language and learning for inclusion* (pp. 125–148). San Diego: Singular Publishing Group.

Shekar, C., & Hegde, M. N. (1996). Cultural and linguistic diversity among Asian Indians: A case of Indian English. *Topics in Language Disorders, 16*(4), 54–64.

Shelton, R., Elbert, M., & Arndt, W. B. (1967). A task for evaluation of articulation change: II. Comparison of task scores during baseline and lesson series testing. *Journal of Speech and Hearing Research, 10,* 578–585.

Shelton, R., Johnson, A., & Arndt, W. (1977). Delayed judgment speech sound discrimination and /r/ or /s/ articulation status and improvement. *Journal of Speech and Hearing Research, 20,* 704–717.

Shibatani, M. (1990). Japanese. In B. Comrie (Ed.), *The world's major languages* (pp. 855–880). New York: Oxford University Press.

Shine, R. (1989). Articulatory production training: A sensory-motor approach. In N. A. Creaghead, P. W. Newman, & W. A. Secord (Eds.), *Assessment and remediation of articulatory and phonological disorders* (2nd ed.). Columbus, OH: Merrill.

Shine, R., & Proust, J. (1982). *Clinical treatment manual: Articulatory production training: A programmed sensory-motor approach.* Greenville, NC: East Carolina University.

Shipley, K. G. (1992). *Interviewing and counseling in communicative disorders: Principles and procedures.* New York: Merrill/Macmillan.

Shipley, K. G., & McAfee, J. (1998). *Assessment in speech–language pathology: A resource manual* (2nd ed.). San Diego, CA: Singular Publishing Group.

Shriberg, L. D. (1975). A response evocation program for /ɝ/. *Journal of Speech and Hearing Disorders, 40,* 92–105.

Shriberg, L. D., & Kent, R. D. (1995). *Clinical phonetics* (2nd ed.). Boston: Allyn & Bacon.

Shriberg, L. D., & Kwiatkowski, J. (1980). *Natural process analysis.* New York: Wiley.

Shriberg, L. D., & Kwiatkowski, J. (1982a). Phonological disorders I: A diagnostic classification system. *Journal of Speech and Hearing Disorders, 47,* 226–241.

Shriberg, L. D., & Kwiatkowski, J. (1982b). Phonological disorders II: A conceptual framework for management. *Journal of Speech and Hearing Disorders, 47,* 242–256.

Shriberg, L. D., & Kwiatkowski, J. (1982c). Phonological disorders III: A procedure for assessing severity of involvement. *Journal of Speech and Hearing Disorders, 47,* 256–270.

Shriberg, L. D., & Kwiatkowski, J. (1983). Computer-assisted natural process analysis (NPA): Recent issues and data. *Seminars in Speech and Lauguage, 4,* 397–406.

Shriberg, L. D., & Kwiatkowski, J. (1990). Self-monitoring and generalization in preschool speech-delayed children. *Language, Speech, and Hearing Services in Schools, 21,* 157–170.

Shriberg, L. D., & Kwiatkowski, J. (1994). Developmental phonological disorders I: A clinical profile. *Journal of Speech and Hearing Research, 37,* 1100–1126.

Shriberg, L. D., & Smith, A. J. (1983). Phonological correlates of middle-ear involvement in speech-delayed children: A methodological note. *Journal of Speech and Hearing Research, 26,* 293–297.

Shriberg, L. D., & Widder, C. (1990). Speech and prosody characteristics of adults with mental retardation. *Journal of Speech and Hearing Research, 33,* 627–653.

Siegel, G. M., Winitz, H., & Conkey, H. (1963). The influence of testing instruments on articulatory responses of children. *Journal of Speech and Hearing Disorders, 28,* 67–76.

Singh, S. (1976). *Distinctive features: Theory and validation.* Baltimore: University Park Press.

Singh, S., & Frank, D. C. (1972). A distinctive feature analysis of the consonantal substitutions pattern. *Language and Speech, 15,* 209–218.

Singh, S., & Polen, S. (1972). Use of distinctive features: Principles and practices. *Acta Symbolica, 3,* 17–25.

Skelly, M., Spector, D., Donaldson, R., Brodeur, A., & Paletta, F. (1971). Compensatory physiologic phonetics for the glossectomee. *Journal of Speech and Hearing Research, 36,* 101–114.

Smit, A. B. (1986). Ages of speech sound acquisition: Comparisons and critiques of several normative studies. *Language, Speech, and Hearing Services in Schools, 17,* 175–186.

Smit, A. B. (1993a). Phonologic error distributions in the Iowa-Nebraska articulation norms project: Consonant singletons. *Journal of Speech and Hearing Research, 36,* 533–547.

Smit, A. B. (1993b). Phonologic error distributions in the Iowa-Nebraska articulation norms project: Word-initial consonant clusters. *Journal of Speech and Hearing Research, 36,* 931–947.

Smit, A. B., Hand, L., Freilinger, J. J., Bernthal, J. E., & Bird, A. (1990). The Iowa articulation norms project and its Nebraska replication. *Journal of Speech and Hearing Disorders, 55,* 779–798.

Smith, B. L., Brown-Sweeney, S., & Stoel-Gammon, C. (1989). A quantitative analysis of reduplicated and variegated babbling. *First Language, 9,* 175–190.

Smith, M. W., & Ainsworth, S. (1967). The effects of three types of stimulation on articulatory responses of speech defective children. *Journal of Speech and Hearing Research, 10,* 333–338.

Smith, N. V. (1973). *The acquisition of phonology: A case study.* Cambridge, UK: Cambridge University Press.

Snow, C. (1977). The development of conversation between mothers and babies. *Journal of Child Language, 4,* 1–22.

Snow, K. (1961). Articulation proficiency in relation to certain dental abnormalities. *Journal of Speech and Hearing Disorders, 26,* 209–212.

Snow, K., & Milisen, R. (1954). The influence of oral versus pictorial representation upon articulation testing results. *Journal of Speech and Hearing Disorders* (Monograph Suppl. 4), 29–36.

Snowling, M., & Stackhouse, J. (1996). Epilogue: Current themes and future directions. In M. Snowling & J. Stackhouse (Eds.), *Dyslexia, speech and language: A practitioner's handbook* (pp. 234–242). London: Whurr.

So, L., & Dodd, B. (1994). Phonologically disordered Cantonese-speaking children. *Clinical Linguistics and Phonetics, 8*(3), 235–255.

Sommers, R. K., Leiss, R. H., Delp, M. A., Gerber, D. F., Smith, R. N., Revucky, M. V., Ellis, D., & Haley, V. A. (1967). Factors related to the effectiveness of articulation therapy for kindergarten, first, and second grade children. *Journal of Speech and Hearing Research, 10,* 428–437.

Spriestersbach, D. C., & Curtis, J. F. (1951). Misarticulation and discrimination of speech sounds. *Quarterly Journal of Speech, 37,* 483–491.

Spring, D. R., & Dale, P. S. (1975). Discrimination of stress in early infancy. *Journal of Speech and Hearing Research, 20,* 224–231.

Square, P., Chumpelik, D., & Adams, S. (1985). Efficacy of the PROMPT system of therapy for the treatment of acquired apraxia of speech. In R. Brookshire (Ed.), *Clinical aphasiology conference proceedings.* Minneapolis, MN: BRK Publishers.

Stackhouse, J. (1992). Developmental verbal dyspraxia: A longitudinal case study. In R. Campbell (Ed.), *Mental lives: Case studies in cognition* (pp. 84–98). Oxford, UK: Basil Blackwell.

Stackhouse, J. (1997). Phonological awareness: Connecting speech and literacy problems. In B. Hodson & M. Edwards (Eds.), *Perspectives in applied phonology* (pp. 157–196). Gaithersburg, MD: Aspen Publishers.

Stampe, D. (1969). The acquisition of phonetic representation. *Papers from the fifth regional meeting of the Chicago Linguistic Society* (pp. 433–444). Chicago: Chicago Linguistic Society.

Stark, R. (1978). Features of infant sounds: The emergence of cooing. *Journal of Child Language, 5,* 379–390.

Stark, R. (1979). Prespeech segmental feature development. In P. Fletcher & M. Garman (Eds.), *Language acquisition.* Cambridge, UK: Cambridge University Press.

Stark, R. (1980). Stages of speech development in the first year of life. In G. Yeni-Komshian, J. Kavanagh, & C. A. Ferguson (Eds.), *Child phonology. Vol. I. Production.* New York: Academic Press.

Stemple, J. C, & Holcomb, B. (1988). *Effective voice and articulation.* Columbus, OH: Merrill.

Stern, D. (1977). *The first relationship.* Cambridge, MA: Harvard University Press.

Stinchfield, S., & Young, E. (1938). *Children with delayed or defective speech: Motor-kinesthetic factors in training*. Stanford, CA: Stanford University Press.

Stockman, I. (1996). Phonological development and disorders in African American children. In A. G. Khami, K. E. Pollock, & J. L. Harris (Eds.), *Communication development and disorders in African American children* (pp. 117–153). Baltimore: Paul H. Brookes.

Stockman, I., & McDonald, E. (1980). Heterogeneity as a confounding factor when predicting spontaneous improvement of misarticulated sounds. *Language, Speech, and Hearing Services in Schools, 11,* 15–29.

Stockwell, R. P., & Bowen, J. D. (1983). *The sounds of English and Spanish*. The Hague: Mouton.

Stoel-Gammon, C. (1984). *Phonetic inventories, 15–24 months: A longitudinal study*. Paper presented at the Third International Congress for the Study of Child Language, July 8–13, Austin, TX.

Stoel-Gammon, C. (1985). Phonetic inventories, 15–24 months: A longitudinal study. *Journal of Speech and Hearing Research, 28,* 505–512.

Stoel-Gammon, C., & Cooper, J. A. (1981). *Individual differences in early phonological and lexical development*. Paper presented at the Second International Congress for the Study of Child Language, August 9–14, Vancouver, BC.

Stoel-Gammon, C., & Cooper, J. A. (1984). Patterns of early lexical and phonological development. *Journal of Child Language, 11,* 247–271.

Stoel-Gammon, C., & Dunn, C. (1985). *Normal and disordered phonology in children*. Austin, TX: PRO-ED.

Stevens, K., & Keyser, S. (1989). Primary features and their enhancement in consonants. *Language, 65,* 81–106.

Strecker, D. (1990). Tai languages. In B. Comrie (Ed.), *The world's major languages* (pp. 747–756). New York: Oxford University Press.

Swank, L. (1994). Phonological coding abilities: Identification of impairments related to phonologically based reading problems. *Topics in Language Disorders, 14,* 56–71.

Swank, L., & Catts, H. (1994). Phonological awareness and written word decoding. *Language, Speech, and Hearing Services in Schools, 25,* 9–14.

Taylor, R., & Shine, R. (1978). *Primary and secondary stress factors influencing the diphthongization and / or monophthongization of the /r/ vowel*. Laboratory research, East Carolina University, Greenville, NC.

Templin, M. C. (1947). Spontaneous versus imitated verbalization in testing articulation in preschool children. *Journal of Speech and Hearing Disorders, 12,* 293–300.

Templin, M. C. (1957). *Certain language skills in children: Their development and interrelationships*. Institute of Child Welfare, Monograph 26. Minneapolis: University of Minnesota Press.

Templin, M. C., & Darley, F. L. (1969). *The Templin-Darley tests of articulation*. Iowa City: Bureau of Education Research and Service, University of Iowa.

Terrel, S., Arensberg, K., & Rosa, M. (1992). Parent-child comparative analysis: A criterion referenced method for the nondiscriminatory assessment of a child who spoke a relatively uncommon dialect of English. *Language, Speech, and Hearing Services in Schools, 23,* 34–42.

Tomblin, J. B., Morris, H. L., Spriestersbach, D. C. (Eds.). (1994). *Diagnosis in speech-language pathology*. San Diego, CA: Singular Publishing Group.

Torgesen, J. K., & Bryant, B. R. (1993). *Phonological awareness training for reading*. Austin, TX: PRO-ED.

Torgesen, J. K., & Bryant, B. R. (1994). *Test of phonological awareness*. Austin, TX: PRO-ED.

Toronto, A. (1977). *Southwestern Spanish articulation test*. Austin, TX: National Education Laboratory Publishers.

Trammell, J., Farrar, C., Francis, J., Owens, S., Shepard, D., Thies, T., Witlin, R., & Faist, L. (1976). *Test of auditory comprehension*. North Hollywood, CA: Foreworks.

Trehub, S. (1976). The discrimination of foreign speech contrasts by infants and children. *Child Development, 47,* 466–472.

Tyler, A., & Watterson, K. (1991). Effects of phonological versus language intervention in preschoolers with both phonological and language impairment. *Child Language and Teaching Therapy, 7,* 141–160.

U. S. Bureau of the Census. (1992). *Statistical abstract of the United States, 1992* (112th ed.). Washington, DC: U. S. Government Printing Office.

U. S. Bureau of the Census. (1996). *Statistical abstract of the United States, 1996* (116th ed.). Washington, DC: U. S. Government Printing Office.

van Keulen, J. E., Weddington, G. T., & DeBose, C. E. (1998). *Speech, language, learning, and the African American child.* Needham Heights, MA: Allyn & Bacon.

van Kleeck, A. (1995). Emphasizing form and meaning repeatedly in prereading and early reading instruction. *Topics in Language Disorders, 16,* 27–49.

Van Riper, C. (1939). *Speech correction: Principles and methods.* Englewood Cliffs, NJ: Prentice-Hall.

Van Riper, C. (1978). *Speech correction: Principles and methods* (6th ed.). Englewood Cliffs, NJ: Prentice-Hall.

Van Riper, C., & Emerick, L. (1984). *Speech correction: An introduction to speech pathology and audiology.* Englewood Cliffs, NJ: Prentice-Hall.

Van Riper, C., & Erickson, R. (1969). A predictive screening test of articulation. *Journal of Speech and Hearing Disorders, 34,* 214–219.

Van Riper, C., & Erickson, R. (1996). *Speech correction: An introduction to speech pathology and audiology* (9th ed.). Boston: Allyn & Bacon.

Van Riper, C., & Irwin, J. (1958). *Voice and articulation.* Englewood Cliffs, NJ: Prentice-Hall.

Velleman, S. L., & Strand, K. (1994). Developmental verbal dyspraxia. In J. E. Bernthal & N. W. Bankson (Eds.), *Child phonology: Characteristics, assessment, and intervention with special populations* (pp. 110–140). New York: Thieme Medical Publishers.

Vihman, M. M. (1998). Early phonological development. In J. E. Bernthal & N. W. Bankson (Eds.), *Articulation and phonological disorders* (4th ed., pp. 63–112). Boston: Allyn & Bacon.

Vihman, M. M., Ferguson, C. A., & Elbert, M. (1986). Phonological development from babbling to speech: Common tendencies and individual differences. *Applied Psycholinguistics, 7,* 3–40.

Vihman, M. M., & Greenlee, M. (1987). Individual differences in phonological development: Ages one to three years. *Journal of Speech and Hearing Research, 30,* 503–521.

Vihman, M. M., Macken, M. A., Miller, R., Simmons, H., & Miller, J. (1985). From babbling to speech: A reassessment of the continuity issue. *Language, 61,* 395–443.

Washington, J., & Craig, H. (1992). Articulation test performance of low-income, African American preschoolers with communication impairments. *Language, Speech, and Hearing Services in the Schools, 23,* 203–207.

Waterson, N. (1981). Child phonology: A prosodic view. *Journal of Linguistics, 7,* 179–211.

Webster, P. E., & Plante, A. S. (1992). Effects of phonological impairment on word, syllable, and phoneme segmentation and reading. *Language, Speech, and Hearing Services in Schools, 23,* 176–182.

Weiner, F. (1979). *Phonological process analysis.* Baltimore: University Park Press.

Weiner, F. (1981). Treatment of phonological disability using the method of meaningful minimal contrast: Two case studies. *Journal of Speech and Hearing Disorders, 46,* 97–103.

Weiner, F., & Bankson, N. (1978). Teaching features. *Language, Speech, and Hearing Services in Schools, 9,* 29–34.

Weiner, P. (1967). Auditory discrimination and articulation. *Journal of Speech and Hearing Disorders, 32,* 19–28.

Weinreich, U. (1953). *Languages in contact.* The Hague: Mouton.

Weiss, C. E., Gordon, M. E., & Lillywhite, H. S. (1987). *Clinical management of articulatory and phonologic disorders* (2nd ed.). Baltimore: Williams & Wilkins.

Welker, G. (1996). *Native American languages* [On-line]: Available FTP: indians.org/welker.americans.htm

Wellman, B., Case, I., Mengert, I., & Bradbury, D. (1931). Speech sounds of young children. *University of Iowa Studies in Child Welfare, 5*(2).

Werker, J., & Tees, R. (1984). Cross-language speech perception: Evidence for perceptual reorganization during the first year of life. *Infant Behavior and Development, 7,* 49–64.

Wertz, R. T., LaPointe, L. L., & Rosenbek, J. C. (1991). *Apraxia of speech in adults: The disorder and its management.* San Diego, CA: Singular Publishing Group.

Weston, A. J., & Irwin, J. V. (1971). Use of paired stimuli in modification of articulation. *Perceptual motor skills, 32,* 947–957.

Whitehurst, G., Fischel, J., Lonigan, C., Valdez-Menchaca, M., Arnold, D., & Smith, M. (1991). Treatment of early expressive language delay: If, when, and how. *Topics in Language Disorders, 11,* 55–68.

Williams, G., & McReynolds, L. (1975). The relationship between discrimination and articulation training in children with misarticulations. *Journal of Speech and Hearing Research, 18,* 401–412.

Williams, J. (1984). Phonemic analysis and how it relates to reading. *Journal of Learning Disabilities, 17,* 240–245.

Willis, W. (1992). Families with African American roots. In E. W. Lynch & M. A. Hanson (Eds.), *Developing cross-cultural competence: A guide for working with young children and their families* (pp. 121–150). Baltimore: Paul H. Brookes.

Wilson, D. K. (1972). *Voice problems in children.* Baltimore: Williams & Wilkins.

Wilson, M. E. (1996). Arabic speakers: Language and culture, here and abroad. *Topics in Language Disorders, 16*(4), 65–80.

Wilson, W. F. (1998). Delivering speech–language and hearing services in the Arab world: Some cultural considerations. In D. E. Battle (Ed.), *Communication disorders in multicultural populations* (2nd ed., pp. 197–210). Boston: Butterworth-Heinemann.

Winitz, H. (1969). *Articulatory acquisition and behavior.* Englewood Cliffs, NJ: Prentice-Hall.

Winitz, H. (1975). *From syllable to conversation.* Baltimore: University Park Press.

Winitz, H. (1984). Auditory considerations in articulation and training. In H. Winitz (Ed.), *Treating articulation disorders: For clinicians by clinicians.* Baltimore: University Park Press.

Winitz, H. (1989). Auditory considerations in treatment. In N. A. Creaghead, P. W. Newman, & W. A. Secord (Eds.), *Assessment and remediation of articulatory and phonological disorders* (2nd ed.). Columbus, OH: Merrill.

Winitz, H., & Irwin, O. C. (1958). Syllabic and phonetic structure of infants' early words. *Journal of Speech and Hearing Research, 1,* 250–256.

Wolfram, W. (1986). Language variation in the United States. In O. Taylor (Ed.), *Treatment of communication disorders in culturally and linguistically diverse populations* (pp. 73–116). San Diego, CA: College-Hill Press.

Wolfram, W. (1991). *Dialects and American English.* Englewood Cliffs, NJ: Prentice-Hall.

Wolfram, W. (1994). The phonology of a sociocultural society: The case of African American vernacular English. In J. E. Bernthal & N. W. Bankson (Eds.), *Child phonology: Characteristics, assessment, and intervention with special populations* (pp. 227–244). New York: Thieme Medical Publishers.

Yavas, M. (Ed.). (1994). *First and second language phonology.* San Diego, CA: Singular Publishing Group.

Yavas, M. (1998). *Phonology: Development and disorders.* San Diego, CA: Singular Publishing Group.

Yavas, M., & Goldstein, B. (1998). Phonological assessment and treatment of bilingual speakers. *American Journal of Speech–Language Pathology, 7,* 49–60.

Yorkston, K. M., Beukelman, D., & Bell, K. R. (1988). *Clinical management of dysarthric speakers.* Austin, TX: PRO-ED.

Yorkston, K. M., Beukelman, D., & Traynor, C. (1984). *Assessment of intelligibility of dysarthric speakers.* Austin, TX: PRO-ED.

Zehel, Z., Shelton, R. L., Arndt, W. B., Wright, V., & Elbert, M. (1972). Item context and /s/ phone articulation test results. *Journal of Speech and Hearing Research, 15,* 852–860.

Zemlin, W. R. (1998). *Speech and hearing science: Anatomy and physiology* (4th ed.). Englewood Cliffs, NJ: Prentice-Hall.

Zuniga, M. E. (1992). Families with Latino roots. In E. W. Lynch & M. J. Hanson (Eds.), *Developing cross-cultural competence* (pp. 151–178). Baltimore: Paul H. Brookes.

Appendixes

551

Appendix A

◆ ◆ ◆ ◆ ◆ ◆ ◆ ◆ ◆ ◆ ◆ ◆ ◆ ◆ ◆ ◆ ◆ ◆ ◆

Muscles and Nerves Involved in the Production of English Consonants

/p/

- Voiceless
- Bilabial
- Stop-plosive

Function	Muscle[a]	Nerve Innervation[b]
Lip compression	orbicularis oris	facial nerve (CN VII)
Velopharyngeal closure	levator veli palatini, superior constrictor, salpingopharyngeus, and palatopharyngeus	vagus nerve (CN X), pharyngeal branch
Mandibular lowering on release	external pterygoid; digastric muscle, anterior belly; and mylohyoid muscle	trigeminal nerve (CN V), mandibular branch
	geniohyoid muscle	C1 spinal nerve

/b/

- Voiced
- Bilabial
- Stop

Function	Muscle	Nerve Innervation
Lip compression	orbicularis oris	facial nerve (CN VII)
Velopharyngeal closure	levator veli palatini, superior constrictor, salpingopharyngeus, and palatopharyngeus	vagus nerve (CN X), pharyngeal branch
Mandibular lowering on release	External pterygoid; digastric muscle, anterior belly; and mylohyoid muscle	trigeminal nerve (CN V), mandibular branch
	geniohyoid muscle	C1 spinal nerve

| Phonation | thyroarytenoid (thyrovocalis), lateral cricoarytenoid, and transverse and oblique interarytenoid | vagus nerve (CN X), laryngeal branch |

/t/

- Voiceless
- Alveolar
- Stop-plosive

Function	Muscle	Nerve Innervation
Lowering of the mandible for lip positioning	digastric muscle, anterior belly; mylohyoid; and external pterygoid	trigeminal nerve (CN V), mandibular branch
	geniohyoid	C1 spinal nerve
Velopharyngeal closure	levator veli palatini, superior constrictor, salpingopharyngeus, and palatopharyngeus	vagus nerve (CN X), pharyngeal branch
Elevation of tongue tip and sides	superior longitudinal, styloglossus	hypoglossal nerve (CN XII)

/d/

- Voiceless
- Alveolar
- Stop-plosive

Function	Muscle	Nerve Innervation
Lowering of the mandible for lip positioning	digastric muscle, anterior belly; mylohyoid; and external pterygoid	trigeminal nerve (CN V), mandibular branch
	geniohyoid	C1 spinal nerve
Elevation of tongue tip and sides	superior longitudinal, styloglossus	hypoglossal nerve (CN XII)
Velopharyngeal closure	levator veli palatini, superior constrictor, salpingopharyngeus, and palatopharyngeus	vagus nerve (CN X), pharyngeal branch
Phonation	thyroarytenoid (thyrovocalis), lateral cricoarytenoid, and transverse and oblique interarytenoid	vagus nerve (CN X), laryngeal branch

/k/

- Voiceless
- Velar
- Stop-plosive

Function	Muscle	Nerve Innervation
Lowering of the mandible for lip positioning	digastric muscle, anterior belly; mylohyoid; and external pterygoid	trigeminal nerve (CN V), mandibular branch
	geniohyoid	C1 spinal nerve
Elevation of tongue dorsum	palatoglossus	spinal accessory (CN XI)
	styloglossus	hypoglossal (CN XII)
Velopharyngeal closure	levator veli palatini, superior constrictor, salpingopharyngeus, and palatopharyngeus	vagus nerve (CN X), pharyngeal branch

/g/

- Voiced
- Bilabial
- Stop

Function	Muscle	Nerve Innervation
Lowering of the mandible for lip positioning	digastric muscle, anterior belly; mylohyoid; and external pterygoid	trigeminal nerve (CN V), mandibular branch
	geniohyoid	C1 spinal nerve
Elevation of tongue dorsum	palatoglossus	spinal accessory (CN XI)
	styloglossus	hypoglossal (CN XII)
Velopharyngeal closure	levator veli palatini, superior constrictor, salpingopharyngeus, and palatopharyngeus	vagus nerve (CN X), pharyngeal branch
Phonation	thyroarytenoid (thyrovocalis), lateral cricoarytenoid, and transverse and oblique interarytenoid	vagus nerve (CN X), laryngeal branch

/m/

- Voiced
- Bilabial
- Nasal

Function	Muscle	Nerve Innervation
Lip compression	orbicularis oris	facial nerve (CN VII)
Phonation	thyroarytenoid (thyrovocalis), lateral cricoarytenoid, and transverse and oblique interarytenoid	vagus nerve (CN X), laryngeal branch

/n/

- Voiced
- Alveolar
- Nasal

Function	Muscle	Nerve Innervation
Lowering of the mandible for lip positioning	digastric muscle, anterior belly; mylohyoid; and external pterygoid	trigeminal nerve (CN V), mandibular branch
	geniohyoid	C1 spinal nerve
Elevation of tongue tip and sides	superior longitudinal, styloglossus	hypoglossal nerve (CN XII)
Phonation	thyroarytenoid (thyrovocalis), lateral cricoarytenoid, and transverse and oblique interarytenoid	vagus nerve (CN X), laryngeal branch

/ŋ/

- Voiced
- Bilabial
- Nasal

Function	Muscle	Nerve Innervation
Lowering of the mandible for lip positioning	digastric muscle, anterior belly; mylohyoid; and external pterygoid	trigeminal nerve (CN V), mandibular branch
	geniohyoid	C1 spinal nerve
Elevation of tongue dorsum	palatoglossus	spinal accessory (CN XI)
	styloglossus	hypoglossal (CN XII)

Phonation	thyroarytenoid (thyrovocalis), lateral cricoarytenoid, and transverse and oblique interarytenoid	vagus nerve (CN X), laryngeal branch

/j/

- Voiced
- Palatal
- Glide

Function	Muscle	Nerve Innervation
Lowering of the mandible for lip positioning	digastric muscle, anterior belly; mylohyoid; and external pterygoid	trigeminal nerve (CN V), mandibular branch
	geniohyoid	C1 spinal nerve
Elevation of tongue dorsum	palatoglossus	spinal accessory (CN XI)
	styloglossus	hypoglossal (CN XII)
Velopharyngeal closure	levator veli palatini, superior constrictor, salpingopharyngeus, and palatopharyngeus	vagus nerve (CN X), pharyngeal branch
Phonation	thyroarytenoid (thyrovocalis), lateral cricoarytenoid, and transverse and oblique interarytenoid	vagus nerve (CN X), laryngeal branch

/w/

- Voiced
- Bilabial-velar
- Glide

Function	Muscle	Nerve Innervation
Lowering of the mandible for lip positioning	digastric muscle, anterior belly; mylohyoid; and external pterygoid	trigeminal nerve (CN V), mandibular branch
	geniohyoid	C1 spinal nerve
Elevation of tongue dorsum	palatoglossus	spinal accessory (CN XI)
	styloglossus	hypoglossal (CN XII)
Velopharyngeal closure	levator veli palatini, superior constrictor, salpingopharyngeus, and palatopharyngeus	vagus nerve (CN X), pharyngeal branch

Phonation	thyroarytenoid (thyrovocalis), lateral cricoarytenoid, and transverse and oblique interarytenoid	vagus nerve (CN X), laryngeal branch
Lip rounding and protrusion	orbicularis oris, mentalis, levator labii inferior, and levator labii superiorus	facial nerve (CN VII)

/l/

- Voiced
- Alveolar
- Liquid

Function	Muscle	Nerve Innervation
Lowering of the mandible for lip positioning	digastric muscle, anterior belly; mylohyoid; and external pterygoid	trigeminal nerve (CN V), mandibular branch
	geniohyoid	C1 spinal nerve
Elevation of tongue tip and sides	superior longitudinal, styloglossus	hypoglossal nerve (CN XII)
Elevation of the tongue blade	transverse lingual	hypoglossal (CN XII)
	palatoglossus	spinal accessory (CN XI)
Velopharyngeal closure	levator veli palatini, superior constrictor, salpingopharyngeus, and palatopharyngeus	vagus nerve (CN X), pharyngeal branch
Phonation	Thyroarytenoid (thyrovocalis), lateral cricoarytenoid, and transverse and oblique interarytenoid	vagus nerve (CN X), laryngeal branch

/r/

- Voiced
- Palatal
- Liquid

Function	Muscle	Nerve Innervation
Lowering of the mandible for lip positioning	digastric muscle, anterior belly; mylohyoid; and external pterygoid	trigeminal nerve (CN V), mandibular branch
	geniohyoid	C1 spinal nerve

Elevation of the tongue blade	transverse lingual	hypoglossal (CN XII)
	palatoglossus	spinal accessory (CN XI)
Positioning of the tongue tip	superior longitudinal	hypoglossal (CN XII)
Velopharyngeal closure	levator veli palatini, superior constrictor, salpingopharyngeus, and palatopharyngeus	vagus nerve (CN X), pharyngeal branch
Phonation	thyroarytenoid (thyrovocalis), lateral cricoarytenoid, and transverse and oblique interarytenoid	vagus nerve (CN X), laryngeal branch
Lip rounding and slight protrusion	orbicularis oris, mentalis, levator labii inferior, and levator labii superiorus	facial nerve (CN VII)

/f/

- Voiceless
- Alveolar
- Fricative

Function	Muscle	Nerve Innervation
Slight retraction and lowering of the mandible	internal pterygoid (retraction); digastric muscle, anterior belly (lowering); mylohyoid (lowering); and external pterygoid (lowering)	trigeminal nerve (CN V), mandibular branch
	geniohyoid (lowering)	C1 spinal nerve
Slight tensing and elevation of the lower lip	buccinator (tension & elevation); risorius (tension & elevation); orbicularis oris, lower portion (tension & elevation); and mentalis (elevation)	facial nerve (CN VII)
Velopharyngeal closure	levator veli palatini, superior constrictor, salpingopharyngeus, and palatopharyngeus	vagus nerve (CN X), pharyngeal branch

/v/

- Voiced
- Alveolar
- Fricative

Function	Muscle	Nerve Innervation
Slight retraction and lowering of the mandible	internal pterygoid (retraction); digastric muscle, anterior belly (lowering); mylohyoid (lowering); and external pterygoid (lowering)	trigeminal nerve (CN V), mandibular branch
	geniohyoid (lowering)	C1 spinal nerve
Slight tensing and elevation of the lower lip	buccinator (tension & elevation); risorius (tension & elevation); orbicularis oris, lower portion (tension & elevation); and mentalis (elevation)	facial nerve (CN VII)
Velopharyngeal closure	levator veli palatini, superior constrictor, salpingopharyngeus, and palatopharyngeus	vagus nerve (CN X), pharyngeal branch
Phonation	thyroarytenoid (thyrovocalis), lateral cricoarytenoid, and transverse and oblique interarytenoid	vagus nerve (CN X), laryngeal branch

/θ/

- Voiceless
- Alveolar
- Fricative

Function	Muscle	Nerve Innervation
Slight lowering of the mandible	digastric muscle, anterior belly; mylohyoid; and external pterygoid	trigeminal nerve (CN V), mandibular branch
	geniohyoid	C1 spinal nerve
Positioning of the tongue tip between the teeth	genioglossus (medial and posterior fibers), longitudinal superior	hypoglossal (CN XII)
Flattening of the tongue	vertical lingual	hypoglossal (CN XII)
Velopharyngeal closure	levator veli palatini, superior constrictor, salpingopharyngeus, and palatopharyngeus	vagus nerve (CN X), pharyngeal branch

| Phonation | thyroarytenoid (thyrovocalis), lateral cricoarytenoid, and transverse and oblique interarytenoid | vagus nerve (CN X), laryngeal branch |

/ð/

- Voiced
- Alveolar
- Fricative

Function	Muscle	Nerve Innervation
Slight lowering of the mandible	digastric muscle, anterior belly; mylohyoid; and external pterygoid	trigeminal nerve (CN V), mandibular branch
	geniohyoid	C1 spinal nerve
Positioning of the tongue tip between the teeth	genioglossus (medial and posterior fibers), longitudinal superior	hypoglossal (CN XII)
Flattening of the tongue	vertical lingual	hypoglossal (CN XII)
Velopharyngeal closure	levator veli palatini, superior constrictor, salpingopharyngeus, and palatopharyngeus	vagus nerve (CN X), pharyngeal branch
Phonation	thyroarytenoid (thyrovocalis), lateral cricoarytenoid, and transverse and oblique interarytenoid	vagus nerve (CN X), laryngeal branch

/s/

- Voiceless
- Alveolar
- Fricative

Function	Muscle	Nerve Innervation
Slight separation of the lips	levator labii superiorus, levator labii inferiorus	facial nerve (CN VII)
Occlusion of the teeth (jaws close together)	internal pterygoid, temporalis, and masseter	facial nerve (CN VII)
Extension and grooving of the tongue tip	genioglossus, anterior fibers (extension), transverse lingual	hypoglossal (CN XII)
Velopharyngeal closure	levator veli palatini, superior constrictor, salpingopharyngeus, and palatopharyngeus	vagus nerve (CN X), pharyngeal branch

/z/

- Voiced
- Alveolar
- Fricative

Function	Muscle	Nerve Innervation
Slight separation of the lips	levator labii superiorus, levator labii inferiorus	facial nerve (CN VII)
Occlusion of the teeth (jaws close together)	internal pterygoid, temporalis, and masseter	facial nerve (CN VII)
Extension and grooving of the tongue tip	genioglossus, anterior fibers (extension), transverse lingual	hypoglossal (CN XII)
Velopharyngeal closure	levator veli palatini, superior constrictor, salpingopharyngeus, and palatopharyngeus	vagus nerve (CN X), pharyngeal branch
Phonation	thyroarytenoid (thyrovocalis), lateral cricoarytenoid, and transverse and oblique interarytenoid	vagus nerve (CN X), laryngeal branch

/ʃ/

- Voiceless
- Alveolar
- Fricative

Function	Muscle	Nerve Innervation
Slight lowering of the mandible	digastric muscle, anterior belly; mylohyoid; and external pterygoid	trigeminal nerve (CN V), mandibular branch
	geniohyoid	C1 spinal nerve
Slight protrusion of the lips	orbicularis oris, mentalis, levator labii superiorus, and levator labii inferiorus	facial nerve (CN VII)
Flattening of the tongue dorsum	vertical lingual	hypoglossal (CN XII)
Depression of the tongue front	genioglossus (anterior fibers), inferior longitudinal, and hyoglossus	hypoglossal (CN XII)
Velopharyngeal closure	levator veli palatini, superior constrictor, salpingopharyngeaus, and palatopharyngeus	vagus nerve (CN X), pharyngeal branch

/ʒ/

- Voiced
- Alveolar
- Fricative

Function	Muscle	Nerve Innervation
Slight lowering of the mandible	digastric muscle, anterior belly; mylohyoid; and external pterygoid	trigeminal nerve (CN V), mandibular branch
	geniohyoid	C1 spinal nerve
Slight protrusion of the lips	orbicularis oris, mentalis, levator labii superiorus, and levator labii inferiorus	facial nerve (CN VII)
Flattening of the tongue dorsum	vertical lingual	hypoglossal (CN XII)
Depression of the tongue front	genioglossus (anterior fibers), inferior longitudinal, and hyoglossus	hypoglossal (CN XII)
Velopharyngeal closure	levator veli palatini, superior constrictor, salpingopharyngeus, and palatopharyngeus	vagus nerve (CN X), pharyngeal branch
Phonation	thyroarytenoid (thyrovocalis), lateral cricoarytenoid, and transverse and oblique interarytenoid	vagus nerve (CN X), laryngeal branch

/tʃ/

- Voiceless
- Alveolar
- Fricative

Function	Muscle	Nerve Innervation
Slight lowering of the mandible	digastric muscle, anterior belly; mylohyoid; and external pterygoid	trigeminal nerve (CN V), mandibular branch
	geniohyoid	C1 spinal nerve
Slight protrusion of the lips	orbicularis oris, mentalis, levator labii superiorus, and levator labii inferiorus	facial nerve (CN VII)
Elevation of the tongue tip, lateral margins, and central apical portion	superior longitudinal, styloglossus	hypoglossal (CN XII)

Velopharyngeal closure	levator veli palatini, superior constrictor, salpingopharyngeus, and palatopharyngeus	vagus nerve (CN X), pharyngeal branch

/ʤ/

- Voiced
- Alveolar
- Fricative

Function	Muscle	Nerve Innervation
Slight lowering of the mandible	digastric muscle, anterior belly; mylohyoid; and external pterygoid	trigeminal nerve (CN V), mandibular branch
	geniohyoid	C1 spinal nerve
Slight protrusion of the lips	orbicularis oris, mentalis, levator labii superiorus, and levator labii inferiorus	facial nerve (CN VII)
Elevation of the tongue tip, lateral margins, and central apical portion	superior longitudinal, styloglossus	hypoglossal (CN XII)
Velopharyngeal closure	levator veli palatini, superior constrictor, salpingopharyngeus, and palatopharyngeus	vagus nerve (CN X), pharyngeal branch
Phonation	thyroarytenoid (thyrovocalis), lateral cricoarytenoid, and transverse and oblique interarytenoid	vagus nerve (CN X), laryngeal branch

/h/

- Voiceless
- Glottal
- Fricative

Function	Muscle	Nerve Innervation
Slight lowering of the mandible	digastric muscle, anterior belly; mylohyoid; and external pterygoid	trigeminal nerve (CN V), mandibular branch
	geniohyoid	C1 spinal nerve
Slight approximation of the vocal folds	thyroarytenoid (thyrovocalis)	vagus nerve (CN X), laryngeal branch

| Velopharyngeal closure | levator veli palatini, superior constrictor, salpingopharyngeus, and palatopharyngeus | vagus nerve (CN X), pharyngeal branch |

[a]Information drawn from Edwards (1997).
[b]Information drawn from Kuehn, Lemme, and Baumgartner (1989).

Appendix B

The International Phonetic
Alphabet (revised 1989)

CONSONANTS

	Bilabial	Labiodental	Dental	Alveolar	Postalveolar	Retroflex	Palatal	Velar	Uvular	Pharyngeal	Glottal
Plosive	p b			t d		ʈ ɖ	c ɟ	k ɡ	q ɢ		ʔ
Nasal	m	ɱ		n		ɳ	ɲ	ŋ	ɴ		
Trill	ʙ			r					ʀ		
Tap or flap				ɾ		ɽ					
Fricative	ɸ β	f v	θ ð	s z	ʃ ʒ	ʂ ʐ	ç ʝ	x ɣ	χ ʁ	ħ ʕ	h ɦ
Lateral fricative				ɬ ɮ							
Approximant		ʋ		ɹ		ɻ	j	ɰ			
Lateral approximant				l		ɭ	ʎ	ʟ			
Ejective stop	pʼ			tʼ		ʈʼ	cʼ	kʼ	qʼ		
Implosive	ɓ			ɗ			ʄ	ɠ	ʛ		

Where symbols appear in pairs, the one to the right represents a voiced consonant. Shaded areas denote articulations judged impossible.

VOWELS

Where symbols appear in pairs, the one to the right represents a rounded vowel.

OTHER SYMBOLS

ʍ Voiceless labial-velar fricative	⊙ Bilabial click		
w Voiced labial-velar approximant	ǀ Dental click		
ɥ Voiced labial-palatal approximant	ǃ (Post)alveolar click		
ʜ Voiceless epiglottal fricative	ǂ Palatoalveolar click		
ʢ Voiced epiglottal plosive	ǁ Alveolar lateral click		
ʡ Voiced epiglottal fricative	ʄ Alveolar lateral flap		
ɕ ʑ Simultaneous ʃ and x	ɕ ʑ Alveolo-palatal fricatives		
ɜ Additional mid central vowel			

Affricates and double articulations can be represented by two symbols joined by a tie bar if necessary.

k͡p t͡s

DIACRITICS

̥ Voiceless	n̥ d̥	̜ More rounded	ɔ̜	ʷ Labialized	tʷ dʷ	̃ Nasalized	ẽ
̬ Voiced	s̬ t̬	̹ Less rounded	ɔ̹	ʲ Palatalized	tʲ dʲ	ⁿ Nasal release	dⁿ
ʰ Aspirated	tʰ dʰ	̟ Advanced	u̟	ˠ Velarized	tˠ dˠ	ˡ Lateral release	dˡ
̤ Breathy voiced	b̤ a̤	̠ Retracted	ī	ˤ Pharyngealized	tˤ dˤ	̚ No audible release	d̚
̰ Creaky voiced	b̰ a̰	̈ Centralized	ë	̴ Velarized or pharyngealized	ɫ		
̼ Linguolabial	t̼ d̼	̽ Mid centralized	ě	̝ Raised	e̝ (ɹ̝ = voiced alveolar fricative)		
̪ Dental	t̪ d̪	̘ Advanced tongue root	e̘	̞ Lowered	e̞ (β̞ = voiced bilabial approximant)		
̺ Apical	t̺ d̺	̙ Retracted tongue root	e̙				
̻ Laminal	t̻ d̻	˞ Rhoticity	ɚ	̩ Syllabic	l̩	̯ Nonsyllabic	e̯

SUPRASEGMENTALS

ˈ Primary stress	ˌ Secondary stress	ˌfoʊnəˈtɪʃən
ː Long	eː	
ˑ Half-long	eˑ	
̆ Extra-short	ĕ	
. Syllable break	ɹi.ækt	
‖ Minor (foot) group		
‖ Major (intonation) group		
‿ Linking (absence of a break)		

TONES AND WORD ACCENTS

LEVEL TONES

˥ Extra-high	
˦ High	
˧ Mid	̄ or ˉ
˨ Low	
˩ Extra-low	
ꜜ Downstep	→ Global rise
ꜛ Upstep	↗ Global fall

CONTOUR TONES

̌ Rise	or ꜒
̂ Fall	꜓
᷄ High rise	
᷅ Low rise	
᷈ Rise fall	etc.

Appendix C

◆ ◆

Definition of Other Phonological Processes

Process	Definition	Examples
Stridency deletion	Deletion of a strident consonant, or substitution of a nonstrident consonant for a strident consonant.	[po] for *sew* [op] for *soap*
Alveolarization	Substitution of an alveolar consonant for a labial or interdental consonant.	[dot] for *boat* [tɪg] for *pig*
Labialization	Substitution of a labial or interdental consonant for an alveolar consonant; other lingual consonants may also be affected.	[bek] for *take* [pɪg] for *dig*
Denasalization	The replacement of a nasal consonant by a nonnasal sound made in the same place of articulation.	[pæt] for *mat* [doz] for *nose*
Metathesis	The reversal of two sounds, which may or may not be adjacent to one another.	[aks] for *ask* [pots] for *post*
Migration	The movement of a sound from one word position to another word position.	[ops] for *soap* [ɪpzɚ] for *zipper*
Glottal replacement	Substitution of a glottal stop for a nonglottal sound usually made in the medial or final position.	[pʔɪ] for *puppy* [joʔ] for *joke*
Apicalization	Substitution of an apical (tongue tip) sound for a labial sound.	[dɔr] for *poor* [dəg] for *bug*
Devoicing of stops	Substitution of a voiceless consonant for a voiced stop.	[pʊk] for *book* [tot] for *goat*
Sound preference substitutions	Substitution of one or two specific phonemes for a group of consonants.	/s/, /z/, /t/, /d/ substituted by /m/

Appendix D

◆ ◆ ◆ ◆ ◆ ◆ ◆ ◆ ◆ ◆ ◆ ◆ ◆ ◆ ◆ ◆ ◆ ◆ ◆ ◆

Passages for Screenings with Older Children and Adults

Adult Passages

Grandfather Passage

You wished to know all about my grandfather. Well, he is nearly ninety-three years old, yet he still thinks as swiftly as ever. He dresses himself in an old black frock coat, usually several buttons missing. A long beard clings to his chin, giving those who observe him a pronounced feeling of the utmost respect. When he speaks, his voice is just a bit cracked and quivers a trifle. Twice each day he plays skillfully and with zest upon a small organ. Except in winter when the snow or ice prevents, he slowly takes a short walk in the open air each day. We have often urged him to walk more and smoke less, but he always answers, "Banana oil." Grandfather likes to be modern in his language.

Rainbow Passage

When the sunlight strikes raindrops in the air, they act like a prism and form a rainbow. The rainbow is a division of white light into many beautiful colors. These take the shape of a long round arch, with its path high above, and its two ends apparently beyond the horizon. There is, according to legend, a boiling pot of gold at one end. People look, but no one ever finds it. When a man looks for something beyond his reach, his friends say he is looking for a pot of gold at the end of the rainbow.

Throughout the centuries men have explained the rainbow in various ways. Some have accepted it as a miracle without physical explanation. To the Hebrews it was a token that there would be no more universal floods. The Greeks used to imagine that it was a sign from the gods to foretell war or heavy rain. The Norsemen considered the rainbow as a bridge over which the gods passed from earth to their home in the sky. Other men tried to explain the phenomenon physically. Aristotle thought the rainbow was caused by reflection of the sun's rays by the rain. Since then physicists have found that it is not reflection, but refraction by the raindrops which causes the rainbow. Many complicated ideas about the rainbow have been formed. The difference in the rainbow depends considerably upon the size of the water drops, and the width of the colored band increases as the size of the drops increases. The actual primary rainbow observed is said to be the effect of superposition of a number of bows. If the red of the second bow falls upon the green of the first, the result is to give a bow with an abnormally wide yellow band, since red and green lights when mixed form yellow. This is a very common type of bow, one showing mainly red and yellow, with little or no green or blue.

Declaration of Independence

We hold these truths to be self-evident, that all men are created equal, that they are endowed by their Creator with certain unalienable rights, that among these are life, liberty and the pursuit of happiness. That to secure these rights, governments are instituted among men, deriving their just powers from the consent of the governed, that whenever any form of government becomes destructive of these ends, it is the right of the people to alter or to abolish it, and to institute new government, laying its foundation on such principles and organizing its powers in such form, as to them shall seem most likely to effect their safety and happiness.

Prudence, indeed, will dictate that governments long established should not be changed for light and transient causes; and accordingly all experience has shown, that mankind are more disposed to suffer, while evils are sufferable, than to right themselves by abolishing the forms to which they are accustomed. But when a long train of abuses and usurpations, pursuing invariably the same object evinces a design to reduce them under absolute despotism, it is their right, it is their duty, to throw off such government, and to provide new guards for their future security.

Children Passages

The Spider's Home

A spider is an amazing animal. It can build its own home, and it doesn't even have to buy wood or a saw. Before the spider begins to build, it looks for the perfect spot. The spider likes to live in a grassy area where lots of insects can get caught in its web. Then the spider eats the insects for dinner. The spider also has to figure out which way the wind is blowing. The wind has to be on the spider's back before it is able to make a house.

After it finds a good place to live, it is ready to spin its webs. The spider has glands in its stomach that produce a silky liquid. It leaps from one side of the house and is carried by the wind to the other side. As it travels through the air, the liquid comes out. As soon as the liquid hits the air, it becomes solid, making a fine, tough thread. The spider uses the first thread as a bridge to travel from one side to the other. Then it continues to build its web strand by strand until its home is complete.

The Toothbrush

Did you know that the toothbrush was invented in a prison? One morning in 1770, a man in an English jail woke up with an idea. He thought it would be better if he could use a brush to clean his teeth, rather than wipe them with a rag. At dinner he took a bone from his meat and kept it. Then he told the prison guard about his idea. The guard gave him some bristles to use for the brush. The prisoner made holes in the bone and stuffed the bristles into the holes. It was a success! The prisoner was so excited about his new invention that he went into the toothbrush business when he got out of jail.

For more than 200 years we have used toothbrushes similar to the one the prisoner invented. Toothbrushes are not made out of bones anymore. They come in all kinds of colors and sizes. The next time you brush your teeth, think about the prisoner in England who invented the toothbrush.

Appendix E

◆ ◆ ◆ ◆ ◆ ◆ ◆ ◆ ◆ ◆ ◆ ◆ ◆ ◆ ◆ ◆ ◆ ◆

Sample Referral Letter
to an Audiologist

1234 Speech Clinic
5050 Avenue Street
Georgetown, CA 90000

May 1, 2000

Feel Good Ear, Nose, and Throat Clinic
Lynn Gonzales, M.A., CCC-A
5067 Lane Street
Georgetown, CA 90000

Re: Stephanie Lindell

Dear Lynn,

Stephanie was seen for a speech and language evaluation at the 1234 Speech Clinic. She has a severe phonological disorder and has difficulty producing many sounds. Her speech intelligibility is approximately 50% to strangers.

During the interview, Mrs. Lindell reported that Stephanie has a history of recurrent ear infections. She indicated that Stephanie's hearing had been screened by her pediatrician but not fully evaluated. Stephanie did not pass the screening administered by her pediatrician.

As part of my assessment, I screened Stephanie's hearing bilaterally at 250, 500, 1,000, 2,000, and 8,000 Hz at 25 db HL. Stephanie failed the hearing screening in both ears. During my assessment I also noticed that she said "huh?" several times and did not appear to hear my instructions on occasion.

I am referring Stephanie for a full audiological evaluation. Her mother indicated that her insurance carrier contracts with your clinic. I have sent a referral for a full audiological evaluation along with my diagnostic report to Stephanie's primary care physician.

Please call (915) 671-0000 if you have any questions.

Sincerely,

Janet Blossom, M.A., CCC-SLP
Speech–Language Pathologist

cc: Mr. and Mrs. Lindell

Appendix F

◆ ◆ ◆ ◆ ◆ ◆ ◆ ◆ ◆ ◆ ◆ ◆ ◆ ◆ ◆ ◆ ◆ ◆

Words and Sentences
for Stimulability Testing

Sound	Initial Position	Medial Position	Final Position	Age of Mastery*
/p/	pot pan pad pipe pack I cook in a pot. Pam is sick. Pack your clothes.	happy copy apple open hippo The boy is happy. I want an apple. The hippo is very big.	dip cup beep soup mop I want a cup of soup. Mop the floor. Get the soap.	2-0
/b/	bag ball bee bike bed The ball is red. I got a new bike. It is time for bed.	bubble labor maybe Bobby obey I like bubble gum. Bobby went home. Maybe he will come.	cab babe mob tub web She is in the tub. I saw a spider web. Mom called me babe.	2-8
/t/	tape tea tan ten Ted Lisa can count to ten. Would you like some tea? She has a very deep tan.	tomato potato guitar hotel detail Tomatoes taste good. Can you play the guitar? He stayed in a hotel.	bait ate boat fat feet Did the dog eat yet? Why were you late? My dad owns a boat.	2-8
/d/	do deck dog dime dam Do you like cake? It cost a dime. The dam is big.	ladder soda loaded padded ready He climbed the ladder. I would like a soda. Are you ready yet?	bed fed head good paid Candy tastes good. He got paid yesterday. Did you hit your head?	2-4

Sound	Initial Position	Medial Position	Final Position	Age of Mastery*
/k/	cup coat cat cab can I bought a new coat. We will take a cab home. Can you play with me?	bacon bucket ticket jacket locket I lost my airline ticket. The bucket is full. I want bacon and eggs.	ache take book make sick Is he sick? I lost my book. Please make a pie.	2-4
/g/	go game gate goat gum Let's play a game. The goat is fat. I like to chew gum.	again soggy foggy organ forget He can play the organ. It is very foggy today. Don't forget to buy ham.	bag pig dog bug big The pig is pink. He caught a bug. The dog is sick.	2-4
/f/	five fat fan fig phone I like to eat figs. He is on the phone. Turn on the fan.	coffee safety waffle infant muffin Do you like coffee? The infant was sick. He ran to safety.	half loaf beef cough cuff I bought a loaf of bread. Beef comes from cows. He ate half the cake.	2-4
/v/	vine vote vase van veil Do not forget to vote! Put the roses in the vase. The keys were in the van.	oven beaver bravo given even Beavers can swim. I liked the movie An elephant is heavy.	save leave shave wave dive Please save me! My dad needs a shave. Wave good-bye.	4-0
/θ/	thin third thought thick thaw He was third in line. I thought you were gone. Thaw out the meat.	author bathtub method toothbrush Kathy The bathtub is clean. Where is my toothbrush? Kathy went home.	bath both booth math path You need to take a bath. I love math. He is behind the booth.	4-0

Sound	Initial Position	Medial Position	Final Position	Age of Mastery*
/ð/	the they that this than They live near. This is your seat. Mike is smaller than Ted.	bother mother feather other weather Please don't bother me. My mother is pretty. The weather is bad.	clothe breathe smooth bathe soothe Don't forget to breathe. It will soothe your cut. He has smooth skin.	4-0
/s/	soap sip sat seed sew Bobby sat on the cake. Did you plant the seed? I don't know how to sew.	assume basic Lassie lasso essay Lassie is a smart dog. Did you write an essay? Don't assume anything.	face boss house loose pass The house is big. The horse was brown. His dog became loose.	3-0
/z/	zip zoo zoom zag zero I like to go to the zoo. What is the zip code? Zebras are striped.	busy cousin diesel dozen frozen My feet feel frozen. She is always busy. Twelve makes a dozen.	boys news has keys noise No news is good news. Please hang the keys. He makes so much noise.	4-0
/ʃ/	ship shoot shop shake shoe The ship set sail. I want a vanilla shake. I love to shop.	action ocean dishes bushy fishing My dad went fishing. Rover has a bushy tail. The ocean is blue.	fish wash push bush cash You must pay cash. Wash your face. He likes to fish.	3-8
/ʒ/		Asia lesion leisure fusion closure I have bad vision. He buried a treasure. Japan is in Asia.	beige rouge massage collage mirage Please massage my neck. It was all a mirage. Her pants are beige.	4-0

Sound	Initial Position	Medial Position	Final Position	Age of Mastery*
/h/	hop he hat ham hot I like turkey and ham. He bought a toy. Rabbits like to hop.	ahead ahoy inhale keyhole beehive I can't find the keyhole. His house is just ahead. Sue is behind Mary.		2-0

/tʃ/	chair
	chip
	chess
	chap
	chin
	He sat in the big chair.
	Do you play chess?
	Sally hurt her chin.
		matches
		achieve
		catcher
		future
		inches
		Don't play with
		   matches!
		Jerry is the catcher.
		The worm is three
		   inches.
			beach
			peach
			catch
			itch
			rich
			I live by the beach.
			The peach was sweet.
			Catch the ball.
				3-8

/dʒ/	job
	joke
	jack
	jeep
	jaw
	Did you take the job?
	He tells bad jokes.
	I bought a jeep.
		digit
		cages
		digest
		agent
		magic
		The birds are in cages.
		He is my insurance
		   agent.
		I like to play magic
		   tricks.
			cage
			page
			stage
			edge
			huge
			I am missing a page.
			He sat by the edge.
			I got stage fright.
				4-0

/w/	wipe wet win wake we Wipe your nose. My clothes are wet. We went on vacation.	away kiwi hallway always aware It's down the hallway. I always check. Kiwi is a green fruit.		2-8

/j/	yell
	yarn
	yolk
	yam
	use
	Don't yell at your
	   brother.
	Did you use my coat?
	The bird is yellow.
		royal
		kayak
		yo-yo
		reuse
		loyal
		I like to play with
		   yo-yos.
		You can reuse that
		   box.
		His friend is loyal.
				2-4

Sound	Initial Position	Medial Position	Final Position	Age of Mastery*
/l/	last loop log leg lap Is your leg broken? I am always last. I sat on my mom's lap.	allow alive daily below chili We get the daily paper. I like chili. He is acting silly.	all bell cell doll mall They are at the mall. The bull looked mean. My doll is lost.	3-4
/r/	run rope rain rake rat I'm afraid of rats. I hate raking leaves. The rope is long.	arrow carry fairy carrot carol I can't carry that bag. I like carrot cake. I lost my earrings.	hair car far door ear Do you live far away? Please lock the door. My ear hurts.	3-4
/m/	mom mad mop man map I can't follow a map. The man is nice. Sue is very mad.	camel comet summer woman mommy I like summer. I saw a comet in the sky. Camels live in the desert.	home ham game lime dim The lime was sour. Let's play a game. Do you like ham?	2-0
/n/	no net nap nut knock Let me take a nap. Please knock first. Nancy is very smart.	bunny any many pony honey My dad bought a pony. The bunny was white. Honey is sweet.	bean can cone fan fun Can I go to the zoo? We had a lot of fun. I like bean soup.	2-0
/ŋ/		hunger bongo jungle singer finger She is a singer. Lions live in the jungle. I cut my finger.	king ring bang song wing The bird hurt his wing. I heard a loud bang. The song was beautiful.	2-0

*Age of mastery is based on Prather et al. (1975) data.

Appendix G

◆ ◆ ◆ ◆ ◆ ◆ ◆ ◆ ◆ ◆ ◆ ◆ ◆ ◆ ◆ ◆ ◆ ◆ ◆ ◆

Worksheet for Traditional Analysis: Types of Errors

Name: _____ Age: _____ Grade: _____

Examiner: _____ School: _____

Teacher: _____ Date: _____

Connected speech: _____ Single words: _____ Formal test: _____

Record Target	Record Errors by Type			Record Stimulability				Select Norms*
Target Sound	Initial Position	Medial Position	Final Position	Stimulable	Isolation/ Syllables	Words	Sentences	Norms

*Norms used = _____

Impression: _____

◆ ◆

Worksheet for Place, Voicing, Manner (PVM) Analysis

Name: _____ Age: _____ Grade: _____

Examiner: _____ School: _____

Teacher: _____ Date: _____

Connected speech: _____ Single words: _____ Formal test: _____

Analysis by Manner of Production

	Produced Correctly (+/−)	Misarticulated (record specific errors)
Nasals		
/m/	_____	_____
/n/	_____	_____
/ŋ/	_____	_____
Stops		
/p/	_____	_____
/b/	_____	_____
/t/	_____	_____
/d/	_____	_____
/k/	_____	_____
/g/	_____	_____
Fricatives		
/f/	_____	_____
/v/	_____	_____
/s/	_____	_____
/z/	_____	_____
/θ/	_____	_____
/ð/	_____	_____
/ʃ/	_____	_____
/ʒ/	_____	_____
/h/	_____	_____

Affricates

/tʃ/   ——————   ————————————————
/dʒ/   ——————   ————————————————

Glides

/j/   ——————   ————————————————
/w/   ——————   ————————————————

Liquids

/r/   ——————   ————————————————
/l/   ——————   ————————————————

Analysis by Place of Articulation

	Produced Correctly (+/−)	Misarticulated (record specific errors)

Bilabials

/m/   ——————   ————————————————
/b/   ——————   ————————————————
/p/   ——————   ————————————————
/w/   ——————   ————————————————

Alveolars

/t/   ——————   ————————————————
/d/   ——————   ————————————————
/s/   ——————   ————————————————
/z/   ——————   ————————————————
/n/   ——————   ————————————————
/l/   ——————   ————————————————

Palatals

/ʃ/   ——————   ————————————————
/ʒ/   ——————   ————————————————
/dʒ/   ——————   ————————————————
/tʃ/   ——————   ————————————————
/j/   ——————   ————————————————
/r/   ——————   ————————————————

Linguadentals

/θ/   ——————   ————————————————
/ð/   ——————   ————————————————

Labiodentals

/f/   ——————   ————————————————
/v/   ——————   ————————————————

Velars

/k/ _____ _____
/g/ _____ _____
/ŋ/ _____ _____

Glottals

/h/ _____ _____

Analysis by Voicing Dimensions

Produced Correctly (+/−)	**Misarticulated** (record specific errors)

Voiced consonants

/m/ _____ _____
/n/ _____ _____
/ŋ/ _____ _____
/b/ _____ _____
/d/ _____ _____
/g/ _____ _____
/v/ _____ _____
/ð/ _____ _____
/z/ _____ _____
/ʒ/ _____ _____
/dʒ/ _____ _____
/r/ _____ _____
/l/ _____ _____
/w/ _____ _____
/j/ _____ _____

Voiceless consonants

/p/ _____ _____
/t/ _____ _____
/k/ _____ _____
/g/ _____ _____
/θ/ _____ _____
/s/ _____ _____
/ʃ/ _____ _____
/tʃ/ _____ _____
/h/ _____ _____

Clinical impressions: _____
_____
_____
_____

Notes: _____
_____
_____
_____

Appendix I

♦ ♦

Worksheet for Identifying Phonological Processes

Name: _____ Age: _____ Grade: _____

Examiner: _____ School: _____

Teacher: _____ Date: _____

Connected speech: _____ Single words: _____ Formal test: _____

Intended Production	Child's Production	Operating Phonological Process(es)
_____	_____	_____
_____	_____	_____
_____	_____	_____
_____	_____	_____
_____	_____	_____
_____	_____	_____
_____	_____	_____
_____	_____	_____
_____	_____	_____
_____	_____	_____
_____	_____	_____
_____	_____	_____
_____	_____	_____
_____	_____	_____
_____	_____	_____
_____	_____	_____
_____	_____	_____
_____	_____	_____
_____	_____	_____
_____	_____	_____
_____	_____	_____
_____	_____	_____
_____	_____	_____
_____	_____	_____
_____	_____	_____
_____	_____	_____
_____	_____	_____
_____	_____	_____
_____	_____	_____

Intended Production	Child's Production	Operating Phonological Process(es)

Frequency of occurrence for each process: _____

_____

_____

Percentage of occurrence for each process (# of actual occurrences divided by total # of opportunities for the process to occur): _____

_____

_____

_____

Clinical impressions: _____

_____

_____

Appendix J

✦ ✦ ✦ ✦ ✦ ✦ ✦ ✦ ✦ ✦ ✦ ✦ ✦ ✦ ✦ ✦ ✦ ✦ ✦

Sample Diagnostic Reports

Sample Diagnostic Report A: Articulation Disorder

Oakenshaw Unified School District
Pupil Personnel Services/Special Education
8679 Main Street
Rosevale, CA 95762

Initial Diagnostic Report

Name: Cassandra Bennett
School: Jefferson Elementary
Grade: 1
Examiner: Adriana Peña-Brooks, M.A., CCC-S

Test date: 10/12/00
Date of birth: 1/8/94
Age: 6–7
Teacher: Mr. Jackson

Referral Information

Cassandra Bennett, a 6-year-old female, was referred for a speech screening by her classroom teacher, Mr. Jackson. He reported that Cassandra's "s" did not sound correct for her age. After a screening was completed, this examiner believed that it was appropriate to perform a more thorough evaluation to assess Cassandra's eligibility for speech and language services.

Background Information and History

A phone interview was conducted with Mrs. Bennett to obtain relevant developmental information and background history. Mrs. Bennett reported that she was also concerned about Cassandra's "s" production. She also indicated that Cassandra has "sounded like this since she started talking."

Cassandra has attended Jefferson Elementary since kindergarten. No prior speech assessments or services were reported. Her developmental history is not remarkable. Mrs. Bennett reported that besides sounding like she always has a cold, Cassandra has enjoyed good health with no diseases of significance.

Family, Social, and Educational History

Cassandra is the first of two children. Mrs. Bennett did not report a family history of communicative disorders. Cassandra attends first grade and is reportedly doing very well in class. She reportedly gets along well with other children. Her classroom teacher characterizes her as "one of the smartest kids in my class." However, he was concerned about the quality of Cassandra's speech.

Assessment Information

Cassandra was very cooperative during the testing process. She put forth an appropriate effort with all the tasks presented. Results are thought to present a valid estimate of competency of the skills tested.

Orofacial Examination. An orofacial examination was performed to assess the structure and function of the oral mechanism as related to speech production. Cassandra's lips and hard palate appeared symmetrical at rest. She was able to perform a variety of labial and lingual tasks. The anterior and posterior faucial pillars were within normal limits. Vertical movement of the pharyngeal wall was observed upon the phonation of /a/. Cassandra had enlarged pharyngeal tonsils. A slight overjet also was noted. The bottom central incisors were partially erupted, which created an open space. Cassandra's erupting lower central incisors were discolored. Diadochokinetic syllable rates were within normal limits.

Hearing Screening. Cassandra's hearing was screened by the school nurse at the beginning of this academic year in August 2000. Results of the screening, as documented in her cumulative folder, were within normal limits. Cassandra passed the hearing screening for the frequencies 250, 500, 1,000, 2,000, and 4,000 at 25 dB HL.

Speech Production and Intelligibility. Cassandra's speech production was assessed with the *Photo Articulation Test–3* (PAT–3) and a conversational speech sample. The PAT–3 assesses the production of all English consonants in the initial, medial, and final positions of words according to types of errors (substitutions, omissions, distortions, additions). An analysis of Cassandra's conversational speech sample and her performance on the PAT–3 revealed the following errors:

Target Sound	Initial	Medial	Final
/s/	Dist[3]/s	Dist[3]/s	Dist[3]/s
/z/	Dist[3]/z	Dist[3]/z	Dist[3]/z
/ʃ/	Dist[1]/ʃ	Dist[1]/ʃ	Dist[1]/ʃ
/ʒ/	Dist[1]/ʒ	Dist[1]/ʒ	Dist[1]/ʒ
/dʒ/			Dist[1]/dʒ
/d/		Dist[1]/d	Dist[1]/d
/t/			Dist[1]/t

Notes: Dist[1] = mild distortion; Dist[2] = moderate distortion; Dist[3] = severe distortion.
Blends: The /s/ component of blends was distorted, as observed in singleton /s/ productions.

Analysis of Cassandra's errors on the speech sample and the PAT–3 revealed that her production of /s/ and /z/ was severely lateralized in all positions of distribution. The consonants /ʃ/, /ʒ/, and /dʒ/ were mildly lateralized. In addition to sibilant distortions, Cassandra demonstrated lateralized production of /d/ in the medial and final positions and distortion of /t/ in the final position of words.

Furthermore, the consonants /ʃ/, /ʒ/, /ʧ/, and /ʤ/ were characterized by the presence of awkward motor movements during their production. While making these sounds, the right side of Cassandra's lower lip deviated down and outward, while the upper and lower lips on the left side made contact and became protruded. Although these movements were also noted during production of /ʧ/, the acoustic quality of that sound remained intact.

Cassandra's speech intelligibility was only mildly affected by her misarticulations. A word-by-word analysis of her conversational speech sample revealed that she was 85% intelligible in unknown conversational contexts. Cassandra was highly stimulable for an improved production of /s/ and /z/ in words using modeling and phonetic placement cues. However, other error consonants were not stimulable during this assessment.

Language Production and Comprehension. Cassandra's conversational speech during the assessment showed essentially normal language and structure. Her mean length of utterance was within normal limits for her age. Based on her responses to the examiner's questions and requests, language comprehension appeared adequate.

Voice and Fluency. Cassandra's speech had normal rate and rhythm. The rate of dysfluencies was within the normal range. Therefore, no further analysis of the dysfluency rate was made.

In conversational speech, Cassandra's resonance was perceptually judged to be hyponasal. During a nasal flutter test, her left naris was perceived to be more obstructed than the right. Audible nasal inspiration was also perceived throughout the examination. Mrs. Bennett indicated during a telephone conversation that Cassandra has "sounded like she's had a cold for a very long time."

Diagnostic Summary and Prognosis

Cassandra Bennett exhibits a mild-moderate articulation disorder characterized by severe lateralization of /s/ and /z/ and mild lateralization of /ʃ/, /ʒ/, /ʧ/, /t/, and /d/. Her speech intelligibility was only mildly affected by her articulation errors. Although a slight overjet was noted during the orofacial examination, it is difficult to determine whether this is a contributing factor to her articulation errors. Research has shown that a high percentage of children with slight malocclusions compensate well and have no associated articulation problems.

Cassandra's prognosis for improvement of her misarticulations and her speech intelligibility is good considering her age, adequate language skills, and stimulability for some of the mispronounced sounds. Also, Cassandra's parents appear to be very supportive and are anxious to follow through with any home assignments.

Recommendations

Cassandra meets eligibility criteria for Language, Speech, and Hearing Services through the school district. Her error productions are atypical in normal development, and she will probably not "outgrow" such sound distortions without clinical intervention. It is recommended that Cassandra receive treatment for her articulation disorder, with an emphasis on improving her production of /s/ and /z/ and other sibilants. It is also recommended that Mrs. Bennett consult with Cassandra's pediatrician regarding her hyponasal quality to rule out any medical problems. Upon Mrs. Bennett's approval, an individualized education plan will be developed for Cassandra.

Adriana Peña-Brooks, M.A., CCC-S
Speech–Language Pathologist, License # XXXX

Sample Diagnostic Report B: Phonological Disorder

University Speech and Hearing Clinic
Central University
Central, California 87665

Initial Diagnostic Report

Name: Jack Lawson
Address: 1400 General Street
City: Universal, California
Telephone number: (000) 120-5678
Referred by: Mother

Birthdate: 8-2-94
Clinic file number: 00000
Date of report: 9-22-00
Diagnosis: Phonological Disorder
Clinician: Susan Lincoln

Background and Presenting Complaint

Jack Lawson, a 6-year-old male, was enrolled in his second semester of speech therapy at the University Clinic on September 15, 2000. Jack's mother served as the informant during this evaluation. The presenting complaint was a severe speech disorder. Mrs. Lawson reported that Jack seems to be "pronouncing words more clearly," is starting to talk more at school, and is using longer sentences. She indicated that she understands approximately 50% of Jack's speech, while others probably understand about 35% when the context of the conversation is known.

History

Birth, Developmental, and Medical History. Mrs. Lawson reported that her pregnancy was full term and that Jack was born by cesarean section. He weighed 6 pounds, 11 ounces. With the exception of recurrent middle ear infections, Jack has enjoyed good health with no diseases of significance. Mrs. Lawson reported that Jack had pressure equalization (PE) tubes placed in his ears at approximately 2 years of age. Middle ear infections were medically treated through antibiotics. According to Mrs. Lawson, a current medical examination revealed that Jack's ears were healthy.

Family, Social, and Educational History. Jack lives with his parents and sister, Karen Lawson. Mrs. Lawson reported that Jack was starting to socialize more with children at school but still tended to play alone. She indicated that Jack does interact with his sister and frequently initiates games to play with her. At the time of this assessment, Jack was attending a day care program at Penter City College. Jack received one semester of speech therapy previously through this clinic. However, there is no other history of speech and language therapy.

Orofacial Examination. An orofacial examination was performed to assess the structural and functional integrity of the oral mechanism. The examination did not reveal anything of clinical significance.

Hearing Screening. A bilateral hearing screening was performed at 25 dB HL for 250, 500, 1,000, 2,000, and 4,000 Hz. Jack responded to all frequencies bilaterally.

Speech Production and Intelligibility. To assess Jack's speech sound production, a conversational speech sample was recorded. In addition, the *Goldman-Fristoe Test of Articulation* (GFTA) Sounds in Words subtest was administered to assess the production of all English consonants in fixed position. The GFTA assesses the production of sounds according to types of errors (omissions, substitutions, additions, distortions) in initial, medial, and final word positions. An analysis of the sample and Jack's performance on the GFTA revealed the following errors:

Target Sound	Initial	Medial	Final
/k/	t/k	t/k	omit
/g/	d/g	d/g	omit
/ŋ/		nd/ŋ	n/ŋ
/s/	p/s	t/s	omit
/z/	d/z	d/z	omit
/v/	b/v	b/v	b/v
/ʃ/	t/ʃ	t/ʃ	omit/ʃ
/ʒ/		d/ʒ	omit
/ʧ/	t/ʧ	t/ʧ	omit
/ʤ/	d/ʤ	d/ʤ	omit
/θ/	f/θ	f/θ	f/θ
/ð/	d/ð	d/ð	d/ð
/r/	w/r	w/r	omit
/l/	w/l	j/l	omit

Blend Errors: k/kl; dw/dr; b/bl; p/pl; fw/fl; kw/kr; tw/sk; t/sl; t/st.

Vowels: No vowel errors were observed.

A phonological process analysis of Jack's speech errors on the *Goldman-Fristoe Test of Articulation* was performed with the *Khan-Lewis Phonological Analysis*. The analysis revealed the following phonological processes in the excessive range of usage:

> deletion of final consonants
> palatal fronting
> velar fronting
> stopping of fricatives and affricates
> cluster simplification
> liquid simplification (liquid gliding and vowelization)

Due to the numerous articulation errors and active phonological processes, Jack was found to be 40% intelligible on a word-by-word basis. Jack's speech intelligibility significantly decreased during episodes of a rapid rate of speech and when the length of his utterances increased.

A phonetic inventory analysis revealed the following productive sounds in Jack's speech, according to initial, medial, and final positions:

> Initial: [m, n, p, b, t, d, f, w, j, h]
> Medial: [m, n, p, b, t, d, f, w, j, h]
> Final: [m, n, p, t, d, b]

Stimulability testing revealed limited stimulability for all of the mispronounced sounds. Jack made closer approximations of all of the sounds in isolation; however, they did not match the target sound.

Language Production and Comprehension. Jack's conversational speech during the assessment showed essentially normal language structure and use except for several missing grammatical morphemes. It is possible that missing grammatical morphemes are due to omission of final consonants. The mean length of utterance (MLU) of his speech sample was 5.7, which is within normal limits for his age.

Voice and Fluency. Although Jack's speech was difficult to understand, he had normal rate and rhythm. The rate of dysfluencies was within the normal ranges. His voice was also judged to be within normal limits.

Diagnostic Summary and Prognosis

Jack Lawson exhibits a severe phonological disorder, which is characterized by several active phonological processes including deletion of final consonants, palatal fronting, velar fronting, stopping of fricatives and affricates, cluster simplification, and liquid simplification (liquid gliding and vowelization). His phonetic inventory was essentially limited to early developing sounds such as stops, nasals, and glides and the fricatives /f/ and /h/. His productive inventory of sounds in the final position of words was limited to [m, n, p, t, d, b], which can help explain the presence of final-consonant deletion. His speech intelligibility was significantly affected by his misarticulations. Jack's phonological disorder may be related to his history of recurrent ear infections during the first two years of his life; however, that cannot be conclusively determined to be the cause of his disorder.

Jack is young, was very cooperative during the assessment, and appears to have excellent family support. However, his prognosis for improved phonological skills and speech intelligibility is judged fair at this time due to the severe nature of his disorder, the significant number of misarticulations and active phonological processes, and his limited stimulability. His prognosis will be reevaluated throughout the course of therapy.

Recommendations

It is recommended that Jack receive speech–language pathology services, with a focus on increasing his phonetic inventory and decreasing the number of active phonological processes. This will likely have a positive effect on his speech intelligibility. As Jack's phonological skills improve, his language may be further evaluated to determine whether morphological features emerge. If they do not, language treatment should be offered.

Submitted by_____

      Susan Lincoln, B.A.
      Student Clinician

Approved by_____

      Adriana Peña-Brooks, M.A., CCC-S
      Speech–Language Pathologist
      Clinical Supervisor

Parents Signature_____

Appendix K

◆ ◆ ◆ ◆ ◆ ◆ ◆ ◆ ◆ ◆ ◆ ◆ ◆ ◆ ◆ ◆ ◆ ◆ ◆ ◆

Baseline Data Sheet

Name: _____ Age: _____ Therapist: _____

Date: _____ Session #: _____ Disorder(s): _____

Potential target behavior: _____

Target Response	Evoked Trials + / – / NR	Modeled Trials + / – / NR	Prompted Trials + / – / NR
1.			
2.			
3.			
4.			
5.			
6.			
7.			
8.			
9.			
10.			
11.			
12.			
13.			
14.			
15.			
16.			
17.			
18.			
19.			
20.			
Percentage Correct			

Appendix L

♦ ♦ ♦ ♦ ♦ ♦ ♦ ♦ ♦ ♦ ♦ ♦ ♦ ♦ ♦ ♦ ♦ ♦ ♦ ♦

Sample Treatment Plans

Sample Treatment Plan 1 (Individualized Education Program for Cassandra Bennett, Sample Diagnostic Report A in Appendix J)

Oakenshaw Unified School District

Individual Education Program-IEP Special Education

Meeting date: 10/20/00   ☑ Initial   ☐ Review   ☐ Triennial
Present program: Regular
Program recommendation: Regular/DIS-LSH (Speech Therapy)
Placement date: 10/21/00
Review date: 10/21/01   **Next triennial date:** 10/12/2003
Written notification of IEP review sent: 10/17/00
Telephone contact date: 10/19/00

Personal Data

Student's name: Cassandra Bennett
Gender: ☐ Male   ☑ Female
Date of birth: 1/8/94
Language of home: English
Language of student: English
English proficiency: ☐ Limited   ☑ Fluent

Grade: 1
School year: 2000–2001
Home school: Jefferson Elementary
School of attendance: Same Track: A
Student identification number: 00000
Student's SS #: XXX-XX-XXX

Present Levels of Performance

Academic: Cassandra is doing very well academically. Reading, writing, and math are at grade level.

Communication: Cassandra's receptive and expressive language skills are age-appropriate. Misarticulations of various sibilants affect the quality of her speech.

Social: Cassandra appears to be a friendly child. She reportedly has many friends.

Self-help/medical needs: Age-appropriate self-help skills. No medical needs.

Committee Members

Administrator: _____

Teacher: _____

Parent: _____

Student: _____

_____

_____

RSP DIS/OTHER SERVICES

☐ RSP Frequency/Duration: _____ Services to begin: _____

☑ LSH Frequency/Duration: _2Xp/wk 30 min ea._ Services to begin: _10-21-00_

☐ AdPE Frequency/Duration: _____ Services to begin: _____

☐ VI Frequency/Duration: _____ Services to begin: _____

☐ Other Frequency/Duration: _____ Services to begin: _____

☐ Other Frequency/Duration: _____ Services to begin: _____

Percentage of Regular Program: 97%

Rationale for Placement

Rationale for placement in special education program/service (check appropriate box)

☐ Attempted modifications to general education have not been successful.

☐ Goals cannot be met in less restrictive environment.

☑ Goals and objectives cannot be met in general education.

☐ Other:

Annual Goals

Age-appropriate articulation skills and improved speech intelligibility

Short-Term Instructional Goals (include evaluation criteria)

1. Teach 90% correct production of /s/ and /z/ at the conversational level in all settings (therapy, home, school, playground, etc.).
2. Teach 90% correct production of /ʃ/ and /ʤ/ at the conversational level in all settings (therapy, home, school, playground, etc.).
3. Teach 90% correct production of /t/ and /d/ at the conversational level in all settings (therapy, home, school, playground, etc.).

Evaluation Procedures

- baseline data
- pre/post tests
- data collection
- SLP tasks
- parent report
- teacher report
- observation
- speech samples

☐ I have been informed of and agree with the above recommended individualized education program recommendation.

☐ I disagree with the above individualized education program and request that my child:

☐ Receive NO special services

☐ Other: _____

Note on abbreviations:

RSP = Resource Specialist
DIS = Designated Instruction Services
LSH = Language, Speech, and Hearing
AdPE = Adaptive Physical Education
VI = Vision Impairment

Sample Treatment Plan 2 (Comprehensive Treatment Program for Jack Lawson, Sample Diagnostic Report B in Appendix J)

University Speech and Hearing Clinic
Central University
Central, California 87665

Treatment Program

Name: Jack Lawson

Date of birth: 8-2-94

Address: 1400 General Streeet

City: Universal, California

Telephone number: (000) 120-5678

Diagnosis: Phonological Disorder

File number: 00000

Semesters in therapy: 2

Date of report: 9-27-00

School: Johnson Elementary

Background Information

Jack Lawson, a 6-year-old male, began his second semester of speech therapy at the University Clinic on September 20, 2000. Jack's speech and language were reevaluated on September 15, 2000. The reevaluation revealed that Jack has made some progress since the initial evaluation last semester on February 12, 2000; however, he continues to exhibit a severe phonological disorder, which is characterized by several active phonological processes including deletion of final consonants, palatal fronting, velar fronting, stopping of fricatives and affricates, cluster simplification, and liquid simplification in the form of liquid gliding and vowelization. Jack's phonetic inventory was limited to early developing sounds, including stops, nasals, glides, and the fricatives /f/ and /h/. His speech intelligibility was 40% on a word-by-word basis. See his folder for a diagnostic report.

Treatment was recommended to increase his phonetic inventory, increase his speech intelligibility, and decrease the number of active phonological processes. Jack's prognosis was judged fair at this time, primarily because of the severe nature of his disorder, the significant number of misarticulations and active phonological processes, and his limited stimulability. He appears to be a cooperative child and seems to have excellent family support. This will probably have a positive effect on his achievement of the goals and objectives.

Target Goals and Objectives

Long-Term Goal. Age-appropriate phonological skills and speech intelligibility for improved communication interactions. Maintenance of the trained articulation and phonological skills across varied audiences, settings, and situations.

Semester Goals. The following goals and objectives were selected for this semester of therapy, which covers a 3-month period from September 20, 2000, to December 20, 2000.

Goal 1: To decrease inappropriate phonological processes
Goal 2: To increase the number of consonants in Jack's phonetic inventory
Goal 3: To increase Jack's speech intelligibility from 40% to 70%

Objectives. The following objectives were developed to support this semester's goals and the long-term goal.

OBJECTIVE #1. Reduction of final-consonant deletion process by directly teaching the correct production of /k/, /ʃ/, and /s/ in word-final position to 90% accuracy. Generalized production of /g/, /ʒ/, and /z/ will be probed and if not produced correctly, will be taught directly.

OBJECTIVE #2. Elimination of the velar-fronting phonological process by directly teaching the correct production of /k/ and /ŋ/ in word-initial and word-final positions to 90% accuracy. Generalized production of /g/ will be probed and if not produced correctly, will be taught directly.

OBJECTIVE #3. Reduction of the stopping phonological process by directly teaching the correct production of /v/, /s/, /ʃ/, /tʃ/ in word-initial position. Generalized production of /z/, /ʒ/, and /dʒ/ will be probed and if not produced correctly, will be taught directly.

Procedures

Base rates will be established for /k/, /ʃ/, /s/, /v/, /g/, /ʒ/, and /z/ (final-consonant deletion); /k/, /g/, and /ŋ/ (velar fronting); and /v/, /s/, /ʃ/, /tʃ/, /z/, /ʒ/, and /dʒ/ (stopping). It should be noted that some of the sound exemplars co-occur across the targeted phonological processes. Generalized production of these phonemes across phonological processes will be assessed. For example, after training /k/ in the final position of words for elimination of final-consonant deletion, generalized production of /k/ to other velars in varied word positions will be probed. If generalized productions are noted, the process of velar fronting will not be directly trained. Training of the process will continue as planned if generalized productions do not occur.

The clinician will use 20 stimulus items per phoneme to measure the production of the target phoneme during modeled and evoked trials. Verbal praise will be given for cooperative behavior during baseline trials.

To reduce or eliminate the final-consonant deletion process, /k/, /ʃ/, and /s/ will initially be taught directly; to eliminate velar fronting, /k/ and /ŋ/ will be taught directly; and to reduce stopping, /v/, /s/, /ʃ/, and /tʃ/ will be taught directly. Treatment for each sound will begin at the word level. If Jack has difficulty imitating the target sounds in words, syllables may be used to teach the sounds. If necessary, phonemes will initially be shaped in isolation. Final-consonant deletion will be the first target to be eliminated. All three final consonants will be initially treated in all treatment sessions. Treatment will systematically move from the word to the phrase and sentence levels. The clinician will use phonetic placement cues, shaping techniques, verbal instructions, modeling, visual feedback, manual guidance, and verbal praise to establish the production of the target phonemes.

When Jack produces the final consonants under training with 90% accuracy in words, probes will be conducted to assess generalized production of untaught phonemes affected by the process (/v/, /g/, /ʒ/, and /z/). An intermixed probe in which words containing taught and untaught phonemes will be used to assess generalized production of untaught final consonants. Training, however, will continue on the selected phonemes at the phrase and sentence levels. Probing of untaught final consonants will be conducted as the treatment moves from the phrase to the sentence level.

Untreated final consonants will be taught if they still are not produced on probes when the initially targeted final consonants have been completed at the sentence level of training. Training will be omitted on the final consonants that are produced on any of the probes without training.

Essentially the same procedure will be used to eliminate the velar fronting and stopping processes. Phonemes selected for initial training will be continued until the sentence level is reached. Periodic probes of untaught phonemes within the process and across the processes that affect the same sound exemplar will be conducted with the intermixed probe procedure. Untaught phonemes will be taught if they are not produced when the initially taught phonemes are produced in sentences.

The clinician will present a picture or an object to evoke each target sound at the word level. The clinician will ask a predetermined question to evoke the target word. The clinician will initially model the correct responses. The clinician will wait 2–3 seconds for Jack's response. The clinician will reinforce Jack's correct responses with verbal praise. Initially, reinforcement will be given on a continuous schedule using primary and social reinforcers. As treatment progresses, an intermittent schedule of reinforcement will be used. Additional reinforcers, including tokens backed up by small gifts, may be used when necessary. Corrective feedback will be given for incorrect responses. Modeling will be discontinued when Jack correctly imitates each sound on five trials. Modeling will be reinstated if errors persist on evoked trials. Minimal or maximal contrasting-pair training will be incorporated into therapy as a specific treatment activity when the client can produce the sound at least at the word level.

Maintenance Program

Jack's parents will observe most, if not all, treatment sessions in the clinic. They will be trained to recognize the correct and incorrect production of phonemes. The clinician will teach Jack's parents to evoke and reinforce the target phonemes at home. The clinician will give Jack's parents a list of target words with which to conduct informal treatment sessions at home. The parents will be asked to record conversational speech samples with Jack and other family members to assess generalized production of phonemes at home.

Treatment will be shifted to nonclinic settings when Jack reaches a 90% accuracy criterion in conversational speech in the clinic setting. Jack will be taken to the campus food court when informal training sessions are conducted. Collaborative efforts will be made with Jack's speech–language pathologist at his school to coordinate services if possible.

Jack will be dismissed from therapy when he reaches a 90% accuracy criterion in the clinic and nonclinic settings in the production of all misarticulated phonemes. This may not be achieved during this semester of therapy. A follow-up session will be scheduled 6 months after dismissal. Upon the initial follow-up, booster treatment will be recommended as needed.

Submitted by:_____
             Joann Johnson, B.A.

Student Clinician

Approved by:_____
               Lucy Masterson, M.A., CCC-SLP
               Clinical Supervisor

I understand the recommended plan of treatment and agree to it.

Client/Parent/Guardian: _____ Date: _____

Note: The style and format for Sample Treatment Plan 2 was based on Hegde (1998a).

Appendix M

♦ ♦ ♦ ♦ ♦ ♦ ♦ ♦ ♦ ♦ ♦ ♦ ♦ ♦ ♦ ♦ ♦ ♦ ♦

Sound-Evoking Techniques for English Consonants

Sound: /p/

Place, Manner, Voicing Features

- Bilabial (lip-lip)
- Stop-plosive (aspirate sound)
- Voiceless

Other Distinctive Features (Chomsky & Halle, 1968)

- Consonantal
- Anterior
- Tense

Articulatory Production

- Lips are shut lightly.

- Soft palate is raised to assist with velopharyngeal closure.

- Tongue is in a neutral position or in the position required for the next sound.

- Oral (air) pressure builds up behind the shut lips.

- Vocal folds are abducted.

- Lips are separated quickly, and breath escapes, creating an explosive sound.

Sound Distribution

- Initial—*pig, pot, pin, pen, pass*
- Medial—*apple, pepper, appointment, apex, appeal*
- Final—*stop, soup, cape, pop, mop*

Developmental Data (age of mastery)

- 4   (Wellman et al., 1931)
- 3½ (Poole, 1934)
- 3   (Templin, 1957)
- 3   (Sander, 1972)
- 2   (Prather et al., 1975)

Frequency of Occurrence

- Delattre, 1965

  - 2.35% of total English consonants
  - 16th in frequency of 24 English consonants
  - 1.45% of total vowels and consonants combined
  - 26th in frequency of 42 sounds (vowels and consonants)

- Shriberg & Kwiatkowski, 1983

  - 3.1% of 24 English consonants
  - 14th in frequency of 24 English consonants

Sound: /b/

Place, Manner, Voicing Features

- Bilabial (lip-lip)
- Stop-plosive
- Voiced

Other Distinctive Features (Chomsky & Halle, 1968)

- Consonantal
- Anterior
- Voiced

Articulatory Production

- Lips are shut lightly.

- Soft palate is raised to assist with velopharyngeal closure.

- Tongue is in a neutral position or in the position required for the next sound.

- Oral (air) pressure builds up behind the shut lips.

- Vocal folds are adducted.

- Lips are separated quickly, and breath escapes, with less force than for /p/.

Sound Distribution

- Initial — *bat, bed, big, be, bay*
- Medial — *robin, baby, bubble, cabin, pebble*
- Final — *cab, tub, rib, robe, herb*

Developmental Data (age of mastery)

- 3   (Wellman et al., 1931)
- 3½   (Poole, 1934)
- 4   (Templin, 1957)
- 4   (Sander, 1972)
- 2–8 (Prather et al., 1975)

Frequency of Occurrence

- Delattre, 1965

  - 3.48% of total English consonants

- 12th in frequency of 24 English consonants
- 2.14% of total vowels and consonants combined
- 18th in frequency of 42 sounds (vowels and consonants)

- Shriberg & Kwiatkowski, 1983

- 3.3% of 24 English consonants
- 13th in frequency of 24 English consonants

Sound-Evoking Techniques for /p/ and /b/

Evoking techniques 1–4 facilitate the production of /p/. To establish /b/, follow the same steps, plus step 5, but instruct the client to add voicing or "turn on the voice box."

Technique 1

- Hold a piece of tissue paper or other lightweight paper in front of the client's lips.

- Instruct the client to: "Close your mouth and fill up your cheeks with air."

- Instruct the client to release the air ("blow") and "try to move the piece of paper."

- Draw attention to the force and explosion characteristics of the sound by directing the client's attention to the movement of the paper.

- Gradually shape the amount of air impounded to a more natural level.

Technique 2

- Hold a piece of tissue paper, other lightweight paper, or the back of the client's hand in front of the client's lips.

- Ask the client to repeat "p" in rapid succession.

- Draw attention to the force and explosion characteristics of the sound by directing the client's attention to the movement of the paper or the sensation of air on the back of the client's hand.

- Manually guide the client's lips for adequate seal if necessary.

Technique 3

- Lightly touch the client's upper and lower lips with a tongue depressor or cotton swab stick.

- Ask the client to bring the lips together to touch the spot you touched.

- Place the client's hand in front of the lips.

- Instruct the client to "blow air" through the closed lips.

- Draw attention to the force and explosion characteristics of the sound by directing the client's attention to the "tickling" sensation on the back of the hand.

- Gradually shape the amount of air released by the client.

Technique 4

- Ask the client to kiss the back of his or her hand loudly.

- Draw attention to the lip seal during the kissing motion.

- Ask the client to gradually make the kissing sounds increasingly more quiet until they are whispered.

- Instruct the client to remove the back of his or her hand and continue the quiet kisses but to blow air out as the kisses are made instead of drawing air in.

Technique 5

- Ask the client to produce [m] or ask the client, "What sound does one make when something tastes really good?—mmmmm . . ."

- Instruct the client to pinch his or her nose shut while producing [m]; airflow will be forced out through the mouth, resulting in [b]. (Manually pinch the client's nose shut if necessary.)

- Focus the client's attention on the new sound (assuming hearing is normal).

Sound: /t/

Place, Manner, Voicing Features

- Lingua-alveolar (tip-ridge)
- Stop-plosive (aspirate sound)
- Voiceless

Other Distinctive Features (Chomsky & Halle, 1968)

- Consonantal
- Coronal
- Anterior
- Tense

Articulatory Production

- Lips are relaxed and slightly parted.

- Soft palate is raised to assist with velopharyngeal closure.

- Tongue tip and blade are raised to contact the alveolar ridge; the sides of the tongue are raised to contact the upper teeth and gums (forming a seal).

- Oral (air) pressure builds up behind the gum-tongue seal.

- Vocal folds are abducted.

- Gum-tongue seal is suddenly opened, and breath escapes, creating an explosive sound.

Sound Distribution

- Initial — *tie, top, tub, table, teacher*
- Medial — *little, after, button, tattoo, city*
- Final — *cat, act, debt, receipt, quit*

Developmental Data (age of mastery)

- 5   (Wellman et al., 1931)
- 4½ (Poole, 1934)
- 6   (Templin, 1957)
- 6   (Sander, 1972)
- 2–8 (Prather et al., 1975)

Frequency of Occurrence

- Delattre, 1965

  - 12.77% of total English consonants
  - 1st in frequency of 24 English consonants
  - 7.85% of total vowels and consonants combined
  - 1st in frequency of 42 sounds (vowels and consonants)

- Shriberg & Kwiatkowski, 1983

  - 11.9% of 24 English consonants
  - 2nd in frequency of 24 English consonants

Sound: /d/

Place, Manner, Voicing Features

- Lingua-alveolar (tip-ridge)
- Stop-plosive
- Voiced

Other Distinctive Features (Chomsky & Halle, 1968)

- Consonantal
- Coronal
- Anterior
- Voiced

Articulatory Production

- Lips are relaxed and slightly parted.

- Soft palate is raised to assist with velopharyngeal closure.

- Tongue tip and blade are raised to contact the alveolar ridge; the sides of the tongue are raised to contact the upper teeth and gums (forming a seal).

- Oral (air) pressure builds up behind the gum-tongue seal.

- Vocal folds are adducted.

- Gum-tongue seal is suddenly opened, and air escapes with less force than for /t/.

Sound Distribution

- Initial — *dog, dad, day, done, double*
- Medial — *body, fading, daddy, shadow, ladder*
- Final — *mud, bread, sand, did, could*

Developmental Data (age of mastery)

- 5 (Wellman et al., 1931)
- 4½ (Poole, 1934)
- 4 (Templin, 1957)
- 4 (Sander, 1972)
- 2–4 (Prather et al., 1975)

Frequency of Occurrence

- Delattre, 1965

  - 5.65% of total English consonants
  - 6th in frequency of 24 English consonants
  - 3.47% of total vowels and consonants combined
  - 9th in frequency of 42 sounds (vowels and consonants)

- Shriberg & Kwiatkowski, 1983

  - 6.4% of 24 English consonants
  - 5th in frequency of 24 English consonants

Sound-Evoking Techniques for /t/ and /d/

These evoking techniques facilitate the production of /t/. To establish /d/, follow the same steps, but also instruct the client to add voicing or "turn on the voice box."

Technique 1

- Demonstrate for the client the placing of the tongue tip firmly against the alveolar ridge.

- Instruct the client to position his or her tongue tip firmly against the alveolar ridge (a mirror can be used to provide the client with visual feedback).

- Direct the client to hold his or her breath briefly, and then instruct the client to quickly lower the tongue while releasing the breath through the mouth.

- Draw the client's attention to the explosive characteristic of the sound.

- Gradually work to shape the amount of air released in the production of this sound.

Technique 2

- Instruct the client to produce [p].

- Ask the client to position the tongue tip between his or her lips and once again attempt to produce [p]. Now that the client has the sound within the vicinity of [t], he or she will be able to receive both tactile and auditory feedback (assuming hearing is normal) of a stoplike sound made with the tongue tip.

- Instruct the client to position the tongue tip against the upper lip only and once again attempt to produce a similar sound.

- Instruct the client to make a similar sound with the tongue tip touching the alveolar ridge.

- *Note:* To evoke [d], develop from [b] instead of [t].

Technique 3

- Place a flavored food upon the client's alveolar ridge by means of a Q-tip.

- Instruct the client to attempt to remove the food by using the tip of the tongue. Once the client has a "feel" for the position of the tongue tip upon the alveolar ridge, proceed with the following steps.

- Ask the client to position the tongue tip upon the alveolar ridge firmly.

- Instruct the client to release the point of contact by lowering the tongue while blowing air out of the mouth.

- Gradually shape the amount of force with which the client expels the air.

Technique 4

- Place a piece of paper or feather in front of the client's mouth.

- Instruct the client to place his or her tongue tip directly behind the front teeth against the gum ridge.

- Instruct the client to blow air out through his or her mouth while quickly lowering the tongue tip.

- Focus the client's attention on the movement of the paper or feather.

- Gradually work to shape the amount of force with which the client expels the air.

Sound: /k/

Place, Manner, Voicing Features

- Lingua-velar (back–soft palate)
- Stop-plosive (aspirate sound)
- Voiceless

Other Distinctive Features (Chomsky & Halle, 1968)

- Consonantal
- High
- Back
- Tense

Articulatory Production

- Lips are relaxed and apart.
- Soft palate is raised to assist with velopharyngeal closure.
- Back of the tongue is raised to contact the soft palate, back molars, and posterior gum ridge, forming a seal.
- Oral (air) pressure builds up behind the seal.
- Vocal folds are abducted.
- Tongue–soft palate seal is opened, and breath escapes, creating an explosive sound.

Sound Distribution

- Initial — *cat, key, kiss, count, quit*
- Medial — *become, account, cookie, echo, buckle*
- Final — *back, cake, talk, sick, bank*

Developmental Data (age of mastery)

- 4 (Wellman et al., 1931)
- 4½ (Poole, 1934)
- 4 (Templin, 1957)
- 4 (Sander, 1972)
- 2–4 (Prather et al., 1975)

Frequency of Occurrence

- Delattre, 1965

  - 4.30% of total English consonants
  - 10th in frequency of 24 English consonants
  - 2.64% of total vowels and consonants combined
  - 15th in frequency of 42 sounds (vowels and consonants)

- Shriberg & Kwiatkowski, 1983

  - 5.1% of 24 English consonants
  - 10th in frequency of 24 English consonants

Sound: /g/

Place, Manner, Voicing Features

- Lingua-velar (back-soft palate)
- Stop-plosive
- Voiced

Other Distinctive Features (Chomsky & Halle, 1968)

- Consonantal
- High
- Back
- Voiced

Articulatory Production

- Lips are relaxed and apart.

- Soft palate is raised to assist with velopharyngeal closure.

- Back of the tongue is raised to contact the soft palate, back molars, and posterior gum ridge, forming a seal.

- Oral (air) pressure builds up behind the seal.

- Vocal folds are adducted.

- Tongue–soft palate seal is opened, and air escapes with less force than for /k/.

Sound Distribution

- Initial—*go, goat, gate, ghost, girl*
- Medial—*ego, wagon, burger, magazine, again*
- Final—*egg, beg, vague, fog, flag*

Developmental Data (age of mastery)

- 4 (Wellman et al., 1931)
- 4½ (Poole, 1934)
- 4 (Templin, 1957)
- 4 (Sander, 1972)
- 2–4 (Prather et al., 1975)

Frequency of Occurrence

- Delattre, 1965

  - 1.57% of total English consonants
  - 19th in frequency of 24 English consonants
  - 0.96% of total vowels and consonants combined
  - 31st in frequency of 42 sounds (vowels and consonants)

- Shriberg & Kwiatkowski, 1983

  - 3.1% of 24 English consonants
  - 15th in frequency of 24 English consonants

Sound-Evoking Techniques for /k/ and /g/

These evoking techniques facilitate the production of /k/. To establish /g/, follow the same steps, but also instruct the client to add voicing or "turn on the voice box."

Technique 1

- Instruct the client to position the tongue tip behind the lower front teeth. (If client is unable to hold this position, a tongue depressor may be used to keep the tongue in place.)

- Instruct the client to "raise" or "hump" the back portion of the tongue until it forms a seal with the roof of the mouth (soft palate); oral pressure may be built up behind this seal.

- Instruct the client to quickly break the seal by lowering the back of the tongue, thus expelling the built-up air.

- Gradually shape the amount of air released by the client.

Technique 2

- Ask the client to produce [t].

- Instruct the client to produce [t] with the tongue tip behind the lower front teeth. With the tongue tip still positioned behind the lower front teeth, proceed with the next step.

- Ask the client to "raise" or "hump" the back of the tongue to the roof of the mouth (the soft palate) and attempt to produce [k].

- *Note:* To evoke [g], develop from [d] instead of [k].

Technique 3

- Instruct the client to produce [i] as in *bee* or *we*.

- Instruct the client to produce a prolonged [i] while raising the back of the tongue until it touches the roof of the mouth (soft palate); once a seal is formed, instruct the client to release the contact. If the resulting sound is more like [g] than [k], instruct the client to turn off his or her voice box.

Technique 4

- Instruct the client to position the tongue tip behind the lower front teeth. If needed, assist client by means of a tongue depressor.

- Model the production of [k] for the client. If needed, shape your hand like the shape of the tongue during the production of [k] in order to aid the client.

- Instruct the client to "raise" or "hump" the back of the tongue to the roof of the mouth (soft palate), forming a seal.

- Instruct the client to allow air to build up behind this seal, and then instruct the client to lower the back of the tongue, thus allowing the built-up air to be released.

Sound: [f]

Place, Manner, Voicing Features

- Labiodental (lip-teeth)
- Fricative
- Voiceless

Other Distinctive Features (Chomsky & Halle, 1968)

- Consonantal
- Anterior
- Continuant
- Tense
- Strident

Articulatory Production

- Mandible is retracted slightly as the lower lip is lightly placed against the bottom edges of the upper teeth.

- Soft palate is raised to assist with velopharyngeal closure.

- Tongue is in a neutral position or in the position required for the next sound.

- Vocal folds are abducted.

- Audible friction is produced as air is directed through the upper teeth–lower lip contact.

Sound Distribution

- Initial—*feet, fudge, fog, phone, fir*
- Medial—*elephant, muffin, coffee, aphasia, after*
- Final—*leaf, laugh, cough, half, roof*

Developmental Data (age of mastery)

- 3 (Wellman et al., 1931)
- 5½ (Poole, 1934)
- 3 (Templin, 1957)
- 4 (Sander, 1972)
- 2–4 (Prather et al., 1975)

Frequency of Occurrence

- Delattre, 1965

  - 2.86% of total English consonants
  - 15th in frequency of 24 English consonants
  - 1.75% of total vowels and consonants combined
  - 23rd in frequency of 42 sounds (vowels and consonants)

- Shriberg & Kwiatkowski, 1983

  - 2.1% of 24 English consonants
  - 16th in frequency of 24 English consonants

Sound: [v]

Place, Manner, Voicing Features

- Labiodental (lip-teeth)
- Fricative
- Voiced

Other Distinctive Features (Chomsky & Halle, 1968)

- Consonantal
- Anterior
- Continuant
- Voiced
- Strident

Articulatory Production

- Mandible is retracted slightly as the lower lip is lightly placed against the bottom edges of the upper front teeth.

- Soft palate is raised to assist with velopharyngeal closure.

- Tongue is in a neutral position or in the position required for the next sound.

- Vocal folds are adducted.

- Audible friction is produced as air is directed through the upper teeth–lower lip contact.

Sound Distribution

- Initial—*vase, verb, vine, vanilla, view*
- Medial—*television, evil, never, river, seven*
- Final—*live, love, dove, five, save*

Developmental Data (age of mastery)

- 5   (Wellman et al., 1931)
- 6½ (Poole, 1934)
- 6   (Templin, 1957)
- 8   (Sander, 1972)
- 4   (Prather et al., 1975)

Frequency of Occurrence

- Delattre, 1965

  - 3.17% of total English consonants
  - 14th in frequency of 24 English consonants
  - 1.95% of total vowels and consonants combined
  - 21st in frequency of 42 sounds (vowels and consonants)

- Shriberg & Kwiatkowski, 1983

  - 1.5% of 24 English consonants
  - 19th in frequency of 24 English consonants

Sound-Evoking Techniques for [f] and [v]

These evoking techniques facilitate the production of [f]. To establish [v], follow the same steps, but also instruct the client to add voicing or "turn on the voice box."

Technique 1

- Instruct the client to bring his or her lower lip in contact with the bottom of the upper front teeth (manual adjustment of this contact may be necessary).

- Instruct the client to blow air out of the mouth between the lower lip and the upper teeth. (Make sure there is no voicing added.)

- Have the client repeat this process with a piece of paper or a feather in front of his or her mouth.

- Use the feather or paper to focus the client's attention on the force of the air emitted.

- Gradually work to shape the force of the air emitted.

Technique 2

- Ask the client to say [ɑ].

- Instruct the client to bring his or her lower lip in contact with the bottom of the upper front teeth while producing a prolonged [ɑ]. (If needed, manually guide the client's lower lip up to contact the bottom of the upper front teeth.)

- Ask the client to once again attempt to produce [ɑ], this time while blowing air out between the lower lip and upper teeth so that audible friction is produced.

- Instruct the client to repeat the above step with his or her voice box turned off.

- *Note:* To facilitate [v], ignore the final step of this evoking technique.

Technique 3

- Ask the client to produce [p].

- Instruct the client to produce [p] while moving the lower lip back until it contacts the bottom of the upper front teeth.

- Instruct the client to keep the lower lip in contact with the bottom of the upper front teeth while blowing air out between the lower lip and the upper front teeth so that audible friction is produced.

- Gradually shape the force of the air emitted.

Technique 4

- Instruct the client to "*gently* bite down" on his or her lower lip.

- Instruct the client to blow air out between the upper teeth and the lower lip. Use a feather or piece of paper positioned in front of the client's mouth to draw the client's attention to the force and direction of the airflow.

Sound: [θ]

Place, Manner, Voicing Features

- Linguadental (tip-teeth)
- Fricative
- Voiceless

Other Distinctive Features (Chomsky & Halle, 1968)

- Consonantal
- Coronal
- Anterior
- Continuant
- Tense

Articulatory Production

- Lips are relaxed and apart.
- Soft palate is raised to assist with velopharyngeal closure.
- Mandible is lowered slightly.

- Tongue tip is placed lightly behind the upper front teeth, or the blade and tip of the tongue are placed in the space between the upper and lower front teeth.

- Vocal folds are abducted.

- Audible friction is produced as air is directed through the tongue-teeth contact.

Sound Distribution

- Initial — *thumb, thigh, thin, thick, theme*
- Medial — *toothbrush, lethal, nothing, pathetic, healthy*
- Final — *teeth, truth, both, mouth, beneath*

Developmental Data (age of mastery)

- 7½ (Poole, 1934)
- 6 (Templin, 1957)
- 7 (Sander, 1972)
- 4 (Prather et al., 1975)

Frequency of Occurrence

- Delattre, 1965

  - 0.97% of total English consonants
  - 20th in frequency of 24 English consonants
  - 0.60% of total vowels and consonants combined
  - 36th in frequency of 42 sounds (vowels and consonants)

- Shriberg & Kwiatkowski, 1983

  - 0.90% of 24 English consonants
  - 21st in frequency of 24 English consonants

Sound: [ð]

Place, Manner, Voicing Features

- Linguadental (tip-teeth)
- Fricative
- Voiced

Other Distinctive Features (Chomsky & Halle, 1968)

- Consonantal
- Coronal
- Anterior
- Continuant
- Voiced

Articulatory Production

- Lips are relaxed and apart.

- Soft palate is raised to assist with velopharyngeal closure.

- Mandible is lowered slightly.

- Tongue tip is placed lightly behind the upper front teeth, or the blade and tip of the tongue are placed in the space between the upper and lower front teeth.

- Vocal folds are adducted.

- Audible friction is produced as air is directed through the tongue-teeth contact.

Sound Distribution

- Initial—*the, this, that, there, then*
- Medial—*bother, mother, clothing, father, other*
- Final—*breathe, bathe, smooth, teethe, clothe*

Developmental Data (age of mastery)

- 6½ (Poole, 1934)
- 7 (Templin, 1957)
- 8 (Sander, 1972)
- 4 (Prather et al., 1975)

Frequency of Occurrence

- Delattre, 1965

  - 4.61% of total English consonants
  - 9th in frequency of 24 English consonants
  - 2.83% of total vowels and consonants combined
  - 13th in frequency of 42 sounds (vowels and consonants)

- Shriberg & Kwiatkowski, 1983

  - 5.3% of 24 English consonants
  - 8th in frequency of 24 English consonants

Sound-Evoking Techniques for [θ] and [ð]

These evoking techniques facilitate the production of [θ]. To establish [ð], follow the same steps, but also instruct the client to add voicing or "turn on the voice box."

Technique 1

- Instruct the client to stick his or her tongue "straight out."

- Instruct the client to *"gently* bite down" on the tongue.

- Instruct the client to slowly retract his or her tongue until only the tongue tip protrudes between the upper and lower front teeth. (If needed, assist client by means of a tongue depressor.)

- Ask the client to blow air over the tongue and through the constriction formed by the tongue and upper front teeth.

Technique 2

- Ask the client to produce [f].

- Instruct the client to push his or her tongue tip forward between the teeth while producing [f]; this will force the lower lip to release contact with the bottom edge of the upper front teeth, allowing the tongue tip to take its place, thus forming [θ].

- Repeat the previous steps until the tongue protrusion is within normal limits. (If needed, manually assist the client with the tongue protrusion.)

Technique 3

- Place a tongue depressor or flavored food directly in front of the client's mouth.

- Instruct the client to touch this item with his or her tongue tip; with the client's tongue extended, proceed with the next step.

- Instruct the client to *"gently* bite down" on the tongue. (If needed, manually raise the client's lower jaw so that both the upper and lower front teeth come in contact with the tongue.)

- Instruct the client to blow air over the tongue and through the constriction formed by the tongue and the upper front teeth.

- Gradually work with the client to achieve the proper amount of tongue protrusion.

Technique 4

- Ask the client to produce [s]. While the client is producing this sound, proceed with the next step.

- Instruct the client to slide the tongue tip forward until it slightly protrudes between the upper and lower front teeth, thus forming [θ].

- Gradually work to get the tongue protrusion within normal limits.

Sound: [s]

Place, Manner, Voicing Features

- Lingua-alveolar (tip-ridge)
- Fricative
- Voiceless

Other Distinctive Features (Chomsky & Halle, 1968)

- Consonantal
- Coronal
- Anterior
- High
- Continuant
- Tense

Articulatory Production

(*Note:* This sound may be produced with the tongue in two different positions.)

- Lips are relaxed and apart.

- Soft palate is raised to assist with velopharyngeal closure.

- Sides of the tongue are against the upper molars.

- (a) Tip of the tongue approximates the lower incisors near the gum ridge while the front of the tongue is both raised toward the alveolar ridge and slightly grooved. OR (b) Tip of the tongue is narrowly grooved and approximates the upper alveolar ridge.

- Vocal folds are abducted.

- Audible friction is produced as air is directed through the groove in the tongue against the upper alveolar ridge and front teeth.

Sound Distribution

- Initial — *city, safe, scent, song, see*
- Medial — *bracelet, eraser, pencil, proceed, upset*
- Final — *dance, kiss, jealous, nice, house*

Developmental Data (age of mastery)

- 5   (Wellman et al., 1931)
- 7½ (Poole, 1934)
- 4½ (Templin, 1957)
- 8   (Sander, 1972)
- 3   (Prather et al., 1975)

Frequency of Occurrence

- Delattre, 1965

  - 7.47% of total English consonants
  - 5th in frequency of 24 English consonants
  - 4.59% of total vowels and consonants combined
  - 7th in frequency of 42 sounds (vowels and consonants)

- Shriberg & Kwiatkowski, 1983

  - 6.9% of 24 English consonants
  - 3rd in frequency of 24 English consonants

Sound: [z]

Place, Manner, Voicing Features

- Lingua-alveolar (tip-ridge)
- Fricative
- Voiced

Other Distinctive Features (Chomsky & Halle, 1968)

- Consonantal
- Coronal
- Anterior
- High
- Continuant
- Voiced
- Strident

Articulatory Production

(*Note:* This sound may be produced with the tongue in two different positions.)

- Lips are relaxed and apart .
- Soft palate is raised to assist with velopharyngeal closure.
- Sides of the tongue are against the upper molars.
- (a) Tip of the tongue approximates the lower incisors near the gum ridge while the front of the tongue is both raised toward the alveolar ridge and slightly grooved. OR (b) Tip of the tongue is narrowly grooved and approximates the upper alveolar ridge.
- Vocal folds are adducted.
- Audible friction is produced as air is directed through the groove in the tongue against the upper alveolar ridge and front teeth.

Sound Distribution

- Initial — *zoom, zebra, zucchini, zipper, zodiac*
- Medial — *lazy, dozen, freezer, visit, scissors*
- Final — *breeze, is, jazz, size, close*

Developmental Data (age of mastery)

- 5 (Wellman et al., 1931)
- 7½ (Poole, 1934)
- 7 (Templin, 1957)
- 8 (Sander, 1972)
- 4 (Prather et al., 1975)

Frequency of Occurrence

- Delattre, 1965

  - 4.90% of total English consonants
  - 7th in frequency of 24 English consonants
  - 3.01% of total vowels and consonants combined
  - 11th in frequency of 42 sounds (vowels and consonants)

- Shriberg & Kwiatkowski, 1983

  - 5.4% of 24 English consonants
  - 7th in frequency of 24 English consonants

Sound-Evoking Techniques for [s] and [z]

Remember, these sounds can be produced with the tongue tip up or down; therefore, follow the client's lead when deciding which way to teach these sounds.

Technique 1 (Tongue Tip Up)

- Instruct the client to raise his or her tongue so that the sides of the tongue come in contact with the inner surface of the upper back teeth.

- Instruct the client to slightly groove the tongue along the midline. (If the client is unable to complete this step, add the following steps: Instruct the client to protrude the tongue and place a drinking straw along the midline; ask the client to slightly raise the sides of the tongue around the straw. Carefully remove the straw from the client's mouth.)

- Instruct the client to place the tip of his or her tongue slightly behind the upper front teeth.

- Instruct the client to bring his or her teeth together.

- Instruct the client to blow air out along the groove of the tongue. *Note:* For [z], instruct the client to add voicing or "turn on the voice box."

Technique 2 (Tongue Tip Up)

- Model for the client protruding the tongue slightly between the front teeth as in [θ]; ask the client to position his or her tongue in a similar fashion.

- Instruct the client to blow air over the tongue and through the constriction formed between the upper front teeth and the tongue, thus producing [θ].

- Push the tip of the client's tongue tip inward by using a thin instrument (tongue blade) in order to change [θ] to [s]. Once the client understands the correct positioning of the tongue, proceed with the next step.

- Instruct the client to repeat the steps without your manual assistance. *Note:* To facilitate [z], develop from [ð] or instruct the client to turn on the voice while saying [θ].

Technique 3 (Tongue Tip Up)

- Ask the client to produce [ʃ].

- Instruct the client to retract his or her lips (smile) and push the tongue slightly forward while producing [ʃ], thus resulting in [s]. *Note:* To facilitate [z], shape from [ð].

Technique 1 (Tongue Tip Down)

- Instruct the client to raise his or her tongue so that the sides of the tongue come in contact with the inner surface of the upper back teeth.

- Instruct the client to lower the tongue tip so that it is placed behind the lower front teeth near the gum ridge.

- Instruct the client to bring the upper and lower front teeth close together, but not touching.

- Instruct the client to blow air out through the mouth, resulting in [s]. *Note:* To facilitate [z], instruct the client to add voicing or "turn on the voice box."

Technique 2 (Tongue Tip Down)

- Ask the client to produce [i].

• Instruct the client to turn off his or her voice box so that [i] is now voiceless. While the client is still producing the voiceless [i], proceed with the next step.

• Instruct the client to gradually close his or her teeth until [s] results. *Note:* To facilitate [z], do not instruct the client to turn off the voice box.

Technique 1 (Tongue Tip Up or Down)

• Instruct the client to place his or her tongue tip behind either the upper or the lower front teeth.

• Instruct the client to draw the tongue tip slightly away from the teeth.

• Instruct the client to close his or her teeth so that they are barely touching. (Manual assistance may be necessary.)

• Place a finger or piece of paper in front of the center of the client's mouth and ask the client to "blow air out over the tongue toward my finger [or the piece of paper]." *Note:* To facilitate [z], instruct the client to add voicing or "turn on the voice box."

Technique 2 (Tongue Tip Up or Down)

• Place a tongue depressor in the client's mouth against either the upper or the lower front teeth and ask the client to use his or her tongue tip to hold it there.

• Ask the client to keep his or her tongue still while the tongue depressor is carefully removed.

• Instruct the client to close his or her teeth.

• Instruct the client to blow air out, resulting in [s]. *Note:* To facilitate [z], instruct the client to add voicing or "turn on the voice box."

Sound: [ʃ]

Place, Manner, Voicing Features

• Lingua-palatal (tip–post ridge)
• Fricative
• Voiceless

Other Distinctive Features (Chomsky & Halle, 1968)

• Consonantal
• Coronal
• High
• Distributed
• Continuant
• Tense
• Strident

Articulatory Production

• Lips are usually protruded and slightly rounded.

- Soft palate is raised to assist with velopharyngeal closure.

- Sides of the tongue are placed against the upper molars; the tip and blade of the tongue are directed toward the lower front teeth, while the broad front surface of the tongue is both raised toward the hard palate and flattened with a wide groove, thus forming a central opening. (This opening is slightly wider and more posterior as compared to /s/.)

- Vocal folds are abducted.

- Audible friction is produced as air is directed through the central opening against the palate, alveolar ridge, and front teeth.

Sound Distribution

- Initial—*she, shop, sugar, sure, shadow*
- Medial—*ocean, issue, dishes, fashion, motion*
- Final—*push, fish, fresh, bush, sash*

Developmental Data (age of mastery)

- 6½ (Poole, 1934)
- 4½ (Templin, 1957)
- 7   (Sander, 1972)
- 3–8 (Prather et al., 1975)

Frequency of Occurrence

- Delattre, 1965

  - 0.88% of total English consonants
  - 21st in frequency of 24 English consonants
  - 0.54% of total vowels and consonants combined
  - 38th in frequency of 42 sounds (vowels and consonants)

- Shriberg & Kwiatkowski, 1983

  - 0.9% of 24 English consonants
  - 20th in frequency of 24 English consonants

Sound: [ʒ]

Place, Manner, Voicing Features

- Lingua-palatal (tip–post ridge)
- Fricative
- Voiced

Other Distinctive Features (Chomsky & Halle, 1968)

- Consonantal
- High
- Continuant
- Coronal
- Distributed
- Voiced
- Strident

Articulatory Production

- Lips are protruded and slightly rounded.

- Soft palate is raised to assist with velopharyngeal closure.

- Sides of the tongue are placed against the upper molars; the tip and blade of the tongue are directed toward the lower front teeth, while the broad front surface of the tongue is both raised toward the hard palate and flattened with a wide groove, thus forming a central opening. (This opening is slightly wider and more posterior as compared to /s/.)

- Vocal folds are adducted.

- Audible friction is produced as air is directed through the central opening against the palate, alveolar ridge, and front teeth.

Sound Distribution

- Initial — does not occur in English
- Medial — *vision, Asia, casual, treasure, decision*
- Final — *beige, garage, corsage, prestige, camouflage*

Developmental Data (age of mastery)

- 6   (Wellman et al., 1931)
- 6½ (Poole, 1934)
- 7   (Templin, 1957)
- 8+ (Sander, 1972)
- 4   (Prather et al., 1975)

Frequency of Occurrence

- Delattre, 1965

  - 0.16% of total English consonants
  - 24th in frequency of 24 English consonants
  - 0.10% of total vowels and consonants combined
  - 41st in frequency of 42 sounds (vowels and consonants)

- Shriberg & Kwiatkowski, 1983

  - <0.1% of 24 English consonants
  - 24th in frequency of 24 English consonants

Sound-Evoking Techniques for [ʃ] and [ʒ]

Evoking techniques 1–3 facilitate the production of [ʃ]. To establish [ʒ], follow the same steps, but also instruct the client to add voicing or "turn on the voice box."

Technique 1

- Ask the client to produce [s]. While the client is producing this sound, proceed with the next step.

- Instruct the client to "pucker" the lips while moving the tongue back until [ʃ] results. *Note:* To facilitate [ʒ], develop from [z].

Technique 2

- Ask the client, "What sound do people make when they want to tell someone to be quiet?" The clinician may raise his or her forefinger up to the lips as if making the common symbol for "shh." This may be enough of a cue to evoke the client's production of [ʃ].

- Shape the sound from this point.

Technique 3

- Instruct the client to raise the sides of his or her tongue so that they come in contact with the inner surface of the upper back teeth.

- Instruct the client to raise the tip and blade of the tongue and place it behind the upper front teeth.

- Instruct the client to slowly slide the tongue along the roof of the mouth to where the bump on the roof of the mouth just begins to go down in the back.

- Once the client's tongue is position, ask the client to lower the tongue slightly. (If needed, direct the tongue down slightly with a tongue depressor.)

- Ask the client to keep this position while puckering his or her lips.

- Instruct the client to blow air out through the mouth.

Technique 4

- Ask the client to produce [i]. While the client is producing this sound, proceed with the next step.

- Instruct the client to "pucker" his or her lips.

- Instruct the client to raise his or her lower jaw slightly. (Manual assistance may be necessary.)

- Instruct the client to blow air out while raising the tongue, resulting in [ʒ]. *Note:* To facilitate [ʃ], instruct the client to produce [i] with the voice off.

Sound: [h]

Place, Manner, Voicing Features

- Glottal
- Fricative
- Voiceless

Other Distinctive Features (Chomsky & Halle, 1968)

- Low
- Continuant

Articulatory Production

(*Note:* There is no set position for the articulators during the production of this sound.)

- Lips assume the position for the next sound.
- Soft palate is raised to assist with velopharyngeal closure.
- Tongue is in a neutral position or in the position required for the next sound.
- Vocal folds are slightly adducted but not close enough to cause phonation.
- Air is directed through the vocal tract with enough force to produce audible friction.

Sound Distribution

- Initial — *who, hat, hurt, heal, honey*
- Medial — *ahead, rehearse, behavior, lighthouse, behind*
- Final — does not occur in English

Developmental Data (age of mastery)

- 3 (Wellman et al., 1931)
- 3½ (Poole, 1934)
- 3 (Templin, 1957)
- 3 (Sander, 1972)
- 2 (Prather et al., 1975)

Frequency of Occurrence

- Delattre, 1965

  - 3.26% of total English consonants
  - 13th in frequency of 24 English consonants
  - 2.01% of total vowels and consonants combined
  - 20th in frequency of 42 sounds (vowels and consonants)

- Shriberg & Kwiatkowski, 1983

  - 4.4% of 24 English consonants
  - 12th in frequency of 24 English consonants

Sound-Evoking Techniques for [h]

Technique 1

- Instruct the client to breathe in through the nose and out through the mouth.

- To direct the client's attention to the emission of the air through the mouth, use a piece of paper placed in front of the client's mouth.

Technique 2

- Model for the client the taking of a deep breath, holding it, and then releasing this breath through the mouth.

- Focus the client's attention on the sound made as the breath is released.

- Instruct the client to follow the modeled example.

- Work with the client until the force of air and audible friction are within normal limits.

Technique 3

- Place a feather or paper strip in front of the client's mouth.

- Instruct the client to open his or her mouth slightly and to relax the tongue.

- Instruct the client to attempt to move the paper or feather by blowing air out of the mouth with a bit of force behind it.

- Work with the client to achieve an acceptable degree of force.

Technique 4

- Instruct the client to part the lips and teeth.

- Ask the client to relax the tongue and lips.

- Instruct the client to cup his or her hand and place it in front of his or her mouth.

- Instruct the client to take a deep breath and then breathe the air out through the mouth into the cupped hand.

Sound: [ʧ]

Place, Manner, Voicing Features

- Alveo-palatal (tip–post ridge)
- Affricate
- Voiceless

Other Distinctive Features (Chomsky & Halle, 1968)

- Consonantal
- Coronal
- High
- Distributed
- Tense
- Strident

Articulatory Production

(*Note:* This phoneme is produced on a single impulse of air.)

- Lips are apart and either slightly rounded or relaxed.

- Soft palate is raised to assist with velopharyngeal closure.

- Sides of the tongue are against the upper molars, while the blade and tip of the tongue are placed just behind the alveolar ridge, thus blocking the airflow briefly.

- Vocal folds are abducted.

- Airflow is blocked briefly and then audibly released by the lowering of the tongue tip and blade, allowing the air to flow through a broad point of constriction that occurs between the front of the tongue and the alveolar ridge.

Sound Distribution

- Initial — *cello, chocolate, cheer, chop, choose*
- Medial — *nature, ritual, teacher, furniture, virtue*
- Final — *rich, preach, such, lunch, watch*

Developmental Data (age of mastery)

- 5   (Wellman et al., 1931)
- 4½   (Templin, 1957)
- 7   (Sander, 1972)
- 3–8 (Prather et al., 1975)

Frequency of Occurrence

- Delattre, 1965

  - 0.63% of total English consonants
  - 23rd in frequency of 24 English consonants
  - 0.39% of total vowels and consonants combined
  - 40th in frequency of 42 sounds (vowels and consonants)

- Shriberg & Kwiatkowski, 1983

  - 0.6% of 24 English consonants
  - 23rd in frequency of 24 English consonants

Sound: [ʤ]

Place, Manner, Voicing Features

- Alveo-palatal (tip–post ridge)
- Affricate
- Voiced

Other Distinctive Features (Chomsky & Halle, 1968)

- Consonantal
- Coronal
- High
- Distributed
- Tense
- Voiced
- Strident

Articulatory Production

(*Note:* This phoneme is produced on a single impulse of air.)

- Lips are apart and either slightly rounded or relaxed.

- Soft palate is raised to assist with velopharyngeal closure.

- Sides of the tongue are against the upper molars, while the blade and tip of the tongue are placed just behind the alveolar ridge, thus blocking the airflow briefly.
- Vocal folds are adducted.
- Airflow is blocked briefly and then audibly released by the lowering of the tongue tip and blade, allowing the air to flow through a broad point of constriction that occurs between the front of the tongue and the alveolar ridge.

Sound Distribution

- Initial—*jam, judge, joke, gentle, gypsy*
- Medial—*soldier, adjust, magic, religion, tragic*
- Final—*fudge, edge, image, page, stage*

Developmental Data (age of mastery)

- 7 (Templin, 1957)
- 7 (Sander, 1972)
- 4 (Prather et al., 1975)

Frequency of Occurrence

- Delattre, 1965

  - 0.88% of total English consonants
  - 22nd in frequency of 24 English consonants
  - 0.54% of total vowels and consonants combined
  - 39th in frequency of 42 sounds (vowels and consonants)

- Shriberg & Kwiatkowski, 1983

  - 0.6% of 24 English consonants
  - 22nd in frequency of 24 English consonants

Sound-Evoking Techniques for [ʧ] and [ʤ]

Evoking techniques 1–4 facilitate the production of [ʧ]. To establish [ʤ], follow the same steps, but also instruct the client to add voicing or "turn on the voice box."

Technique 1

- Ask the client to produce [ʃ], or to evoke this sound, ask, "What sound does one make to request that someone be quiet?"—Shh! While the client is producing this sound, proceed with the next step.

- Instruct the client to raise the tip of the tongue to the roof of the mouth so that he or she can feel the "bump" behind the upper front teeth.

- Remind the client to "pucker" his or her lips, and then instruct the client to lower the tongue tip while forcing air out of the mouth, resulting in [ʧ].

Technique 2

- Instruct the client to raise his or her tongue tip and blade to the roof of the mouth right behind the upper front teeth.

- Instruct the client to slide the tongue back along the roof of the mouth to the bumpy portion of the roof and then the slight decline. Once the client finds the place where the bump begins to decline, instruct the client to keep the tip of the tongue there, and proceed with the next step.

- Instruct the client to "pucker" the lips and to lower the tongue tip while forcing air out of the mouth.

Technique 3

- Instruct the client to place the tip of his or her tongue against the roof of the mouth right behind the two upper front teeth.

- Instruct the client to then slide the tongue tip back slightly to the bump on the roof of the mouth. (It may be necessary to push the tongue tip back to this position by means of a tongue depressor.)

- Instruct the client to "pucker" his or her lips.

- Instruct the client to make the sneezing sound (*choo!*) by slightly lowering the tongue tip while forcing built-up air pressure out of the mouth.

Technique 4

- Instruct the client to produce the following phrase, in which [t] is followed by [ʃ]: "That ship is at shore?" Other phrases the clinician may use are *what shall, that shell, what shape, that ship.* Instruct the client to hold the [t] briefly and then "explode" into the [ʃ], thus forming [tʃ].

- Work with the client to shape the [tʃ] sound from these sentences and phrases. *Note:* To facilitate [dʒ], work from phrases such as *meet you, had you, found you, could you.*

Sound: [m]

Place, Manner, Voicing Features

- Bilabial (lip-lip)
- Nasal
- Voiced

Other Distinctive Features (Chomsky & Halle, 1968)

- Consonantal
- Sonorant
- Anterior
- Nasal
- Voiced

Articulatory Production

- Lips are shut lightly.

- Tongue is in a neutral position or in the position required for the next sound.

- Velopharyngeal port is open.

- Vocal folds are adducted.

- Air is directed through the open velopharyngeal port, the nasal cavity, and out the nostrils.

Sound Distribution

- Initial—*maybe, mine, me, mud, man*
- Medial—*lemon, grammar, command, famous, hammer*
- Final—*calm, home, thumb, jam, dime*

Developmental Data (age of mastery)

- 3 (Wellman et al., 1931)
- 3½ (Poole, 1934)
- 3 (Templin, 1957)
- 3 (Sander, 1972)
- 2 (Prather et al., 1975)

Frequency of Occurrence

- Delattre, 1965

  - 4.74% of total English consonants
  - 8th in frequency of 24 English consonants
  - 2.91% of total vowels and consonants combined
  - 12th in frequency of 42 sounds (vowels and consonants)

- Shriberg & Kwiatkowski, 1983

  - 5.9% of 24 English consonants
  - 6th in frequency of 24 English consonants

Sound-Evoking Techniques for [m]

Technique 1

- Instruct the client to bring his or her lips together, breathe in deeply through the nose, and then release the breath out the nose.

- Ask the client to say "Ah."

- Instruct the client to close his or her lips, breathe in deeply through the nose, and then let air out through the nose while saying "Ah."

Technique 2

- Ask the client to take a deep breath through the mouth, close the mouth, and expel the air through the nose. (If working with a child, you may take turns doing this with the child so that it becomes more like a game.)

- Instruct the client to repeat the previous step, but also instruct him or her to add voicing or hum while expelling the air through the nose.

Technique 3

- Ask the client to produce [bʌ].

- Instruct the client to produce the same sound with his or her mouth closed, letting the air flow through the nose.

- Draw attention to the nasal emission by placing a mirror under the nose.

Technique 4

- Instruct the client to bring his or her lips together and hum, or ask the client, "What does one say when something tastes really good?"—Mmmmm!

- These suggestions may result in the correct production of [m].

Sound: [n]

Place, Manner, Voicing Features

- Lingua-alveolar (tip-ridge)
- Nasal
- Voiced

Other Distinctive Features (Chomsky & Halle, 1968)

- Consonantal
- Sonorant
- Coronal
- Anterior
- Nasal
- Voiced

Articulatory Production

- Lips are relaxed and slightly apart.

- Sides of the tongue are against the upper teeth and gums, while the tip and blade of the tongue are raised to contact the alveolar ridge.

- Velopharyngeal port is open.

- Vocal folds are adducted.

- Air is directed through the open velopharyngeal port, the nasal cavity, and out the nostrils.

Sound Distribution

- Initial—*name, number, none, knock, knife*
- Medial—*banana, funny, dinosaur, tunnel, wonder*
- Final—*sun, can, balloon, skin, listen*

Developmental Data (age of mastery)

- 3   (Wellman et al., 1931)
- 4½ (Poole, 1934)

- 3   (Templin, 1957)
- 3   (Sander, 1972)
- 2   (Prather et al., 1975)

Frequency of Occurrence

- Delattre, 1965

  - 11.46% of total English consonants
  - 2nd in frequency of 24 English consonants
  - 7.04% of total vowels and consonants combined
  - 3rd in frequency of 42 sounds (vowels and consonants)

- Shriberg & Kwiatkowski, 1983

  - 12.0% of 24 English consonants
  - 1st in frequency of 24 English consonants

Sound-Evoking Techniques for [n]

Technique 1

- Ask the client to place his or her tongue in position for [d].

- Instruct the client to close his or her mouth, breathe in deeply through the nose, and hold the breath briefly.

- Instruct the client to let the air out through the nose while attempting to produce [d].

Technique 2

- Instruct the client to produce [ɑ]. While the client is producing this sound, proceed with the next step.

- Instruct the client to raise both sides of the tongue to contact the inner surface of the back teeth and to place the front of the tip of the tongue behind the upper front teeth.

- This should block the airflow through the oral cavity and send it through the nose, resulting in [n].

Technique 3

- Use a visual aid such as a mirror to instruct the client to place his or her tongue tip against the alveolar ridge. With the client's tongue in place, proceed with the next step.

- Instruct the client to breathe in and out through his or her nose.

- Keeping the tongue in position, instruct the client to breathe in through the nose and then breathe out through the nose with the addition of voicing.

Technique 4

- Lightly touch the client's upper gum ridge (alveolar ridge) with a tongue depressor or cotton swab.

- Ask the client to raise the tip of the tongue to contact the spot you touched.

- Instruct the client to breathe in through the nose and breathe out through the nose with the "voice box" turned on.

Sound: [ŋ]

Place, Manner, Voicing Features

- Lingua-velar (back–soft palate)
- Nasal
- Voiced

Other Distinctive Features (Chomsky & Halle, 1968)

- Consonantal
- Sonorant
- High
- Back
- Nasal
- Voiced

Articulatory Production

- Lips are relaxed and apart.

- Back of the tongue is raised against the lowered soft palate, back molars, and posterior gum ridge.

- Velopharyngeal port is open.

- Vocal folds are adducted.

- Air is directed through the open velopharyngeal port, the nasal cavity, and out the nostrils.

Sound Distribution

- Initial — does not occur in English
- Medial — *hunger, stronger, jinx, donkey, singer*
- Final — *ring, bang, wrong, laughing, evening*

Developmental Data (age of mastery)

- 4½ (Poole, 1934)
- 3 (Templin, 1957)
- 6 (Sander, 1972)
- 2 (Prather et al., 1975)

Frequency of Occurrence

- Delattre, 1965

  - 2.20% of total English consonants

- 17th in frequency of 24 English consonants
- 1.35% of total vowels and consonants combined
- 27th in frequency of 42 sounds (vowels and consonants)

- Shriberg & Kwiatkowski, 1983

- 1.6% of 24 English consonants
- 17th in frequency of 24 English consonants

Sound-Evoking Techniques for [ŋ]

Technique 1

- Ask the client to breathe in and out through his or her nose, and use a mirror to focus the client's attention on the nasal emission.

- Instruct the client to attempt to produce [g] with his or her mouth closed, thus directing the air out of the nostrils and forming [ŋ].

Technique 2

- Ask the client to place the tongue tip directly behind the lower front teeth. (If necessary, a tongue depressor may be used to keep the tongue in place.)

- Instruct the client to "hump" or "raise" the back of the tongue, as in the production of [k] and [g].

- Instruct the client to breathe out of the nose while voicing or with the voice box turned on.

Technique 3

- Instruct the client to produce [i].

- Ask the client now to produce a prolonged [i] while raising the back of the tongue so that it forms a seal with the roof of the mouth, resulting in [ŋ].

- Repeat the above steps while focusing the client's attention on the tongue placement and nasal emission.

Technique 4

- Instruct the client to produce [m], hum, or attempt to say "Ah" with the mouth closed. Choose the method that is easiest for the client—this will allow the client to become familiar with the voicing and nasal emission that accompany this sound.

- Demonstrate for the client the tongue position for [ŋ], then instruct the client to "hump" or "raise" the back of his or her tongue while resting the tip of the tongue behind the lower front teeth.

- Instruct the client to once again hum or attempt to say "Ah" without moving the tongue from its position, resulting in [ŋ].

Sound: [j]

Place, Manner, Voicing Features

- Lingua-palatal
- Glide
- Voiced

Other Distinctive Features (Chomsky & Halle, 1968)

- Consonantal
- Sonorant
- High
- Distributed
- Continuant
- Voiced

Articulatory Production

- Lips are relaxed or in the position for the next sound.

- Soft palate is raised to assist with velopharyngeal closure.

- Tongue is shifted forward in the oral cavity and the sides of the tongue are placed against the upper teeth; the tip and blade of the tongue are raised toward the alveolar ridge (approximating the position for /i/).

- The "glide" portion of this sound occurs as the tongue is moved into position for the next sound.

- Vocal folds are adducted.

- Air is directed through the oral cavity.

Sound Distribution

- Initial — *yellow, young, year, yogurt, you*
- Medial — *million, canyon, onion, lawyer, coyote*
- Final — does not occur in English

Developmental Data (age of mastery)

- 4   (Wellman et al., 1931)
- 4½   (Poole, 1934)
- 3½   (Templin, 1957)
- 4   (Sander, 1972)
- 2–4 (Prather et al., 1975)

Frequency of Occurrence

- Delattre, 1965

  - 2.01% of total English consonants
  - 18th in frequency of 24 English consonants
  - 1.23% of total vowels and consonants combined
  - 28th in frequency of 42 sounds (vowels and consonants)

- Shriberg & Kwiatkowski, 1983

  - 1.6% of 24 English consonants
  - 18th in frequency of 24 English consonants

Sound-Evoking Techniques for [j]

Technique 1

- Instruct the client to make a quick, tight [ʒ] or to say [ʒ] several times quickly. This will often result in [j]. If not, also instruct the client to slightly lower the tip of the tongue.

Technique 2

- Instruct the client to relax the tongue, allowing it to lie flat in the mouth.

- Instruct the client to open his or her mouth. Then *gently* tap the middle portion of the tongue with a tongue depressor and ask the client to slightly raise the area touched.

- Instruct the client to breathe while voicing.

Technique 3

- Ask the client to produce [i].

- Instruct the client now to produce a prolonged [i] quickly followed by [u], resulting in [iju]. After the client establishes [iju], proceed with the next step.

- Instruct the client to "make the [i] silent," which will result in [ju].

Technique 4

- Ask the client to produce [ð]. While the client is producing [ð], proceed with the next step.

- Instruct the client to retract the tongue straight back from its starting position until the tip is even with the back portion of the alveolar ridge. (Assist the client with retracting the tongue a proper distance.)

- Instruct the client to slightly lower the tip of the tongue and continue breathing out with the voice on, thus forming [j].

Sound: [w]

Place, Manner, Voicing Features

- Bilabial (also referred to as labial-velar)
- Glide
- Voiced

Other Distinctive Features (Chomsky & Halle, 1968)

- Consonantal
- Sonorant
- High
- Back
- Rounded

- Distributed
- Continuant
- Voiced

Articulatory Production

- Lips are rounded and slightly protruded.

- Soft palate is raised to assist with velopharyngeal closure.

- Body of the tongue is moved posteriorly and raised toward the palate while the front of the tongue is placed low in the oral cavity (approximating the position for /u/).

- The "glide" portion of this sound occurs as the tongue is moved into position for the next sound.

- Vocal folds are adducted.

- Air is directed through the oral cavity.

Sound Distribution

- Initial — *wood, wire, wake, one, water*
- Medial — *beware, reward, driveway, power, awhile*
- Final — does not occur in English

Developmental Data (age of mastery)

- 3   (Wellman et al., 1931)
- 3½ (Poole, 1934)
- 3   (Templin, 1957)
- 3   (Sander, 1972)
- 2–8 (Prather et al., 1975)

Frequency of Occurrence

- Delattre, 1965

  - 3.15% of total English consonants
  - 11th in frequency of 24 English consonants
  - 1.94% of total vowels and consonants combined
  - 17th in frequency of 42 sounds (vowels and consonants)

- Shriberg & Kwiatkowski, 1983

  - 4.9% of 24 English consonants
  - 11th in frequency of 24 English consonants

Sound-Evoking Techniques for [w]

Technique 1

- Ask the client to produce [u].

- Instruct the client to produce a prolonged [u] quickly followed by [ə], resulting in [uwɑ]. After the client establishes [uwɑ], proceed with the next step.

- Instruct the client to "make the [u] silent," which will result in [wɑ].

Technique 2

- Instruct the client to raise the back of his or her tongue toward the roof of the mouth, but make sure it does not touch. (If needed, assist by means of a tongue depressor.)

- Instruct the client to round the lips and bring them close together.

- Instruct the client to breathe out while voicing or with the voice box on.

Technique 3

- Ask the client to produce [bʌ] (a child may be asked to make the sound used to scare someone: "Boo!").

- Instruct the client now to round his or her lips and place them close together.

- Instruct the client to attempt to say [bʌ], resulting in [wʌ].

Technique 4

- Ask the client to produce [u].

- Instruct the client to produce a prolonged [u] while both rounding and placing the lips close together, often resulting in [w].

Sound: [r]

Place, Manner, Voicing Features

- Alveo-palatal (post tip–ridge)
- Glide
- Voiced

Other Distinctive Features (Chomsky & Halle, 1968)

- Vocalic
- Consonantal
- Sonorant
- Coronal
- Rounded
- Continuant
- Voiced

Articulatory Production

- Lips are usually rounded, or they may take the position required for the next sound.

- Soft palate is raised to assist with velopharyngeal closure.

- Sides of the tongue are against the upper molars, while the front of the tongue is raised toward the palate; tip of the tongue approximates the alveolar ridge (retroflex *r*) or points down toward the lower teeth.

- The "glide" portion of this sound occurs as the tongue is moved into position for the next sound.

- Vocal folds are adducted.
- Air is directed through the oral cavity.

Sound Distribution

- Initial—*wreath, write, rope, ran, room*
- Medial—*around, berry, orange, pirate, carrot*
- Final—*car, appear, chair, core, hair*

Developmental Data (age of mastery)

- 5   (Wellman et al., 1931)
- 7½   (Poole, 1934)
- 4   (Templin, 1957)
- 6   (Sander, 1972)
- 3–4 (Prather et al., 1975)

Frequency of Occurrence

- Delattre, 1965

    - 8.32% of total English consonants
    - 3rd in frequency of 24 English consonants
    - 5.11% of total vowels and consonants combined
    - 5th in frequency of 42 sounds (vowels and consonants)

- Shriberg & Kwiatkowski, 1983

    - 6.7% of 24 English consonants
    - 4th in frequency of 24 English consonants

Sound-Evoking Techniques for [r] and [ɚ], and [ɝ]

Technique 1

- Instruct the client to place his or her tongue tip slightly behind the upper front teeth. (Manual assistance may be necessary.)

- Instruct the client to "curl the tongue backward" without touching the roof of the mouth with the tongue.

- Instruct the client to round the lips slightly while breathing out with the voice on, resulting in [r].

Technique 2

- Ask the client to produce [ɚ].

- Ask the client to produce [ɚ] quickly followed by a vowel such as [i].

- Instruct the client to produce these vowels together several times, resulting in [ɚri]. After the client establishes [ɚri], proceed with the next step.

- Instruct the client to "make the [ɚ] silent," resulting in [ri].

Technique 3

- Ask the client to place the tongue in position for [d].

- Instruct the client to slightly lower the tip of the tongue.

- Instruct the client to retract the tongue, resulting in the curling of the back of the tongue.

- Instruct the client to slightly round his or her lips while breathing out with the voice box turned on.

Technique 4

- Ask the client to growl like a tiger (*grrr!*), or ask the client, "What sound does a race car make?"—Rrrrr! These cues may result in the correct production or [r].

Sound: [l]

Place, Manner, Voicing Features

- Alveolar (tip-ridge)
- Lateral
- Voiced

Other Distinctive Features (Chomsky & Halle, 1968)

- Vocalic
- Consonant
- Sonorant
- Coronal
- Anterior
- Lateral
- Continuant
- Tense
- Voiced

Articulatory Production

- Lips are relaxed and apart, or they may take on the position required for the next sound.

- Soft palate is raised to assist with velopharyngeal closure.

- Tip of the tongue is placed in contact with the alveolar ridge, and the sides of the tongue are lowered to create openings on both sides of the tongue.

- Vocal folds are adducted.

- Air is directed around the sides of the tongue as it travels through the oral cavity.

Sound Distribution

- Initial—*love, little, leap, lungs, lemon*
- Medial—*follow, eleven, family, salad, jelly*
- Final—*ball, uncle, shovel, hill, oil*

Developmental Data (age of mastery)

- 4   (Wellman et al., 1931)
- 6½ (Poole, 1934)
- 6   (Templin, 1957)
- 6   (Sander, 1972)
- 3–4 (Prather et al., 1975)

Frequency of Occurrence

- Delattre, 1965

  - 7.69% of total English consonants
  - 4th in frequency of 24 English consonants
  - 4.72% of total vowels and consonants combined
  - 6th in frequency of 42 sounds (vowels and consonants)

- Shriberg & Kwiatkowski, 1983

  - 5.3% of 24 English consonants
  - 9th in frequency of 24 English consonants

Sound-Evoking Techniques for [l]

Technique 1

- Place a tongue depressor under the tip and blade of the client's tongue and lift the tongue tip and blade behind the upper front teeth.

- Instruct the client to breathe out while voicing, resulting in [l].

Technique 2

- Using a tongue depressor, cotton swab, or flavored food, touch the place on the client's alveolar ridge where the tongue tip makes contact for the production of [l].

- Instruct the client to place his or her tongue at the spot you touched. Once there, instruct the client to breathe, allowing the air to flow around the sides of the tongue.

- Instruct the client to turn on the voice box and repeat the previous step.

Technique 3

- Ask the client to produce [ɑ]. While the client is producing this sound, proceed with the next step.

- Instruct the client to place his or her tongue tip behind the upper front teeth, resulting in [l]. (If needed, use a tongue depressor to raise the tip of the tongue behind the upper front teeth.)

Technique 4

- Ask the client to position the tongue as if producing [ð].

- Instruct the client to lower the jaw slightly.

- Instruct the client to slide the tongue tip up the back side of the front teeth to the alveolar ridge behind the two front teeth.

- Instruct the client to lower the sides of the tongue slightly.

- Instruct the client to breathe out while voicing, resulting in [l].

Note: In addition to the author's clinical experience, the information for this appendix was drawn from various sources, including Bleile (1995), Chomsky and Halle (1968), Delattre (1965), Edwards (1997), Garbutt and Anderson (1980), Medlin (1975), Nemoy and Davis (1980), Poole (1934), Prather et al. (1975), Sander (1972), Shriberg and Kwiatkowski (1983), Stemple and Holcomb (1988), Templin (1957), and Wellman et al. (1931).

Appendix N

♦ ♦

Treatment Recording Sheet

Name: _____ Therapist: _____

Age: _____ Date: _____ Session #: _____

Disorder(s): _____ Target behavior: _____

Criterion: _____

Target Responses	1	2	3	4	5	1	2	3	4	5	1	2	3	4	5	1	2	3	4	5

Percent correct: _____

Appendix O

♦ ♦ ♦ ♦ ♦ ♦ ♦ ♦ ♦ ♦ ♦ ♦ ♦ ♦ ♦ ♦ ♦ ♦ ♦

Probe Recording Sheet

Name: _____ Age: _____ Therapist: _____

Date: _____ Session #: _____ Disorder(s): _____

Target behavior: _____

Target Responses	Correct (+) / Incorrect (−)
1.	
2.	
3.	
4.	
5.	
6.	
7.	
8.	
9.	
10.	
11.	
12.	
13.	
14.	
15.	
16.	
17.	
18.	
19.	
20.	

Percent correct: _____

Glossary

◆ ◆ ◆ ◆ ◆ ◆ ◆ ◆ ◆ ◆ ◆ ◆ ◆ ◆ ◆ ◆ ◆ ◆ ◆

abducted: Open, drawn apart; as in *abducted vocal folds*. See also *adducted*.

accessory nerve XI: Classified as a cranial nerve, it is both a cranial and a spinal nerve that supplies the muscles of the pharynx, soft palate, head, and shoulders.

acoustic: Pertaining to sound.

acoustics: A branch of phonetics, which pertains to the study of the science of sound. It includes the study of the origin, transmission, modification, and effects of sound vibrations.

acoustic nerve VIII: See *vestibular acoustic nerve VIII*.

acoustic phonetics: Branch of phonetics dedicated to the study of the science of sound. See *acoustics*.

acoustic reflex: Reflexive contraction of the tensor tympani and the stapedius muscles triggered by loud sounds and noises.

Adam's apple: The lay term for the thyroid notch in the larynx.

adaptation: In articulation, the process by which sounds are affected by or take on the properties of other surrounding sounds. The perceptual property of the sound may be unaffected.

addition: A form of articulation error; a superfluous sound that does not belong in a word (e.g., "biga" for *big*).

adducted: Closed or nearly closed, as in *adducted vocal folds*.

advanced word forms: Words used by a young child that have an advanced pronunciation in comparison to the rest of the child's phonological system. The use of such forms may disappear as the child's phonological system matures. Synonym: *progressive idioms*.

afferent: The flow of information toward the cell body.

affricates: A group of consonants with the characteristics of stops and fricatives.

age of customary production: The age at which approximately 50% of children can be expected to produce a particular singleton sound.

age of mastery: The age at which approximately 90% of children can be expected to produce a particular singleton sound.

air conduction: Sound traveling through the medium of the air; air-conducted sound reaches the cochlea through the outer and middle ear.

allographs: Different letters (alphabetic symbols) and letter combinations that can be used to represent the same sound (phoneme) in a specific language.

allophones: Variations of a phoneme.

allophonic variations: Articulatory or perceptual variations of the same phoneme, often caused by the sound's phonetic environment. Such variations do not change the meaning of a word.

alveolar process: The outer edges of the maxillary bone (upper jaw) that house the molar, bicuspid, and cuspid teeth.

alveolar ridge: A ridge on the maxilla that overlies the roots of the teeth, most often located behind the upper anterior teeth. In most people it serves as the point of articulation for English sounds /s/, /z/, /t/, /d/, /n/, /l/.

alveolar sounds: Consonant sounds /s/, /z/, /t/, /d/, /n/, /l/ made by placing the tongue against the alveolar ridge.

alternating motion rates: Alternating repetitive movements of the tongue. Part of diadochokinetic testing by successive repetition of the same syllable sequence (e.g., /pʌ pʌ pʌ pʌ/, /tʌ tʌ tʌ tʌ/, and /kʌ kʌ kʌ kʌ/).

amplitude: Magnitude or range of movement of sound waves; the greater the amplitude, the louder the sound is perceived.

anatomy: Structure of an organism. The science pertaining to the structure of organisms.

aneurysm: Circumscribed dilation of an artery. Formed by a stretching of its walls; can be suggestive of a condition in which the weakened blood vessel may burst.

ankyloglossia: Limited movement of the tongue tip due to an abnormally short lingual frenulum; also known as tongue-tie.

anoxia: Lack of or deficiency of oxygen; a potential cause of brain damage.

antecedent event: A stimulus presented *before* a target response is produced or attempted.

anterior feature: Distinctive feature characteristic of sounds made in the front region of the mouth, generally at the alveolar ridge or forward. See *distinctive features*.

anticipatory substitution: Sound substitution created by the coarticulatory effects of a sound that follows the target sound.

aperiodic: Sound vibrations (or other events) that do not repeat themselves at regular intervals; aperiodic sound is perceived noise.

aphasia: An acquired language disorder due to brain damage or disease; a variety of difficulties in formulating, expressing, and understanding language.

aphonia: Loss of voice.

applied phonetics: A branch of phonetics dedicated to the practical application of the knowledge gained from experimental, articulatory, acoustic, and perceptual phonetics.

apraxia: A disorder of sequenced movements of body parts in the absence of muscle weakness, incoordination, or paralysis; an acquired motor programming disorder. See also *oral apraxia, limb apraxia,* and *apraxia of speech.*

apraxia of speech: A sensorimotor disorder of speech, characterized by impaired ability to position the speech muscles and sequence the muscle movements (respiratory, laryngeal, and oral) necessary for volitional production of sounds and words.

approximants: Sounds produced by an "approximating" contact between the two articulators that form them; includes liquids and glides.

aprosody: Loss of the melody of speech (prosody). A less severe form is referred to as dysprosody (disordered prosody).

arresting sound: A consonant sound that closes a syllable.

articulation: In speech, movement of the speech mechanism to produce the sound of speech. One of the four basic processes involved in speech production.

articulation disorders: Problems in producing speech sounds.

articulator-bound features: Sound features produced by the action of a single articulator.

articulator-free features: Sound features produced by the actions of multiple articulators.

articulators: Organs of the speech production mechanism; help produce meaningful sound by interrupting the flow of exhaled air or by narrowing the space for its passage. The articulators include the lips, tongue, velum, jaw, hard palate, alveolar ridge, and teeth.

articulatory phonetics: A branch of phonetics that focuses on how a speaker of a language makes speech sounds.

arytenoid cartilages: Two small, pyramid-shaped cartilages capable of various kinds of movements; the vocal folds move accordingly because of their attachment to the arytenoids.

assessment: In articulation, the process that is followed and the procedures that are used to identify the presence or absence of an articulation or phonological disorder.

assimilation: The effect one speech sound has on another when produced in close sequence, such that the sounds become more like each other. The effect can be so extensive that it can be perceptually identified. See also *progressive assimilation* and *regressive assimilation*.

association fibers: Neural fibers that connect different parts of the brain within the two hemispheres.

ataxia: Disturbed balance and abnormal gait caused by damage to the cerebellum.

ataxic dysarthria: A motor speech disorder associated with ataxia. See also *dysarthria*.

athetosis: A neurological disorder characterized by slow, involuntary, writhing, and "worm-like" movements.

atrophy: Degeneration or wasting away of muscle, tissues, or organs. Muscular atrophy often occurs in paralysis.

audible nasal emission: Noise that can be heard of the air escaping through the nose.

audiogram: A graph that shows the results of various hearing tests.

audiologist: A specialist in the study of hearing and in the assessment and rehabilitation of hearing impairment.

audiology: The study and understanding of normal and disordered hearing and the rehabilitation of individuals with hearing loss.

audiological evaluation: Procedures used to measure hearing ability. Such procedures most often include but are not limited to pure-tone air- and bone-conduction thresholds; speech reception and discrimination scores; and discrimination of speech in the presence of noise.

audiological screening: A quick procedure performed to determine the need for further audiological evaluation. Testing is typically restricted to 500, 1,000, 2,000, and 4,000 Hz at 20–25 dB and performed in a quiet but not soundproof environment.

auditory bombardment: Procedure by which a child is provided with amplified auditory stimulation for a particular sound that is being taught.

auditory training: A rehabilitative process of training a person with hearing loss to listen to amplified sounds, recognize their meanings, and distinguish one sound from another.

aural rehabilitation: An educational process designed to improve the communicative abilities of a person with hearing loss; it includes auditory training, counseling, and speech–language therapy.

auricle: The most visible part of the outer ear, also known as the pinna.

automatic speech: Linguistic material often produced with minimal volitional control; may include such utterances as consecutive numbers, days of the week, expletives, verses, prayers, songs, and various kinds of common expressions.

autonomic nervous system: A system of nerves divided into sympathetic and parasympathetic branches that controls many involuntary functions of the body.

babbling: The playful vocal sounds that babies produce beginning at about 6 to 7 months of age.

back feature: A distinctive feature that characterizes sounds made in the back part of the oral cavity; the body of the tongue is retracted from the neutral position /ə/ during the production of sounds containing the back distinctive feature.

basal ganglia: Structures deep within the brain that help integrate motor impulses.

baselines: Measures of a client's target behaviors or treatment objectives before those behaviors are taught; they help the clinician establish client improvement, clinical effectiveness, and professional accountability.

base rating: The process followed by a clinician to obtain baseline measures of a client's target behaviors before those behaviors are taught. See also *baselines*.

basilar membrane: The floor of the cochlea, containing the organ of Corti and its several thousand hair cells that respond to sound.

behavioral principles: Concepts and procedures of operant conditioning and learning; frequently used in the treatment of communication disorders.

Bernoulli effect: Increased velocity and decreased pressure when gasses or liquids move through a constricted passage.

bifid uvula: A split uvula suggesting that there may be a cleft underneath the tissue covering the palate.

bifurcation: Division or forking into two branches. The trachea bifurcates into two bronchi.

bilabial: Involving both lips; bilabial sounds are produced primarily by the two lips.

bilateral: On both sides, as in *bilateral cleft lip* or *bilateral hearing loss*.

bilingual: Of two languages; often refers to a person who speaks two languages.

binary classification system: A (+) and (−) value system that identifies whether a specific feature is present or absent in a sound. See also *distinctive features*.

blends: Two or more consonant sounds made next to each other with no vowel separation (e.g., /tr/, /pl/, /str/). See also *cluster*.

bone conduction: A process of conducting sound through bone vibrations.

bound morpheme: A morpheme that cannot convey meaning by itself; for example, the regular plural *s* in the word *cats*. A bound morpheme is attached to a free morpheme for meaning.

brain stem: The collective term for the medulla, the pons, and the midbrain structures of the central nervous system.

breathiness: The voice quality that results when air escapes through partially open vocal folds.

broad phonetic transcription: The act of writing a phoneme into special phonetic symbols enclosed between virgules (slash marks); it can be interpreted only by someone familiar with the phonology of the language transcribed (e.g., /bot/ for *boat*; /ʃɪp/ for *ship*).

Broca's aphasia: Nonfluent, predominantly expressive aphasia. Associated with a lesion in the third frontal convolution of the dominant hemisphere. Characterized by problems with initiation of sound sequences in words and restricted grammar and vocabulary. Verbal output is often limited to expression of high-frequency content words. Auditory comprehension is relatively spared, allowing the individual to communicate information through yes-no or multiple-choice questions; writing is often affected.

Broca's area: A center for motor speech control within the frontal lobe of the language-dominant hemisphere in the brain.

bronchi: Primary divisions of the trachea that penetrate the lungs, one for the right lung and the other for the left lung; they serve to transport air to and from the lungs.

buccinator: A large, flat muscle that makes up most of the cheeks.

bulbar palsy: Paresis and atrophy of the muscles of the lips, tongue, mouth, and larynx as a result of lesions in the motor centers of the medulla oblongata.

canonical babbling: Term used in reference to the combined stages of reduplicated and variegated babbling.

carryover: The regular use of newly learned speech or language skills in everyday situations.

cartilage: Tough connective tissues, as in the *thyroid cartilage,* which is one of the cartilages of the larynx.

cavity: A hollow space within the body; a structure within the body containing other structures, as in the *oral cavity,* which contains the tongue, hard palate, soft palate, and so forth.

centering diphthongs: Diphthongs in which one of the stressed vowels combines with schwar /ɚ/. Synonym: *rhotic diphthongs.*

central nervous system: The brain and the spinal cord.

cerebellum: A structure below the brain and behind the brain stem that regulates equilibrium, body posture, and coordinated fine motor movements.

cerebral hemispheres: The two halves of the brain divided by the longitudinal or intrahemispheric fissure.

cerebral palsy: Brain damage suffered during infancy or the prenatal period and the resulting paralysis and problems of physical growth, locomotion, communication, and sensory problems.

cerebrospinal fluid: A clear fluid that surrounds and cushions the cerebrum.

cerebrum: The biggest of the central nervous system structures and the most important for speech, language, and hearing.

chronic otitis media: The permanent rupture of the tympanic membrane with or without middle ear disease.

Class I malocclusion: Misalignment of some individual teeth while the two arches are normally aligned.

Class II malocclusion: The upper jaw is protruded and the lower jaw is retracted or receded.

Class III malocclusion: The upper jaw is receded and the lower jaw is protruded.

cleft palate: Failure of the premaxilla to fuse with the maxillary bone and/or failure of the palatine process to fuse at the midline.

closed syllable: Vowel followed by a singleton consonant or consonant cluster.

closed-syllable word: A word that ends in a singleton consonant or consonant cluster (e.g., *pot, stop, must, last*).

cluster: Two or more consonant sounds made next to each other with no vowel separation. See also *blends.*

cluster reduction: Omission of one or more consonants of a cluster (e.g., "top" for *stop*).

cluster simplification: Omission or substitution of one or more sound segments in a consonant cluster. Can be considered a phonological process if it occurs frequently in a child's phonological system.

coarticulation: Articulatory movements for one phone that are carried over into the production of previous or subsequent phones; influence of one phone on another in perception or production.

cochlea: The main inner ear structure of hearing; it looks like the shell of a snail and is filled with a fluid called endolymph.

cochlear implant: An electronic device that is surgically placed in the cochlea and other parts of the ear of a deaf person and delivers the sound directly to the acoustic nerve endings in the cochlea.

coda: Consonant segment or consonant cluster that follows the nucleus (vowel or diphthong) of a syllable.

code switching: Changing from one language or dialect to another during a conversation.

cognates: Consonants produced in the same place and manner, except that one is voiceless and the other is voiced; in phonetic transcription they are typically written in pairs, with the voiceless sound given first (e.g., /p-b/, /wh-w/, /f-v/, /t-d/, /s-z/, /k-g/, /ʃ-ʒ/, /ʧ-ʤ/, /θ-ð/).

cognitive model of development: Theory proposing that children actively test hypotheses regarding phonological constraints and systems.

commissural fibers: The fibers that connect the two hemispheres of the brain.

communication: A form of social behavior; exchange of information.

communication board: An apparatus used by a person with limited verbal expression to communicate his or her needs, thoughts, and ideas. The apparatus may contain the letters of the alphabet, numbers, or commonly used words and phrases.

compensatory articulation: Correct or markedly improved production of sounds through unusual methods of articulation by a child with defective speech structures.

complementary distribution: Sounds that cannot be interchanged in a certain position; allophones that together cover all possible positional occurrences but do not appear in the same linguistic environment.

complete cleft of the palate: Total separation of the two palatal shelves of the hard palate.

complex tone: In acoustics, a sound wave characterized by combined pure tones; it has more than one pitch and contains components of different frequencies.

conductive hearing loss: Diminished conductance of sound to the middle or inner ear due to the abnormalities of the external auditory canal, the eardrum, or the ossicular chain of the middle ear.

congenital disorder: A disorder noticed at the time of birth or soon thereafter.

congenitally deaf: A person who is born deaf.

consonant: A conventional speech sound made by certain movements of the articulatory muscles that alter, interrupt, or obstruct the expired airstream; defined according to manner of production, place of articulation, and voicing dimensions.

consonantal feature: A distinctive feature applied to sounds that have a marked constriction along the midline region of the vocal tract. Includes all consonant sounds except /h/, /w/, and /j/.

consonant deletion: A phonological process that describes the omission of initial or final consonants of words; a phonological problem. See also *final-consonant deletion* and *initial-consonant deletion*.

consonant harmony: An assimilation phonological process that affects manner of production or place of articulation; includes labial assimilation, velar assimilation, nasal assimilation, and alveolar assimilation.

consonant sequence reduction: The omission of one or more sound segments from two or more adjoining consonants.

contextual testing: A special assessment procedure that helps identify a facilitative phonetic context for correct production of a particular phoneme.

contiguous assimilation: A type of assimilation in which the affected sound and the sound that caused the change are adjacent to each other, with no interfering sound between them.

continuant: Distinctive feature applied to sounds made with an incomplete point of constriction; flow of air is not entirely stopped. Continuant sounds are /w/, /f/, /v/, /θ/, /ð/, /s/, /z/, /l/, /ʃ/, /ʒ/, /j/, /r/.

contralateral: Refers to the opposite side, as in *contralateral motor control*. See also *ipsilateral*.

contrast therapy approach: A cognitive-linguistic approach to the treatment of articulation and phonological disorders; incorporates structured activities to increase awareness of the semantic distinction between the error production and the target.

coronal feature: A distinctive feature used in reference to sounds made with the tongue blade raised above the neutral position required for the production of /ə/. Includes consonants /θ/, /ð/, /t/, /d/, /s/, /z/, /n/, /l/, /ʃ/, /ʒ/, /tʃ/, /dʒ/, /r/.

corrective feedback: A treatment procedure by which a client is provided with specific verbal, visual, or written feedback about the acceptability of a response immediately after the response is made.

cranial nerves: Nerves that emerge out of holes (foramina) in the base of the skull; they play a major role in speech production.

craniofacial anomalies: Birth defects of the skull and face.

Creutzfeldt-Jakob disease: Transmissible disease of the brain characterized by spongiform encephalopathy (sponge-like appearance of the brain), progressive vacuolation (empty spaces) in the gray matter, and the death of nerve cells.

cricoarytenoid joint: A joint that connects the arytenoids to the cricoid cartilage and permits circular and sliding movements.

cricoid cartilage: A cartilage of the larynx and also the top ring of the trachea.

cricothyroid joint: A joint that connects the cricoid with the thyroid cartilage; permits back-and-forth movements.

cricothyroid muscle: A muscle that lengthens and tenses the vocal folds.

criterion of performance: The level of accuracy (e.g., 80% correct) in the production of a target behavior taught in treatment.

cross-sectional method: A research method in which many subjects, selected from different age levels, are studied simultaneously for a relatively brief duration. See also *longitudinal method*.

cued speech: Speech produced with manual cues that represent the sound of speech; it supplements and improves speech reading.

deaf: A person whose hearing loss typically exceeds 70 dB and who cannot hear or understand conversational speech under normal circumstances.

decibel (dB): A basic unit to measure the intensity of sound; it is ⅒ of a bel, the basic unit of measurement named after Alexander Graham Bell.

dementia: General mental deterioration due to neurological or psychological factors. Among the symptoms associated with dementia are disorientation, impaired memory, impaired judgment, and deteriorating intellect.

denasalization: Substitution of an oral sound for a nasal sound (e.g., "tep" for *ten*); a problem of articulation.

dependent variable: Behaviors taught to clients by clinicians; effects of a behavior or event studied by scientists.

developmental apraxia of speech (DAS): A childhood motor speech disorder affecting the motor programming of the articulators; it primarily affects articulation and prosody. Also termed *developmental verbal dyspraxia*.

diacritical markers: Special symbols used in narrow phonetic transcription to depict the articulatory or perceptual features of a phone.

diadochokinetic syllable rates: The speed at which a speaker can repeat selected syllables (e.g., pʌ-tə-kə).

diadochokinetic testing: A special procedure used to evaluate the client's ability to rapidly alternate and sequence repetitive articulatory movements; helps assess the functional and structural integrity of the lips, jaw, and tongue through rapid repetitions of syllables.

diagnosis: A clinical judgment about the presence or absence of a disorder; also a description of the severity and nature of the disorder.

dialect: Variation of speech within a specific language. Every dialect may have its own unique phonologic, semantic, morphologic, syntactic, and pragmatic characteristics.

diaphragm: A thick dome-shaped muscle that separates the stomach from the thorax, important for respiration.

diencephalon: A structure of the brain stem; it includes the thalamus and the hypothalamus.

diphthong: A combination of two pure vowels. See also *monophthong*.

diplegia: Paralysis of *either* the legs *or* the arms.

diplophonia: The production of two tones due to the simultaneous vibration of the ventricular vocal folds and the true vocal folds.

discontinuity theory: Theory indicating that speech sounds are not shaped out of the early vocalizations found in the babbling stage.

discrete trial: Structured opportunity to produce a selected target behavior.

discriminative stimuli: Persons, objects, and physical settings that are associated with a reinforced response; the response is more likely to occur in the presence of such stimuli.

distinctive feature approach: An articulation-phonological treatment approach based on the distinctive features or phonemic contrasts of sounds; the goal of treatment is to establish missing distinctive features that create contrasts between words.

distinctive features: Unique characteristics that distinguish one phoneme from another.

distortions: Imprecise productions of speech sounds.

doubling: A phonological process characterized by reduplication or doubling of a syllable; often alters a single-syllable word form into a multisyllable production (e.g., [dada] for *dog* and [baba] for *ball*).

Down syndrome: A particular genetically inherited condition of mental retardation.

duration: A property of sound; a measure of time during which vibrations are sustained. Vowels have longer duration than consonants.

dysarthria: A group of motor speech disorders due to paralysis, weakness, or incoordination of speech muscles caused by central or peripheral nerve damage. There are seven types of dysarthria: flaccid, ataxic, spastic, hypokinetic, hyperkinetic, unilateral upper motor neuron, and mixed.

dysphonia: A general term for a disordered voice.

dysprosody: Disordered prosody. See also *aprosody*.

echoic: An imitative verbal response; the stimulus and the response are the same.

echolalia: "Parrotlike" repetition of what is heard; an early sign of autism.

efferent nerves: Nerves that conduct impulses from the central nervous system to the peripheral organs.

electromyography: A technique of sensing, amplifying, and recording electrical activity of the muscles.

elicited responses: Reflexive responses triggered by stimuli; for example, the dilation of the pupil in response to light. See also *evoked responses*.

endolymph: A kind of fluid that fills the cochlea.

endoscopes: Mechanical devices used to illuminate and examine internal organs by conducting light to and from an organ via thin fiberoptic tubes that are inserted either through the mouth (oral endoscopy) or through the nose (nasal endoscopy).

epilepsy: A seizure disorder caused by an excessive electrical discharge of damaged or abnormal brain cells resulting in convulsion in the body.

esophagus: The flexible tube through which food reaches the stomach.

etiology: The study of causes of diseases and disorders.

eustachian tube: Also known as the auditory tube, it connects the middle ear with the nasopharynx and helps maintain a balanced air pressure within and outside the middle ear.

evoked responses: Responses that are not imitated, not reflexive, but learned; they are produced in relation to various discriminative stimuli.

evoked trial: A structured opportunity for the production of the target behavior; certain stimuli are arranged so that the target response is likely to occur.

exemplar: A response that illustrates the target behavior.

expansions: Elaborations of a child's utterance to make it longer and grammatically more correct.

experimental phonetics: A branch of phonetics dedicated to the development of scientific methods for the study of speech sounds.

external auditory meatus: Also known as the ear canal, it is a muscular tube that resonates the sound that enters it.

extrapyramidal system: A neural pathway that carries motor impulses from the brain to various muscles via several relay stations (hence also known as the indirect system). See also *pyramidal system*.

extrinsic muscles of the larynx: Laryngeal muscles with at least one attachment to structures other than the larynx. See also *intrinsic muscles of the larynx.*

facial nerve VII: A cranial nerve that controls a variety of facial expressions and movements.

facilitative phonetic context: A surrounding sound or group of sounds that has a positive influence on the production of a misarticulated sound.

feature geometry: A theory of phonology purporting that feature combinations of a sound segment are hierarchically organized.

final-consonant deletion: A phonological process affecting the production of final consonants. Patterned deletion of consonant sounds in the final position of words.

finger spelling: A form of sign language in which the words are spelled in the air with the fingers.

fistula: A minute opening left after cleft palate surgery.

fissures: Relatively deep valleys of the brain that form boundaries of broad divisions of the cerebrum. See also *gyrus.*

flaccid dysarthria: A type of dysarthria associated with disorders of the lower motor neuron. Speech is characterized by marked hypernasality and nasal emission; breathiness may be present during phonation; audible inspiration may be perceived; consonant production is imprecise.

flaccid paralysis: Muscles that are too soft and flabby, caused by a lesion in the lower motoneurons.

foot: In the metric theory of phonology, a timing unit that consists of a stressed syllable and one or more unstressed syllables.

foramina: An opening or hole.

fossilized word forms: See *frozen word forms.*

free morpheme: A morpheme that can stand alone and mean something. See also *bound morpheme.*

frenulum: A small cord of tissue that extends from the floor of the mouth to the midline inferior surface of the tongue blade; if too short, it may restrict the elevation and extension of the tongue, which may or may not affect articulation.

frequency: In reference to sound, the number of times a cycle of vibration repeats itself within a second.

frequency of occurrence: In articulation and phonology, the number of times a particular phonological process occurs.

fricatives: A category of speech sounds that are produced by severely constricting the oral cavity and forcing the air through the point of constriction.

frontal lobe: The largest of the four lobes of the cerebrum, containing the primary motor cortex and Broca's area, which is especially important for speech production.

fronting: Substituting sounds produced in the front of the mouth for sounds produced in the back of the mouth; classified as a phonological process that occurs in both normally developing children and children with phonological disorders.

frozen word forms: Words that children continue to mispronounce despite the development of a more advanced phonological system; such words are likely related to names of familiar people or pets and are used often. Synonym: *regressive idioms.*

functional articulation disorders: Disorders that do not have a demonstrable organic or neurological cause.

functional unit: A class or a group of verbal responses that have similar stimulus conditions and consequences.

fundamental frequency: The average rate at which given vocal folds vibrate, or the lowest frequency component of a complex tone.

generalization: The production of untrained (new) behaviors following training of similar behaviors, or the production of trained behaviors when shown new stimuli not used in training.

glides: Speech sounds that are produced by gradually changing the shape of the articulators.

glossectomy: The surgical removal of the tongue and floor of the mouth.

glossopharyngeal nerve IX: A cranial nerve that supplies the tongue and pharynx.

glottal sounds: Sounds that are produced by keeping the vocal folds open and letting the air pass through; because this results in friction noise, glottals are also fricatives.

glottis: An opening that results when the vocal folds are abducted.

gyrus: A ridge on the cortex; the cortex has many *gyri* (plural).

hair cells: Hairlike structures (*cilia*) found on the organ of Corti; they respond to sound vibrations.

hard of hearing: Term used to describe a person with a hearing loss within the range of 25 dB to 75 dB; a person who is hard of hearing has some useful hearing.

hard palate: The roof of the mouth and the floor of the nasal cavity. The point of constriction for several sounds including /ʃ/, /ʒ/, /ʤ/, /ʧ/.

harshness: Roughness of the voice; undesirable vocal quality due mainly to irregular vibrations of the vocal folds.

hearing level: The lowest intensity of a sound necessary to stimulate the auditory system.

hearing screening: A brief testing procedure that separates those who have normal hearing from those who must be tested in detail (because they are suspected to have hearing loss).

hemiplegia: Paralysis of either the left or the right half of the body.

hertz (Hz): The name for cycles per second.

high feature: Distinctive feature term referring to sounds made with the tongue elevated above the neutral position required for /ə/. The high-consonant sounds are /ʃ/, /ʒ/, /j/, /ʧ/, /ʤ/, /k/, /g/, /ŋ/.

high-amplitude sucking method: A scientific method of studying speech discrimination in young infants by measuring their sucking rates when various sound syllables are presented.

hoarse: A voice quality that includes both breathiness and harshness.

homonymy: The loss of linguistic contrast between two or more words due to the presence of phonological processes.

hyoid bone: A U-shaped bone that floats under the jaw; the muscles of the tongue and various muscles of the skull, larynx, and jaw are attached to this bone.

hyperkinesia: Increased (exaggerated or too much) body movement.

hypernasality: Excessive nasal resonance on nonnasal speech sounds.

hypoglossal nerve XII: A cranial nerve that innervates the tongue.

hypokinesia: Reduced (diminished or too little) range and force of muscle movements.

hyponasality: Too little nasal resonance on the nasal sounds of a language; may result from a cold or other condition obstructing the nasal passages.

hypothalamus: A structure within the diencephalon of the central nervous system; it helps integrate the actions of the autonomic nervous system and controls emotional experiences.

hypothesis of discontinuity: See *discontinuity theory.*

idiopathic: Of unknown cause or origin.

idiosyncratic processes: Phonological processes that are unique to an individual child and are not common in the normal course of development.

imitation: In articulation therapy, the client's response to the clinician's model of the target production.

immediate imitation: In articulation therapy, the client's immediate imitation of the modeled target response.

inappropriate communicative behaviors: A client's typical behaviors in place of appropriate speech–language behaviors; in articulation therapy, a client's sound substitutions, omissions, or distortions; in phonological therapy, a child's absence of distinctive features or use of phonological processes.

incomplete cleft palate: The partial fusing of the two palatal shelves of the hard palate.

incus: The second and middle bone of the ossicular chain in the middle ear. See also *malleus* and *stapes.*

independent analysis: In articulation-phonological assessment, a description of the client's speech production errors without reference to the adult model; most clinically useful with very young children or children with significantly decreased speech intelligibility.

individualized education program: Federally and state-mandated program for children with disabilities and special needs who qualify for special education services in the public school system.

Individuals with Disabilities Education Act: Federal legislation that demands the provision of special education services to children with disabilities and special needs in the public schools; includes children with speech and language disorders.

information-getting interview: One of the first steps of a formal speech–language assessment, during which the clinician collects important background information from the client or the client's parents.

initial-consonant deletion: A phonological process affecting the production of initial consonants; patterned deletion of consonant sounds in the initial position of words.

instructions: In speech–language treatment, verbal stimuli that help facilitate a client's actions (i.e., production of the target sound or behavior).

intelligibility: How understandable a person's speech is to family members, strangers, and other listeners.

intensity: Magnitude of sound; sounds that are perceived as louder are greater in intensity.

interdental sound: Sound made by lightly placing the tip of the tongue between the upper and lower central incisors; English interdental sounds include voiced /ð/ and voiceless /θ/.

interfering behaviors: Verbal and nonverbal behaviors that interrupt the treatment process. Such behaviors include crying, off-seat behavior, excessive verbal interruptions, and inattention to task.

internal auditory meatus: The opening through which the auditory nerve exits the inner ear.

International Phonetic Alphabet (IPA): A set of phonetic symbols, each of which stands for only one speech sound.

interrupted feature: Distinctive feature term applied to sounds produced by complete blockage of the airstream at their point of constriction; such sounds are the stops /t/, /d/, /k/, /g/, /p/, /b/ and the affricates /ʧ/, /ʤ/.

intervocalic: In articulation, singleton consonants or consonant blends that occur between vowels or diphthongs.

intonation: System within a language relating to pitch, stress, and juncture of the spoken language; pattern of pitch and stress in the flow of a person's speech.

intrinsic muscles of the larynx: Muscles that begin and end within the larynx and include the thyroarytenoid, the cricothyroid, the posterior cricoarytenoid, the lateral cricoarytenoid, and the interarytenoid muscles. See also *extrinsic muscles of the larynx*.

ipsilateral: On the same side of the body. See also *contralateral*.

jargon: In speech and language development, verbal behavior by young children that begins at about 10 months out of the variegated babbling stage; productions are characterized by strings of sounds and syllables with a variety of stress and intonational patterns. Often overlaps with the early period of meaningful speech. Also called *conversational babble* and *modulated babble*.

juncture: A suprasegmental device that helps make semantic or grammatical distinctions in speech, including brief pauses to signal what might be represented by punctuation marks in written English.

kinesthetic cues: In articulation therapy, visual or verbal cues that focus on the position of the articulators or their correct pattern of movements to teach the correct production of a speech sound.

key words: A word or words in which a typically misarticulated sound is made correctly; can be used in therapy to stabilize the production of the sound across words.

labiodental sounds: Sounds that are produced by the lips and teeth.

labyrinth (of the temporal lobe): A fluid-filled system of interconnecting canals and passages that houses structures of the inner ear.

language: A system of symbols and codes in communication; a form of social behavior shaped and maintained by a verbal community.

language assessment: A process of observation and measurement of a client's language behaviors; typically, it precedes the development of a language treatment program.

language sampling: A procedure of recording a person's language behaviors under relatively normal conditions and, whenever possible, with the help of conversational speech; part of a language assessment.

laryngologist: A medical specialist who treats throat problems.

laryngopharynx: The structure above the larynx and below the oropharynx.

larynx: A tubelike structure in the neck that includes various muscles along with the vocal folds, cartilages, and membranes.

lateral cricoarytenoid muscle: A paired muscle that brings the vocal folds together (an adductor).

laterals: Sounds that are produced by letting air escape through the sides of the tongue; English /l/ is a lateral.

lax vowels: Vowel sounds that are made without added muscle tension and have a short duration. The vowels typically described as lax include /ɪ/, /ɛ/, /æ/, /ʊ/, /ɑ/, /ɚ/, /ə/, /ʌ/.

levator veli palatini: A paired muscle that elevates the soft palate.

limb apraxia: The inability of some patients to move a limb voluntarily that cannot be accounted for by muscle weakness, incoordination, or paralysis.

linear phonological theories: Theories presuming that phonological properties are linear strings of segments and that sound segments are a bundle of independent features or characteristics.

lingua-alveolar sounds: Sounds produced by raising the tip of the tongue to make contact with the alveolar ridge, which is immediately behind the front teeth.

linguadental sounds: Sounds produced by the tongue as it makes contact with the upper teeth.

linguapalatal sounds: Sounds produced by the tongue as it comes in contact with the hard palate, which is located just behind the alveolar ridge.

linguavelar sounds: Sounds produced by the back of the tongue as it raises to make contact with the velum (soft palate).

linguistic-based approaches: In articulation-phonological therapy, treatment programs or approaches with the underlying philosophy that children's production errors result from phonological processes or rules of the adult system that have not yet been learned or fully acquired, or have been suppressed.

linguistics: The study of language, its structure, and the rules that govern that structure.

linguists: Professionals who specialize in linguistics.

liquids: Speech sounds produced with the least restriction of the oral cavity; also called semivowels. English /r/ and /l/ are liquids.

longitudinal fissure: A fissure that divides the cerebrum into the left and right hemispheres.

longitudinal method: A procedure of studying one or a few subjects for an extended period of time to document changes in selected variables. Children's acquisition of language may be studied longitudinally. See also *cross-sectional method.*

long-term goals: Broadly defined speech and language behaviors that a client needs to learn in order to improve his or her overall communication competence.

loudness: A perceived characteristic of sound. Loudness is determined by the intensity of the sound signal; loudness of phonation or speech is determined by the degree of subglottal air pressure.

low feature: Distinctive feature term used to describe sounds made with the tongue lowered for the neutral position of /ə/. In American English, only the consonant /h/ has the low feature.

lower motor neuron damage: Neurological damage to the nerve fibers that descend from the central nervous system and exit the neuraxis (brain and spinal cord) to communicate with the cranial and spinal nerves.

maintenance procedures: Treatment procedures used to enhance the client's use of the target behaviors in extraclinical settings across time.

malleus: The first bone of the ossicular chain located in the middle ear and attached to the tympanic membrane. See also *incus* and *stapes.*

malocclusions: Deviations in the shape and dimensions of the upper and lower jaw bones, the positioning of individual teeth, and the relation between the two jaws.

mandible: The lower jaw, which forms the floor of the mouth and houses the lower set of teeth.

mandibular process: Two of a number of bulges that develop during the third week of embryonic growth; this process results in the mandible, lower lip, and the chin.

manner of production: The degree of and type of constriction of the vocal tract while producing certain speech sounds.

manual guidance: Any procedure in which the clinician uses his or her hands and fingers to physically guide and shape a correct response from a client.

marginal babbling: Infant vocal productions characterized by CV and VC syllable sequences that begin at about 4 months of age.

mastication: The act of chewing.

maxillae: A pair of large facial bones that form a major portion of the hard palate and the upper jaw.

maxillary processes: Two of a number of bulges that develop during the third week of embryonic growth; they give rise to the face, mouth, cheeks, and the sides of the upper lip.

mean length of utterance (MLU): The average length of a speaker's utterances as measured in terms of morphemes.

meatus: An anatomical channel or passageway between confining walls within the body.

medulla: The uppermost portion of the spinal cord, which enters the cranial cavity; it controls breathing and other vital functions of the body.

meningitis: An infectious disease that destroys the layers of the membrane (meninges) that surround and protect the brain.

metalinguistics: The study of the conscious awareness of language as a tool and the ability to reflect on language.

metaphonological: A subcomponent of metalinguistics; the ability to reflect on sounds and words.

metric theory: A nonlinear phonological theory that suggests a hierarchy based on feet, syllables, and segments; emphasizes the syllable structure and stress patterns of words in a language.

metathesis: A phonological process characterized by the reversal of two sounds in a word that may or may not be adjacent to each other (e.g., [pots] for *post*).

metathetic error: The reversal of two sounds within a word that may or may not be adjacent to each other.

midbrain: Also known as the *mesencephalon,* it is a narrow structure that lies above the pons and links the higher centers of the brain with the lower centers.

minimal pairs: Morphemes that are similar except for one sound (e.g., *mit / sit, hot / pot, bake / bait*).

mixed nerves: Nerve fibers that carry sensory as well as motor impulses.

modeled trial: A prearranged opportunity for the production of a target behavior during which the clinician provides a model and the client is instructed to imitate the modeled production.

modeling: A treatment procedure used to facilitate a target production; the clinician models the target behavior and the client is instructed to imitate the clinician.

modulated babble: See *jargon.*

monolingual: Refers to the use or knowledge of one language.

monophthong: Term used in reference to pure vowels.

monoplegia: Paralysis of only one limb.

morpheme: The smallest meaningful unit of a language.

morphology: The study of word structures.

morphophonemics: Sound alterations that result from joining one morpheme with another; morphophonemic rules specify how sounds are produced in combination in morphemes.

moto-kinesthetic cues: Cues provided by the clinician to teach the placement of sounds. The clinician touches and manipulates the client's articulators to facilitate correct production of the target sound. Moto-kinesthetic cues are often accompanied by auditory and visual cues.

moto-kinesthetic method: A procedure of teaching the correct production of speech sounds; the clinician manually moves the articulators to provide motor and kinesthetic feedback to the client.

motor-based approaches: In articulation therapy, treatment programs or approaches that focus on teaching the motor behaviors associated with the production of speech sounds; often considered "traditional" articulation treatment approaches.

motor nerves: Nerve fibers that carry impulses for movement from the brain to the muscles.

motor speech disorders: Also known as neurogenic speech disorders; result from central or peripheral nervous system damage. Apraxia of speech and dysarthria are considered motor speech disorders.

motor unit: Neurological terms referring to the motor nuclei, cranial nerve, myoneural junction, and muscle, which together constitute the motor unit.

multilingual: Refers to more than two languages; a multilingual person is one who uses three or more languages.

multiple-phoneme approach: A highly structured motor-based articulation approach developed to meet the needs of children with multiple articulation errors; key features of the multiple phoneme approach are the simultaneous teaching of multiple phonemes, a systematic application of behavioral principles, and an analysis of sound production in conversational speech.

multiple sclerosis: A neurological disorder characterized by progressive and deteriorating muscular disability produced by an overgrowth of the myelin sheath surrounding the nerve tracts; paralysis, muscular tremors, and dysarthria may be associated to varying degrees depending on the site of lesion.

myoelastic-aerodynamic theory of phonation: A theory that states that vocal fold vibrations are due to air pressure, the difference between positive and negative pressure, and the elasticity of the muscles.

myofunctional therapy: Treatment aimed at correcting a tongue thrust or myofunctional imbalance.

McDonald's sensorimotor approach: A motor-based articulation therapy approach with the underlying philosophy that the syllable is the basic unit of training and that certain phonetic contexts can be used to facilitate correct production of the error sound.

narrow phonetic transcription: A detailed form of recording a speech sound or utterance using the symbols of the International Phonetic Alphabet and special diacritic markers; transcription enclosed in brackets to highlight the allophonic features or variations of a phoneme (e.g., [kʰout] for *coat* would indicate an aspirated production of the /k/ sound).

nasals: Speech sounds with nasal resonance added to them; produced while keeping the velopharyngeal port open.

nasal emission: Excessive airflow through the nose that can often be measured and perceived; heard most frequently during the production of voiceless plosives and fricatives; typically indicative of an incomplete seal between the oral and the nasal cavities; often associated with cleft palate speech and some types of dysarthria.

nasal feature: A distinctive feature applied to sounds resonated in the nasal cavity. The nasal sounds include /m/, /n/, and /ŋ/.

nasopharynx: The section of the pharynx that lies just behind the nasal cavities.

natural phonology: A theoretical explanation of articulatory and phonological development; describes universal phonological processes evident in children's speech and considers those processes as innate mechanisms of simplifying the adult productions.

nerve cells: Specialized cells that make up the central nervous system; basic building blocks in the CNS responsible for receiving, transmitting, and synthesizing information; each nerve cell consists of a single axon, a cell body, dendrite(s), and many terminal knobs.

nervous system: An organization of nerves according to some structural, spatial, and functional principles.

neurologist: A medical specialist who diagnoses and treats disorders of the nervous system.

neuron: A single nerve cell. See also *nerve cells*.

neuropathology: The nature of a disease or damage and the structural and functional changes in the nervous system that result from disease processes.

neurotransmitter: A chemical substance that activates the receptive sites of nerve cells and helps generate the electrical nerve impulses necessary for stimulation of the nerve cell body.

noncontiguous assimilation: A type of assimilation in which the assimilated sound and the sound causing the assimilation are separated by an intervening sound.

nonreflexive vocalizations: Infant vocal productions that are nonreflexive in nature; includes such productions as cooing, vocal play, marginal babbling, reduplicated babbling, variegated babbling, and jargon.

nonlinear phonological theory: In phonology, the theoretical assumption that there is some sort of hierarchy that helps organize segmental and suprasegmental phonological properties or units; among several such proposed theories are the metric theory and feature geometry theory.

nonphonemic diphthong: Diphthongs that do not contrast meaning in words when they are interchanged with their pure-vowel counterpart; the only two American English nonphonemic diphthongs are /ei/ and /ou/.

nonreduplicated babbling: See *variegated babbling*.

nonverbal corrective feedback: A treatment procedure by which corrective feedback is provided through nonverbal means such as facial expressions, gestures, and other signals.

norms: Standards or patterns derived from a representative sampling of median achievement of a large group; a range of statistical information against which individual performance can be compared.

nucleus: 1. The controlling center of the neuron. 2. The vowel or diphthong that follows the initial consonant or blend in a syllable.

obturator: A prosthetic device used to cover the cleft of the hard palate and help achieve better velopharyngeal closure.

obstruents: Distinctive feature term used for consonants that are made with complete closure or narrow constriction of the oral cavity so that the airstream is stopped or friction noise is produced; obstruents include stops, fricatives, and affricates.

occipital lobe: One of the four lobes of the cerebral cortex; located at the lower back portion of the head just above the cerebellum; primarily concerned with vision.

occlusion: The manner in which the upper and lower dental arches meet each other.

omission: An absence of a required sound in a word position; a type of articulation error.

onset: One of the components of the syllable; the consonant or consonant cluster that initiates the syllable.

open syllable: A syllable that ends in a vowel or a diphthong.

open-syllable word: A word that ends with an open syllable. See also *open syllable*.

operant: A class of behaviors that can be increased or decreased by arranging certain consequences for them.

operant conditioning: A procedure of creating, increasing, or decreasing behaviors by arranging certain stimulus conditions and immediate consequences.

oral apraxia: An inability to move the muscles of oral structures for nonspeech purposes in the absence of muscle weakness, incoordination, or paralysis. See also *apraxia of speech* and *limb apraxia*.

oral astereognosis: An inability to discriminate among and identify the types, locations, and sensations of various objects in the oral cavity.

oral form recognition: The ability to identify and discriminate among the locations and sensations of objects placed in the mouth with no visual information. Synonym: *oral stereognosis*.

orbicularis oris: The muscle that makes up the lips.

organ of Corti: The inner ear's structure of hearing; it contains the hair cells that respond to sound.

organic: Relating to an organ or structure of the body.

organic articulation disorder: An inability to produce correctly all or some of the standard sounds of a language as a result of anatomical, physiological, or neurological causes.

orofacial examination: A procedure conducted to rule out gross organic problems of the face and mouth that may be associated with disorders of communication.

orthodontics: The study and treatment of deviations of dental structures.

orthodontist: A dental specialist who moves the oral structures with the help of specially constructed devices.

ossicular chain: A set of three tiny bones (the malleus, incus, and stapes) found in the middle ear; the chain that conducts sound to the inner ear.

otitis media: An infection of the middle ear; a frequent cause of conductive hearing loss in children.

oval window: An opening to, and a part of, the inner ear.

paired-stimuli approach: A motor-based articulation treatment approach that depends on the identification of a key word to teach correct production of a target sound in other contexts; a highly structured approach that capitalizes on operant principles and progresses sequentially from words to sentences to conversation; because a single speech sound is the target at any one time, this approach is most suited for children who have sound distortions or a few articulation errors.

palatine bone: A part of the hard palate.

palatine process: The central, platelike portion of the maxillary bones; embryonically identified as the secondary palate, it forms the major portion of the roof of the mouth and the hard palate.

palatoglossus: A muscle that lowers the soft palate and elevates the dorsum of the tongue.

palatogram: An impression made by the tongue on an artificial palate.

palatopharyngeus: A muscle that lowers the soft palate and moves the pharyngeal walls inward.

palilalia: A speech disorder in which a word, phrase, or sentence is said repeatedly with increasing speed and declining distinctiveness; often associated with Parkinson's disease.

palsy: Paralysis.

paraphasia: A word substitution problem found frequently in aphasic persons who can speak fluently and grammatically.

paraplegia: Paralysis of the legs only.

parietal lobe: One of the four lobes of the cerebral cortex; it lies behind the frontal lobe and integrates such body sensations as pain, touch, and temperature.

Parkinson's disease: A degenerative disease of the nervous system whose symptoms include rigidity of posture, hand tremors, and speech disorders (hypokinetic dysarthria).

partial assimilation: In articulation, a physiological occurrence in which a sound takes on some of the characteristics of a neighboring sound.

pattern analysis: In articulation-phonological assessment, the clinician's attempt to identify any patterned or systematic modifications in the client's speech production errors.

percentage of occurrence: When conducting a phonological process analysis, the actual percentage with which the child uses a particular phonological process; calculated by determining the number of times the child uses a particular phonological process and dividing that number by the total number of opportunities for occurrence of the process.

perception: The process by which people select, organize, integrate, and interpret sensory information into a meaningful and coherent picture of the world around them.

perceptual phonetics: A branch of phonetics that studies the perception of sounds by the listener, including sound awareness and sound interpretation.

perilymph: The fluid that fills the canals that lie within the inner ear.

periodic: The patterned repetition of the vibrations of a complex tone, which is a sound that consists of different frequencies. See also *complex tone.*

peripheral hearing problems: Reduced hearing ability due to pathologies in the outer, middle, or inner ear (excluding the auditory nerve).

peripheral nervous system: A collection of nerves that are outside the skull and the spinal column; includes the cranial nerves, the spinal nerves, and portions of the autonomic nerves.

pharyngeal flap operation: A surgical procedure to reduce hypernasality due to a short velum. A muscular flap is raised from the back wall of the throat and attached to the soft palate.

pharyngeal fricatives: Consonant sounds produced by lingual-pharyngeal contact and an unusual tongue configuration; often an associated compensatory error in children with cleft palate.

pharyngoplasty: A set of surgical procedures used to improve the functioning of the velo-pharyngeal mechanism by implanting various substances (including Teflon) into the pharyngeal wall to make it bulge.

pharynx: The throat.

phonate: To produce sound.

phonation: One of the four basic speech processes. The production of voice through vocal fold vibration.

phone: In the study of speech production, a single speech sound represented by a single symbol in a phonetic system.

phoneme: A group or family of very closely related speech sounds that vary slightly in their production but are sufficiently similar acoustically that the listener perceives them as the same sound. For example, whether *t* in *cat* is aspirated or unaspirated, the listener perceives the sound as /t/.

phonemic awareness: A person's underlying knowledge that words are created by sounds and sound combinations. Synonym: *phonological awareness.*

phonemic diphthong: A diphthong that cannot be reduced to its pure-vowel components without affecting the meaning of the words in which they occur.

phonemic inventory: In a phonological analysis, an inventory of sounds that a child uses contrastively to signal a difference in the meanings of words.

phonemic transcription: Recording of a speech sound or speech unit into phonemic symbols, which are enclosed between virgules (slash marks); such recording indicates the phoneme to which the sound belongs. Synonym: *broad transcription.*

phonemics: Study of the sound system and sound differences in a language.

phonetics: Study of speech sounds, their production and acoustic properties, and the written symbols used to represent their production.

phonetic inventory: A person's repertoire of speech sounds; sounds that a person can produce with appropriate articulation although not always contrastively.

phonetic transcription: See *narrow phonetic transcription.*

phonetic placement method: A procedure of teaching a target sound by describing and demonstrating in front of a mirror how that sound is produced correctly.

phonological awareness: See *phonemic awareness.*

phonological disorders: Errors of many phonemes that form patterns or clusters.

phonological knowledge approach: A linguistic-based phonological treatment approach that assumes that children's knowledge of the phonological rules of the adult system is reflected in their productions; in essence, the greater the consistency of correct sound production across varied contexts, the higher the level of phonological knowledge. The initial stages of therapy would focus on sounds that reflect the least knowledge.

phonological process analysis: In articulation-phonological assessment, the classification of sound errors according to operating phonological processes; the frequency of occurrence and percentage of occurrence of common phonological processes and idiosyncratic processes are calculated.

phonological processes: Many ways or patterns of simplifying difficult sound productions by omissions or substitutions.

phonology: The study of speech sounds, sound patterns, and the rules used to create words with those sounds.

phonotactics: Rules for how sounds can be combined to form syllables and how those sounds can be distributed; some rules vary across languages.

phrase: An utterance that is grammatically incomplete (e.g., "The boy").

physical prompts: In articulation therapy, visual signs or gestures that help a client visualize correct production of the target sound.

physical stimulus generalization: In articulation-phonological therapy, a client's production of the target sounds in untrained words.

pinna: See *auricle.*

pitch: A sensation determined by the frequency of sound vibration; the greater the frequency, the higher the perceived pitch.

place of articulation: One of three factors used to classify consonants; refers to the place of articulatory contact or constriction.

plosive sound: A stop consonant produced when the impounded air pressure behind the point of constriction is released through the oral cavity; not all stop consonants are plosive in nature.

pons: The structure that bridges the two halves of the cerebellum.

positive reinforcement: A method of increasing a response by presenting something desirable immediately after that response is made; a frequently used positive reinforcer is verbal praise.

posterior cricoarytenoid muscle: A muscle that pulls the vocal folds apart (an abductor).

postvocalic: A consonant or consonant blend produced after a vowel or a diphthong; postvocalic sounds terminate the syllable.

pragmatics: The study of the rules that govern the use of language in social situations.

prefix: A morpheme added at the beginning of a base morpheme.

prelingual: The period before the acquisition of language, as in *prelingually deaf.*

prelinguistic: Refers to a period before the acquisition of language, as in *prelinguistic speech.*

premaxilla: The front portion of the maxillary bone.

presbycusis: A common type of sensorineural hearing loss among the elderly.

pressure: Force, distributed over a certain area.

pressure consonants: Consonant sounds produced with a buildup of intraoral pressure, which include fricatives, stops, and affricates.

prevocalic: In speech production, a consonant or consonant blend occurring before a vowel or diphthong; prevocalic sounds initiate the syllable.

primary auditory cortex: An area within the temporal lobe concerned with hearing.

primary motor cortex: An area within the frontal lobe that controls voluntary movement.

primary palate: An embryonic structure from which the upper lip and the alveolar process evolve.

probe procedure: A clinical procedure used to assess the generalized production of the trained target behavior to untrained sounds, words, sentences, audiences, settings, and so forth.

prognosis: A statement about the future course of a disorder when certain therapeutic steps are taken or when nothing is done.

programmed learning: A method of mastering various skills by the systematic use of operant conditioning principles.

progressive assimilation: A type of assimilation in which a sound takes on the articulatory or acoustic qualities of a preceding sound.

progressive idioms: See *advanced word forms*.

projection fibers: Neural pathways to and from the brain stem and spinal cord on the one hand and the sensory and motor areas of the cortex on the other hand.

prompts: "Hints" or "cues" used in treatment to draw a target response from a client.

prosodic view of development: In speech and language development, a view that pays attention to words as the initial learning units. It states that children's acquisition of phonological skills begins with a mastery of certain initial words, which are schemata of adult forms.

prosody: Variations in rate, pitch, loudness, stress, intonation, and rhythm of continuous speech.

prosthesis: A device developed and fitted to compensate for missing or deformed structures.

protowords: Consistent sound patterns produced by young children that are semantically potent (carry meaning) but are not modeled after any adult words.

pseudobulbar palsy: Paralysis of the muscles of mastication, articulation, and swallowing as a result of neurological damage to both hemispheres of the brain.

punisher: In behavior modification terms, any stimulus that decreases a behavior when it is presented upon the behavior's occurrence.

punishment: A procedure designed to decrease the frequency of selected behaviors by arranging an immediate consequence for those behaviors.

pure tone: A tone of single frequency.

pure-tone audiometry: Audiometry in which tones of various frequencies and intensities are used as auditory stimuli in the measurement of a person's hearing ability.

pure vowels: Vowel sounds that maintain a relatively unchanged quality across the syllables in which they are produced.

pyramidal system: A bundle of nerve fibers that originate in the motor cortex and travel to the brain stem; it is the primary pathway of impulses for voluntary movement. (Also called the direct system.) See also *extrapyramidal system*.

quadriplegia: Paralysis of all four limbs.

range of motion: The limitations within which a motion or movement may occur.

raspberries: In speech and language development, bilabial fricative sounds produced by young infants in the vocal play stage.

real words: See *true words*.

recurrent laryngeal nerve: A branch of the cranial nerve X (vagus); it moves down the chest cavity and then reverses its course back to the laryngeal and pharyngeal areas; it innervates many intrinsic laryngeal muscles and palatal muscles.

reduplicated babbling: Infant vocal productions in which a series of consonant-vowel syllables are repeated (e.g., *ma-ma, pa-pa, bo-bo*); such productions begin at about 7 months of age.

referent: An object, event, person, or abstraction represented by a symbol, verbal or otherwise.

reflexive vocalizations: Automatic responses produced by an infant that reflect his or her physical state, including crying, burping, coughing, and hiccuping.

register: A variation of language use depending on a particular speaking situation.

regressive assimilation: A type of assimilation in which a sound takes on some or all of the articulatory or acoustic features of a following sound.

regressive idioms: See *frozen word forms.*

regressive substitution: Sound substitution in which a phoneme is affected by a sound that occurs earlier in the word; a speech characteristic of verbal apraxia.

reinforcer: An event that follows a response and thereby makes that response more likely in the future.

relational analysis: In articulation-phonological assessment, a comparison of a child's productions to the adult target forms within a specific linguistic community. Such a comparison helps the clinician identify the types of errors according to substitutions, additions, omissions, and deletion; the absence of any phonological rules or distinctive features; and the presence of active phonological processes.

releasing sound: A consonant sound that begins the syllable.

reliability: The consistency with which an event is repeatedly measured.

resonance: Forced vibration of a structure that is related to the source of sound; vibration of cavities below and above the larynx (source of sound).

respiration: One of the four basic speech processes. This system provides the air supply necessary for vocal fold vibration and speech production.

response cost: Taking a reinforcer away from a child every time a particular response is made in order to decrease such a response.

rhotic: Distinctive feature term used for the /r/ consonant and its various allophonic variations.

rhotic diphthongs: See *centering diphthongs.*

rhyme: A collective term for the nucleus and coda components of a syllable.

rib cage: Also known as the thoracic cage; a cylinder-like structure of 12 ribs that houses vital organs including the heart and the lungs.

Rochester method: A means of communication that combines finger spelling and oral speech.

round feature: Distinctive feature term applied to sounds made with the lips rounded or protruded; includes the consonants /r/ and /w/ and the vowels /u/, /ʊ/ /o/, /ɔ/, and /ɝ/.

schwa: Name for the neutral vowel /ə/.

schwar: Name for the vowel /ɚ/.

screening: A brief procedure that helps determine whether a person should be assessed at length or not.

secondary palate: Hard palate.

semantics: The study of the meaning of language.

semicircular canals: Structures of the inner ear responsible for maintaining balance (equilibrium).

semivowel: A consonant sound made by maintaining the vocal tract briefly in the vowel-like position needed for the following vowel in a syllable; term used for /w/, /j/, and sometimes /l/ and /r/.

sensorineural hearing loss: Diminished hearing due to damaged hair cells of the cochlea or the auditory portion of the cranial nerve VIII. See also *conductive hearing loss.*

sensorimotor approach: Motor-based articulation approach based on the assumption that the syllable is the basic unit of training and that environmental phonetic contexts can be used to facilitate correct production of the target sound. The goal is to increase the client's auditory, tactile, and proprioceptive awareness of the motor patterns in speech production. Synonym: *McDonald's sensorimotor approach.*

sensory-perceptual training: A step typically included in the traditional articulation therapy approach; the goal is to increase the client's awareness of his own sound errors by incorporating ear-training activities such as sound identification and discrimination.

sensory nerves: Those cranial nerves that carry sensory information from a sense organ to the brain.

septum: The structure that divides the nasal cavities.

sequential bilingualism: Learning a second language after one language has been mastered.

sequential motion rates: Rapid movements from one articulatory posture to another by repetition of different syllable chains. Part of diadochokinetic testing by repetitive movement of the syllable sequence /pʌtəkə/.

serous otitis media: A disease of the middle ear, in which it becomes inflamed and filled with thick or watery fluid.

shaping: See *successive approximation.*

short-term objectives: In articulation-phonological therapy, the sounds, phonological rules, and other behaviors selected for training that support the long-term goals or final target behaviors.

sibilants: Distinctive feature term applied to high-frequency consonant sounds that have a more strident quality and longer duration than most other consonants; most phoneticians classify /s/, /z/, /ʃ/, /ʒ/, /ʧ/, /ʤ/ in this category.

silent nasal emission: Inaudible leakage of air through the nose during the production of nonnasal speech sounds.

simultaneous bilingualism: The linguistic process of learning two languages at the same time.

soft palate: A flexible muscular structure at the juncture of the oropharynx and the nasopharynx; also known as the velum, it may be lowered to open the velopharyngeal port or raised to close it.

soft neurological signs: Mild neurological abnormalities that are undetectable or difficult to identify during specialized testing (e.g., CT scan). Neurological damage may be presumed based on some abnormal behaviors (e.g., fine-motor problems).

sonorant: A consonant sound produced with a relatively unobstructed flow of air at the point of constriction: /m/, /n/, /ŋ/, /l/, /r/, /j/, and /w/.

sound: Waves of disturbance in the molecules of a gas, a liquid, or a solid created by the vibrations of an object and the sensation felt by the hearing mechanism due to those vibrations.

sound approximation: Production of a misarticulated sound that approaches the target or standard production of that phoneme.

spastic dysphonia: A voice disorder caused by very tight closure (adduction) of the vocal folds and characterized by a strangled, squeezed, choppy, harsh, and breathy voice.

spastic paralysis: A form of paralysis due to lesions in the upper motoneurons characterized by too rigid muscles.

spasticity: Increased tone or rigidity of muscles.

spectogram: Photograph of the pressure waves of a particular sound.

spectrum: Pattern of physical energy across a frequency range for a particular sound.

speech: Production of phonemes; articulated sounds and syllables. See also *language.*

speech–language pathologist: A specialist in the study, assessment, and treatment of speech–language (communication) disorders.

speech–language pathology: The study of human communication and its disorders and the assessment and treatment of those disorders.

speech perception: The identification of speech sounds from acoustic cues.

speech reading: A method of understanding speech by looking at the face of the speaker; a skill used by people with hearing loss to understand speech.

stapedius muscle: A small muscle attached to the stapes in the middle ear; in response to loud sounds, it normally contracts to stiffen the ossicular chain.

stapes: One of the three bones of the ossicular chain in the middle ear. See also *incus* and *malleus.*

startle reflex: An infant's automatic response to loud sound, involving sudden movement that suggests a jumping response.

stimulability: The extent to which a misarticulated sound can be produced correctly by imitation or other cues.

stops: Speech sounds produced by completely stopping the airflow; also known as stop-plosives.

stopping: Phonological process term used to describe patterned substitutions of stop consonants for fricatives and affricates.

stress: A suprasegmental device that gives prominence to certain syllables within a sequence of syllables.

stress-timed languages: Languages across the world in which stressed syllables tend to be produced at regular intervals, including English, German, Russian, and Arabic.

stridents: Consonant sounds that are made by forcing the airstream through a small opening, which results in intense noise: /f/, /v/, /s/, /z/, /ʃ/, /ʒ/, /ʧ/, /ʤ/.

submucous cleft: An opening in the palate that is covered by the mucous membrane.

substitution: The production of a wrong sound in place of a right one.

successive approximation: A treatment technique for establishing a target behavior not in the client's repertoire; the client's target responses are progressively shaped to match the final target behavior. Synonym: *shaping.*

suffix: A morpheme added at the end of a word.

sulcus: A shallow valley on the surface of the brain; the brain has many *sulci* (plural). See also *fissures.*

supplementary motor cortex: An area of the frontal lobe that is thought to be involved in the motor planning of meaningful speech.

suprasegmentals: The prosodic features of a language, including stress, intonation, timing, duration, and juncture.

syllabic speech sound: A vowel sound that creates the syllable; sometimes refers to consonants that take on a syllable-forming status (e.g., /l/ in the second syllable of the word *handle*).

syllable: The combination of a consonant and a vowel.

syllable-timed languages: Languages across the world in which syllables (stressed and unstressed) are produced at regular intervals; includes such languages as French, Italian, Greek, Spanish, Turkish, and Hindi.

syllable word shapes: Organization of consonants and vowels in a syllable (e.g., CVC = consonant, vowel, consonant; CCVC = consonant, consonant, vowel, consonant).

synapse: The juncture at which the neurons communicate with each other.

synaptic cleft: The tiny gap (space) between two neurons.

syntax: The arrangement of words to form meaningful sentences; a part of grammar.

target behavior: A behavior that a client is taught and expected to learn.

temporal bone: One of the four lobes of the cerebral cortex; it contains the primary auditory cortex and Wernicke's area.

temporomandibular joint: The joint between the mandible and the temporal lobe.

tense feature: Distinctive feature term applied to sounds that are made with a relatively greater degree of tension or contraction at the root of the tongue, including the consonants /p/, /t/, /k/, /tʃ/, /dʒ/, /ʃ/, /f/, /s/, /l/, /θ/ and vowels /i/, /e/, /o/, /u/, /ʌ/, /ɝ/.

tensor veli palatini: A pair of muscles that stretch the soft palate.

tensor tympani: A muscle in the middle ear that tenses the eardrum.

thalamus: A part of the diencephalon that lies above the brain stem; the thalamus integrates sensory information and relays it to various parts of the cerebral cortex.

threshold of hearing: An intensity level at which a tone is faintly heard at least 50% of the time it is presented.

time-out: A procedure used to decrease the frequency of an error response; every time an error response is made, a brief period of no reinforcement or silence is imposed.

tongue thrust: A pattern of deviant or reverse swallow in which the tongue pushes against the teeth.

total assimilation: In articulation, a physiological occurrence in which a sound takes on all of the characteristics of a neighboring sound. In essence, the sound becomes identical to a neighboring sound (e.g., the *k* of *cat* totally assimilating to the *t* that follows to produce "tat").

total communication: A method of communication that simultaneously uses speech, manual signs, and finger spelling.

trachea: A tube formed by a ring of cartilages leading to the lungs.

traditional treatment approach: A classic approach to the treatment of articulation disorders. A highly structured program that progresses from sensory perceptual training to production training and then from the sound in isolation to the maintenance of learned behaviors in nonclinical settings across time.

training broad approach: An articulation-phonological treatment approach in which several target sounds are taught at the same time.

transfer: The extension of newly learned behaviors from one setting (usually the clinical setting) to various other settings.

treatment objectives: The skills selected for training.

treatment procedures: Special techniques a clinician uses to effect changes in client behaviors.

trigeminal nerve V: A cranial nerve that supplies many structures of the face; controls jaw and tongue movements.

true words: Words used by young children that have semantic consistency and closely match adult production in their phonological and articulatory features. Synonym: *real words.*

tympanic membrane: The thin, semitransparent, cone-shaped eardrum, which is highly sensitive to sound.

underlying processes: The deep phonological patterns in children's production errors.

unilateral: One sided.

unilateral cleft: A cleft on one side of the alveolar ridge and the lip.

unrounded vowels: Vowels made without lip rounding: /i/, /ɪ/, /ɛ/, /e/, /ɑ/, /æ/, /ɚ/, /ə/, /ʌ/.

utterance: An isolated unit of verbal expression preceded and followed by silence. An utterance may be made up of a single word, phrase, clause, or sentence.

vagus nerve X: A cranial nerve that supplies many organs including the larynx, the pharynx, the base of the tongue, and the external ear.

validity: The degree to which a test or other measuring instrument measures what it claims to measure.

variegated babbling: Infant vocalizing that typically begins at about 9 months of age; it is characterized by the production of vowel, consonant-vowel, and some consonant-vowel-consonant syllable combinations, with varying consonants and vowels from one syllable to another.

velar fronting: Phonological process characterized by the substitution of alveolar consonants for velar sounds; typical substitutions include *d* / *g, t* / *k,* and *n* / ŋ; however, others may be observed.

velocity: Quickness or speed of motion.

velopharyngeal closure: The physiological act of closing the nasal cavity from the oral cavity so that air is directed through the mouth rather than the nose; closure is achieved by intricate upward, backward, and lateral movements of the velum and various pharyngeal muscles.

velopharyngeal port: The structure that connects the oral and nasal passages; it may be closed or opened by various muscle actions.

velum: The soft palate; formed by muscles that help raise or lower it.

ventricles: The small spaces in the skull that are filled with cerebrovascular spinal fluid.

verbal apraxia: Difficulty in initiating and executing the movement patterns necessary to produce speech when there is no paralyis, weakness, or incoordination of speech muscles; thought to be due to the brain's disturbed motor planning.

verbal corrective feedback: Verbal information provided to a client when a target or other behavior is inadequate, inappropriate, or unacceptable.

verbal prompt: A verbal "hint" or "cue" used to draw a target response from a client; it may include the use of vocal emphasis and the provision of verbal information (e.g., "When you make your *s,* remember that your tongue stays inside your mouth").

vestibular acoustic nerve VIII: The vestibular branch of this cranial nerve, which is concerned with balance, body position, and movement.

vestibular system: An inner ear structure containing three semicircular canals; the system is concerned with balance, body position, and movement.

virgules: Slash marks used to enclose phonemic symbols.

visually reinforced head-turn method: A method to study speech perception in infants and young babies.

vocal emphasis: A treatment technique by which a clinician increases his or her vocal intensity to highlight a target behavior; in articulation therapy, a clinician would say the target sound more loudly or prolong production of the target sound.

vocal folds: A pair of thin muscles in the larynx whose vibrations are the source of voice. Also termed *vocal cords*.

vocalic: Distinctive feature term used for sounds made without marked constriction of the vocal tract; includes all vowels and the consonants /l/ and /r/.

vocalis muscles: The vibrating parts of the vocal folds; also known as the thyroarytenoid muscles.

voiced sounds: Sounds made with vocal fold vibration.

voiceless sounds: Sounds made without vocal fold vibration.

voicing: The presence of vocal fold vibrations in the production of speech sounds. Also termed *voice*.

volitional speech: Speech productions made under voluntary control.

vowel: A speech sound produced with an unrestricted passage of the airstream through the oral cavity; a syllable-forming sound.

vowel quadrilateral: A schematic representation of the tongue positions for the four extreme points of vowel production /i/, /u/, /æ/, and /ɑ/.

Wernicke's area: A center in the temporal lobe thought to be responsible for both understanding and formulating speech.

Index

◆ ◆ ◆ ◆ ◆ ◆ ◆ ◆ ◆ ◆ ◆ ◆ ◆ ◆ ◆ ◆ ◆ ◆ ◆ ◆

About the Authors

Adriana Peña-Brooks, M.A., is a speech–language pathologist with Elk Grove Unified District in Elk Grove, California, where she works with children in kindergarten through sixth grade with varying speech and language disorders. Prior to her position with Elk Grove Unified, she was an instructor and clinical supervisor at California State University, Fresno, where she taught both undergraduate- and graduate-level courses. She has also worked extensively with adults with neurogenic-based speech, language, cognitive, and swallowing disorders. Mrs. Peña-Brooks has presented various workshops at the local, state, and national levels.

M. N. (Giri) Hegde is a professor of communicative sciences and disorders at California State University, Fresno. He holds a master's degree in experimental psychology from the University of Mysore, India, and a post-master's diploma in medical psychology from Bangalore University, India. His doctoral degree in speech–language pathology is from Southern Illinois University in Carbondale, Illinois.

Dr. Hegde is a specialist in research methods, fluency disorders, language, and treatment procedures in communicative disorders. He has made many professional and scientific presentations to national and international audiences on a wide variety of topics in communicative disorders. He has published many research articles and over 18 books on a wide range of subjects in speech–language pathology. He has received numerous state and national professional accolades and honors, including the ASHA Fellow Award.